# Essentials of Pediatric Hematology/Oncology Nursing

## A CORE CURRICULUM

### THIRD EDITION

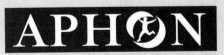

ASSOCIATION of PEDIATRIC
HEMATOLOGY/ONCOLOGY NURSES

Copyright © 2008
Association of Pediatric
  Hematology/Oncology Nurses
4700 W. Lake Avenue
Glenview, IL 60025-1485
All rights reserved.

**EDITOR**

**Nancy E. Kline, PhD RN CPNP FAAN**
Director, Center for Evidence-Based Practice and Research
Department of Nursing
Memorial Sloan-Kettering Cancer Center
New York, NY

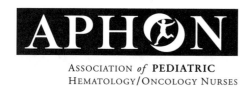

ASSOCIATION *of* **PEDIATRIC**
HEMATOLOGY/ONCOLOGY NURSES

## Staff

**Executive Director:** Karen Nason, CAE
**Managing Editor**: Katherine Wayne
**Graphic Designer:** Robert Stoeck
**Associate Editor:** June Won
**Assistant Editor:** Katie Hamill
**Editorial Assistants:** Amy Hastings and Cori Mohr

**Copyright © 2008 Association of Pediatric Hematology/Oncology Nurses**
All rights reserved. No part of this book, except for brief quotations embodied in critical articles and reviews, may be used or reproduced in any manner whatsoever without written permission.

Printed in the United States of America

Association of Pediatric Hematology/Oncology Nurses
4700 W. Lake Avenue
Glenview, IL 60025-1485

Library of Congress Catalog Number: 2008935438
ISBN 978-0-9666193-3-1

*Note:* As new scientific information becomes available through basic and clinical research, recommended treatments and drug therapies undergo changes. The authors, editors, and publisher have done everything possible to make this book accurate, up-to-date, and in accord with the standards accepted at the time of publication. The recommendations contained herein reflect APHON's judgment regarding the state of general knowledge and practice in the field as of the date of publication. Any practice described in this book should be applied by the healthcare practitioner in accordance with professional standards of care used in regard to the unique circumstances that may apply in each situation. The reader is advised always to check product information (package inserts) for changes and new information regarding dosage and contraindications before administering any drug. Caution is especially urged when using new or infrequently ordered drugs or treatments. Figures and tables in the book are used as examples only. They are not meant to be all-inclusive, nor do they represent endorsement of any particular institution by APHON. Any mention of specific products and opinions related to those products do not indicate or imply endorsement by APHON. The authors, editors, and publisher are not responsible for errors or omissions or for consequences from application of this book, and make no warranty, expressed, or implied in regard to the contents of this book.

## Editor

**Nancy E. Kline, PhD RN CPNP FAAN**
Director, Center for Evidence-Based Practice and Research
Department of Nursing
Memorial Sloan-Kettering Cancer Center
New York, NY

## Section Editors

**Wendy L. Hobbie, MSN RN CRNP**
Associate Program Director Cancer Survivorship Program
The Children's Hospital of Philadelphia
Philadelphia, PA

**Mary C. Hooke, PhD RN CPON®**
Clinical Nurse Specialist
Children's Hospitals and Clinics of Minnesota
Minneapolis, MN

**Cheryl Rodgers, MSN RN CPNP CPON®**
Clinical Instructor
Baylor College of Medicine
Pediatric Nurse Practitioner
Texas Children's Hospital
Houston, TX

**Joan O'Brien Shea, MSN RN CPON®**
Education Coordinator
General Clinical Research Center
Children's Hospital Boston
Boston, MA

# Contributors

**Sameeya N. Ahmed-Winston, MSN RN CPNP**
Pediatric Nurse Practitioner
Bone Marrow Transplant Clinic
Texas Children's Hospital
Houston, TX

**Pat Wills Alcoser, MSN RN CPON®**
Pediatric Nurse Practitioner
Bone Marrow Transplant Clinic
Texas Children's Hospital
Houston, TX

**Arlene L. Androkites, MSN RN CPNP**
Pediatric Oncology Nurse Practitioner
Dana-Farber Cancer Institute
Boston, MA

**Christina Baggott, MN APRN-BC PNP CPON®**
Pediatric Nurse Practitioner
Lucile Packard Children's Hospital at Stanford
Palo Alto, CA

**Diane E. Baniewicz, MSN RN CRNP**
Nurse Practitioner, Division of Oncology
Children's Hospital of Philadelphia
Philadelphia, PA

**Karyn J. Brundige, MSN RN ARNP CPNP**
Pediatric Hematology/Oncology Nurse Practitioner
Children's Hospital and Regional Medical Center
Seattle, WA

**Claire A. Carlson, BSN RN**
Research Nurse/Nurse Coordinator, Cancer Survivorship Program
Children's Hospital of Philadelphia
Philadelphia, PA

**Christine Chordas, MSN RN CPNP**
Pediatric Nurse Practitioner
Dana-Farber Cancer Institute
Boston, MA

**Susanne B. Conley, MSN RN CRNP**
Clinical Nurse Specialist
Dana-Farber Cancer Institute
Boston, MA

**Teresa M. Conte, MSN RN CNAA CPON®**
Adjunct Faculty
Villanova University
Villanova, PA

**Rebecca D'Amore, MSN RN CPNP CPON®**
Pediatric Nurse Practitioner
Memorial Sloan-Kettering Cancer Center
New York, NY

**Linda D'Andrea, MSN RN CS CCRN CPON®**
Pediatric Nurse Practitioner
Memorial Sloan-Kettering Cancer Center
New York, NY

**Deborah Diotallevi, MS RN CPNP**
Pediatric Nurse Practitioner
Memorial Sloan-Kettering Cancer Center
New York, NY

**Judith M. Doell, MSN RN FNP CPON®**
Clinical Nurse Specialist, Oncology Clinic
Children's Hospital of Philadelphia
Philadelphia, PA

**Tracy Douglas, MSN RN PNP**
Pediatric Nurse Practitioner, Division of Neuro-Oncology, Department of Oncology
St. Jude Children's Research Hospital
Memphis, TN

**Eileen Duffey-Lind, MSN RN CPNP**
Pediatric Oncology Nurse Practitioner
Dana-Farber Cancer Institute
Boston, MA

**Debra A. Eshelman-Kent, MSN RN CPNP**
Pediatric Nurse Practitioner
Children's Medical Center–Dallas
Dallas, TX

**Angela M. Ethier, PhD RN CNS CPN CT**
Houston, TX

**Elisa S. Frederick, MSN RN PNP CS**
Pediatric Oncology Nurse Practitioner
Jimmy Fund Clinic/Dana-Farber Cancer Institute
Boston, MA

**Rhonda Fritz, MSN RN CPNP**
Hemophilia Nurse Practitioner
Children's Hospital Boston/Boston Hemophilia Center
Boston, MA

**Elizabeth A. Gilger, MSN RN APRN-BC CPON®**
Pediatric Nurse Practitioner
St. Jude Children's Research Hospital
Memphis, TN

**Sara Gonzalez, MS RD LD**
Clinical Dietician
Texas Children's Hospital
Houston, TX

**Kathy M. Harney, RN PNP**
Nurse Practitioner—Thrombophilia/Anticoagulation Service,
  Division of Hematology/Oncology
Children's Hospital Boston
Boston, MA

**Jane Hennessy, MPH RN CNP-AC**
Pediatric Nurse Practitioner
Children's Hospitals and Clinics of Minnesota
Minneapolis, MN

**Ruth Anne Herring, MSN RN CPNP CPON®**
Pediatric Nurse Practitioner, Vannie E. Cook, Jr. Children's
  Cancer and Hematology Clinic
Texas Children's Cancer Center and Hematology Service
McAllen, TX

**Joy Hesselgrave, MSN RN CPON®**
Clinical Specialist
Texas Children's Hospital
Houston, TX

**Wendy L. Hobbie, MSN RN CRNP**
Associate Program Director Cancer Survivorship Program
The Children's Hospital of Philadelphia
Philadelphia, PA

**Marilyn J. Hockenberry, PhD RN-CS PNP FAAN**
Director, Center for Research and Evidence-Based Practice
Professor, Department of Pediatrics
Baylor College of Medicine
Nurse Scientist
Texas Children's Hospital
Director of Nurse Practitioners
Texas Children's Cancer Center
Houston, TX

**Judith Ann Holloway, BSN RN CPON®**
Legacy Emanuel Children's Hospital
Portland, OR

**Mary C. Hooke, PhD RN CPON®**
Clinical Nurse Specialist
Children's Hospitals and Clinics of Minnesota
Minneapolis, MN

**Eufemia Jacob, PhD RN**
Assistant Professor
University of California-Los Angeles
Los Angeles, CA

**Nancy E. Kline, PhD RN CPNP FAAN**
Director, Center for Evidence-Based Practice and Research
Department of Nursing
Memorial Sloan-Kettering Cancer Center
New York, NY

**Ruth Landers, MSN RN CPNP CPON®**
Pediatric Nurse Practitioner
Arkansas Children's Hospital
Little Rock, AR

**Wendy Landier, MSN RN CPNP CPON®**
Clinical Director, Center for Cancer Survivorship
City of Hope National Medical Center
Duarte, CA

**Deborah J. Lee, BSN RN CPNP CPON®**
Education Coordinator, Bone Marrow Transplant
Texas Children's Hospital
Houston, TX

**Lauri A. Linder, MS APRN CPON®**
Assistant Professor, Clinical
University of Utah College of Nursing
Salt Lake City, UT

**Catherine Fiona Macpherson, PhD RN CPON®**
Staff Nurse
Children's Hospital and Regional Medical Center
Lecturer
University of Washington School of Nursing
Seattle, WA

**Linda Madsen, MS RN CNP CPON®**
CNP
Children's Hospitals and Clinics of Minnesota
Minneapolis, MN

**Kathleen McCarthy, BSN RN**
Head Research Nurse
Texas Children's Hospital
Baylor College of Medicine
Houston, TX

**Robin McCune, RN CPN CPON®**
Pediatric Hematology/Oncology Clinician
Medical City Children's Hospital
Dallas, TX

**Julie McMahon, MSN RN CPNP-AC CPON®**
Pediatric Nurse Practitioner, Pediatric Observation Unit
Memorial Sloan-Kettering Cancer Center
New York, NY

**Kathleen Meeske, PhD RN**
Director, Health Outcomes and Cancer Control Research
Childrens Hospital Los Angeles
Los Angeles, CA

**Rebecca A. Monroe, MSN RN CPNP CPON®**
McKinney, TX

## Contributors

**Revonda B. Mosher, MSN RN CPNP CPON®**
Pediatric Nurse Practitioner, Division of Pediatric Hematology-Oncology
Sinai Hospital of Baltimore
Baltimore, MD

**James E. Munn, MS RN**
Program and Nurse Coordinator, Hemophilia and Coagulation Disorders Program
University of Michigan
Ann Arbor, MI

**Colleen Nixon, BSN RN CPON®**
Clinical Educator, Inpatient Hematology/Oncology
Children's Hospital Boston
Boston, MA

**Robbie Norville, MSN RN CPON®**
Clinical Nurse Specialist
Texas Children's Cancer Center and Hematology Service
Houston, TX

**Suzanne L. Nuss, PhD RN APRN-CNS**
Clinical Nurse Specialist
The Nebraska Medical Center
Omaha, NE

**Janice Nuuhiwa, MSN RN CNS CPON®**
Staff Development Specialist
Children's Memorial Hospital
Chicago, IL

**Susan K. Ogle, MSN RN CRNP**
Oncology Clinic Nurse Manager/Cancer Survivorship Nurse Practitioner
Children's Hospital of Philadelphia
Philadelphia, PA

**Joan O'Hanlon-Curry, MS RN CPNP CPON®**
Administrative Nurse Manager/Pediatric Nurse Practitioner
The Children's Hospital at Montefiore
Bronx, NY

**Jill E. Brace O'Neill, MS RN-CS PNP**
Pediatric Nurse Practitioner
David B. Perini, Jr. Quality of Life Clinic/Dana-Farber Cancer Institute
Boston, MA

**Janice Post-White, PhD RN FAAN**
Research Consultant, Complementary and Alternative Medicine
Adjunct Associate Professor
University of Minnesota School of Nursing
Minneapolis, MN

**Elaine Pottenger, MS RN CNS CPNP**
Pediatric Nurse Practitioner
Memorial Sloan-Kettering Cancer Center
Chicago, IL

**Joanne Quillen, MSN RN CRNP CPON®**
Neuro-Oncology Nurse Practitioner
Children's Hospital of Philadelphia
Philadelphia, PA

**Debbie Reid, BSN RN CPON®**
Education Manager
Childrens Hospital Los Angeles
Los Angeles, CA

**Maureen M. Reilly, BSN RN**
Research Nurse/Nurse Coordinator, Cancer Survivorship Program
Children's Hospital of Philadelphia
Philadelphia, PA

**Deborah L. Robinson, MSN APRN BC PNP CPON®**
Advanced Practice Nurse, Pediatric Hematology/Oncology
St. Louis Children's Hospital, Washington University
St. Louis, MO

**Lona Roll, MSN RN**
Clinical Nurse Specialist Pediatric Hematology/Oncology
CHRISTUS Santa Rosa Childrens Hospital
San Antonio, TX

**Cheryl Rodgers, MSN RN CPNP CPON®**
Clinical Instructor
Baylor College of Medicine
Pediatric Nurse Practitioner
Texas Children's Hospital
Houston, TX

**Susanne Rosenberg, BSN RN CPON®**
RN Staff Nurse
St. Louis Children's Hospital
St. Louis, MO

**Carol Rossetto, MSN RN CPNP CPON®**
Pediatric Nurse Practitioner
Memorial Sloan-Kettering Cancer Center
New York, NY

**Kathleen Ruccione, MPH RN FAAN**
Nursing Administrator/Director, HOPE Program
Center for Cancer and Blood Diseases
Childrens Hospital Los Angeles
Los Angeles, CA

**Vicki K. Schaefers, MSN RN CNP-AC CPON®**
Acute Care Pediatric Nurse Practitioner
Children's Hospitals and Clinics of Minnesota
Minneapolis, MN

**Beth Ann Savage, MSN CPNP CPON®**
Pediatric Advanced Practice Nurse
University of Medicine and Dentistry of New Jersey
The Cancer Institute of NJ
New Brunswick, NJ

**Tamara E. Scott, MSN CPNP CPON®**
Pediatric Hematology/Oncology Nurse Practitioner
Kaiser Permanente Medical Center
Sacramento, CA

**Rita Secola, MSN RN CPON®**
Clinical Manager
Childrens Hospital Los Angeles
Los Angeles, CA

**Joan O'Brien Shea, MSN RN CPON®**
Education Coordinator
General Clinical Research Center
Childrens Hospital Boston
Boston, MA

**Kristin Stegenga, PhD RN**
Nurse Researcher
Children's Mercy Hospital
Kansas City, MO

**Cynthia A. Stutzer, MS RN**
Clinical Nurse Specialist, Oncology
British Columbia Children's Hospital
Vancouver, BC, Canada

**Christine Sullivan, MSN RNC PNP**
Pediatric Nurse Practitioner, Pediatric Oncology
UMass Memorial Medical Center
Worcester, MA

**Roseann Tucci, MSN RN CPNP**
Nurse Practitioner
Memorial Sloan-Kettering Cancer Center
New York, NY

**Leticia Valdiviez, MSN RN CNS CPON®**
Clinical Nurse Specialist
Children's Memorial Hospital
Chicago, IL

**Joetta D. Wallace, MSN RN FNPC CPON®**
Pediatric Nurse Practitioner
Miller Children's Hospital
Long Beach, CA

**Cynthia Walsh, MA RN CPON®**
Assistant Nurse Manager, Hematology/Oncology
Children's Hospitals and Clinics of Minnesota
Minneapolis, MN

**Melody Ann Watral, MSN RN CPNP CPON®**
Pediatric Nurse Practitioner, Pediatric Neuro-Oncology
Duke University Medical Center
Durham, NC

**Branlyn E. Werba, PhD**
Pediatric Psychologist, Division of Oncology
Children's Hospital of Philadelphia
Philadelphia, PA

**Elizabeth H. Whittam, MS RNC FNP**
Nurse Practitioner, Adult Survivor Program, Pediatrics
Memorial Sloan-Kettering Cancer Center
New York, NY

# Reviewers

**Sarah J. Bottomley, MSN RN CPNP**
Pediatric Nurse Practitioner-Endocrine
M.D. Anderson Cancer Center
Houston, TX

**Michael E. Comeau, MS RN AOCN®**
Clinical Nurse Specialist, Pediatrics Jimmy Fund Clinic
Dana-Farber Cancer Institute
Boston, MA

**Deborah S. Echtenkamp, MSN RN CPON®**
Pediatric Hematology/Oncology Clinical Nurse Specialist
Medical City Children's Hospital
Dallas, TX

**Lindsay A. Gainer, MSN RN**
Nurse Manager
Hematopoetic Stem Cell Transplant Unit
Children's Hospital Boston
Boston, MA

**Lisa Morrissey, MSN RN CNE-BC CPON®**
Nurse Manager, Inpatient Hematology/Oncology
Children's Hospital Boston
Boston, MA

**Jill E. Brace O'Neill, MS RN-CS PNP**
Pediatric Nurse Practitioner
David B. Perini Jr. Quality of Life Clinic, Dana-Farber Cancer Institute
Boston, MA

# Table of Contents

## Section I. Pediatric Hematology/Oncology Nursing Practice

History and Philosophy of Pediatric Oncology Nursing ..................................................2
*Marilyn J. Hockenberry*

Standards of Pediatric Oncology Nursing ..................................................4
*Revonda B. Mosher*

Association of Pediatric Hematology/Oncology Nurses ..................................................6
*Joetta D. Wallace*

## Section II. Pediatric Cancers

Overview of Childhood Cancer ..................................................10
*Christina Baggott*

Epidemiology of Childhood Cancer ..................................................10
*Kathleen Ruccione and Kathleen Meeske*

Leukemia ..................................................15
*Kathleen McCarthy*

Non-Hodgkin's Lymphoma ..................................................20
*Arlene L. Androkites*

Hodgkin's Lymphoma ..................................................25
*Arlene L. Androkites*

Central-Nervous-System Tumors ..................................................28
*Melody Ann Watral*

Neuroblastoma ..................................................32
*Linda D'Andrea*

Osteosarcoma ..................................................36
*Judith Ann Holloway*

Ewing's Sarcoma of Bone and Soft Tissue and Peripheral Primitive Neuroectodermal Tumors ..................................................40
*Rebecca D'Amore*

Tumors of the Kidney ..................................................43
*Eileen Duffey-Lind*

Rhabdomyosarcoma ..................................................48
*Julie McMahon*

Retinoblastoma ..................................................52
*Diane Baniewicz*

Rare Tumors of Childhood ..................................................54
*Elisa S. Frederick*

## Section III. Overview of Hematology

Origin of Blood Cells ..................................................62
*Jane Hennessy and Tamara E. Scott*

Anemia ..................................................64
*Jane Hennessy*

Neutropenia ..................................................65
*Jane Hennessy and Tamara E. Scott*

Thrombocytopenia ..................................................67
*Jane Hennessy*

## Section IV. Childhood Cancer Treatment

Diagnostic and Staging Procedures ..................................................70
*Nancy E. Kline*

History of Chemotherapy . . . . . . . . . . . . . . . . . . . . . . . . . . . . . . . . . . . . . . . . . . . . . . . . . . . . . . . . . . . . . 73
*Christine Sullivan*

Clinical Trials . . . . . . . . . . . . . . . . . . . . . . . . . . . . . . . . . . . . . . . . . . . . . . . . . . . . . . . . . . . . . . . . . . . . . 74
*Elizabeth A. Gilger*

Chemotherapy . . . . . . . . . . . . . . . . . . . . . . . . . . . . . . . . . . . . . . . . . . . . . . . . . . . . . . . . . . . . . . . . . . . . 75
*Christine Sullivan*

Guidelines for Safe Handling of Chemotherapy . . . . . . . . . . . . . . . . . . . . . . . . . . . . . . . . . . . . . . . . . 89
*Susanne B. Conley*

Administration of Vesicants . . . . . . . . . . . . . . . . . . . . . . . . . . . . . . . . . . . . . . . . . . . . . . . . . . . . . . . . . 90
*Linda Madsen*

Surgery . . . . . . . . . . . . . . . . . . . . . . . . . . . . . . . . . . . . . . . . . . . . . . . . . . . . . . . . . . . . . . . . . . . . . . . . . . 92
*Carol Rossetto*

Radiation Therapy . . . . . . . . . . . . . . . . . . . . . . . . . . . . . . . . . . . . . . . . . . . . . . . . . . . . . . . . . . . . . . . . 94
*Joy Hesselgrave and Christine Chordas*

Hematopoietic Stem-Cell Transplantation . . . . . . . . . . . . . . . . . . . . . . . . . . . . . . . . . . . . . . . . . . . . . 98
*Robbie Norville*

Biologic Response Modifiers . . . . . . . . . . . . . . . . . . . . . . . . . . . . . . . . . . . . . . . . . . . . . . . . . . . . . . . 108
*Robin McCune*

Cell and Gene Therapy . . . . . . . . . . . . . . . . . . . . . . . . . . . . . . . . . . . . . . . . . . . . . . . . . . . . . . . . . . . 112
*Robbie Norville*

Complementary and Alternative Treatments . . . . . . . . . . . . . . . . . . . . . . . . . . . . . . . . . . . . . . . . . . 115
*Janice Post-White*

## Section V. Side Effects of Treatment

Bone-Marrow Suppression . . . . . . . . . . . . . . . . . . . . . . . . . . . . . . . . . . . . . . . . . . . . . . . . . . . . . . . . 122
*Pat Wills Alcoser*

Impairment of the Immune System . . . . . . . . . . . . . . . . . . . . . . . . . . . . . . . . . . . . . . . . . . . . . . . . . 123
*Pat Wills Alcoser*

Central-Nervous-System Complications . . . . . . . . . . . . . . . . . . . . . . . . . . . . . . . . . . . . . . . . . . . . . 126
*Linda Madsen*

Ototoxicity . . . . . . . . . . . . . . . . . . . . . . . . . . . . . . . . . . . . . . . . . . . . . . . . . . . . . . . . . . . . . . . . . . . . . 130
*Wendy Landier*

Endocrine Abnormalities . . . . . . . . . . . . . . . . . . . . . . . . . . . . . . . . . . . . . . . . . . . . . . . . . . . . . . . . . 131
*Rebecca A. Monroe*

Cardiac and Pulmonary Complications . . . . . . . . . . . . . . . . . . . . . . . . . . . . . . . . . . . . . . . . . . . . . . 132
*Vicki Schaefers*

Gastrointestinal Complications . . . . . . . . . . . . . . . . . . . . . . . . . . . . . . . . . . . . . . . . . . . . . . . . . . . . 134
*Ruth Landers and Joan O'Hanlon-Curry*

Renal and Bladder Complications . . . . . . . . . . . . . . . . . . . . . . . . . . . . . . . . . . . . . . . . . . . . . . . . . . 140
*Ruth Anne Herring*

Skin Changes . . . . . . . . . . . . . . . . . . . . . . . . . . . . . . . . . . . . . . . . . . . . . . . . . . . . . . . . . . . . . . . . . . . 142
*Robbie Norville*

Musculoskeletal Complications . . . . . . . . . . . . . . . . . . . . . . . . . . . . . . . . . . . . . . . . . . . . . . . . . . . . 143
*Sameeya N. Ahmed-Winston*

Nutritional Complications . . . . . . . . . . . . . . . . . . . . . . . . . . . . . . . . . . . . . . . . . . . . . . . . . . . . . . . . 145
*Cheryl Rodgers*

Growth and Developmental Complications . . . . . . . . . . . . . . . . . . . . . . . . . . . . . . . . . . . . . . . . . . 146
*Deborah J. Lee*

Pain . . . . . . . . . . . . . . . . . . . . . . . . . . . . . . . . . . . . . . . . . . . . . . . . . . . . . . . . . . . . . . . . . . . . . . . . . . . 148
*Eufemia Jacob*

Oncologic Emergencies . . . . . . . . . . . . . . . . . . . . . . . . . . . . . . . . . . . . . . . . . . . . . . . . . . . . . . . . . . . 153
*Rita Secola and Debbie Reid*

# Table of Contents

## Section VI. Supportive Care

Psychological Preparation and Support for Painful Procedures .............................................. 162
*Catherine Fiona Macpherson*

Sedation for Painful Procedures. ........................................................................................ 164
*Catherine Fiona Macpherson*

Central Venous Access Devices ......................................................................................... 165
*Joetta D. Wallace*

Nutritional Support .......................................................................................................... 169
*Cheryl Rodgers and Sara Gonzalez*

Treatment of Infections. .................................................................................................... 173
*Pat Wills Alcoser*

Blood Product Support. .................................................................................................... 178
*Teresa M. Conte*

## Section VII. Psychosocial Issues

Development of Infants (Birth–1 Year) .............................................................................. 186
*Mary C. Hooke*

Development of Toddlers (1–3 Years) ................................................................................ 187
*Mary C. Hooke*

Development of Preschoolers (4–6 Years) .......................................................................... 188
*Mary C. Hooke*

Development of School-Age Children (7–12 Years) ........................................................... 189
*Linda Madsen*

Development of Adolescents (13–18 Years). ....................................................................... 191
*Linda Madsen*

Development of Young Adults (18–25 Years) ..................................................................... 194
*Linda Madsen and Mary C. Hooke*

Family Systems ................................................................................................................ 197
*Lona Roll*

Family Resources ............................................................................................................. 199
*Suzanne L. Nuss*

Cultural Care ................................................................................................................... 202
*Jane Hennessy*

Spirituality ....................................................................................................................... 205
*Kristin Stegenga*

School Reentry and Attendance ......................................................................................... 205
*Lauri A. Linder*

Professional Nurse-Patient Relationships. ........................................................................... 208
*Cynthia Walsh*

## Section VIII. Patient and Family Education

Teaching by Developmental Level. ..................................................................................... 216
*Wendy Landier*

Family Education ............................................................................................................. 219
*Judith M. Doell*

Critical Learning Periods. .................................................................................................. 222
*Judith M. Doell*

The Pediatric Hematology/Oncology Nurse as Educator. .................................................... 224
*Judith M. Doell*

## Section IX. Care for the Terminally Ill Child and the Family

Children and Death ........................................................... 228
*Angela M. Ethier*

Physical Care of the Terminally Ill Child ................................... 229
*Janice Nuuhiwa*

Psychosocial Care of the Terminally Ill Child .............................. 233
*Janice Nuuhiwa*

Bereavement .................................................................. 235
*Rebecca A. Monroe*

Professionals' Grief, Distress, and Bereavement ............................ 237
*Cynthia A. Stutzer*

Moral Distress ............................................................... 239
*Cynthia A. Stutzer*

Ethical Dilemmas in Terminal Care .......................................... 241
*Kristin Stegenga*

Legal Concerns in Terminal Care ............................................ 243
*Kristin Stegenga*

## Section X. Late Effects of Childhood Cancer

Definition and Overview ..................................................... 246
*Wendy L. Hobbie*

Central Nervous System ..................................................... 246
*Joanne Quillen*

Hypothalamic-Pituitary Axis ................................................. 253
*Deborah Diotallevi and Elaine Pottenger*

Thyroid Function ............................................................ 255
*Deborah Diotallevi and Elaine Pottenger*

Vision and Hearing .......................................................... 256
*Debra A. Eshelman-Kent*

Head and Neck .............................................................. 258
*Maureen M. Reilly and Claire A. Carlson*

Cardiovascular System ...................................................... 260
*Joanne Quillen*

Respiratory System .......................................................... 261
*Claire A. Carlson and Maureen M. Reilly*

Gastrointestinal and Hepatic System ........................................ 263
*Claire A. Carlson and Maureen M. Reilly*

Genitourinary System ....................................................... 265
*Debra A. Eshelman-Kent*

Reproductive System: Testes ................................................ 267
*Susan K. Ogle and Wendy L. Hobbie*

Reproductive System: Ovaries ............................................... 268
*Susan K. Ogle and Wendy L. Hobbie*

Musculoskeletal System ..................................................... 269
*Debra A. Eshelman-Kent*

Hematopoietic System ...................................................... 271
*Jill E. Brace O'Neill*

Immune System ............................................................. 272
*Jill E. Brace O'Neill*

Second Malignant Neoplasms ................................................ 273
*Elizabeth H. Whittam*

# Table of Contents

Psychosocial Effects: Personal-Emotional .................................................. 275
*Branlyn E. Werba*

Psychosocial Effects: Political-Social ........................................................ 276
*Branlyn E. Werba and Wendy L. Hobbie*

Psychosocial Effects: Educational Issues ................................................... 277
*Branlyn E. Werba*

Promoting Health After Childhood Cancer .............................................. 278
*Roseann Tucci*

## Section XI. Hematology

Autoimmune Hemolytic Anemia .............................................................. 286
*Karyn J. Brundige*

Sickle-Cell Disease ..................................................................................... 288
*Beth Ann Savage*

Thalassemia ................................................................................................ 292
*Beth Ann Savage*

Glucose-6-Phosphate Dehydrogenase Deficiency .................................... 294
*Deborah L. Robinson*

Hereditary Spherocytosis ........................................................................... 296
*Susanne Rosenberg*

Bone-Marrow-Failure Syndromes ............................................................. 297
*Joan O'Brien Shea*

Shwachman-Diamond Syndrome ............................................................. 302
*Teresa M. Conte*

Chronic Neutropenia ................................................................................. 304
*Karyn J. Brundige*

Immune Thrombocytopenic Purpura ....................................................... 307
*Phaedra Truglia*

Evans Syndrome ......................................................................................... 309
*Karyn J. Brundige*

Thrombosis and Thrombophilia ............................................................... 312
*Kathy M. Harney*

Hemolytic-Uremic Syndrome ................................................................... 314
*Leticia Valdiviez*

Paroxysmal Nocturnal Hemoglobinuria ................................................... 317
*Colleen Nixon*

Hemophilia ................................................................................................. 320
*Rhonda Fritz*

Von Willebrand Disease ............................................................................. 323
*James E. Munn*

**Index** .................................................................................................... 329

# Acknowledgments

The third edition of the *Essentials of Pediatric Hematology/Oncology Nursing: A Core Curriculum* has a new face, a new title, and a remarkable amount of new information. This edition not only incorporates pertinent updates on the pediatric oncology content, but also includes an entirely new section containing 16 chapters of hematology content. More than 70 APHON members, along with other experts in the field of pediatric hematology/oncology nursing, participated in this work, and their dedication and contributions to a truly exceptional resource is evident. It is our hope and intent that this reference text is of benefit to every pediatric hematology/oncology nurse, and it is to the patients we care for that we dedicate this book.

Nancy E. Kline, Editor

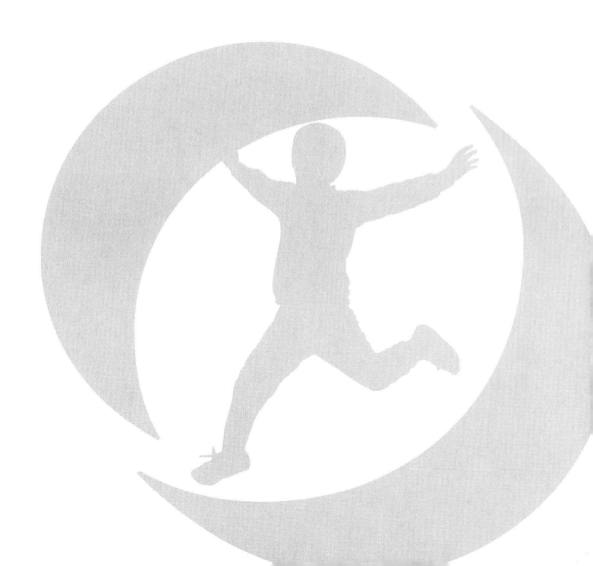

# Section I  Pediatric Hematology/Oncology Nursing Practice

Nancy E. Kline

## Section Outline

**History and Philosophy of Pediatric Oncology Nursing**

**Standards of Pediatric Oncology Nursing**

**Association of Pediatric Hematology/Oncology Nurses**

# History and Philosophy of Pediatric Oncology Nursing

*Marilyn J. Hockenberry*

Few situations in nursing exceed the challenges of caring for a child with cancer. To accomplish this in today's complex healthcare environment, nurses caring for children with cancer must keep pace with advances in treatment and technology. Childhood cancer care requires skilled nurses to manage disease-related and treatment-related side effects, coordinate supportive care, administer chemotherapy, and prepare the child and the family for invasive procedures and complex treatment schedules. Expert pediatric oncology nurses are able to evaluate the child's condition using their extensive knowledge of childhood cancer, develop a plan of care in collaboration with other healthcare professionals, provide direct nursing care management, and evaluate the child's progress based on specific patient outcomes. As more children are treated in the outpatient or home environment, nurses have become coordinators of care in these settings. As a result, even though some treatment still necessitates hospitalization, pediatric oncology nurses support outpatient treatment when possible.

As a pediatric specialty that involves the care of children of all ages (i.e., from infancy through adolescence), pediatric oncology nursing requires a strong foundation in the normal growth and development of children and the principles of family-centered care. Within an oncology discipline, pediatric nurses acquire knowledge of a practice that must include cancer screening, follow-up of late effects, assessment for second malignancies, and prevention of adult cancers. Even though more children are either living with or cured of cancer than die from it, pediatric oncology nurses still must be specialized in pain management and end-of-life care in order to provide support and comfort to children who will not survive.

## History of Childhood Cancer Treatment

The first pediatric cancer unit in the United States was established in 1939 at the Memorial Sloan-Kettering Cancer Center in New York. St. Jude Children's Research Hospital was the first facility devoted exclusively to pediatric malignancies (Foley & Fergusson, 2002). The discovery in the 1940s that folic acid antagonists produced temporary remission in children with acute leukemia marked the first documented progress made in the treatment of childhood cancer. In the 1950s and 1960s, single chemotherapy agents were used to treat childhood cancer, resulting in modest successes. During the late 1960s, combinations of chemotherapy agents were found to be more successful than single-drug therapy. By the 1970s, childhood leukemia was responding dramatically to combination chemotherapy. During this period, prophylactic treatment to the central nervous system (CNS) in children with leukemia resulted in the landmark discovery that CNS disease could be prevented, resulting in improved survival.

Wilms' tumor is another example of early success in the treatment of childhood cancer. Forty years ago, cure rates for children with Wilms' tumor, the most common kidney cancer, reached only 20% at the best treatment centers. Today, 90% of children with Wilms' tumor are cured. Similar successes are found with other childhood cancers; more than 80% of children with cancer surpass the 3-year survival mark (Gurney & Bondy, 2006).

Rapid discoveries and improvements in cure rates were made possible through national cooperative studies. The Children's Cancer Group (CCG) and Pediatric Oncology Group (POG) were established in 1955 with the support of the National Cancer Institute. Major cancer centers and children's hospitals participated in these study groups from the very beginning, and most children with cancer were enrolled in protocol studies. As a result, findings from national cancer clinical trials were rapidly disseminated. The impact of cooperative studies in pediatrics prompted the development of multi-drug chemotherapy, while emphasizing the need to develop individualized combinations of modalities as well.

In the 1970s, it became evident that different tumors responded differently to the same treatment therapies. For example, although radiation therapy was appropriate for Ewing's sarcoma, it was not effective for osteogenic sarcoma. Protocols were adjusted accordingly. The effect of this knowledge reached far beyond the pediatric oncology specialty. This relatively small field in oncology influenced the development of treatment trials for adults with cancer. The successes of the pediatric oncology national study groups in discovering the use of combination chemotherapy, developing adjunct therapies, and organizing treatment through cooperative trials paved the way for future progress in treating all types of cancer.

Since the development of the two pediatric oncology cooperative groups more than 50 years ago, nurses have played crucial roles within the organizations (Ruccione, Hinds, Wallace, & Kelly, 2005). Networks among pediatric oncology nurses were created to facilitate nursing contributions to the disease committees throughout both CCG and POG. Nurses participated as members of protocol, disease, and scientific committees and contributed to concept design, trial analysis, and publications. Nurses were instrumental in developing patient and family teaching tools and were involved in writing treatment guidelines, assisting with the completion of protocol roadmaps, and serving as resources for other professionals within the cooperative groups (Ruccione et al.).

In 1998, CCG, POG, the National Wilms Tumor Study Group, and the Intergroup Rhabdomyosarcoma Study Group (IRSG) formed a unified group named the Children's Oncology Group (COG). Pediatric oncology nurses still continue their important roles within COG. Recently, COG nursing leaders have taken an active role in structuring nursing research within the cooperative group. This initiative is paving the way for nursing researchers to play significant roles in collaborative research studies within the specialty.

## History of Pediatric Oncology Nursing

Nursing was originally generic in practice; that is, nurses cared for all patients, regardless of age or diagnosis. It was not until the early 20th century that nurses began to specialize in the type of care provided. Oncology nursing was recognized as a specialty with the development of the first academic course devoted exclusively to cancer nursing at Teacher's College at Columbia University in 1947 (Craytor, 1982). At that time, the nurses who took care of children with cancer were pediatric nurses who had no formal training in oncology. Care of a child with cancer was short in duration and focused on helping a family and child face certain death. Children were most commonly diagnosed with leukemia and often bled to death due to the unavailability of component blood therapies such as platelets and packed red blood cells. Intravenous therapies were temporary and difficult to administer; there were no central lines or parenteral nutrition. The nurse's role focused on supporting nutritional needs (nurses themselves often cooked special foods for the child), managing infections with limited antibiotics, assessing for the constant threat of infection, and supporting the family and the child. Struggling to prevent or treat infection with first-generation antibiotics involved working in reverse isolation with patients who had fever and neutropenia. Children frequently died of overwhelming infection.

It was not until the mid-1970s that pediatric oncology nursing became recognized as a distinct subspecialty. With the advent of combination therapies in the late 1960s and 1970s, patients developed specific care needs. In addition, the increased survival of children treated for cancer required extensive nursing knowledge of the diagnosis and treatment of cancer, side-effect management, and supportive-care strategies.

In 1974, the Association of Pediatric Oncology Nurses (APON) was formed by a group of nurses who met at the Association for the Care of Children's Health Conference in 1973 (Greene, 1983). APON was based on the philosophy that pediatric oncology nursing is a specialty that requires specific knowledge and expertise in the care of children who have cancer. Children with cancer are not small adults, but individuals who have special and unique needs. Childhood cancers are significantly different from adult cancers. They are generally systemic rather than organ-based, requiring distinctly different treatment regimens. Today, pediatric oncology nursing is recognized as a distinct subspecialty within pediatrics as well as within oncology. This distinction was formalized with the development of specialty certification in pediatric oncology nursing in 1993 (Foley & Fergusson, 2002).

## Philosophy of Pediatric Oncology Nursing

Pediatric oncology nurses are essential contributors to the successful treatment and cure of children with cancer. As such, pediatric oncology nurses recognize the importance of family-centered care, collaborative practice, and excellence in clinical care that begins at diagnosis and continues through survivorship, sometimes until after a child's death. Above all, pediatric oncology nurses realize the meaning hope can give. The philosophy of family-centered care is central to pediatric oncology nursing practice. The recognition that the family is the constant in a child's life is key to successful pediatric nursing practice. This philosophy is exemplified by nursing care that is planned with the family and the child. Family-centered care begins at the time of diagnosis with the child included in decisions as is age appropriate.

Pediatric oncology nursing thrives on team collaboration. It is believed that the best care is provided to patients with cancer and their families when all members of the patient care team are actively involved. A commitment to family-centered care requires the family and the child, as age appropriate, to be involved in all decisions made by the patient care team. Focus on the child and the family's ability to maintain as normal a lifestyle as possible during treatment requires collaboration among all involved in the decision making. Placing the child and the family at the center of care allows nurses to provide individualized care that provides an optimal chance for cure within the context of the child and the family's unique environment.

Pediatric oncology nurses provide care for a patient population that has an expectation of survival and probable cure. Within the past 20 years, pediatric cancer has become a chronic disease that has increased the scope of practice for the pediatric oncology nurse. Care for survivors of childhood cancer is now a major focus of nursing practice within the specialty. At the same time, the pediatric oncology nurse must be competent in providing care for the child and the family in the event the child will not survive cancer.

Despite the dramatic improvements in survival rates for children with cancer, the family's needs are tremendous as they cope with a serious physical illness and the fear that the child will not be cured. For pediatric oncology nurses, support of children and their families is based on the belief that communication promotes understanding and clarity; with understanding, fear diminishes; in the absence of fear, hope emerges; and in the presence of hope, anything is possible.

## References

Craytor, J. K. (1982). Highlights in education for cancer nursing. *Oncology Nursing Forum, 9*(4), 51–59.

Foley, G. V., & Fergusson, J. H. (2007). History, issues, and trends. In C. R. Baggott, K. P. Kelly, D. Fochtman, & G. V. Foley (Eds.), *Nursing care of children and adolescents with cancer* (3rd ed., pp. 2–23). Glenview, IL: Association of Pediatric Hematology/Oncology Nurses.

Greene, P. E. (1983). The Association of Pediatric Oncology Nurses: The first ten years. *Oncology Nursing Forum, 10,* 59–63.

Gurney, J. G., & Bondy, M. L. (2006). Epidemiology of childhood cancer. In P. A. Pizzo & D. G. Poplack (Eds.), *Principles and practice of pediatric oncology* (5th ed., pp. 1–13). Philadelphia: Lippincott, Williams & Wilkins.

Ruccione, K. S., Hinds, P. S., Wallace, J. D., & Kelly, K. P. (2005). Creating a novel structure for nursing research in a cooperative clinical trials group: The children's oncology group experience. *Seminars in Oncology Nursing, 21*(2), 79–88.

# Standards of Pediatric Oncology Nursing

*Revonda B. Mosher*

In 1978, the Association of Pediatric Oncology Nurses (APON), in collaboration with the American Nurses Association, published the first pediatric oncology nursing standards, *Standards of Pediatric Oncology Nursing Practice*. In 1987 and 2000, the standards were revised, under the titles *Scope of Practice and Outcome Standard of Practice for Pediatric Oncology Nurses* and *Scope and Standards of Pediatric Oncology Nursing Practice*, respectively. The latest edition, *Pediatric Oncology Nursing: Scope and Standards of Practice,* was published in 2007. Future iterations of this document will incorporate hematology nursing practice in congruence with the change in the name of the association (from the Association of Pediatric Oncology Nurses to the Association of Pediatric Hematology/Oncology Nurses) that occurred in 2007.

Nursing standards are rules or definitions of what a nurse does to provide competent care. Standards of nursing care have three components: professional standards of practice, standards of professional performance, and specialty practice guidelines. *Pediatric Oncology Nursing: Scope and Standards of Practice* is an example of specialty practice guidelines. Within the *Scope and Standards*, standards of care and of professional performance are outlined for the pediatric oncology nurse and the pediatric oncology advanced practice registered nurse (APRN). The standards are critical for guiding pediatric oncology nurses in delivering high-quality nursing care. The comprehensive standards are summarized as follows.

## Standards of Care for the Pediatric Oncology Nurse

**Standard 1. Assessment:** Collection and documentation of data regarding the child and the family. Assessment in the areas of physical care, growth and development, psychosocial care at various points in the treatment process, education, palliative care, long-term survival, and prevention and early detection are included in the data collection process.

**Standard 2. Diagnosis: Determination of the diagnosis by using assessment data from nursing and other disciplines.** Individual problems and appropriate interventions can be identified once diagnoses are known.

**Standard 3. Outcomes Identification: Identification of outcomes to help the nurse, child, and family work toward mutual goals of care.** Expected outcomes may include adequate education, optimal growth and development, optimal physical and emotional health, minimal symptom distress, prevention of toxicity, early detection of secondary malignancies, limited late effects, or an improved quality of life for children dying from cancer.

**Standard 4. Planning: Prescription of interventions that will achieve the expected outcomes.** The plan of care incorporates current knowledge of pediatric and oncology nursing. The child and the family are active participants in achieving outcomes. The financial, social, spiritual, and cultural domains of the family are considered essential to the plan of care.

**Standard 5. Implementation: Implementation of the plan of care to meet the expected outcomes of the child and the family.** The nurse works with other healthcare professionals to implement a plan of care that will improve the child's health status and quality of life and optimize family functioning.

**Standard 5a. Coordination of Care: Communication across the care continuum is maintained to ensure appropriate and safe care for patients.** The nurse communicates across disciplines and settings to facilitate care transition and documents pertinent information in the medical record.

**Standard 5b. Health Teaching and Health Promotion: Ongoing education is provided to maintain optimal health and prevent illness.** Hematology/Oncology nurses are in a unique position to interact on a regular basis with patients to educate and reinforce optimal lifestyle behaviors for healthy living.

**Standard 6. Evaluation: Measurement of the child and the family's progress toward expected outcomes.** The evaluation process may include revising the diagnosis, expected outcomes, and plan of care if the expected outcomes have not been attained.

## Standards of Professional Performance of the Pediatric Oncology Nurse

**Standard 7. Quality of Practice: Active participation in improving the quality, safety, and effectiveness of nursing care.** The pediatric oncology nurse integrates new knowledge, technology, and scientific advances in both basic and behavioral sciences into the care of children with cancer.

**Standard 8. Education: Demonstration of competency in pediatric oncology nursing practice and maintenance of current knowledge.** The rapid expansion of knowledge requires the pediatric oncology nurse to be committed to lifelong learning, which may include seeking opportunities to learn and obtaining certification to demonstrate professional development.

**Standard 9. Professional Practice Evaluation: Self-evaluation in relation to practice standards and legal statutes and regulations.** The pediatric oncology nurse acquires the required competencies needed to provide quality care. The nurse is able to identify his or her strengths and weaknesses and initiate methods to improve his or her performance.

**Standard 10. Collegiality: Contribution to the professional development of peers, colleagues, and others.** The pediatric oncology nurse is a leader in sharing knowledge of pediatric oncology nursing and serves as both a formal and an informal preceptor or mentor. The nurse identifies the learning needs of others and fosters their professional development, contributing to improved care for children with cancer.

**Standard 11. Collaboration: Collaboration with children, families, and the multidisciplinary team to provide care to the child with cancer.** The nurse collaborates with other team members whose unique abilities can contribute to the care of the child with complex and intensive needs. This collaboration may include referrals to community and home-based resources.

**Standard 12. Ethics: Recognition of the rights of children and families and decision making in accordance with ethical principles.** The nurse advocates for the rights of children with cancer and designs interventions that are in agreement with ethical principles. The nurse applies basic principles of autonomy, beneficence, nonmaleficence, justice, and veracity; identifies resources available; maintains confidentiality; reports unethical practices; and maintains therapeutic nurse-patient relationships.

**Standard 13. Research: Participating, reviewing, and integrating research in the development of knowledge to be used in clinical practice and decision making.** The nurse participates in and reviews research and utilizes research findings. The nurse ensures that protocol requirements are met for children who are enrolled in clinical trials (most children with cancer are). The nurse identifies clinical questions for scientific inquiry.

**Standard 14. Resource Utilization: Skillful management of the care environment, ensuring that it is safe, effective, and cost-effective.** The nurse uses appropriate resources so that safe, effective care can be delivered in a cost-effective way. Decisions regarding benefits and cost of treatment are made by identifying resources, prioritizing actions, and delegating responsibility when needed so that desired outcomes are met.

**Standard 15. Leadership: Serving as leader, role model, and mentor of colleagues and students in clinical setting.** The nurse acts as a leader by coordinating care, fostering a learning environment, encouraging others to succeed, addressing changes in practice to decrease errors, and participating in professional organizations.

## Standards of Care for the Pediatric Oncology Advanced Practice Registered Nurse

The pediatric oncology APRN complies with the standards of care and professional performance of the clinical nurse while blending the roles of pediatric and oncology APRN. Like the standards for the clinical nurse, the APRN standards address the areas of assessment, diagnosis, outcome identification, planning, implementation, and evaluation.

**Standard 1. Assessment: Collection of data and use of assessment skills to determine the physical, emotional, cultural, and social needs of the child and the family as well as their general well-being.** The APRN assesses the child in the areas of physical care, growth and development, psychosocial care, education, palliative care, long-term survival, and prevention and early detection. The data include physical assessment and history, as well as diagnostic, imaging, and laboratory tests.

**Standard 2. Diagnosis: Analysis of assessment data to identify actual and potential diagnoses.** The APRN develops differential diagnoses and validates them with the child and the family and with members of the healthcare team. The APRN utilizes critical thinking, advanced clinical skills, and complex data obtained during the history taking and assessment of the child to make a diagnosis.

**Standard 3. Outcomes Identification: Development of individualized expected outcomes in collaboration with the multidisciplinary team when appropriate.** Focused expected outcomes help the child return to optimal health or experience a peaceful death. The APRN uses critical thinking skills, evidence-based research findings, clinical guidelines, and advanced clinical knowledge to develop measurable and realistic outcomes.

**Standard 4. Planning: Formulation and implementation of a prioritized plan of care, including interventions based on the diagnoses to achieve desired outcomes.** The APRN prescribes interventions that reflect advanced clinical knowledge and research findings. The plan should include strategies to meet the multiple needs of complex patients.

**Standard 5. Implementation: Implementation of the plan of care using the various components of the APRN's role (coordination, health teaching and promotion, consultation, prescriptive authority and treatment, and referral).** The APRN prescribes and implements plans of care that are within the scope of his or her practice and consults with colleagues as needed.

**Standard 5a. Coordination of Care: Development, implementation, and facilitation of the plan of care promotes optimal patient outcomes.** The APRN works closely with other healthcare providers to develop and communicate a multidisciplinary plan of care.

**Standard 5b. Health Teaching and Health Promotion: Continual patient and family education is required to restore and maintain health.** By providing continuity of care, the APRN is in a unique position to develop an ongoing rapport with the patient and family and become a reliable source of health information.

**Standard 5c. Consultation: Consultation with authoritative sources is needed to manage complex patient care.** Advanced nursing education positions the APRN to provide the patient, family, and community with health and disease-related information.

**Standard 5d. Prescriptive Authority and Treatment: The ability to accurately and independently prescribe medications and perform procedures promotes continuity of care.** Advanced education and expanded role functions allow the APRN to appropriately diagnose and treat disease within their individual scope of practice according to institutional, state, and federal regulations.

**Standard 6. Evaluation: Evaluation of the response to the plan and interventions, and monitoring of the progress toward achievement of expected outcomes.** The APRN evaluates responses to interventions and revises plans and interventions as needed.

## Standards of Professional Performance for the Pediatric Oncology Advanced Practice Registered Nurse

**Standard 7. Quality of Practice: Evaluation of quality of care in terms of clinical outcomes and the effectiveness of clinical (RN) and advanced pediatric oncology nursing (APRN) practice.** The APRN develops and evaluates standards of care, analyzes outcome data, participates in quality improvement activities, and collaborates with the healthcare team to improve patient care outcomes.

**Standard 8. Education: Acquisition and maintenance of current knowledge and skills in the area of pediatric oncology nursing and related disciplines.** Continuing educational opportunities and research and evidence-based findings enhance nurses' performance and knowledge of nursing issues.

**Standard 9. Professional Practice Evaluation: Accountability to oneself, the public, and the profession to provide competent and culturally sensitive care.** Self-evaluation includes soliciting feedback from peers, colleagues, other healthcare members, and the child and the family to identify personal strengths, weaknesses, and learning needs to develop performance goals.

**Standard 10. Collegiality: Develop collegial relationships with many disciplines to ensure quality of care for children with cancer and their families.** The APRN is a model of expert practice, a mentor to other RN's and colleagues, and part of an interdisciplinary team. The APRN contributes to development of the nursing and APRN role and improved health care for children and families.

**Standard 11. Collaboration: The APRN promotes collaboration with the multidisciplinary team to care for the child and the family.** The APRN facilitates multidisciplinary and interdisciplinary collaboration, as well as collaboration with the Children's Oncology Group and other research organizations to contribute to improvement in the care of children with cancer.

**Standard 12. Ethics: Respect for the rights of all children and families; conformity to ethical principles when making decisions and designing interventions.** The APRN models the basic ethical principles of autonomy, beneficence, nonmaleficence, justice, and veracity. The APRN maintains confidentiality, ensures institutional review board regulations are followed, adheres to institutional policy and procedures related to biomedical or organizational ethics, and addresses advance directives in persons 18 years of age or older. Equal care is delivered to all children regardless of race, culture, ethnicity, socioeconomic status, or ability to pay.

**Standard 13. Research: Contribution to nursing knowledge through utilization of research findings and maintenance of an evidence-based practice.** The APRN promotes research by encouraging evidence-based practices, developing researchable ideas, collaborating with others to develop research proposals, participating in clinical trials research, and protecting the rights of research participants.

**Standard 14. Resource Utilization: Strategies identified and implemented to wisely utilize healthcare resources in caring for children with cancer across the continuum of care.** The APRN uses appropriate resources, develops innovative solutions, and then evaluates strategies to ensure high-quality, cost-effective care.

**Standard 15. Leadership: Service as a leader, role model, and mentor for the professional development of peers, colleagues, staff, and students.** Leadership skills are developed by contributing to the professional development and education of others and by participating in professional and specialty organizations. The APRN shares knowledge by presenting or publishing in his or her area of expertise and advocating in various arenas for the needs of children with cancer and their families.

## Summary

Pediatric oncology nursing involves caring for children with cancer across a continuum of care, from diagnosis to cure or a peaceful death. The care is delivered in many settings: inpatient and outpatient settings, the home, the school, the community, and, possibly, a hospice setting. The child must be cared for within the context of the family and community from which he or she comes. This is a principal core value in family-centered care.

The facilitation of family-centered care by the pediatric oncology nurse and the pediatric oncology APRN provide the healthcare team and the family with an environment of mutual respect, quality care, and satisfactory outcomes, regardless of the outcome of the disease in the child. Pediatric oncology nurses who support the values of family-centered care and the scope and standards of pediatric oncology nursing practice are contributing to improvements in the care of children and families with cancer.

# Association of Pediatric Hematology/Oncology Nurses

*Joetta D. Wallace*

In 1973, four pediatric oncology nurses attending an Association of the Care of Children's Health (ACCH) conference envisioned the formation of an association specifically for their own specialty. At a meeting on November 3, 1974, the first members of the new group adopted a name—the Association of Pediatric Oncology Nurses (APON), elected their first officers, began developing bylaws, and founded a newsletter (Heiney & Wiley, 1996). Despite the significant amount of time and energy expended to establish the structure of the organization, the meeting participants also discussed educational offerings to improve the care of children with cancer (Heiney & Wiley). APON was officially incorporated on April 15, 1976, with 85 charter members. One of the premises for the development of APON was the recognition of the unique characteristics and needs of the nurse caring for the pediatric oncology patient.

In 2001, APON revised its structure, and the primary objectives of encouraging membership volunteerism and promoting efficiency of operations and product development were established. The vision statement created during APON's developmental stages was revised in 2001 to reflect changes within the organization and the healthcare industry. It now reads, "Children and adolescents with cancer and blood disorders and their families will receive the highest quality of care" (APON, 2003). In support of this vision, the following mission statement also was developed: "APON will provide and promote expertise in pediatric hematology/oncology nursing to its members and the public at large" (APON). The organization recognizes the nurse's role in caring for children and adolescents along the trajectory of their disease, including issues related to late effects of disease and treatments, which also includes palliative and supportive care. In 2006, the membership voted to reflect this change in scope of care and added "Hematology" to the association's name, which also acknowledged that most members care for hematology as well as oncology patients, thereby changing the organization's name to the Association of Pediatric Hematology/Oncology Nurses (APHON, 2007).

As of early 2008, APHON membership has surpassed 2,700, and the organization projects an annual budget of approximately $1.5 million. There are 38 local chapters in the United States and Canada and more than 100 international members. APHON's newsletter, *APHON Counts,* provides quarterly updates to members.

## Structure of APHON

APHON is governed by an elected board of directors, consisting of a president, president-elect or past president, secretary, treasurer, and three board members (directors-at-large). Standing APHON committees include Conference, Education Provider, Local Chapter, Nominations, and Steering. With the exceptions of the Nominations and Steering committees, committee membership is voluntary, and committee chairs are appointed by the president. The Nominations committee is elected by the general membership, and the chairperson of this committee is elected by the committee members. Steering committee members are appointed by the board of directors; this committee directs the organization's short-term projects to ensure that volunteers' time is used effectively. APHON's home office, managed by Association Management Center (an association management firm), is located in Glenview, IL.

The 38 local chapters operate under policies and procedures developed at the national level and are required to offer a minimum of four educational offerings each year. These educational programs, including many 1- or 2-day conferences held by local chapters, significantly increase the quality of local professionals' understanding of children and adolescents with cancer and blood disorders and their families. Local chapters are the key to the continued success of APHON and are the roots that keep the organization standing firm.

APHON members and other interested parties can keep up-to-date on APHON activities and conference highlights by visiting APHON's Web site, www.aphon.org. APHON members can discuss benchmarking and practice issues and concerns on the PracticeNET message boards. The Web site also contains educational materials and links to the Web sites of other organizations of interest to pediatric hematology/oncology nurses.

## Conferences

APHON holds a national conference each year in late September or early October. The annual conference is always highly rated and is an excellent opportunity for networking as well as education. To make it possible for different chapters to host at a regional level, the conference rotates to cities in different regions of the country (e.g., East, Midwest, West) each year. Conference attendance exceeds 700 attendees and is enjoyed by nurses and other healthcare professionals in the field.

The primary objective of the conference is to provide education to pediatric hematology/oncology nurses—an objective that is vital to APHON's overall mission of pursuing excellence in the care of children and adolescents diagnosed with cancer and blood disorders. In 1996, APHON was accredited by the American Nurses Credentialing Center's Commission on Accreditation as a provider of continuing nursing education. APHON's national conference has become a major forum for the presentation of research and clinical practice innovations.

## Publications

In 1984 the first issue of the bimonthly *Journal of the Association of Pediatric Oncology Nurses (JAPON)* was published. The journal was renamed the *Journal of Pediatric Oncology Nursing (JOPON)* in 1989, when Philadelphia-based publisher W.B. Saunders Company assumed publishing responsibilities. As of July 2003, *JOPON* is published by SAGE Publications in Thousand Oaks, CA. APHON's newsletter, *APHON Counts,* is published quarterly.

APHON has a wealth of publications developed by members for patient and family education, including *When Your Child Has Cancer,* a CD-ROM program in both English and Spanish; *Pediatric Tumor Series: Handbooks for Families,* which includes *Central Nervous System Tumors, Ewing's Sarcoma Family of Tumors, Germ Cell Tumors, Neuroblastoma, Osteosarcoma, Rhabdomyosarcoma, Retinoblastoma,* and *Wilms' Tumor* booklets. Families also can benefit from APHON's *Cancer Treatment Fact Sheets,* in English and Spanish, which include information about 71 different drugs particular to the treatment of pediatric cancer.

In addition, APHON has an extensive print and electronic publications collection designed for nurses and other healthcare providers. The third edition of *Nursing Care of Children and Adolescents with Cancer,* one of APHON's premier publications, was published by W.B. Saunders in 2002. In 2007, APHON acquired the copyright, and the book's fourth edition is in production at the time of this printing. APHON's *Essentials of Pediatric Hematology/Oncology Nursing: A Core Curriculum,* is now in its third edition and includes additional hematology content. APHON's *Pediatric Oncology Nursing: Scope and Standards of Practice* (2007) is the first edition that APHON has published on its own and is considered to be the national standard for pediatric oncology nursing practice.

The APHON *Foundations* series of CD-ROMs provide an overview of specific nursing issues involved in caring for children and adolescents with cancer and blood disorders and include the following: *APON's Foundations of Pediatric Hematology/Oncology Nursing: A Comprehensive Orientation and Review Course* (2003); *APON/PBMTC's Foundations of Pediatric Blood and Marrow Transplantation: A Core Curriculum* (2005); and *APHON's Foundations of Pediatric Hematology Nursing: A Comprehensive Orientation and Review* (2007). A booklet addressing pain management issues, *Pain Management in Children with Cancer,* is also available. Information about all of these publications can be found on APHON's Web site, www.aphon.org.

## Certification

APHON has two levels of certification available for its members. The Pediatric Chemotherapy and Biotherapy Program is an extensive, 2-day program that provides a national standard for the nurse administering chemotherapy and biotherapy to children and adolescents. There are more than 5,300 APHON chemotherapy/biotherapy providers and almost 300 nurses who are trained instructors for the course.

The second level of professional certification is provided in partnership with the Oncology Nursing Certification Corporation (ONCC). Certification validates a nurse's expertise to supervisors, clients, colleagues, and the general public. Most institutions recognize certification through career ladder advancement. Accrediting bodies such as the American College of Surgeons and American Nurses Credentialing Center Magnet Recognition Program assess nursing certification when recognition is given to an institution. The first certification examination was offered in 1993, and today there are more than 1,500 certified pediatric oncology nurses (CPON®s) in the country. Certification is maintained by meeting continuing education requirements every 4 years.

An APHON member who holds CPON® certification sits as an elected member of the ONCC board of directors. The APHON board also has a liaison to ONCC, appointed by the president. ONCC conducts ongoing item-writing sessions and role-delineation surveys to ensure the examination reflects the most current practice. APHON members are invited to participate in these exercises.

## APHON's Professional Involvement

APHON supports its vision through educational endeavors and the support of professional nursing practice. With such a global vision, APHON cannot operate alone and must work in cooperation with other organizations. These organizations include, but are not limited to, the Children's Oncology Group, Oncology Nursing Society, Oncology Nursing Certification Corporation, National Coalition for Cancer Research, CancerSource.com, the American Nurses Association, the American Cancer Society, the American Society of Pediatric Hematology/Oncology, the Association of Pediatric Oncology Social Workers, Candlelighters, and the Leukemia/Lymphoma Society.

APHON represents experts in the care of pediatric hematology/oncology patients within the nursing profession. APHON is a small organization by virtue of the relatively rare incidence of childhood cancer; however, by joining their voices with others, APHON members can be a significant influence in the discipline and profession. APHON has developed and published several position statements on topics important to its membership. APHON also signed numerous letters to Congress, in partnership with other organizations that share APHON's vision and mission, stating its positions on proposed or necessary legislation.

APHON's founders believed that the highest standards of nursing practice are achieved through education, research, certification, advocacy, and affiliation (Heiney & Wiley, 1996). APHON celebrated 30 years of service in 2006 and remains committed to this mission.

**References**

Association of Pediatric Oncology Nurses. (2003). *About APON*. Retrieved August 22, 2003, from www.apon.org.

Association of Pediatric Hematology/Oncology Nurses. (2007). *About APHON*. Retrieved December 30, 2007, from www.aphon.org.

Heiney, S. P., & Wiley, F. M. (1996). Historical beginnings of a professional nursing organization dedicated to the care of children and adolescents with cancer and their families: The Association of Pediatric Oncology Nurses from 1974–1993. *Journal of Pediatric Oncology Nursing, 13,* 196–203.

# Section II  Pediatric Cancers

**Nancy E. Kline**

## Section Outline

**Overview of Childhood Cancer**

**Epidemiology of Childhood Cancer**

**Leukemia**

**Non-Hodgkin's Lymphoma**

**Hodgkin's Lymphoma**

**Central-Nervous-System Tumors**

**Neuroblastoma**

**Osteosarcoma**

**Ewing's Sarcoma of Bone and Soft Tissue and Peripheral Primitive Neuroectodermal Tumors**

**Tumors of the Kidney**

**Rhabdomyosarcoma**

**Retinoblastoma**

**Rare Tumors of Childhood**
Nasopharyngeal Carcinoma
Fibrosarcoma
Malignant Hepatic Tumors
Germ-Cell Tumors
Synovial Sarcoma
Alveolar Soft-Part Sarcoma

**Bibliography**

## Overview of Childhood Cancer

*Christina Baggott*

Children comprise approximately 2% of all cancer cases in the United States. The types of malignancies in the pediatric population are vastly different from those that affect adults. The most common types of cancer among adults include prostate, breast, lung, and colon cancers. Children tend to develop leukemias, brain tumors, and a variety of solid tumors. Although some adult cancers have associated risk factors that could be avoided, such as smoking and exposure to the sun, very few environmental factors have been linked to pediatric malignancies. Pediatric oncology represents only a small segment of the discipline of oncology; however, many advances in the diagnosis and treatment of cancer have resulted from treating pediatric malignancies.

Cancer is the leading cause of death from disease in U.S. children. In 2004, the mortality rates of children with cancer were 2.4 per 100,000 in children 1–4 years old and 2.5 per 100,000 in children 5–14 years old. In comparison, cancer is the second leading cause of death from disease in adults (second to heart disease), with an overall mortality rate of 187.4 per 100,000 individuals (Miniño, Heron, & Smith, 2006).

Most recently, cancer incidence and treatment in adolescents and young adults have become of interest and concern in pediatric oncology. The incidence of cancer among adolescents and young adults represents only 2% of all invasive cancers. However, the malignancy rate in this age group (15–29 years old) is three times higher than that in children younger than 15 years (Bleyer, Budd, & Montello, 2006). The most common cancers among the 15–19-year-old population in the United States are Hodgkin's lymphoma, germ-cell tumors, central-nervous-system (CNS) tumors, Non-Hodgkin's lymphoma, thyroid cancer, malignant melanoma, and acute lymphocytic leukemia (ALL). This pattern is different than what has been seen in both younger and older patient populations. Many of the common malignancies in children younger than 5 years are virtually absent in the 15–19-year-old group. Similarly, cancers that predominate in adults are unusual among adolescents.

Survival rates for children younger than 15 years have increased at a rate of 1.5% per year. Similar improvements have been noted in the survival rates of adults older than 50 years. Adolescents and young adults between 15 and 24 years of age, however, have experienced increases in survival of less than 0.5% per year (Bleyer et al., 2006). A partial explanation for the relative lack of progress in curing the adolescent population at the same rate as that realized in the younger pediatric population is the lack of participation in clinical trials. Between 1997 and 2003 the rate of 15–19-year-old cancer patients participating in clinical trials was estimated at 10%–15%. This rate is roughly one-quarter of the clinical trial participation rate of children younger than 15 years (Bleyer et al.). The National Cancer Institute (NCI) and pediatric and adult cooperative groups sponsored by the NCI have launched a national initiative to increase the number of adolescents and young adults in clinical trials.

Leukemia is the most common malignancy in children, and the most common type of leukemia is ALL, which represents 75% of all pediatric leukemia cases. Although the presenting signs of the various types of leukemia may be similar, the treatment and the response to treatment of childhood leukemias vary greatly.

CNS tumors are the most common types of solid tumors in children. Not all brain tumors are malignant by histology, but even a benign tumor can have devastating effects on a child. The treatment for brain tumors in children often presents difficulties because therapies such as radiation may have debilitating effects on the developing brain.

Lymphoma, including Non-Hodgkin's lymphoma and Hodgkin's lymphoma, is a malignancy common to both children and adults. However, the subtypes of lymphoma and their treatments in the two populations often differ.

Many pediatric solid tumors usually develop only in the pediatric population; in rare instances they may occur in adults. These tumors include neuroblastoma, Wilms' tumor, rhabdomyosarcoma, retinoblastoma, osteosarcoma, and Ewing's sarcoma.

Some of the factors leading to improved cure rates in pediatric oncology patients include the use of combination chemotherapy, multimodal treatment for childhood solid tumors, improvements in nursing and supportive care, development of research centers for comprehensive childhood cancer treatment, cooperation among treatment institutions and the development of cooperative study groups, recognition of the psychological effects of cancer treatment, and continued follow-up of pediatric oncology patients to track trends in the late effects of cancer treatment. Young children are particularly prone to long-term sequelae of cancer therapy. The endeavor to cure cancer with aggressive therapy must be carefully balanced with the potential for lifelong adverse consequences.

### References

Bleyer, A., Budd, T., & Montello, M. (2006). Adolescents and young adults with cancer: The scope of the problem and criticality of clinical trials. *Cancer, 107,* 1645–1655.

Miniño, A. M., Heron, M. P., & Smith, B. L. (2006). Deaths: Preliminary data for 2004. *National Vital Statistics Reports.* Retrieved September 23, 2007, from www.cdc.gov/nchs/data/nvsr/nvsr54/nvsr54_19.pdf.

## Epidemiology of Childhood Cancer

*Kathleen Ruccione and Kathleen Meeske*

### Incidence and Mortality

Pediatric and adolescent cancer cases comprise a small proportion of overall cancer cases both in the United States and worldwide. Approximately 12,400 individuals younger than 20 years old are diagnosed with cancer each year in the United States, in contrast with the approximately 1.4 million adults who are diagnosed annually. Incidence is determined from reports contributed by cancer registries in several metropolitan areas and states that participate in the NCI's Surveillance Epidemiology and End Results (SEER) program. Data from the most recently published SEER monograph shaped the trends depicted in **Table 2-1**. Recently, important differences in type of cancer, incidence, and survival among individuals in the 15–30-year-old age group

# Section II Pediatric Cancers

> **Table 2-1. Recent Trends in Childhood Cancer Incidence and Mortality**
>
> - Overall incidence increased from the mid-1970s, but rates in the past decade have been relatively stable. There seemed to be a slight leveling off or a slight decline during 1990–1995.
> - Most experts now attribute the small increases that were seen in the incidence of CNS tumors, leukemia, and neuroblastomas in recent years to changes in diagnostic technology, reporting, and classification.
> - When all sites were combined, overall cancer incidence was higher for males than for females.
> - If incidence data were divided into four groups by age, the highest incidence was among the youngest and oldest, compared with the two intermediate age groups.
> - If incidence data were examined year by year, the highest rates were in infants.
> - The majority of cancers (57%) were leukemia, CNS tumors, or lymphoma.
> - Incidence rates for African American children were lower than for European American children overall and for many of the specific disease sites. Hispanic and Asian American children had rates intermediate to those for European Americans and African Americans. The lowest incidence rates were among American Indian children.
> - Survival rates have improved dramatically with newer, more effective treatments. Overall survival is now estimated at 80%, although there is variation according to tumor type. Cancer remains the leading cause of death from disease in childhood.
>
> Adapted from material in *Cancer incidence and survival among children and adolescents: United States SEER Program 1975–1995*, by L. A. G. Ries, M. A. Smith, J. G. Gurney, M. Linet, T. Tamra, J. L. Young, et al. (Eds.), 1999, Bethesda, MD: National Cancer Institute (NIH Pub. No. 99-4649).

have been recognized, and cancer in the adolescent and young adult population is receiving increased attention. There is a significant difference in the incidence and distribution of cancer diagnoses for 15–19-year-olds as compared to older adults and individuals younger than 15 years of age. For people younger than 20 years of age, survival rates have improved dramatically with newer, more effective treatment. Overall survival is now estimated at 80%, although survival rates vary according to the type of cancer. Cancer remains the leading cause of death from disease in childhood.

Individual cancer types vary considerably by sex, age, and race; grouping them together masks these differences. Specific information about the epidemiology of individual types of childhood cancer is presented within the sections on these malignancies.

## Patterns of Cancer in Children and Adolescents

In addition to differences in incidence and mortality, cancer in children and adolescents also differs from cancer in adults in sites of origin, type of tissue involved, latency, opportunities for prevention and early detection, treatment response, and prognosis. Characteristics of childhood cancers compared with cancers in adults are listed in **Table 2-2**. Adult cancers usually are grouped by primary site, but pediatric cancers are better tabulated by their histologic type and primary site. The International Classification of Childhood Cancer (ICCC) was developed to meet this purpose. Highest rates are for groups I (leukemia), II (lymphoma), and III (CNS).

## Risk Factors for Cancer in Children and Adolescents

The specific stages that lead to the development of any childhood cancer are still unknown despite considerable epidemiologic research. Epidemiologists look for associations between environmental exposures or host (i.e., genetic) characteristics that increase the likelihood of developing a disease. These characteristics or exposures are risk factors. Various exposures have been investigated as risk factors for childhood cancer, but it is likely that no one factor, no single exposure or genetic trait, determines whether a person will develop cancer. Current understanding is that it is probably the interaction of many factors that produces cancer, a concept referred to as multiple causation or *multifactorial etiology*. In this view, cancer develops because of the predisposing characteristics of the person who is interacting with the environment. In pediatrics, this picture is even more complex because characteristics and exposures of the child's mother and father may play a role (though not yet well understood) in the development of the child's cancer.

The concept of multiple causation is useful when the results of epidemiologic studies are interpreted. For example, laboratory and epidemiologic studies may indicate that exposure to a certain chemical can cause leukemia, but not all children exposed to that chemical will develop leukemia. Additional studies will be needed to determine what other factors must interact with chemical exposure to cause the disease.

The SEER Pediatric Monograph includes summaries of current knowledge of the causes of the various childhood cancers; they are categorized as (a) known risk factors, (b) factors for which evidence is suggestive but not conclusive, and (c) factors for which evidence is inconsistent or limited. Some examples of known risk factors for childhood cancer are shown in **Table 2-3**. In addition to identifying factors that increase the risk of cancer, epidemiologists are conducting studies to identify protective factors that decrease the risk of cancer.

## Genes and the Human Genome

Human cells have 23 pairs of chromosomes; normally, one chromosome of each pair comes from the mother and the other comes from the father. Each chromosome contains a very long (unfolded, it would be 6 feet long) twisted molecule called deoxyribonucleic acid (DNA). The DNA macromolecule contains two chains of sugar and phosphate molecules. Each sugar molecule is attached to another kind of molecule called a *base*. The bases are purines (adenine and guanine) or pyrimidines (cytosine and thymine) known as A, G, C, T, respectively. In a chromosome, a stretch of DNA that stores the instructions for making a protein

### Table 2-2. Features of Childhood and Adult Cancers

| Characteristic | Childhood Cancer | Adult Cancer |
| --- | --- | --- |
| Frequency | Rare (<1% of all cancers) | Frequent (>1% of all cancers) |
| Ethnic predisposition | Incidence higher in White Americans | Incidence higher in African Americans |
| Type of cancer | Leukemias and sarcomas (non-ectodermal embryonal tissue) more common | Carcinomas derived from epithelial tissue more common |
| Presentation | Often metastatic at diagnosis | Often only local disease at diagnosis |
| Preventable | Not at this time | Screening available for some cancers (e.g., mammography, colonoscopy, prostate specific antigen) |
| Cooperative group treatment protocols for standard therapy | Widely available for children | Not generally available for adults |
| Prognosis | Overall 5-year survival rate 70%–90% | Overall 5-year survival rate <60% |

is a gene; each chromosome has thousands of genes. The protein-production instructions are spelled out in four-letter codes, using varying sequences of A, G, C, and T. The beauty of the DNA structure is not only that it can produce the proteins needed for life, but also that it is self-reproducing (i.e., it can copy itself). To do that, it unzips into two ladders that are reverse images of each other. Each half then rebuilds itself, using components stored in the cell. The finished copies are identical because As can bond only with Ts, and Gs can bond only with Cs.

The human genome, the full set of instructions to make a person, contains approximately 3 billion base pairs. In 2000, scientists announced that they had made a draft of the map of virtually all the base pairs in the 23 chromosomes in the human genome. Now scientists are working to understand the function of genes and their proteins, mapping single nucleotide *polymorphisms*, which essentially are "misspellings" in the ACGT code, and studying the epigenome, which controls how and when genes are expressed. Emerging discoveries in these areas may transform medicine through new treatment strategies and new possibilities for disease prevention.

## Genes Associated with Cancer Susceptibility

Recent discoveries in molecular biology are helping to solve the cancer puzzle, showing how normal cellular control mechanisms malfunction to cause cancer and lay the groundwork for genetic testing and new approaches to treatment. For some time, it has been known that when a parent transmits a cancer-associated gene mutation, there is an increased susceptibility to familial cancer. Inherited cancer susceptibility syndromes account for only about 5% of newly diagnosed cancer cases in the United States each year. For the majority of childhood cancer cases, there is no evidence of familial cancer susceptibility. For that reason, epidemiologists are increasingly focusing their research on gene-environment interactions.

Current understanding is that cancer is a genetic disease in the sense that something in the genes must go awry for cancer to develop. Three classes of genes play major roles in triggering cancer: oncogenes, tumor suppressor genes, and DNA damage response (repair) genes. When these genes are functioning correctly, they choreograph the life cycle of the cell and the intricate steps by which the cell enlarges and divides. Today, all oncology nurses must have a working knowledge of genetics in order to understand new information about cancer causes and new treatment approaches.

### Oncogenes

Proto-oncogenes have a role in normal cell division and growth through a signaling process that orchestrates the cell cycle. If they are mutated, proto-oncogenes become carcinogenic oncogenes. Changes produced by specific oncogenes cause the cell cycle to go out of control. An example of an oncogene in pediatric cancer is N-myc, which is involved in neuroblastoma and glioblastoma.

### Tumor Suppressor Genes

Oncogenes' effects have been likened to a car's accelerator sticking in acceleration mode. In contrast, tumor suppressor gene malfunction can be equated to the loss of a car's braking system. Normal tumor suppressor genes keep cell growth in check. When these genes are damaged or missing, the cell ignores inhibitory signals and grows out of control.

The first human tumor suppressor gene was identified in a pediatric tumor: retinoblastoma, the malignancy Knudson was studying when he proposed the "two-hit hypothesis" (Knudson, 1971). Cells have two copies (i.e., alleles) of every gene, providing a built-in safety mechanism if a normal tumor-suppressing gene is missing or inactive. Losing a functioning copy of a gene is called *loss of heterozygosity* (LOH). What the two-hit hypothesis proposed was that in the hereditary form of retinoblastoma, the first "hit" occurs in a germ-cell. That hit predisposes cells—specifically retinal cells—to develop a tumor after another mutation occurs. In nonhereditary retinoblastoma, both hits occur later in the development of the retina, and there is no constitutional predisposition to malignancy that can be passed on to future generations. The two-hit hypothesis was confirmed by laboratory experiments that showed that deletion of an Rb gene results in LOH, which predisposes cells to tumor development. It is currently understood that the two-hit hypothesis, which may have more than two steps, applies to all malignancies that have hereditary and nonhereditary forms.

### DNA Repair, or Damage Response, Genes

These caretaker genes ensure that each DNA strand is copied correctly during cell division. If these genes are mutated, cancer can

# Section II Pediatric Cancers

### Table 2-3. Risk Factors for Cancer in Children and Adolescents

**Examples of Known Risk Factors**

*Prenatal*

- Prenatal diagnostic irradiation—modest ↑ risk of childhood leukemia
- DES exposure in utero— ↑ risk of clear-cell adenocarcinoma of vagina
- Transplacental transmission of certain maternal cancers (very rare)—melanoma, lymphoma, bronchogenic carcinoma

*Postnatal*

- Radiation (WWII atomic bomb exposure)
  — ↑ risk of leukemia or solid tumors in exposed children
- Radiation for thymus enlargement or ringworm (1940s and 1950s)
  — ↑ risk of leukemia or solid tumors of head/neck
- Chemotherapy/radiation
  — ↑ risk of second malignant neoplasms
- Viral—nasopharyngeal carcinoma and some lymphomas associated with Epstein-Barr virus

**Examples of Possible Risk Factors**

*Inconclusive or inconsistent findings*

- In utero exposures: antinausea medications, barbiturates, antibiotics, marijuana, frequent alcohol use, nitrosamine-containing substances.
- Exposure to pesticides, electromagnetic fields, motor vehicle exhaust

Adapted from material in "Biologic basis of cancer in children and adolescents" by K. S. Ruccione, 2007, in *Nursing Care of Children and Adolescents with Cancer* (3rd ed., pp. 24–63), ed. C. R., Baggott, K. P. Kelly, D. Fochtman, & G. V. Foley, Glenview, IL: Association of Pediatric Hematology/Oncology Nurses.

---

result from accumulations of mutations in critical growth-regulating genes, including proto-oncogenes and tumor suppressor genes. Some examples of disorders associated with faulty DNA repair genes and an increased risk of cancer are Bloom syndrome, ataxia-telangiectasia, Fanconi anemia, and hereditary nonpolyposis colon cancer.

## Hallmarks of Cancer

An understanding of the dynamic interactions between tumor cells and other cells and substances in their vicinity, and how they modulate each other, has opened a new view of cancer as a disease of the cell's microenvironment. Cancer results from genetic mutations in a cell. These mutations can change the amount or the activity of proteins involved in regulating cell life. The transformation from normal cell to malignant cell is a progressive multistep process, involving a succession of genetic changes. In this process, a cancer acquires the ability to circumvent normal control mechanisms and manipulate its local environment. Hanahan and Weinberg (2000) proposed that there are six essential alterations in normal cell physiology that collectively dictate malignant growth (**Figure 2-1**).

### Self-Sufficiency in Growth Signals

In normal cells, growth-stimulating signals communicate from outside the cell to deep within its interior. This happens when one cell secretes proteins known as growth factors that move through spaces between cells and bind to specific receptors. A succession of other proteins relays the signal until it reaches the nucleus, alerting the cell to go through its growth cycle. Recent research that focused on these normal cell activities has helped explain what happens in malignant tumors.

A hallmark of cancer is that cancer cells are not dependent on normal mechanisms to move from a quiescent state into an active proliferative state. The concept is that tumors are complex tissues in which cancer cells have hijacked normal endothelial cells and fibroblasts and forced them to release growth-stimulating signals. In this model, immune cells attracted to sites of malignant cells may promote, rather than eliminate, the cancer. Thus, cancer cells do not rely on normal growth signals.

### Insensitivity to Antigrowth Signals

Another characteristic of cancer is the overstimulation of a cell's growth-promoting mechanisms combined with its normal braking systems being evaded or ignored. An important discovery

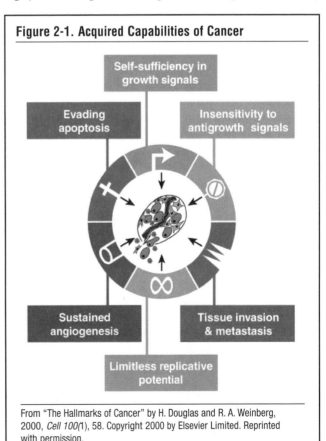

Figure 2-1. Acquired Capabilities of Cancer

From "The Hallmarks of Cancer" by H. Douglas and R. A. Weinberg, 2000, *Cell 100*(1), 58. Copyright 2000 by Elsevier Limited. Reprinted with permission.

was that there is a destination point in the cell's nucleus that promotes or inhibits growth; this has been called the cell clock. In normal cells, the cell clock programs the events of the cell cycle through various molecules. Two molecules important in this process are cyclins and cyclin-dependent kinases (CDKs). In almost every malignancy, the cell clock is malfunctioning.

### Evading Apoptosis
A cell's ability to elude an important cellular defense against runaway cell growth contributes to cancer development. *Apoptosis* refers to a backup system that tells the cell to destroy itself if something essential is damaged or if controls are deregulated. Evading apoptosis allows tumors to grow and also may make them more resistant to treatment.

### Limitless Replicative Potential
Counters within cells, called *telomeres*, keep track of how many times cells reproduce themselves as a defense against uncontrolled growth. Telomeres are located in DNA segments at the end of chromosomes. In normal cells, telomeres shorten a bit every time chromosomes are replicated. When they shrink below a certain threshold length, an alarm signals the cell to enter senescence and stop reproducing. With cancer, however, the malignant cell's ability to produce an enzyme called telomerase, which replaces telomeric segments, permits the cell to reproduce endlessly.

### Sustained Angiogenesis
*Angiogenesis* is the proliferation of new capillaries. When cells are functioning normally, angiogenesis is activated during menstruation, placental nourishment of the fetus, and wound healing. Tumors also can switch on angiogenesis, which increases their blood supply and enables them to expand. Tumors can produce growth factors such as the vascular endothelial growth factor (VEGF) and basic fibroblast growth factor (bFGF). Their actions are counterbalanced by angiogenesis inhibitors such as angiostatin or endostatin. Regulatory molecules moving between cells and their microenvironment relay signals that change the balance of angiogenesis inducers and inhibitors, thereby activating an "angiogenic switch." Close proximity to capillaries is necessary for cells to survive, and tumors cannot expand beyond 1–2 mm$^3$ unless new blood vessel growth occurs. In cancer, angiogenesis is literally the lifeblood of the malignancy.

### Tissue Invasion and Metastasis
When cancer spreads, it is because some cells in the tumor have mutated with the characteristics for successful metastasis. Such cells disregard the normal tissue barrier of the *extracellular matrix* (ECM), the structure that provides support for the development and organization of tissues. These mutated cells have alterations in the proteins that are involved in tethering cells to their surroundings. The proteins include cell-cell adhesion molecules, which are involved in mediating cell-to-cell interactions; integrins, which are involved in linking cells to the ECM structure; and proteases, which are enzymes that can facilitate invasion of cancer cells into nearby tissue, across blood vessel walls, and through normal epithelial cell layers. Together, these substances play a role in degrading the ECM, which permits cancer cells to untether from the tumor and to establish themselves in other tissue. Local invasion starts the multistep process of metastasis, known as the metastatic cascade. Angiogenesis is essential in this process. If clinically significant metastases are to develop, every step of the cascade must be completed. Particular types of primary tumors metastasize preferentially to specific anatomic sites. The capacity for tissue invasion and metastasis in cancer is deadly; metastatic disease is responsible for most deaths caused by cancer.

## Common Patient and Family Concerns
There are still no definitive, clear, cause-and-effect answers for parents who want to know exactly what caused their child's cancer. Many parents of children with cancer form theories about the origin of their child's cancer as they search for its cause and meaning. It can be helpful to discuss these ideas and to reassure parents that this searching for answers is a normal part of the process of adjusting to the cancer diagnosis.

Another common area of parental concern is the possibility that the child's cancer was part of a cancer cluster. Although several clusters have been investigated, such studies have taught us very little about the causes of cancer; more has been learned from epidemiologic and laboratory research. Researchers conducting more recent epidemiologic studies are collecting direct evidence of exposure (e.g., carcinogenic effects on DNA) and are searching for inherited variations in genes that would predispose children to cancer. Pediatric hematology/oncology nurses are in a key position to facilitate patient and family participation in these studies. As biologic science advances, and especially as particular genes are implicated in specific childhood cancers, different challenges will emerge: Nurses may find themselves needing to learn and understand the ethical, legal, and social issues in predictive genetic testing and having to help parents who may be struggling with "genetic guilt." Fortunately, resources are increasingly available for nursing education, as well as patient/family education, in the rapidly evolving field of epidemiology and genetics.

## Nursing Assessment and Interventions
Understanding the biologic basis of cancer and all of its implications for young people and their families is a critical challenge for pediatric oncology nurses in the 21st century. As recent discoveries become integrated into clinical practice, nurses will care for patients and families who need well-informed, sensitive, and ethical nursing assessments and interventions with regard to the epidemiology and biology of cancer.

### Goal
The patient, as appropriate for age and developmental level, and family will be adequately informed about the diagnosis and epidemiologic/biologic factors related to the cancer.

**Assessment:**
- Assess the learning styles of the patient and family. (See Section VIII, "Patient and Family Education.")
- Assess the patient's and the family's knowledge of, and prior experience with, cancer.
- Assess the patient's and the family's knowledge of risk factors (e.g., environmental exposures, genetic factors) related to the cancer.
- Assess the family's sources of information on risk factors related to cancer (e.g. Internet, friends and relatives, television).
- Update and maintain the family's medical history. This is

particularly relevant for nurses who practice in ambulatory settings, especially in posttreatment clinics. Special attention should be given to cancers that may have developed in first-, second-, and third-degree relatives.

**Interventions:**
- Communicate with the patient and the family in a style that is appropriate for them. If their perspective on cancer is based on what they have seen in adult friends and relatives, it may be helpful to discuss the important differences between cancer in children and adults.
- Provide the patient and family with honest, compassionate answers to their questions and concerns. Help them formulate questions as needed and guide them to appropriate resources.
- Provide the patient and family with appropriate informational resources. Use the most current version of the SEER Pediatric Monograph, or the Children's Oncology Group (COG) Epidemiology Committee materials, or both as a basis for discussing risk factors related to the cancer.
- Inform the patient and family about pertinent epidemiology and biology studies that may be recruiting patient participants.
- Encourage families that are at increased risk for hereditary cancer syndromes to provide medical documentation of family members' cancers for confirmation purposes. Collaborate with the medical team to refer these individuals for genetic counseling and possible genetic predisposition testing as appropriate.

## Goal
The patient and the family will adequately cope with information that has been provided about the epidemiology/biology of the disease.

**Assessment:**
- Assess the family's communication and coping styles in general. (See Section VIII, "Patient and Family Education.")
- Assess the family's response to information presented about any known risk factors related to the cancer.
- Assess the family's response to genetic aspects (if any) of the cancer.
- Assess the patient's and the family's concept of why the cancer occurred (i.e., their explanation for the cancer and its meaning in their lives).

**Interventions:**
- Encourage the patient and family to share their beliefs about the cause of the cancer, acknowledging and validating that forming a theory about why the cancer happened is a normal reaction to a cancer diagnosis.
- Provide emotional support.
- Ensure that the family is aware of when and how to contact members of the healthcare team.
- Encourage the family to discuss news reports about cancer epidemiology/risk factors with the healthcare team.
- Anticipate the need for referral services (e.g., genetic counseling, social work, chaplain).
- Anticipate that survivors will have questions and concerns about cancer risk in their offspring as they think about starting a family.

## Expected Patient and Family Outcomes
The child, the family, or both can do the following:
- Name the type of malignancy and describe any known risk factors related to it.
- Use informational and support resources appropriately.
- Identify available resources for genetic counseling and testing if relevant.
- Determine whether participation in epidemiologic and/or biologic studies is appropriate.
- Verbalize how and when to contact the healthcare team with concerns or questions.

### References
Hanahan, D., & Weinberg, R. A. (2000). The hallmarks of cancer. *Cell, 100,* 57–70.

Knudson, A. G. (1971). Mutation and cancer: Statistical study of retinoblastoma. *Proceedings of the National Academy of Sciences, 68,* 820–823.

# Leukemia

*Kathleen McCarthy*

## Definition
*Leukemia* is a malignant disorder of the blood and blood-forming organs, including the bone marrow, lymph nodes, and spleen.

## Pathophysiology
The hematopoietic system is composed of undifferentiated pluripotent stem cells. Signals from the hematopoietic microenvironment regulate the proliferation and differentiation of the stem cells into mature elements (e.g., red blood cell, granulocyte, monocyte, lymphocyte, or platelet). Malignant stem cells result in cells that lose the ability to regulate cell division and to differentiate to mature functioning cells. Immature cells (i.e., blasts) accumulate in the marrow spaces, peripheral vasculature, and organs. Normal cell proliferation is then blocked because of the lack of space and nutrients in the marrow. Presenting symptoms, which include anemia, neutropenia, and thrombocytopenia, are a direct result of the replacement of normal cells with leukemia cells. An accumulation of leukemia cells in other organs and tissues also may cause symptoms.

Acute lymphoblastic leukemia (ALL) results from abnormalities in differentiation and proliferation in the lymphoid cell lineage. Synonyms for ALL include acute lymphocytic, lymphoid, lymphoblastic, and precursor B and precursor T leukemia. Acute myelogenous leukemia (AML) results from abnormalities in differentiation and proliferation of the myeloid/erythroid or megakaryocytic cell lines. AML also is referred to as acute nonlymphoblastic, myeloid, or myeloblastic leukemia. Chronic myeloid leukemia (CML) results from an abnormality in proliferation of myeloid cells.

## Classification
Classification of leukemia has become a complex but essential process that uses morphology, immunophenotypic, molecular genetic, and cytogenetic features. Previous classification was

derived from the French-American-British Cooperative Group (FAB) classification system that was based primarily on a morphologic and biochemical system. A classification scheme developed by the World Health Organization (WHO) is based on a more comprehensive system that utilizes morphology, immunophenotyping, cytogenetic, and clinical features (**Table 2-4**). The identification of leukemia subtypes has therapy and prognosis implications. The three major classifications of childhood leukemia are

- ALL, which accounts for 75%–80% of childhood leukemia
- AML, which accounts for 15%–20% of childhood leukemia
- CML, which accounts for less than 5% of childhood leukemia.

## Morphology

Morphology is based on the descriptive appearance of the blood and bone marrow cells under the light microscope. Determination of whether the blast cells are myeloid or lymphoid can often be made.

## Immunophenotyping

Normal hematopoietic cells undergo changes in the expression of cell surface antigens as they mature in the bone marrow. Monoclonal antibodies have been developed that react with lineage-specific and stage-specific lymphoid and myeloid activation and differentiation antigens. These antibodies help confirm the differentiation between ALL and AML. Each monoclonal antibody is identified with a classification number with the prefix CD. The most common antigen for ALL is CD10, which is positive in 80% of ALL patients. These patients have a more favorable prognosis than those who are CD10 negative.

## Biochemical Markers

Leukemia cells have different reactions when exposed to certain chemicals. Lymphoid and myeloid leukemia differentiation can be made, and further identification of various cell types is possible with some chemicals.

## Cytogenetics

Cytogenetic abnormalities are found in more than 90% of patients with ALL. Abnormalities exist both in the number of chromosomes (known as ploidy, also measurable as a DNA index) and structure (i.e., translocations or deletions). These abnormalities can be detected by conventional chromosome analysis methods but often are found with reverse transcriptase polymerase chain reaction (RT-PCR) and fluorescence in situ hybridization (FISH), which are more sensitive techniques.

Aberrations in chromosome number (i.e., ploidy) are associated with prognosis. Leukemia cells can be described as diploid (containing 46 chromosomes), hyperdiploid (more than 46 chromosomes), hypodiploid (less than 46 chromosomes), and pseudodiploid (46 chromosomes with structural change). Hyperdiploidy is associated with a good prognosis, whereas hypodiploidy and pseudodiploidy are associated with poor outcomes. Trisomies 4 and 10 are associated with a low risk of treatment failure.

Both ALL and AML are associated with common translocations that hold prognostic significance. Common translocations associated with ALL are TEL-AML1, BCR-ABL, and MLL. TEL-AML1 is the most common abnormality (occurring in 20%–30% of cases), and occurs when the TEL gene on chromosome 12p13 fuses with the AML1 gene on chromosome 21q22; it is associated with a favorable outcome. MLL arrangement t(4;11) is located on chromosome 11q23. This translocation, the most common within this subtype is found in infant ALL and is associated with a poor prognosis despite intensive therapy. Philadelphia chromosome-positive (Ph+) leukemia expresses the BCR-ABL protein and is characterized by the presence of t(9;22); (q34;q11) translocation. Ph+ leukemia can be ALL or CML, depending where the breakpoint on chromosome 22 occurs. In CML, the translocation can be detected in multiple cell lines. Ph+ ALL occurs in 2%–3% of cases and responds poorly to conventional chemotherapy. In CML, 99% of cases are characterized by the presence of t(9;22).

AML is a highly molecular heterogeneous disease with many chromosome abnormalities. Because so many changes occur, it has been difficult to assign prognostic significance. Recent advancements in subtype classification have shown implications in predicting outcomes and therapy decisions. Translocation may continue even when the child is considered in remission and can be indicative of an impending relapse. Common translocations associated with AML include PML/RARA, AML1-ETO, and Inv (16). PML/RARA, t(15;17); (q22;q12), is observed in M3 AML (acute promyelocytic leukemia) and is associated with the best prognosis of all AML subgroups. AML1-ETO, t(8;21), is the most common abnormality seen in AML (8%–13%) and carries an average-to-good prognosis (**Table 2-5**). The presence of trisomy 21 (Down syndrome) is the single-best predictor of favorable outcome in AML.

### Table 2-4. French-American-British (FAB) Classification for Leukemia

**FAB categories for acute myelogenous leukemia (AML)**

| | |
|---|---|
| M0 | Minimally differentiated AML |
| M1 | Myelogenous leukemia without maturation |
| M2 | Myelogenous leukemia with maturation |
| M3 | Promyelocytic leukemia |
| M4 | Myelomonocytic leukemia |
| M5 | Monoblastic/monocytic leukemia |
| M6 | Erythroleukemia |
| M7 | Megakaryoblastic leukemia |

**World Health Organization (WHO) categories for AML**

AML with recurrent cytogenetic translocations
AML with multilineage dysplasia
AML and myelodysplastic syndrome, therapy related
AML not otherwise categorized
Acute leukemia with ambiguous lineage

| FAB categories for acute lymphoblastic leukemia (ALL) | WHO categories for ALL |
|---|---|
| L1 | Precursor B-cell ALL |
| L2 | Precursor T-cell acute lymphoblastic leukemia |
| L3 | Burkitt-cell leukemia |

### Table 2-5. Common Chromosomal Abnormalities and Influence on Prognosis

| Disease | Chromosomal Abnormality | Prognosis |
|---|---|---|
| Precursor B-cell ALL | hyperdiploidy | favorable |
| | hypodiploidy | unfavorable |
| | t(12;21) | favorable |
| | trisomy 4 and 10 | favorable |
| | t(4;11) | unfavorable |
| AML | t(8/21) | favorable |
| | inv(16) | favorable |
| | t(15/17) | favorable |
| | t(4/11) | unfavorable |

*Note.* ALL = acute lymphoblastic leukemia; AML= acute myelogenous leukemia.

## Incidence and Etiology

Despite concerted efforts to determine the cause of leukemia, its etiology remains unknown. However, there are known factors that increase the risk for the development of leukemia.

### Acute Lymphoblastic Leukemia

There are 4,900 new cases of ALL per year in the United States, and ALL accounts for 75%–80% of all cases of childhood leukemia (40% of all childhood cancers). The peak age of onset is between 2 and 6 years. ALL affects more Caucasian and Hispanic children than children of African descent and more males than females. Male predominance is greater in T-cell disease. There also is a higher incidence of ALL in Western and industrialized nations.

Environmental exposure to ionizing radiation has been associated with ALL development. The following genetic factors are associated with the disease:
- trisomy 21, also known as Down syndrome (20 times the risk over unaffected children)
- Fanconi anemia, Diamond-Blackfan anemia
- ataxia telangiectasia, Klinefelter syndrome, Shwachman syndrome, Bloom syndrome
- older maternal age at birth
- maternal history of fetal loss
- a sibling with ALL (2–4 times the risk of an only child; monozygotic twins less than 7 years of age have a 25% chance of developing ALL once one twin does).

### Acute Myelogenous Leukemia

AML accounts for 15% of all cases of childhood leukemia in the United States, with 1,000 children diagnosed per year. Peak incidence is in the neonatal period. Frequency of AML remains stable with a slight increase during adolescence. It is more common in the Hispanic population, with a higher incidence in African Americans than in Caucasians. The subtype acute promyelocytic leukemia (APML) has a higher incidence in the Hispanic population.

The following genetic factors are associated with disease:
- trisomy 21, also known as Down syndrome (greatest occurrence less than 3 years of age; thereafter, incidence is the same as with ALL)
- Fanconi anemia, aplastic anemia, Bloom syndrome, Diamond-Blackfan anemia
- neurofibromatosis
- Myelodysplastic syndrome (monosomy 7)
- sibling with AML (2–4 times the risk over an only child); twins less than 6 years of age have a 20%–25% chance of developing AML once one twin does).

## Environmental Exposure

The following environmental factors are associated with the disease:
- certain drugs and chemicals (e.g., alkylating agents, epipodophyllotoxins, nitro-soureas, benzenes, herbicides, pesticides)
- ionizing radiation
- prenatal maternal cigarette smoke exposure
- prenatal maternal alcohol use
- advanced maternal age
- petroleum product exposure.

## Clinical Presentation

Patients may present with one or more of the following symptoms (**Table 2-6**):
- abnormal complete blood count (CBC)
- bruising, petechiae, epistaxis
- fatigue

### Table 2-6. Presenting Signs and Symptoms of Leukemia

| Acute Lymphoblastic Leukemia | Acute Nonlymphoblastic Leukemia |
|---|---|
| Anemia: malaise, fatigue, and pallor | Lymphadenopathy |
| Thrombocytopenia: gingival, cutaneous, or nasal bleeding | Fever |
| Neutropenia: fever | Pallor |
| Hepatosplenomegaly | Anorexia, weight loss |
| Central-nervous-system disease (<10% of cases at diagnosis): increased intracranial pressure, headache, vomiting, and visual disturbances | Weakness, fatigue |
| | Sore throat, recurrent infections |
| Bone pain (23% of cases present with bone pain) | Other respiratory symptoms |
| | Gastrointestinal symptoms: abdominal pain, nausea, and vomiting |
| Lymphadenopathy | Gingival hypertrophy |
| | Chloromas |

- pallor, anemia
- weight loss, anorexia
- malaise, irritability
- lymphadenopathy
- hepatosplenomegaly
- bone pain, especially in lower extremities
- abdominal pain
- signs and symptoms of infection, often have a history of upper respiratory infection (URI) within past 1–2 months
- painless testicular swelling (in ALL)
- chloroma, subcutaneous nodules, infiltration of gingival (in AML).

## Diagnostic

A diagnostic includes disease staging to determine the classification of leukemia before beginning therapy. Diagnosis is made through the use of a history, physical examination, and bone marrow aspirate.

The history should include a review of the medical history, current illnesses, duration of symptoms (e.g., pain, fatigue, infection, fever, bleeding, and central nervous system (CNS) symptoms, including headache, vision changes, or facial palsy), prior exposures, and familial history of malignancies. A psychosocial assessment also should be done. The physical examination should note liver/spleen size from costal margin, presence of testicular swelling, and lymphadenopathy.

A chest X ray is done to rule out anterior mediastinal mass and to evaluate airway status before sedation for bone marrow aspirate/biopsy.

CBC and differential may reveal a low, normal, or high white blood cell count and peripheral blasts that may or may not be present on differential. Platelets may be low or normal.

Bone marrow aspiration can reveal more than 25% blasts (cytogenetics, immunophenotyping, morphology, and special stains are done to differentiate the type of leukemia). Bone marrow biopsy can reveal the cellularity of the marrow (as indicated should the aspirate be of poor quality or yield).

Lumbar puncture is done to rule out CNS disease for cell count, cytology (if blasts are present in the differential, it is an indication of CNS disease), glucose, and protein. If diagnosis of leukemia has already been established, the lumbar puncture often can be performed in conjunction with the first intrathecal chemotherapy treatment.

Evaluations prior to chemotherapy are essential. Baseline liver enzymes should be taken to evaluate the hepatic ability to metabolize chemotherapeutic agents. Blood chemistries, including potassium, calcium, phosphorous, magnesium, blood urea nitrogen (BUN), and LDH levels should be taken. These values can reach critically abnormal values with the start of chemotherapy (i.e., tumor lysis syndrome). High uric acid and creatinine levels often are associated with renal failure. LDH provides an estimate of tumor burden.

## Prognostic Considerations

Symptoms at presentation, and diagnostic methods for defining subtypes of leukemia, allow the patient to be classified according to a risk group (**Table 2-7**).

With ALL, the risk group classification will determine therapy.

**Table 2-7. Favorable Prognostic Factors in AML**

Age >2 years
White blood cells <50,000
Female
Absence of extramedullary disease
Presence of t(8;21), inv(16), or normal chromosomes
Down syndrome

*Note.* AML= acute myelogenous leukemia.

**ALL:** 75%–85% of children are cured of the disease.
**AML:** 45%–50% of children are cured of the disease

## Treatment and Prognosis

### ALL

Principles of treatment include
- use of CNS prophylaxis—either cranial irradiation or intrathecal chemotherapy
- use of combination chemotherapy to maintain remission
- observation of tumor for lysis syndrome
- understanding of prognostic features at diagnosis to determine therapy; the three most important factors are
  - age at diagnosis (children 2–10 years old are likely to have the most favorable prognosis)
  - initial leukocyte count (less than 50,000/mm$^3$ most favorable)
  - speed of response to treatment.

**Induction therapy:** The goal is to eliminate leukemic blasts and obtain a remission bone marrow (less than 5% blasts) with normal peripheral count (absolute neutrophil count more than 1,000/mm$^3$ and platelet count more than 100,000/mm$^3$). Therapy usually consists of weekly vincristine, a corticosteroid such as prednisone or dexamethasone, and asparaginase. Patients at higher risk often receive an anthracycline (e.g., doxorubicin, duanorubicin). Intrathecal cytarabine or methotrexate (MTX), or both, also will be given. This therapy produces a remission rate of 98% after 4–5 weeks of treatment. Prevention of tumor lysis syndrome is a major concern.

**Consolidation therapy:** Induction chemotherapy kills much of the leukemia, but an even greater reduction of leukemia cells is needed to ensure eradication of the disease. Chemotherapy agents often include asparaginase, high-dose or intermediate-dose MTX, vincristine, doxorubicin, corticosteroid, cytarabine, oral MTX, and mercaptopurine.

**CNS prophylactic therapy:** Intrathecal MTX or triple intrathecal (i.e., MTX, cytarabine, and hydrocortisone) chemotherapy is used during induction, consolidation, and maintenance therapies. The use of prophylaxis therapy decreases the likelihood of CNS relapse to less than 5%. Patients with high-risk features such as lymphoblasts in their cerebrospinal fluid (CSF) at diagnosis, elevated CSF leukocyte count, physical signs of CNS leukemia, or T-cell disease may receive craniospinal irradiation, usually during consolidation therapy.

**Maintenance therapy:** The goal is to maintain remission. This therapy usually continues for 2–3 years and includes daily mercaptopurine (Purinethol) and MTX, usually with intermittent doses of vincristine and a corticosteroid. CNS prophylaxis continues throughout maintenance.

## AML

Assessment of patients receiving therapy includes the following:
- Observe or monitor for bleeding due to thrombocytopenia and disseminated intravascular coagulation.
- Observe for fever, neutropenia, and infection.
- Observe for tumor lysis syndrome (much less common than with ALL).
- Observe for leukoreduced if the white blood count is more than 200,000.

**Induction chemotherapy:** This therapy comprises a combination of three to seven or more drugs in a highly intensive regimen, except for acute promyelocytic leukemia, which utilizes retinoic acid as a differentiation agent and lower doses of chemotherapy. Dosages must be high enough to achieve bone marrow aplasia, and supportive care using broad spectrum antibiotics and antifungal prophylaxis should be included in initial therapy. Active drugs include cytarabine, doxorubicin, thioguanine (6-TG), prednisone, and etoposide (VP-16).

**Postremission therapy:** Therapy is of shorter duration than for ALL—usually 6 months of intensive induction-like courses.

Allogeneic bone marrow transplantation is usually recommended if there is a matched related donor, especially for high-risk patients in first remission.

**CNS prophylaxis:** Twenty percent of patients who do not receive CNS treatment will relapse. CNS leukemia at diagnosis does not adversely affect long-term prognosis. CNS is treated with intrathecal chemotherapy before each cycle of therapy.

**Minimal residual disease:** Minimal residual disease (MRD) is detected using polymerase chain reaction (PCR) probes and other DNA markers contained in leukemic cells. MRD can be quantified, thereby providing an estimate of the number of leukemia cells to normal bone marrow cells. An elevated MRD present during therapy suggests a poor prognosis and increased risk of relapse.

## Recurrent Disease

### ALL

There is a 15%–20% relapse rate for ALL. If relapse occurs while a patient is receiving therapy, prognosis is extremely poor. Those who relapse more than 12 months after completion of therapy have a better chance at long-term survival. Treatment includes intensive chemotherapy—usually with drugs not used in previous therapy. Allogeneic stem-cell transplant should be considered.

### Extramedullary Relapse

CNS relapse occurs in 10% of patients. Treatment includes intrathecal therapy and craniospinal irradiation with systemic chemotherapy. Testicular relapse, seen in 2%–5% of patients, is treated with testicular radiation and chemotherapy.

### AML

A patient has a 25% chance of a second remission if relapse occurs while receiving chemotherapy and a 50% chance of achieving a second remission if relapse occurs after completing chemotherapy. Whenever possible, allogeneic bone marrow transplantation should be used. Autologous transplantation may be considered.

## Nursing Assessment and Interventions

### Goal

The patient will experience minimal complications related to the diagnosis of leukemia.

**Assessment:**
- Assess presenting symptoms and determine the type of leukemia.
- Obtain a complete history, including the incidence and duration of symptoms (e.g., pain, fatigue, infection, bleeding, neurological changes), predisposing factors (e.g., exposure to radiation, cytotoxic drugs, genetic abnormalities), and pertinent family history.
- Perform a complete physical examination, and assess for pallor, petechiae, bleeding, signs of infection, rash, lymphadenopathy, hepatosplenomegaly, and neurological changes.
- Review laboratory findings.
- Review radiological imaging studies (e.g., chest X ray).
- Review surgical and pathology reports as indicated.
- Assess the child's degree of pain and discomfort.

**Interventions:**
- Provide comfort measures.
- Provide pain medication as needed.
- Monitor for tumor lysis syndrome (i.e., maintain strict intake and output of fluids and monitor serum chemistries). (See Section V, "Side Effects of Treatment.")
- Administer leukoreduced blood products and chemotherapy as indicated.
- Take measures to prevent tumor lysis syndrome; provide intravenous (IV) hydration with alkalization and allopurinol.
- Explain all tests, procedures, and results to the patient and the family.

### Goal

The patient will experience minimal complications related to treatment.

**Assessment:**
- Assess the child for signs of toxicity related to specific chemotherapy agents. (See the discussion of chemotherapy in Section IV, "Childhood Cancer Treatment.")
- Assess the child for toxicity if he or she has had radiation therapy. (See the discussion of radiation therapy in Section IV, "Childhood Cancer Treatment.")
- Assess the child for signs of infection.
- Assess the child for evidence of fatigue, bleeding, pain, and nutritional deficits.
- Monitor fluids and electrolytes.
- Determine which type of IV access is needed.
- Assess for signs and symptoms of emergency complications.
- Assess for the patient's response to therapy (i.e., a decreased number of blasts in peripheral blood, decrease in the size of enlarged nodes, or hepatosplenomegaly; decrease in blast cells in bone marrow).

**Interventions:**
- Refer the child for central IV access as needed.
- Provide comfort measures.
- Administer pain medication as needed.
- Provide instruction on proper mouth care, nutrition, and hygiene.

- Educate the family about neutropenia, anemia, thrombocytopenia, the signs and symptoms of infection, and fever precautions.
- Obtain cultures and radiological examinations as ordered, when infection is suspected, and initiate antibiotics if indicated. (See Section V, "Side Effects of Treatment.")
- Provide alternative methods of nutrition (e.g., oral supplements, nasogastric [nasogastric] and parenteral supplements).
- Review all findings of laboratory studies and radiological studies with the patient and the family.

### Goal
The patient and the family will be adequately informed regarding diagnosis, disease, and treatment.
**Assessment:**
- Assess the patient's and the family's level of knowledge about the diagnosis and disease.
- Assess their level of knowledge about treatment (e.g., surgery, radiation therapy, chemotherapy).
- Assess their learning styles. (See Section VIII, "Patient and Family Education.")
- Assess how well they understand the role of the multidisciplinary team in treating children with leukemia.

**Interventions:**
- Communicate with the patient and the family in an appropriate style.
- Provide them with appropriate educational resources and review the material with them.
- Ensure that the family is aware of when and how to contact the healthcare team.
- Encourage the patient and the family to ask questions about the diagnosis, disease, and treatment.
- Clarify the information provided by various members of the multidisciplinary team.

### Goal
The patient and family will cope adequately with the diagnosis.
**Assessment:**
- Assess the family's communication and coping styles in general.
- Assess the family's adjustment to the diagnosis.

**Interventions:**
- Give honest answers to questions from the patient and the family.
- Provide emotional support.
- Anticipate the need for referral for services (e.g., social work, chaplain, child life, Candlelighters, American Cancer Society, Leukemia Society).
- Offer age-appropriate "hospital play."
- Offer to help the patient and the family contact another family who has experience with a similar malignancy to exchange information.

### Expected Patient and Family Outcomes
The child, the family, or both can
- Describe the type of leukemia and the plan of care.
- List the expected and the possible toxic side effects of therapy.
- Outline methods for preventing infection.
- Describe the schedule of treatment, procedures, and follow-up care.
- Describe available community resources.
- Demonstrate the skills needed to care for the child at home.
- Verbalize how and when to contact the healthcare team if problems or questions arise.

## Non-Hodgkin's Lymphoma

*Arlene L. Androkites*

### Definition
*Non-Hodgkin's lymphoma* (NHL) originates in the cells and organs of the immune system. The cells of the immune system are diverse in morphologic and immunologic features. A malignant transformation occurs in the cells of the immune system and their precursors. The cells of origin are undifferentiated lymphoid cells that cause systemic changes much like childhood leukemias.

### Pathophysiology
NHL is believed to result from genetic aberrations that influence cellular proliferation, differentiation, and cell death (i.e., apoptosis), which are essential for a normal immune response. Cytogenetic studies are associated with recurrent, nonrandom chromosome translocations characteristic of the various subtypes of NHL. Children with Wiskott-Aldrich syndrome, ataxia-telangiectasia, or other inherited or acquired immunodeficiency syndromes are at increased risk for NHL. The role of Epstein-Barr virus (EBV) is unclear but is thought to precede or occur concomitantly with B-cell transformation, which is associated with Burkitt's lymphoma (BL).

### Four Types of Histology
Histologic classification of NHL attempts to identify the malignant cell of origin that will help clinicians understand the biologic behavior of the tumor. NHL is divided into T- and B-cell lymphomas, with subdivisions specific to precursor characteristics. The World Health Organization (WHO) classification system defines the histologic classification system for NHL as lymphoblastic lymphoma (LL), BL and Burkitt-like lymphoma (BLL), diffuse large B-cell lymphoma, and anaplastic large-cell lymphoma (ALCL).

### Lymphoblastic Lymphoma
Lymphoblastic lymphoma accounts for one-third of all childhood lymphomas. More than 85%–90% are derived from immature T cells undergoing differentiation in the thymus, and about 10%–15% express the phenotype of pre-B cells, accompanied by multiple cytogenetic abnormalities. Approximately 70% of patients with T-cell LL present with a mediastinal mass. Compression-related symptoms include dyspnea, stridor, wheezing, dysphagia, and swelling of the head and neck. Neck, supraclavicular, and axillary lymphadenopathy may be present. T-cell disease commonly spreads to the bone marrow, the central nervous system (CNS), and gonads. If the marrow has more than

25% blasts, the patient is considered to have acute lymphoblastic leukemia. LL of B-cell origin commonly presents as localized disease of bone, lymph nodes, and skin.

### Burkitt's Lymphoma or Burkitt-Like Lymphoma

BL and BLL account for about 40% of all childhood NHL. BL is characterized by the chromosomal translocation of B-cell immunoglobulin genes. The most common translocation is t(8;14; q24;q11), which involves the gene for immunoglobulin heavy chain. The abdomen and pelvis are common sites of disease. Patients may present with a rapidly enlarging mass, abdominal pain, intussusception, intestinal obstruction, or intestinal perforation. Complete excision of the tumor is indicated and associated with improved outcome. Other sites of disease include peripheral lymph nodes, bone, and bone marrow. CNS involvement is present in approximately 10% of all cases.

Endemic BL is common in Africa and New Guinea, where 50% of all childhood cancers are NHL. Endemic BL is associated with a number of distinctive features, including jaw involvement and EBV infection.

### Diffuse Large B-Cell Lymphoma

Diffuse large B-cell lymphoma has basophilic cytoplasm, large nuclei, and prominent nucleoli. These lymphomas are a heterogeneous group of tumors, which can be seen at the genetic level. Primary mediastinal tumors have been shown to be molecularly different from other diffuse large B-cell lymphomas. Patients with mediastinal tumors have superior outcomes compared to those with disseminated disease. These tumors express various B-cell markers, such as CD19, CD20, CD22, and CD 79a. One-half to two-thirds of the cases express surface immunoglobulin. Pediatric cases differ from adult cases in distinct subtypes and translocations.

Two-thirds of all patients present with advanced disease, commonly in the abdomen. Lymph node involvement is more common in diffuse large B-cell lymphoma than it is in BL. Bone marrow, mediastinal, and CNS disease are uncommon.

### Anaplastic Large-Cell Lymphoma

ALCL is uncommon and accounts for approximately 8%–12% of pediatric NHL and approximately 30%–40% of all pediatric large-cell lymphomas. This lymphoma presents with a population of cells that have anaplastic features consisting of kidney-shaped nuclei often with an eosinophilic region near the nucleus. These lymphomas often express null cell or T-cell antigens. CD30 (Ki-1) antigen is also expressed.

More than 90% of pediatric ALCL cases feature anaplastic lymphoma kinase (ALK) protein gene rearrangements. Large-cell lymphomas that lack ALK expression are associated with a worse prognosis. Most cases present with peripheral, intrathoracic, or intraabdominal lymph nodes. Bone involvement is common and also can be a primary site for disease. Hepatosplenomegaly, fever, and weight loss also are presenting symptoms. Cases involving bone marrow, lymph nodes, and skin carry a poor prognosis. CNS involvement is rare.

## Incidence and Etiology

In developed countries, lymphomas (including Hodgkin's and NHLs) rank third in incidence after acute leukemia and brain tumors, and comprise 15% of all childhood cancers. NHL is more common than Hodgkin's disease in children younger than 10 years old; however, the incidence of Hodgkin's disease is almost twice that of NHL in children between 15 and 19 years of age. There are approximately 750–800 new cases of childhood NHL each year in the United States. The incidence is three to four times higher in males than females and in children younger than 15 years of age. NHL is uncommon in children younger than 5 years old, but the incidence increases steadily in children older than 10 years. Age-specific incidence of NHL varies according to histologic subtype.

There is an increased incidence of lymphoma in children with congenital immunodeficiency syndromes such as Wiskott-Aldrich syndrome, severe combined immunodeficiency (SCIDS), X-linked lymphoproliferative disease, and ataxia-telangiectasia, as well as in those with acquired immunodeficiency syndrome (AIDS). Increased incidence of NHL also is associated with immunosuppression after solid organ and stem cell transplants, particularly T-cell-depleted stem cell transplantation.

## Clinical Presentation

Clinical features typically are determined by the initial sites of disease and the degree to which the tumor has spread. In addition to symptomatology correlating to the primary site, a child may have systemic symptoms of fever, malaise, weight loss, anorexia, and night sweats. Almost two-thirds of patients will initially present with locally advanced or metastatic disease.

### Abdomen

Symptoms may include abdominal pain, nausea, vomiting, change in bowel habits, abdominal distension, palpable mass, intussusception, obstructive jaundice, and gastrointestinal (GI) bleed. In addition to intestinal sites, tumors may be present in the liver, spleen, kidneys, pancreas, and ovaries.

### Mediastinum

Symptoms may include dysphagia, subtle cough, wheezing, stridor, dyspnea, orthopnea, pericardial effusion, superior vena cava (SVC) syndrome with distended neck veins, head and neck edema, inferior vena caval obstruction, pericardial tumor or effusion, or cardiac tamponade.

### Head and Neck

Symptoms may include cervical lymphadenopathy, jaw swelling, unilateral tonsillar enlargement, nasal obstruction, snoring, rhinorrhea, or cranial nerve palsies.

### CNS (Rare)

Symptoms may include headache, vomiting, irritability, or papilledema.

### Bone Marrow

Symptoms may include pallor, anemia, or thrombocytopenia.

### Other Presentation Sites

Symptoms may involve breast, testicular, skin, pharyngeal, nasopharyngeal, adrenal gland, epidural, thyroid, salivary gland, orbital, bone, muscle, or lung parenchyma.

## Diagnostic

Given the rapidity of tumor growth, diagnostics should be performed as promptly as possible in order to prevent life-threatening complications that result from the tumor mass. BL is the fastest-growing tumor in humans, with a doubling time of 24 hours. Tumor lysis syndrome is mostly seen in children with BL and precursor T-cell lymphoblastic lymphoma. The diagnostic evaluation includes determining the extent of disease before therapy is started. This evaluation should include the following:

- A complete history of the current illness, including the incidence and duration of symptoms such as pain, fatigue, bleeding, and neurological changes; existence of predisposing factors such as genetic abnormalities, previous solid organ or bone marrow transplant, family history, risk factors for human immunodeficiency virus (HIV), and/or exposure to radiation, cytotoxic drugs, and immunosuppressive medications
- A complete physical examination, including possible detection of pallor, petechiae, signs of infection, rash, lymphadenopathy, hepatosplenomegaly, neurological changes, other masses (especially abdominal), and respiratory symptoms
- Laboratory studies, including CBC with differential, reticulocyte count, liver function studies, lactate dehydrogenase, urinalysis, hepatic and renal studies, erythrocyte sedimentation rate, and electrolytes. Alterations of potassium, calcium, phosphorous, and magnesium levels may be seen in acute tumor lysis syndrome. Testing to rule out other diagnoses, including alpha-fetoprotein, CA 125, or urinary catecholamines, should be done.
- Bilateral bone marrow aspiration and biopsy. (Patients with more than 25% blasts are diagnosed with acute leukemia.)
- Surgical biopsy of the involved site. Open biopsy of a node or mass is ideal because it permits sufficient tissue for histologic, morphologic, cytogenetic, immunophenotypic, molecular, and enzymatic studies. If it is not possible to obtain open biopsy because of the patient's condition (e.g., respiratory distress from a large mediastinal mass), a fine needle aspiration or biopsy of a mass or pleural fluid or cerebrospinal fluid (CSF) is recommended. A diagnostic tap of pleural fluid or ascites often contains malignant cells in LL and BL and may spare the need for a more invasive procedure.
- Chest X ray
- Chest computed tomography (CT) scan, if chest X ray is abnormal or suspicious. A chest CT scan is especially important to assess the airway prior to any invasive procedure in a child with a mediastinal mass.
- Thoracic ultrasound for monitoring thoracic tumor
- Abdominal ultrasound that includes liver, spleen, kidneys, abdomen, and pelvis
- Bone scan, Gallium scan, or positron emission tomography (PET) scan
- Head and neck CT scan or magnetic resonance imaging (MRI) study, or both, depending on the disease site
- If indicated, lumbar puncture with examination of CSF, MRI for detection of CNS disease, or endoscopy.

## Staging

The majority of childhood lymphomas are high grade, in contrast with adult NHL, which is primarily low and intermediate grade. Prompt staging of a patient's disease is paramount because of the aggressive and rapid growth rate of NHL. In addition, accurate staging is crucial because it dictates the intensity and duration of therapy, and, therefore, has an impact on prognosis. Staging systems describe the tumor, its primary site, and sites of spread or metastases. Pediatric NHL historically has been staged according to the Murphy Ann Arbor System. The St. Jude Children's Research Hospital staging system is most commonly used today (**Table 2-8**). Patients are staged with limited-stage disease (one or two masses on one side of the diaphragm), or with extensive intrathoracic or intraabdominal disease. Histologic classification is considered for patients with advanced-stage disease.

## Prognostic Considerations

The 5-year, event-free survival rates for children with NHL are 85%–95% for children with early stage NHL and 70%–90% for children with advanced-stage disease. CNS-directed therapy for

---

**Table 2-8. St. Jude Children's Research Hospital Staging System for Non-Hodgkin's Lymphoma**

**Stage I**

A single tumor (extranodal) or single anatomic area (nodal) with the exclusion of mediastinum or abdomen

**Stage II**

A single tumor (extranodal) with regional node involvement

Two or more nodal areas on the same side of the diaphragm

Two single (extranodal) tumors with or without regional node involvement on the same side of the diaphragm

A primary gastrointestinal tract tumor, usually in the ileocecal area, with or without involvement of associated mesenteric nodes only

**Stage III**

Two single tumors (extranodal) on opposite sides of the diaphragm

Two or more nodal areas above and below the diaphragm

All the primary intrathoracic tumors (mediastinal, pleural, and thymic)

All extensive primary intraabdominal disease*

All paraspinal or epidural tumors, regardless of the other tumor site(s)

**Stage IV**

Any of the above with initial CNS or bone marrow involvement††

* A distinction is made between apparently localized GI tract lymphoma and more extensive intraabdominal disease. Stage II disease typically is limited to a segment of the gut plus or minus the associated mesenteric nodes only, and the primary tumor can be completely removed grossly by segmental excision. Stage III disease typically exhibits spread to para-aortic and retroperitoneal areas by implants and plaques in mesentery or peritoneum or by direct infiltration of structures adjacent to the primary tumor. Ascites may be present, and complete resection of all gross tumor is not possible.

† If marrow involvement is present initially, the number of abnormal cells must be 25% or less in an otherwise normal marrow aspirate with normal peripheral blood picture.

From *Nursing Care of Children and Adolescents with Cancer* (3rd ed., p. 539), ed. C. R. Baggott, K. P. Kelly, D. Fochtman, & G. V. Foley, 2007, Glenview, IL: Association of Pediatric Hematology/Oncology Nurses.

LL and BL has increased overall survival. The addition of radiation therapy, however, does not improve overall survival. Classification systems based on biology, immunology, and molecular biology of NHLs, improvements in imaging and staging systems, advances in supportive care, and application of chemotherapy have contributed to improvement in the outcome for children with NHL.

## Treatment

Initial treatment may focus on managing the presenting symptoms that are associated with marrow involvement, mediastinal and intraabdominal tumors, and biochemical disturbances (e.g., hyperuricemia, acute tumor lysis syndrome). Before a patient receives chemotherapy, his or her chemistries must be stabilized because the chemotherapy could exacerbate such abnormalities, thereby potentially placing the patient at further risk.

Surgery is necessary for staging and if a resection is needed, as with emergency situations or when a complete resection of an isolated GI tumor is possible. In the case of resection, however, surgery may delay chemotherapy because it puts patients at risk for fistula and perforation after the surgery. A second surgery also may be indicated, particularly with patients who are not responding to chemotherapy and who are being treated as low risk.

Radiation has no "routine" role as a therapeutic modality for childhood NHL. The exception is when emergency situations such as airway, intestinal, or spinal obstructions mandate immediate reduction in tumor size. Cranial radiation therapy (XRT) may be used for patients with T-cell LL.

## Multiagent Chemotherapy

The primary therapeutic modality for childhood NHL is chemotherapy, regardless of stage or site(s) of the disease. The tumor responds to many different agents. Many children with NHL receive intrathecal agents such as MTX (Mexate) or cytarabine (cytosine arabinoside), or both for CNS prophylaxis.

## Histology and Staging as Determinants of Treatment Protocol

### Limited-Stage Disease (Stages I and II)

Children with Stage I or II NHL have an excellent prognosis, with a 5-year, disease-free survival rate of 85%–95%. BL, BLL, and large B-cell lymphoma typically are treated similarly, given their similar histology as B-cell lymphomas. Such patients have overall survival rates of approximately 90% when treated with multiagent, intensive chemotherapy for 3–6 months. Regimens include these chemotherapeutic agents: cyclophosphamide (Cytoxan), vincristine (Oncovin), MTX, prednisone, and Adriamycin. Newer protocols include high-dose MTX in initial therapy and other agents such as etoposide, ifosfamide, and high-dose Ara-C.

**Lymphoblastic lymphoma:** LL is optimally treated with chemotherapeutic regimens similar to ALL protocols—three-phase multiagent therapy (8–10 agents) involving induction, consolidation, and maintenance, which typically spans 15–36 months. CNS prophylaxis also is given. Patients with limited disease have an 80%–90% overall survival rate, and patients with extensive disease have an overall survival rate of 60%–80%.

**Anaplastic large-cell lymphoma:** ALCL is a recently identified subtype; therefore, standard therapy has yet to be determined. Children with ALCL also have an 80%–90% overall survival rate and are treated with protocols similar to those used for B-cell lymphomas. Protocols used for LL, Hodgkin's disease, and adult "diffuse aggressive lymphomas" also have been used for ALCL. Effective treatment for Stage I and II disease includes three cycles of cyclophosphamide, doxorubicin, vincristine, and prednisone (CHOP) without radiation therapy. Vinblastine is also used in randomized trials during the consolidation phase of therapy.

**CNS prophylaxis:** CNS prophylaxis is used for most NHLs, except for those diseases in which CNS spread is uncommon and for patients who have minimal disease that does not involve the head, neck, or epidural regions. CNS therapy typically includes MTX alone or MTX and Ara-C. In some institutions, patients with T-cell LL receive cranial radiation.

### Advanced-Stage Disease (Stages III and IV)

**Burkitt's lymphoma:** Cyclophosphamide, high-dose MTX, cytarabine, and, more recently, ifosfamide and etoposide are used to treat advanced stages of BL. Among patients treated for more than 6 months, 80% are cured.

**Lymphoblastic lymphoma:** LL is treated similarly to high-risk ALL, with 2 years of multiagent systemic chemotherapy, intrathecal therapy, and cranial XRT with a 5-year, disease-free survival rate of 80%.

**Large-cell lymphoma and recurrent disease:** Large-cell lymphomas and recurrent disease are treated with vincristine, prednisone, and doxorubicin, substituting MTX after the cumulative dose is reached. These approaches have resulted in a 2-year, disease-free survival rate of 70%–80%. The addition of monoclonal antibodies such as rituximab to intensive chemotherapy regimens will likely increase survival rates.

The prognosis generally is grave for children who relapse. Although "salvage" therapy may be effective, many clinicians feel that a more aggressive initial approach is warranted and that limited stages should be treated with the same intensive and prolonged regimen used to treat advanced-stage disease. As a result, some chemotherapeutic agents that were initially considered to be salvage therapy now are used for initial therapy. Ifosfamide, carboplatinum, and etoposide (ICE) chemotherapy is sometimes used for palliation, but it is unlikely to benefit patients who were previously treated with these agents.

Often an attempt is made to treat chemosensitive disease using high-dose chemotherapy, ideally with agents that the child has not been exposed to previously. Patients who have responsive-relapsed disease, even in the absence of complete remission, are then candidates for stem cell transplantation. Such patients have a 50% disease-free survival rate at 5 years. Conditioning therapy regimens have included both total body irradiation (TBI)-containing regimens and chemotherapy-only regimens—particularly for patients who have already received XRT. No clear-cut advantage to either approach has been determined. ALCL patients generally do not have favorable outcomes with autologous stem-cell transplant and may benefit from repetitive chemotherapy agents or use of single-agent vinblastines such as vincristine, cis-retinoic acid, or alpha-interferon. The role of allogeneic transplant currently is being explored with the theoretical premise that there will be a graft-versus-tumor effect.

## Nursing Assessment and Interventions

### Goal
The patient will experience minimal complications related to lymphoma.

**Assessment:**
- Know the type of lymphoma being treated and its presenting symptoms.
- Obtain a complete history, including the incidence and duration of symptoms (e.g., pain, fatigue, infection, bleeding, neurological changes), predisposing factors (e.g., exposure to radiation, cytotoxic drugs, genetic abnormalities), and pertinent family history.
- Perform a complete physical examination and assess for pallor, petechiae, bleeding, signs of infection, rash, lymphadenopathy, hepatosplenomegaly, neurological changes, and masses.
- Review the laboratory findings.
- Review radiological imaging studies, as indicated.
- Review surgical and pathology reports, as indicated.
- Assess the child's degree of pain.

**Interventions:**
- Provide comfort measures.
- Provide pain medication as needed.
- Monitor for tumor lysis syndrome (i.e., strict intake and output and monitoring serum chemistries; see Section V, "Side Effects of Treatment.")
- Administer blood products and chemotherapy as needed.
- Monitor for signs of tumor lysis syndrome by providing IV hydration with alkalization and allopurinol.
- Explain all tests, procedures, and results to the patient and the family.

### Goal
The patient will experience minimal complications related to treatment.

**Assessment:**
- Assess the child for toxicity related to specific chemotherapy agents.
- Assess the child for toxicity related to radiation therapy, if used.
- Assess for signs of infection.
- Assess the child for evidence of fatigue, bleeding, pain, and nutritional deficits.
- Monitor intake and output of fluids and electrolytes.
- Determine which type of IV access is needed.
- Assess the child for emergent complications.
- Assess the child for response to therapy (e.g., decrease in the size of enlarged nodes or hepatosplenomegaly, absence of disease in bone marrow).

**Interventions:**
- Refer the child for additional IV access as needed.
- Provide comfort measures.
- Give pain medication as needed.
- Provide instruction on proper mouth care, nutrition, and hygiene.
- Educate the family about neutropenia, anemia, thrombocytopenia, the signs and symptoms of infection, and fever-related precautions.
- Obtain cultures and radiological examinations as ordered, when infection is suspected, and initiate antibiotics if indicated.
- Provide alternative methods of nutrition (e.g., oral supplements, nasograstric (NG) or parenteral supplements).
- Review all laboratory findings and radiological studies with the patient and the family, as appropriate.

### Goal
The patient and the family will be adequately informed regarding diagnosis, disease, and treatment.

**Assessment:**
- Assess the level of knowledge of the patient and the family about the diagnosis and disease.
- Assess the patient's and the family's level of knowledge about treatment (i.e., surgery, radiation therapy, chemotherapy).
- Assess their learning styles.
- Assess their understanding of the role of the multidisciplinary team in treating children with lymphoma.

**Interventions:**
- Communicate with the patient and the family in an appropriate style.
- Provide them with appropriate educational resources and review the materials with them.
- Confirm that the family knows the members of the healthcare team, as well as when and how to contact them.
- Encourage the patient and the family to ask questions about the patient's diagnosis, disease, and treatment.
- Clarify information provided by various members of the multidisciplinary team.

### Goal
The patient and the family will adequately cope with the diagnosis.

**Assessment:**
- Assess the family's general communication and coping styles.
- Assess the family's adjustment to the diagnosis.

**Interventions:**
- Provide emotional support.
- Anticipate the need for referral for services (e.g., social work, chaplain, Candlelighters, American Cancer Society, Leukemia Society).
- Offer age-appropriate "hospital play."
- Offer to introduce a contact family who has dealt with a similar malignancy to talk with the patient and the family.

## Expected Patient and Family Outcomes
The child, the family, or both can do the following:
- Describe the type of lymphoma and the plan of care.
- List the expected and possible toxic side effects of therapy.
- Outline methods to prevent infections.
- Describe the schedule of treatment, procedures, and follow-up care.
- Describe available community resources.
- Demonstrate the skills needed to care for the child at home.
- Explain how and when to contact the healthcare team if problems or questions arise.

# Hodgkin's Lymphoma

*Arlene L. Androkites*

## Definition
*Hodgkin's lymphoma* is a malignancy that involves the spleen and lymphatic system. Thomas Hodgkins first described the disease in 1932.

## Pathophysiology
Hodgkin's lymphoma is often characterized by the presence of binucleate or multinucleated giant cells, as first described by Sternberg in 1898 and again by Reed in 1902. The classic Reed-Sternberg cell has a bilobed nucleus with two large, prominent nucleoli that give the cell an owl's eye appearance. The presence of these cells is critical in establishing the diagnosis of Hodgkin's lymphoma in the majority of cases. These malignant cells account for 0.1%–10% of the tumor's total cell population, making Hodgkin's lymphoma unique. Most of the tumor instead is composed of inflammatory cells and fibrosis, which result from cytokine release.

## Histologic Subtypes
The World Health Organization (WHO) histologic classification of Hodgkin's lymphoma has been adopted universally. This system, which is largely based on the Rye classification, divides Hodgkin's lymphoma into two broad classes: classical Hodgkin's lymphoma (cHL) and nodular lymphocyte predominant Hodgkin's lymphoma (NLPHL). NLPHL consists of cells with large, multilobed nuclei that are termed "popcorn cells." cHL, the hallmark of which is the Reed-Sternberg cell, is further divided into the following four subtypes, which are differentiated based on tissue structure, fibrosis, and inflammatory process and are equally responsive to treatment.

### Nodular Sclerosis Hodgkin's Lymphoma (NSHL)
The most common cHL subtype, NSHL accounts for 45% of all cases in children up to 8 years of age and 80% of all cases in older children and adolescents. The disease often involves the lower cervical, supraclavicular, and mediastinal lymph nodes. The lymph node capsule appears thickened, and the lymphoid tissue appears nodular. The radiographic appearance of these nodes slowly returns to normal with treatment.

### Mixed Cellularity Hodgkin's Lymphoma (MCHL)
This subtype occurs in approximately 30% of all cases and is seen most commonly in children 10 years of age or younger. Frequently, the disease is advanced, with extranodal involvement. The lymph node usually is diffusely effaced and contains numerous Reed-Sternberg cells in an inflammatory background of lymphocytes, plasma cells, eosinophils, histiocytes, and malignant reticular cells.

### Lymphocyte-Rich Classical Hodgkin's Lymphoma (LRCHL)
This subtype affects approximately 5% of patients with Hodgkin's lymphoma. LRCHL usually presents as localized disease and contains Reed-Sternberg cells within a background of mostly small B lymphocytes.

### Lymphocyte-Depleted Hodgkin's Lymphoma (LDHL)
This is a rare subtype of Hodgkin's lymphoma that is associated with patients with HIV. It is linked with late-stage, extensive disease that is widespread in bones and bone marrow and is characterized by many Reed-Sternberg cells, few lymphocytes, and diffuse fibrosis and necrosis.

### Nodular Lymphocyte-Predominant Hodgkin's Lymphoma (NLPHL)
This class closely resembles the LRCHL subtype and affects mostly males 10 years of age and younger. Patients often present with localized disease and are asymptomatic.

## Incidence and Etiology
Hodgkin's lymphoma accounts for 6% of all childhood cancers, with a significant male-to-female dominance of 4:1 in children up to 8 years of age. This difference decreases with age and is almost equal by age 10 and older, with a 1.3:1 ratio noted. Hodgkin's lymphoma has a unique age distribution that differs based on geography, ethnicity, and socioeconomic status. In industrialized countries, the early age peak occurs in the mid to late 20s, and the second peak occurs after age 50. In developing countries, the early peak occurs before adolescence. Three distinct forms of Hodgkin's lymphoma have emerged: a childhood form (14 years of age and younger), a young adult form (ages 15–34), and an older adult form (ages 55–74), with a low incidence among children younger than age 5. There is an increased incidence of the childhood form of Hodgkin's lymphoma in children of lower socioeconomic status. In contrast, there is an increased incidence of the young adult form of Hodgkin's lymphoma seen in families of higher socioeconomic status. Although it is rare, Hodgkin's lymphoma can be genetic. There is an increased incidence in children with immunologic disorders, whether caused by genetics, infection, or iatrogenic agents. Epstein-Barr virus (EBV) has been associated with Hodgkin's lymphoma and has been found in Reed-Sternberg cells of some patients. Approximately 15%–25% of adolescents and young adults have EBV-positive Hodgkin's lymphoma.

## Clinical Presentation
Patients with Hodgkin's lymphoma may present with a variety of symptoms or be completely asymptomatic. The majority of patients, approximately 80%, will present with painless adenopathy, usually in the supraclavicular or cervical area. The affected lymph nodes are characteristically firm with a rubbery texture and may be sensitive to palpation. Approximately two-thirds of patients present with mediastinal involvement, which may cause symptoms as a result of pressure on the trachea and bronchi. Of the total number of U.S. children and adolescents with Hodgkin's lymphoma, 80%–85% of them only have involvement of lymph nodes or the spleen, or both, making them Stages I thru III. The remaining 15%–20% will present with Stage IV, noncontinuous extranodal involvement to the lung, bones, liver, and/or bone marrow.

As many as 25% of patients may have systemic symptoms. These may include fatigue, fever, weight loss, and night sweats. Sometimes these symptoms are nonspecific. Other times they are constitutional and correlate with prognosis. These are referred to as *B symptoms* and include the following: unexplained fever higher than 38 °C for more than 3 days, unexplained weight loss of 10% within 6 months of diagnosis, and drenching night sweats. The presence of any of the above places the patient in the B category when staging. When B symptoms are absent, the disease category is referred to as A when staging. Pruritus also can be observed, but it occurs more commonly in patients with advance-stage disease and may be mild to severe.

## Ann Arbor Staging Classification for Hodgkin's Lymphoma (revised in 1989)

### Stage I
Involvement of a single lymph node region (I), or a single lymph node region with extension from the node to an adjacent extralymphatic region (IE).

### Stage II
Involvement of two or more lymph node regions on the same side of the diaphragm (II), or two or more lymph node regions on the same side of the diaphragm with extension from those regions to an extralymphatic adjacent organ (IIE).

### Stage III
Involvement of lymph node regions on both sides of the diaphragm (III), or lymph node regions on both sides of the diaphragm with extension to an adjacent extralymphatic organ (IIIE), involvement of the spleen (IIIS+), or both (IIIE+S).

### Stage IV
Noncontiguous involvement of one or more extralymphatic organs or tissues with or without associated lymph node involvement.

## Diagnostic
Diagnostic evaluation begins with a thorough history and physical examination. Lymph node chains are assessed for size and measured. Evaluation of a child with suspected Hodgkin's lymphoma may include the following:
- a complete blood count with differential, which may or may not be normal
- sedimentation rate, which may be elevated
- comprehensive metabolic panel, including liver function tests and an alkaline phosphatase
- serum copper and ferritin, which may be elevated
- lymph node biopsy
- chest radiograph with measurement of mediastinal mass to thoracic chest cavity ratio—it is important to determine bulky disease, which refers to lymphadenopathy measuring greater than or equal to 33% of the maximum intrathoracic cavity
- CT or MRI scan, or both, for evaluating disease of the chest, neck, abdomen, and pelvis
- bone marrow biopsy for all children except those with stages IA/IIA disease
- bone scan
- gallium scan
- positron emission tomography scan (preferred to the Gallium scan)
  Surgical staging with lymph-node sampling is not common.

## Prognostic Considerations
Approximately 90%–95% of children with Hodgkin's lymphoma can be cured. Favorable prognostic indicators are generally characterized by localized nodal involvement in the absence of B symptoms and bulky disease.

Unfavorable prognosis has been associated with advanced stage of disease, the presence of B symptoms, bulky disease, extra-nodal disease, male gender, and elevated sedimentation rate.

## Treatment
The goal of treatment is to cure disease while preventing toxicity such as radiation-related organ dysfunction, infertility, musculoskeletal abnormalities, and secondary neoplasms or leukemias.

The treatment plan depends on the child's age, disease stage, and clinical presentation. Treatment rarely includes radiation therapy alone; sometimes chemotherapy alone is warranted, but most often combined-modality treatment is used, including low-dose involved field radiation therapy and combination multiagent chemotherapy regimens.

### Chemotherapy
Multiple agents in lower total cumulative doses are used in an attempt to minimize toxicities related to specific agents. Cycles are generally repeated every 21–28 days. Patients are reevaluated after several cycles to determine their response to treatment; modifications are made to the regimen as needed.

Commonly used chemotherapy regimens are as follows:
- VAMP—Vincristine, adriamycin, MTX, and prednisone
- COPP—Cyclophosphamide, vincristine, procarbazine, and prednisone
- ABVD—Adriamycin, bleomycin, vinblastine, and dacarbazine
- OPPA (used in females)—Vincristine, prednisone, procarbazine, and adriamycin
- OEPA (used in males)—Vincristine, etoposide, prednisone, and adriamycin
- COPP/ABV—Cyclophosphamide, vincristine, prednisone, procarbazine, adriamycin, bleomycin, and vinblastine
- ABVE-PC—Adriamycin, bleomycin, vincristine, etoposide, prednisone, and cyclophosphamide
- BEACOPP (advanced stage)—Bleomycin, etoposide, adriamycin, cyclophosphamide, vincristine, prednisone, and procarbazine.

Low-dose, involved field radiation therapy (LD-IFRT) is used to achieve local control and minimize damage to noncancerous tissue.

## Refractory or Recurrent Disease
Most relapses occur within 3 years of diagnosis; although relapses have been reported as long as 10 years after diagnosis, these are rare. Overall long-term survival in these patients ranges from 30% to 90% and is dependent on several factors. The type of treatment selected and the prognosis will depend heavily on the therapy received at the time of the initial diagnosis as well as the duration of time since the relapse. Salvage chemotherapy may be attempted with combination regimens consisting of agents not commonly used in the initial treatment such as cytarabine, carboplatin, cisplatin, ifosfamide, etoposide, vinorelbine, gemcitabine, and

vinblastine. Treatment also may include radiation in low or higher doses. For high-risk patients including children with refractory disease, those who relapse within 1 year of completing therapy, or those who experience multiple relapses, a myeloablative treatment regimen followed by autologous hematopoietic stem call transplantation is the treatment of choice and results in progression free survival rates of 30%–65%.

## Nursing Assessment and Interventions

### Goal
The patient will experience minimal complications related to the onset of the tumor.
**Assessment:**
- Review the patient's type and stage of Hodgkin's lymphoma.
- Assess the presenting symptoms and obtain a complete history, including the incidence and duration of symptoms (e.g., lymphadenopathy, fevers, weight loss, night sweats, pain, fatigue, infection, bleeding, neurological changes), predisposing factors (e.g., exposure to radiation, cytotoxic drugs, genetic abnormalities), and family history.
- Perform a complete physical examination to determine the presence of enlarged lymph nodes, pallor, petechiae, signs of infection, rash, hepatosplenomegaly, and neurological changes.
- Review the laboratory findings.
- Review radiological imaging studies, as indicated.
- Review surgical and pathology reports, as indicated.
- Assess the child's degree of pain.

**Interventions:**
- Provide comfort measures.
- Provide pain medication as needed.
- Monitor serum chemistries for tumor lysis syndrome, provide IV hydration with alkalinization and allopurinol, and strictly monitor intake and output.
- Monitor for signs of respiratory compromise.
- Monitor for signs of superior vena cava syndrome.
- Monitor for signs of abdominal complications.
- Administer blood products and chemotherapy as needed.

### Goal
The patient will experience minimal complications related to treatment.
**Assessment:**
- Assess for toxicity related to specific chemotherapy agents. (See the discussion of chemotherapy in Section IV, "Childhood Cancer Treatment.")
- Assess for toxicity related to radiation therapy. (See the discussion of radiation therapy in Section IV, "Childhood Cancer Treatment.")
- Assess for complications related to any surgery performed. (See the discussion of surgery in Section IV, "Childhood Cancer Treatment.")
- Assess for signs of infection.
- Assess for evidence of fatigue, bleeding, pain, and nutritional deficits.
- Monitor intake and output of fluids and electrolytes.
- Determine which type of IV access is needed.
- Assess for the possibility of emergency complications.
- Assess for a response to therapy (i.e., decrease in the size of the mass or enlarged lymph nodes, decrease in sedimentation rate, improved weight, and resolution of pruritis).

**Interventions:**
- Provide comfort measures.
- Provide pain medication, as needed.
- Provide medication to relieve pruritis.
- Provide instruction on proper mouth care, nutrition, and hygiene.
- Educate the family regarding neutropenia, anemia, thrombocytopenia, the signs and symptoms of infection, and fever precautions.
- Obtain cultures as ordered and when infection is suspected, and initiate antibiotics if indicated.
- Provide alternative methods of nutrition (e.g., oral supplements, nasogastric or parenteral supplements).
- Obtain and review laboratory and radiological studies with the patient and the family.

### Goal
The patient and the family will be adequately informed regarding diagnosis, disease, and treatment.
**Assessment:**
- Assess the level of knowledge of the patient and the family about the diagnosis and disease.
- Assess the patient's and the family's level of knowledge about treatment (i.e., surgery, radiation therapy, chemotherapy).
- Assess the learning styles of the patient and the family. (See Section VIII, "Patient and Family Education.")
- Assess how well the patient and the family understand the role of the multidisciplinary team in treating children with Hodgkin's lymphoma.

**Interventions:**
- Communicate with the patient and the family in an appropriate style.
- Provide the patient and the family with appropriate educational resources and review the material with them.
- Ensure that the family is aware of when and how to contact the healthcare team.
- Encourage the patient and the family to ask questions related to the diagnosis, disease, and treatment.
- Clarify information provided by various members of the multidisciplinary team.

### Goal
The patient and the family will cope adequately with the diagnosis.
**Assessment:**
- Assess the family's communication and coping styles.
- Assess the family's adjustment to the diagnosis.

**Interventions:**
- Provide the patient and the family with honest answers.
- Provide emotional support.
- Anticipate the need for referral services (e.g., social work, child life, chaplain).
- Refer patients and their families to outside services and information through the Leukemia and Lymphoma Society or the National Cancer Institute, or both.

- Offer to introduce a contact family who has dealt with a similar malignancy to talk with the patient and the family.

## Expected Patient and Family Outcomes
The child, the family, or both can do the following:
- Describe Hodgkin's lymphoma and the plan of care.
- List the expected and possible toxic side effects of therapy.
- Outline methods to prevent infection.
- Describe the schedule of treatment, procedures, and follow-up care.
- Describe available community resources.
- Demonstrate the skills needed to care for the child at home.
- Explain how and when to contact the healthcare team if problems or questions arise.

# Central-Nervous-System Tumors

*Melody Ann Watral*

## Brain Tumor

### Definition
A tumor in the regions of the brain that can be malignant or benign, based upon the microscopic appearance of the mass, is defined as a *brain tumor*.

### Pathophysiology
**Astrocytomas:** These tumors account for 50% of all pediatric brain tumors and are classified according to the degree of anaplasia. The World Health Organization's 2007 classification system for astrocytomas is as follows:
- Grade I—Pilocytic or subependymal giant-cell astrocytomas
- Grade II—Pilomyxoid, diffuse, or pleomorphic astrocytomas
- Grade III—Anaplastic astrocytomas
- Grade IV—Glioblastoma multiforme, giant-cell glioblastoma or gliosarcoma (Louis, Ohgaki, Wiestler, & Cavenee, 2007).

Grades III and IV tumors have higher mitotic activity, and Grade IV tumors have vascular changes and necrosis.

Fifteen percent to twenty-five percent of astrocytomas occur in the cerebellum (the majority have a low-grade histology), 25% occur in the cerebral hemispheres (with an equal distribution of low-grade and malignant histology), 20% develop in the brainstem (the majority have a malignant histology), 5% are tumors of the optic pathway (the majority with a low-grade histology), and 7% occur in the hypothalamus (the majority have a low-grade histology).

**Brainstem glioma (anaplastic astrocytoma or glioblastoma of the brainstem):** There is a rapid onset of symptoms in this type of tumor. It appears as a diffuse tumor on magnetic resonance imaging (MRI). Less than 10% of patients will survive longer than 18 months from the time of diagnosis. The tumor is surgically inoperable in the majority of cases. (See Section IV, "Childhood Cancer Treatment," for exceptions.)

**Medulloblastoma:** This tumor type, which accounts for 20% of all pediatric brain tumors, is the most common malignant primary central-nervous-system (CNS) tumor. It is a highly cellular, small, round, blue cell tumor and usually arises in the cerebellum or in the fourth ventricle. It grows aggressively and may metastasize through the CNS and extraneurally into the bone marrow and viscera.

**Ependymoma:** This type of tumor accounts for 9% of all primary pediatric brain tumors. Two-thirds of the cases occur as infratentorial lesions, often in the posterior fossa, with the remaining cases occurring supratentorially. The WHO (2007) system classifies this tumor type as follows:
- Grade I—Subependymomas (i.e., benign, slow growing) and myxopapillary ependymomas (a variant with favorable prognosis)
- Grade II—Classic ependymomas
- Grade III—Anaplastic ependymomas, which may develop through malignant progression from low-grade ependymomas, but typically show anaplastic features on the first biopsy.

**Craniopharyngioma:** Six percent to nine percent of all pediatric tumors are of this type. This tumor arises from the sella, which is adjacent to the pituitary gland, the hypothalamus, and the optic nerve.

### Incidence and Etiology
An estimated 3,410 new cases of childhood primary brain tumors were expected to be diagnosed in the United States in 2005. At least 2,590 of the cases occurred in children younger than 15 years of age. Tumors of the CNS are the second most common neoplasm and the most common solid tumor in children. Sixty percent are in the posterior fossa (i.e., infratentorial tumors such as cerebellar astrocytomas, medulloblastomas, ependymomas) and 40% are supratentorial (e.g., astrocytomas, hypothalamic and optic pathway tumors, craniopharyngiomas). The causes are unknown. Possible sites of oncogenesis include chromosome 17 in medulloblastoma and astrocytoma tumors and chromosome 10 in glioblastoma tumors.

### Clinical Presentation
Diagnosis often is difficult to establish; symptoms often mimic common childhood illnesses and vary, depending upon the location and growth rate of the tumor (**Figure 2-2**). A sudden onset of symptoms tends to occur in more aggressive (malignant) tumors. A slow, indolent course and incidental radiological finding tend to indicate slowly growing (benign) tumors.

Posterior fossa symptoms (i.e., headache, vomiting, ataxia, nystagmus, diplopia) most commonly are caused by increased intracranial pressure (ICP). Cranial nerve deficits are associated with brain stem involvement either from tumor, infiltration, and compression on the surrounding structures, or from hydrocephalus. Supratentorial symptoms include hemiparesis, seizures, visual changes, and intellectual problems. Midline tumors in the hypothalamus/pituitary region present with visual changes, endocrine abnormalities, and increased ICP.

ICP may result from the mass effect exerted by the tumor on the surrounding structures or from the obstruction of cerebrospinal fluid (CSF) flow. The "classic triad" of symptoms from elevated ICP are morning headaches, lethargy, and nausea and/or vomiting (headaches usually improve after vomiting). However, most initial signs of increasing ICP are subacute, including declining academic performance, personality changes, fatigue, and

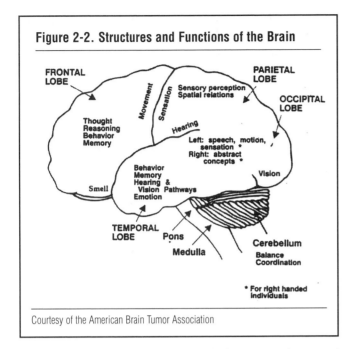

Figure 2-2. Structures and Functions of the Brain

Courtesy of the American Brain Tumor Association

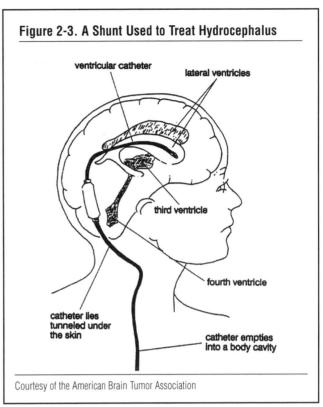

Figure 2-3. A Shunt Used to Treat Hydrocephalus

Courtesy of the American Brain Tumor Association

complaints of vague intermittent headaches. Signs of increased ICP in younger children include increased irritability, increased head circumference, bulging fontanel(s), and the "sun setting" sign (limited upward gaze and a forced downward deviation of the eyes), which may be seen in infants with ICP.

When possible, the mass lesion responsible for the increased ICP should be removed. An external ventricular drain may be placed for CSF diversion after surgery. A ventriculoperitoneal (VP) shunt may be required to treat persistent hydrocephalus that does not resolve after tumor resection or biopsy (**Figure 2-3**). An endoscopic anterior third ventriculostomy (i.e., establishing an opening in the floor of the third ventricle to reestablish CSF pathways) may eliminate the need for a permanent VP shunt.

## Diagnostic

The diagnostic includes an evaluation of the extent of the disease before therapy is started. An evaluation should include the following:
- a complete history of the current illness—specifically, the incidence and duration of symptoms such as pain, fatigue, weakness, and neurological changes (e.g., developmental delay or regression, morning vomiting, headache, seizures, visual changes, ataxia); predisposing factors (e.g., exposure to radiation, cytotoxic drugs, genetic abnormalities); and family history.
- a physical examination that includes growth and development, cranial nerve examination, gait, strength, sensory examination, coordination, deep tendon reflexes, head circumference, and mental status.
- MRI of the brain—the gold standard test—which has replaced computed tomography (CT) scans in most cases.
- MRI of the spine—before surgery if there is an infratentorial tumor.
- magnetic resonance angiography if there is concern about the vascularity of the tumor.
- positron emission tomography (PET) scan, which may be used to evaluate the metabolic activity of the tumor.
- bone marrow aspirates and bone scan, which are done only in cases of medulloblastoma.

## Prognostic Considerations
- The tumor's rate of cell growth is a consideration (high-grade tumors have a poorer prognosis).
- Surgical accessibility allows for more than 95% of patients with low-grade tumors to be cured and for improved survival in patients with high-grade tumors when more than 95% of the tumor is removed.
- Deep tumors, even those that are histologically benign, have significant sequelae.
- Infants with malignant tumors have a poor prognosis.
- Younger children tend to recover deficits after surgery to a fuller extent than do older children.

## Treatment and Prognosis

Surgery is the primary treatment, with the goal being maximal surgical resection. Advances in surgical techniques in the past decade are responsible for maximal surgical resection with lower morbidity. MRI and stereotactic, or MRI computer-guided surgery permit surgeons to plan an approach that minimizes injury to the adjacent brain tissue. Intraoperative electrophysiological monitoring of the motor strip and motor pathways identify the tumor's location in relation to other tissue. Surgical procedures are performed in stages, and second-look operations keep the surgeon involved throughout all stages of the illness.

Posterior fossa syndrome, which can occur after surgery, can include different signs and symptoms such as mutism or speech disturbances, dysphagia, decreased motor function, cranial nerve palsies, and emotional lability. Signs and symptoms occur 24–100+ hours after surgery. Recovery may take weeks or months, depending upon the severity of the symptoms.

**Radiation therapy:** Radiation therapy, the oldest treatment for brain tumors, is used to treat malignant tumors or deep benign lesions with a large amount of residual disease. Radiation therapy affects the ability of cells to continue dividing by targeting the cells' DNA. Improved technology (i.e., three-dimensional imaging utilizing CT and MRI and focused irradiation) has improved accuracy while causing minimal damage to normal tissue.

Radiation therapy is delayed in children younger than 3 years old because of its detrimental effects on the developing brain. Use of local field or cranial-spinal radiation therapy is dependent upon the histological findings. Standard radiation therapy, with approximately 200 cGy per treatment to a total of 5,500–6,000 cGy to the local field, is given once daily. Spinal doses are usually 2,400 cGy.

**Hyperfractionated radiation treatment:** This treatment consists of 100 cGy given twice daily at least 6 hours apart, which permits a higher total dose (usually 7,200 cGy) and a lower ultimate morbidity.

**Chemotherapy:** Chemotherapy is a standard treatment for certain brain tumors and is given with, or as an adjuvant treatment to, radiation therapy. Clinical studies by the Children's Oncology Group and the Pediatric Brain Tumor Consortium have tested specific chemotherapy agents against histologically malignant and benign tumors.

Chemotherapy agents most commonly used to treat pediatric brain tumors include vincristine (Oncovin), carmustine (BCNU), lomustine (CCNU), carboplatin (CBDCA), cisplatin (Platinol), etoposide (VP-16), cyclophosphamide (Cytoxan), thiotepa (Thiotepa), temozolomide (Temodar), and irinotecan (CPT-11). High-dose chemotherapy followed by autologous peripheral stem-cell rescue has replaced radiotherapy in patients who are diagnosed with highly malignant tumors (with minimal residual disease) before 3 years of age.

**Biologic agents:** Monoclonal antibodies are immunoglobins produced in the laboratory that bind to a specific target on the cancer cell, having an antitumor effect. Angiogenesis inhibitors may prevent the formation of blood vessels from surrounding tissue to a solid tumor, thus limiting the nutritional supply of the tumor.

**Supportive care:** Supportive care should focus on the risk of increased ICP. Hydration is aimed at maintaining an isovolumic state to avoid fluid and electrolyte shifts that could result in brain edema. Maintenance fluids are administered with mannitol (Osmitrol) and furosemide (Lasix) to maintain diuresis and fluid balance.

## Treatment for Specific Types of Brain Tumors

**Low-grade astrocytoma of the cerebellum:** The goal is gross total resection (i.e., greater than 95% removal). If that total is not achieved with the first surgery, another operation may be performed. Surgically accessible tumors of this type can be cured with gross total resection alone. The recurrence rate is very low. Patient progress is followed with periodic MRI scans.

**Low-grade astrocytoma (supratentorial):** A gross total resection, if possible, has the best prognosis and is usually obtainable in frontal, parietal, and temporal tumors. Chemotherapy or local field radiation is given to midline tumors that are not completely resected.

**Low-grade (exophytic) astrocytomas of the brainstem:** This type of tumor, which accounts for less than 20% of all brainstem tumors, is often located in the medulla (based upon MRI appearance). Surgical debulking of exophytic brainstem tumors may be possible, but there is a significant risk of lower cranial nerve problems after surgery, which can affect swallowing and breathing. Local field radiation therapy has been used with older children with good results. Children younger than 3 years of age with large residual disease are given chemotherapy.

**High-grade astrocytoma (supratentorial):** The prognosis is poor for this type of tumor. Gross total resection offers the best prognosis. Chemotherapy and focal radiation therapy are given after surgery. High-dose chemotherapy with autologous peripheral stem-cell rescue may be effective for patients with minimal residual disease.

**High-grade astrocytoma of the brainstem:** This tumor has a rapid onset of symptoms (e.g., increased ICP, cranial nerve deficits, hemiparesis) and a diffuse appearance on MRI, involving multiple levels of the brainstem. Morbidity from surgery outweighs its advantages. Treatment consists of local standard fraction or hyperfractionated radiation therapy with or without adjunctive chemotherapy or biologic therapy. Overall survival in patients with diffuse pontine gliomas is less than 10%; the median survival time is 18 months from diagnosis, despite radiation therapy, with or without chemotherapy or biologic therapy.

**Medulloblastoma:** The presenting symptoms associated with medulloblastoma are related to increased ICP (i.e., morning headaches with forceful or projectile vomiting). Hydrocephalus occurs secondary to mass effect and obstruction of CSF flow from the fourth ventricle. Surgical resection is the initial treatment. MRI of the spine, CSF sampling, and bone scan studies are done to determine the extent of the disease. The best prognosis is associated with gross total resection without metastatic disease at diagnosis. Cranial-spinal radiation is used in children older than 3 years of age. Chemotherapy is given during and after radiation therapy. High-dose chemotherapy, with autologous bone marrow/peripheral stem-cell rescue, is administered in children younger than 3 years of age. The overall, average, long-term survival rate is 60%–65% and has been reported as high as 70% in patients who are considered "good-risk" at diagnosis.

**Ependymoma:** Approximately 60%–75% of ependymomas are found in the posterior fossa (fourth ventricle); 25%–40% of ependymomas are supratentorial. The best prognosis is associated with gross total surgical resection, which is difficult in the fourth ventricle because of its close proximity to the brainstem. Radiation (focal or cranial-spinal) with or without chemotherapy is used after surgery. Prognosis is dependent upon histology, the degree of metastatic disease, and the extent of surgical resection, which is the most significant prognostic indicator.

**Craniopharyngioma:** Surgical resection is the primary treatment for this type of tumor; however, gross total removal is difficult because of its proximity to the hypothalamus, pituitary gland, and optic chiasm. Surgical morbidity (i.e., hypothalamic or pituitary dysfunction, neurocognitive dysfunction, visual problems, and psychosocial problems) and mortality are significant. Focal radiation therapy, intracystic radioactive implants, and chemotherapy are used to treat recurrent or residual tumor. Gross total resection is associated with long-term survival but often results in significant morbidity.

## Recurrent Disease

Disease commonly recurs in infants and in patients with malignant astrocytomas and subtotally resected low-grade tumors. Late recurrence is most frequently associated with medulloblastoma. Patients should be evaluated for possible surgical debulking, radiation therapy (if it has not been previously administered), or experimental chemotherapy or biologic agent therapy. Placement of a ventriculoperitoneal shunt may be required if hydrocephalus is present. High-dose chemotherapy, followed by autologous peripheral stem-cell rescue, is used for patients with recurrent malignant tumors and minimal residual disease. Pain management and supportive care should be given as needed, and patients should be referred to a hospice.

### Reference

Louis, D. N., Ohgaki, H., Wiestler, O. D., & Cavenee, W. K. (2007). World Health Organization Classification of Tumors of the Central Nervous System. Retrieved May 26, 2008, from www.brainlife.org/who/2007_classification.htm.

## Spinal-Cord Tumors

### Definition

*Spinal-cord tumors* are intramedullary tumors within the spinal-cord.

### Pathophysiology

Of these tumors, 60% are astrocytomas, 16% are ependymomas, and the remainder consist of metastatic medulloblastomas, dermoid tumors, and lipomas. The majority of spinal-cord tumors have low-grade histology, but exceptions are anaplastic astrocytoma and glioblastoma multiforme (GBM) tumors.

### Incidence and Etiology

Spinal-cord tumors account for 4%–6% of all pediatric CNS tumors. They occur most frequently in children who are between 10 and 16 years of age. The incidence in males and females is equal.

### Clinical Presentation

Symptoms, which may be present for months before a tumor is diagnosed, include spine deformities, pain, motor weakness, and sensory disturbances (e.g., paresthesias, dysesthesias, radiculopathy, and, rarely, sphincter dysfunction).

### Diagnostic

An MRI will reveal an intramedullary tumor that is either extensive or focal in nature. Radiographs may detect scoliosis, along with a diffusely widened spinal canal.

### Prognostic Considerations

The majority (85%–90%) of spinal-cord tumors in children are not fatal. High-grade astrocytomas account for only 10%–15% of all spinal-cord tumors. These tumors are not responsive to current aggressive surgical, radiation, and chemotherapy regimens. Patients with deficits before surgery have a greater risk that those deficits will persist after surgery or any adjunctive treatment. Younger children tend to recover postoperative deficits more completely than do older children.

### Treatment and Prognosis

Early diagnosis of spinal-cord tumors is an important factor in the treatment and prognosis. Surgical resection, which has the goal of achieving a radical—or even total—excision when technically possible, is desirable. Ependymomas are clearly demarcated from the adjacent normal spinal-cord and are more easily resected than most tumors. Low-grade astrocytomas that have an interface between the normal spinal-cord and tumor are more easily removed than most tumors. The use of intraoperative sensory and motor-evoked potentials by electrophysiological monitoring can facilitate surgical resection. Ideally, surgery should be performed by a pediatric neurosurgeon in a large tertiary care center.

Radiation therapy often is used. The use of chemotherapy to treat malignant spinal-cord tumors has been limited. Physical and occupational therapy are often necessary after surgery.

### Recurrent Disease

Surgical resection may be possible for recurrent disease. Radiation therapy may be administered after surgery.

### Nursing Assessment and Interventions

#### Goal

The patient will experience minimal complications related to the onset of the tumor.

**Assessment:**
- Know the type of brain or CNS tumor, location of the tumor, and presenting symptoms.
- Assess the presenting symptoms and obtain a complete history, including incidence and duration of symptoms (e.g., pain, fatigue, weakness, developmental delay, morning vomiting, headache, seizures, ataxia), predisposing factors (e.g., exposure to radiation, cytotoxic drugs, genetic abnormalities), and family history.
- Perform a complete physical examination that includes growth and development, cranial nerve examination, gait, strength, sensory examination, deep tendon reflexes, head circumference, and mental status.
- Review laboratory findings.
- Review radiological imaging studies, as indicated.
- Review surgical and pathology reports, as indicated.
- Assess the child's degree of pain.

**Interventions:**
- Provide comfort measures.
- Provide pain medication as needed.
- Explain all tests, procedures, and results to the patient and the family.

#### Goal

The patient will experience minimal complications related to treatment.

**Assessment:**
- Assess the child for toxicity associated with specific chemotherapy agents. (See the discussion of chemotherapy in Section IV, "Childhood Cancer Treatment.")
- Assess the child for toxicity associated with radiation therapy, if it was given. (See the discussion of radiation therapy in Section IV, "Childhood Cancer Treatment.")

- Assess the child for toxicities associated with specific biologic response modifiers (BRMs). (See the discussion of BRMs in Section IV, "Childhood Cancer Treatment.")
- Assess the child for complications associated with surgery if surgery has been performed. (See the discussion of surgery in Section IV, "Childhood Cancer Treatment.")
- Assess for signs of infection.
- Assess the child for evidence of fatigue, bleeding, pain, and nutritional deficits.
- Monitor fluid intake and electrolytes.
- Determine which type of IV access the patient needs.
- Assess for the possibility of emergency complications.
- Assess for response to therapy (i.e., decrease in size of mass, evaluation of any metastatic disease).

**Interventions:**
- Refer the child for central IV access as needed.
- Provide comfort measures.
- Provide pain medication, as needed.
- Provide instruction on proper mouth care, nutrition, and hygiene.
- Educate the family regarding neutropenia, anemia, thrombocytopenia, signs and symptoms of infection, and fever precautions.
- Obtain cultures and radiological examinations as ordered, when infection is suspected, and initiate antibiotics if indicated.
- Provide alternative methods of nutrition (e.g., oral supplements, nasogastric and parenteral supplements).
- Review all findings of laboratory and radiological studies with the patient and the family.

### Goal
The patient and the family will be adequately informed regarding the diagnosis, disease work-up, and treatment.

**Assessment:**
- Assess the level of knowledge of the patient and the family about the diagnosis and disease work-up.
- Assess their level of knowledge about treatment (i.e., surgery, radiation therapy, chemotherapy, biologic response modifiers).
- Assess their learning styles. (See Section VIII, "Patient and Family Education.")
- Assess how well they understand the role of the multidisciplinary team in treating children with CNS tumors.

**Interventions:**
- Communicate with the patient and the family in an appropriate style.
- Provide them with appropriate educational resources and review the material with them.
- Determine that the family is aware of when and how to contact the healthcare team.
- Encourage the patient and the family to ask questions related to the diagnosis, disease work-up, and treatment.
- Clarify the information provided by various members of the multidisciplinary team.

### Goal
The patient and the family will cope adequately with the diagnosis.

**Assessment:**
- Assess the family's communication and coping styles in general.
- Assess the family's adjustment to the diagnosis.

**Interventions:**
- Give the patient and the family honest answers to their questions.
- Provide emotional support.
- Anticipate the need for referral services (e.g., social work, chaplain, Candlelighters, American Cancer Society, Leukemia Society, American Brain Tumor Association, and Pediatric Brain Tumor Foundation of the United States).
- Offer the child age-appropriate "hospital play."
- Offer to introduce a contact family who has dealt with a similar malignancy to talk with the patient and the family.

## Expected Patient and Family Outcomes
The child, the family, or both can do the following:
- Describe the type of brain or CNS tumor and the plan of care.
- List the expected and possible toxic side effects of therapy.
- Outline methods for preventing infection.
- Describe the schedule of treatment, procedures, and follow-up care.
- Describe available community resources.
- Demonstrate the skills needed to care for the child at home.
- Explain how and when to contact the healthcare team if problems or questions arise.

# Neuroblastoma

*Linda D'Andrea*

## Definition
*Neuroblastoma* is a malignancy of the sympathetic nervous system. It develops from neural crest cells and is usually found in the form of a mass in the neck, chest, and/or abdomen, most often arising from the adrenal gland. It has diverse clinical, genetic, and biological characteristics, which can result in a wide range of prognostic outcomes from spontaneous regression of the tumor to metastatic disease.

## Pathophysiology
A neuroblastoma is a solid soft mass with microscopic nests of small tumor cells separated by fibrovascular septa with areas of hemorrhage, calcification, and necrosis. It is composed of small round cells with blue granules and has a varied spectrum of maturation, including neuroblastoma or ganglioneuroblastoma (malignant forms), and ganglioneuroma (the most mature/benign form, without metastatic potential).

Electron microscopy and immunohistochemistry help differentiate neuroblastoma from other small, round, blue-cell tumors such as rhabdomyosarcomas. Pseudorosettes can be seen in 15%–50% of cases. Depending upon its size and location, this tumor can cause clinical effects as it enlarges.

The biology of each individual tumor coupled with the child's age at diagnosis can have distinctive prognostic implications and are key factors in developing an appropriate treatment plan. Having multiple copies of the N-*myc* oncogene, referred to as N-*myc* amplification (less than 10 copies), is associated with advanced stages of disease, rapid tumor progression, and a poor prognosis. A gene called TrkA may be associated with cell differentiation and tumor regression. High-TrkA expression is associated with a biologically and clinically favorable group, infants up to 1 year of age and stages 1, 2, and 4S; whereas a lack of TrkA expression and a high expression of the TrkB gene are associated with unfavorable neuroblastoma (stage 4). A loss of heterozygosity and of "neuroblastoma suppressor genes" has been linked to a deletion of chromosomes 1p and 11q and a gain of 17q.

Tumors that are hyperdiploid (i.e., DNA index [DI] greater than 1) are more likely to reflect lower-stage disease and favorable biology, whereas tumors that are diploid (i.e., DI of 1) are more likely to have advanced disease and less-favorable outcomes.

## Incidence and Etiology

Neuroblastoma is the most common extracranial solid tumor in children, accounting for approximately 8% of all childhood cancers. The incidence in the United States from 1975 to 2000 was 10.2 per million children younger than age 15, with approximately 650 new cases diagnosed per year. It is the most common malignancy in infants, accounting for 50% of all malignancies in newborns. The phenomenon of spontaneous tumor regression and maturation of the tumor make it difficult to know its precise incidence, which may actually be higher. Neuroblastoma is slightly more common in boys than girls (1.1:1.0) and in Caucasians than in other races. The average age at diagnosis of a child with neuroblastoma is 2 years, with almost 90% of children being diagnosed by age 5; a diagnosis after age 10 is rare.

Known as the "silent tumor," neuroblastoma presents with widespread metastatic disease at diagnosis in 60% of patients. Increased incidence has been reported in patients with neurofibromatosis Type I, Hirschsprung disease, and central hypoventilation (Ondine's curse).

Although neuroblastoma usually occurs sporadically, 1%–2% of patients report a family history of the disease. A small subset of patients have familial transmission through an autosomal dominant gene, with an increased incidence among siblings and identical twins. Mass screenings for early detection that use urine catecholamines have been attempted in other countries, but they were problematic because of issues such as specimen collection, unreliability of test results, lack of access to all infants, infants lost to follow-up, consumption of healthcare resources, and the subjection of infants to cancer treatment that may not be necessary. Screening studies at 6 months of age or younger, therefore, are not thought to reduce the incidence of late-appearing, advanced-stage disease.

## Clinical Presentation

Signs and symptoms of neuroblastoma can be generalized or specific to the tumor location and metastatic sites. Tumors can occur anywhere along the sympathetic nervous system. In more than 50% of the cases, the primary site of disease arises from the adrenal gland, 30% of tumors will occur in the abdomen (nonadrenal), and almost 15% will be thoracic in origin. A thoracic primary tumor is generally associated with localized disease (i.e., stages 1–3), whereas an adrenal primary tumor is associated with stages 4 and 4S. Other disease sites include the head, posterior mediastinum, pelvis, and neck. Sites of metastatic disease include the lymph nodes, bone, bone marrow, liver, and subcutaneous tissue. Rarely does disease spread to the lung and brain except as a manifestation of relapsing or end-stage disease.

If metastases to bone or bone marrow, or both, are present, the patient may have malaise, low-grade fever, or may limp. Catecholamine secretion may produce flushing, periods of excessive sweating, and irritability and may contribute to hypertension, although the more likely cause of hypertension in neuroblastoma patients is the pressure placed on the renal artery by the presence of a tumor and the resulting activation of the renin-angiotensin system. Subcutaneous tumors may appear as hardened bluish nodules that can be seen or palpated; they have been described as a "blueberry muffin" sign. Periorbital lesions with proptosis and periorbital ecchymoses can be present and have been mistaken for signs of child abuse. A tumor in the intervertebral ganglion tends to grow into intervertebral foramena, forming a dumbbell-shaped mass that may produce symptoms of cord compression that include paralysis, weakness in the extremities, incontinence, and pain. This is an oncologic emergency, and early recognition is imperative because cord compression can result in permanent paralysis.

High thoracic and cervical masses can be associated with Horner syndrome (seen in 2.4% of diagnosed patients), which consists of unilateral ptosis, myosis, and anhydrosis.

Several unique paraneoplastic syndromes have been associated with predominantly localized neuroblastoma, which presents at an early age. Opsomyoclonus (i.e., myoclonic jerking and random eye movement) and cerebellar ataxia have been observed in 1.3% of patients.

Approximately 5% of patients have symptoms related to the secretion of vasoactive intestinal polypeptide (VIP) by the tumor, which causes intractable diarrhea that can result in hypokalemia and dehydration. Most tumors secreting VIP are mature histologically (ganglioneuroblastoma or ganglioneuroma), and patients with these tumors almost always have favorable outcomes.

The signs and symptoms of neuroblastoma can vary and often can go overlooked for some time. This factor, coupled with the generally young age of patients at onset, contributes to the high percentage of patients diagnosed with stage 4 metastatic disease.

## Diagnostic

A diagnostic work-up for neuroblastoma includes an evaluation of the primary tumor as well as the full extent of disease before the initiation of therapy. This evaluation should include the following:

- complete history of the current illness, including symptoms of increased catecholamines (e.g., hypertension, flushing, periods of excessive sweating, irritability); weight loss, anorexia, cachexia, and diarrhea; pain, limping, refusal to walk or use extremities; symptoms associated with pressure to surrounding systems such as changes in bowel or bladder function due to compression

- complete physical examination that includes observation for periorbital ecchymosis or proptosis, or both; bluish, movable cutaneous or subcutaneous nodules (almost exclusively in infants); abdominal mass that may cross midline, hepatomegaly, or pelvic mass; lymph nodes; paralysis; extremity weakness
- computed tomography and/or magnetic resonance imaging with gadolinium to identify the location(s) of disease as well as information about the size and extension of a solid tumor
- bone scan to assess for metastases to the bones
- laboratory studies, including a complete blood count with a differential; elevated ferritin is present in patients with advanced disease and is associated with poor prognosis; elevated serum lactate dehydrogenase (LDH) is also seen in stage 4 disease and can be used as a prognostic indicator
- urinary catecholamines (i.e., vanillymandelic acid and homovanillic acid), which are elevated in 90%–95% of cases
- bone marrow aspirate and biopsy (biopsies are positive in 11%–30% of samples in which aspirate yielded negative results)
- biopsy of tumor tissue to confirm the diagnosis and to determine the patient's N-*myc* and ploidy (DNA index or DI) status
- Metaiodobenzylguanidine (MIBG) scan, which often is sensitive to neuroblastoma and is extremely useful in determining metastatic disease
- positron emission tomography scan to assess metastatic disease that is not sensitive to MIBG.

## Staging

This is the process that determines the location of disease at diagnosis. A cooperative group effort to develop a universal staging system known as the International Neuroblastoma Staging System (INSS) has been in effect for the last 20 years (**Table 2-9**). It is currently in the process of being revised a third time based on improved understanding of this unique cancer.

## Prognosis

When evaluating prognosis in neuroblastoma, several factors must be taken into account, including the INSS stage, the child's age at the time of diagnosis, the N-*myc* status of the patient, and, in some cases, the tumor histology and DNA ploidy.

### Low Risk
- Stages 1 and 2
- Stage 4S (younger than 1 year of age)
- Greater than 90% event-free survival.

### Intermediate Risk
- Stage 3
- Stage 4 (younger than 1 year of age)
- Stage 4S with large liver metastasis or diploid DNA index
- 80%–85% 5-year, event-free survival.

### High Risk
- Stage 4 (older than 1 year of age)
- N-*myc* amplification regardless of age or stage
- Overall 5-year survival, 30%–40%
- Several studies report survival of 40%–60%.

**Table 2-9. International Neuroblastoma Staging System (INSS)***

| Stage | Description |
|---|---|
| 1 | Localized tumor with complete gross excision, with or without microscopic residual disease; representative ipsilateral lymph nodes negative for tumor microscopically (nodes attached to and removed with the primary tumor may be positive). |
| 2A | Localized tumor with incomplete gross excision; representative ipsilateral nonadherent lymph nodes negative for tumor microscopically. |
| 2B | Localized tumor with or without complete gross excision, with ipsilateral nonadherent lymph nodes positive for tumor. Enlarged contralateral lymph nodes must be negative microscopically. |
| 3 | Unresectable unilateral tumor infiltrating across the midline, with or without regional lymph node involvement; or localized unilateral tumor with contralateral regional lymph node involvement; or midline tumor with bilateral extension by infiltration (unresectable) or by lymph node involvement. The midline is defined as the vertebral column. Tumors originating on 1 side and crossing the midline must infiltrate to or beyond the opposite side of the vertebral column. |
| 4 | Any primary tumor with dissemination to distant lymph nodes, bone, bone marrow, liver, skin, and/or other organs (except as defined for stage 4S). |
| 4S | Localized primary tumor (as defined for stage 1, 2A, or 2B), with dissemination limited to skin, liver, and/or bone marrow (limited to infants less than 1 year of age). Marrow involvement should be minimal (<10% of total nucleated cells identified as malignant by bone biopsy or by bone marrow aspirate). More extensive bone marrow involvement would be considered to be stage 4 disease. The results of the MIBG scan (if performed) should be negative for disease in the bone marrow. |

Source: Data from National Cancer Institute NCI – PDQ
*Combines features of the previously used POG and CCG systems

## Treatment

Treatment for patients with neuroblastoma is based on staging and risk factors at the time of diagnosis and can range from observation or surgery alone to multimodal therapy used in intermediate- and high-risk neuroblastoma. Patients with intermediate-risk neuroblastoma may receive chemotherapy and undergo surgical resection, whereas high-risk patients receive much more extensive therapy in four phases: (1) induction chemotherapy, (2) primary site, local control (i.e., surgery and radiation therapy), (3) high-dose marrow ablative therapy, and (4) management of minimal residual disease.

### Observation Alone

Observation alone may be indicated for patients younger than 1 year of age with stage 4S disease and favorable biology. Patients should be observed for spontaneous regression of the disease. Treatment in these patients is no longer recommended.

### Surgery

Surgery has a pivotal role in the diagnosis, management, and curing of neuroblastoma. It may consist of a biopsy to confirm diagnosis, debulking, or gross total resection of the primary tumor.

Surgery alone is curative in low-stage disease (i.e., stages 1 and 2) with 5-year, event-free survival greater than 90%.

## Chemotherapy

Chemotherapy is a key modality in the management of neuroblastoma patients who have intermediate- or high-risk disease. Intermediate-risk therapy generally consists of lower dose chemotherapy for 4–8 cycles. In contrast, high-risk patients will receive high-dose induction chemotherapy, including cyclophosphamide, adriamycin, vincristine, cisplatin, and etoposide.

## Radiation Therapy

Neuroblastoma cells are very radioresponsive; therefore, radiation therapy has an important role in the treatment of neuroblastoma. Radiation therapy is administered to the primary site after surgical resection and to potentially any metastatic sites that have not completely resolved with chemotherapy alone. It also may be used before surgery to alleviate an emergency situation caused by the presence of the tumor, including proptosis, respiratory or cardiac compromise, or cord compression. Radiation therapy also has a role in the palliative care of patients, when indicated.

## Bone Marrow Transplant/High-Dose Chemotherapy with Stem-Cell Rescue (HDC/SCR)

Children with high-risk disease may receive intensive short-term chemotherapy, with or without total body irradiation (TBI), followed by the infusion of purged or unpurged stem cells. In a tandem transplant this process is repeated using the same or different agents, with TBI only being done with the second treatment, if at all. Agents commonly used in this treatment may consist of two to three of the following: carboplatin, etoposide, melphalan, cyclophosphamide, and thiotepa.

## Immunotherapy

The use of immunotherapy in the treatment of high-risk neuroblastoma has been shown to be effective, especially with minimal residual disease. A monoclonal antibody that is produced from the white cells of mice (3F8) attaches to the neuroblastoma-specific cell surface ganglioside GD2 and is used in conjunction with cytokines. This process serves as a signal to the patient's own immune system to attack and kill neuroblastoma cells. Ch 14.18 is a human-mouse chimeric monoclonal antibody (mAb) that is being used in the same way but has not been shown to have a clear impact on outcomes as of yet. Studies on both antibodies are ongoing.

## Retinoid Compounds

The use of isotretinoin has become a standard of care for high-risk patients and is used to treat minimal residual disease by inducing apoptosis and differentiation.

## Recurrent and Refractory Disease

The treatments for recurrent and refractory disease can consist of high- or low-dose conventional and unconventional chemotherapy, as well as other innovative options, depending on the goal of treatment and the extent of relapse. Patients with low- or intermediate-risk disease with a local relapse may undergo a second surgery. This alone may be curative or it may be done with or without chemotherapy or radiation, or both. However, it is the patients with recurrent or refractory disease after treatment for high-risk disease who remain the greatest challenge and who historically have had little chance of a cure (0%–10%). Current approaches for these patients may include the following.

### Cytotoxic Agents

Cyclophosphamide, topotecan, and irinotecan have proven results against refractory and recurrent disease.

### Targeted Delivery of Radionuclides

This consists of delivering radionuclides directly to neuroblastoma cells, which are known to be radiation-sensitive, by attaching them to MIBG, somatostatin analogs, or anti-GD2 monoclonal antibodies. These treatments may require a stem-cell rescue.

### Retinoid Compounds

The use of fenretinide, a synthetic retinoid that induces cytotoxicity in neuroblastoma cell lines, has shown promise in the treatment of retinoic acid-resistant cells.

## Nursing Assessment and Interventions

### Goal

The patient will experience minimal complications related to the onset of tumor.

**Assessment:**
- Determine the type of malignancy and the location and extent of disease.
- Obtain a complete history, including symptoms associated with catecholamines (i.e., hypertension, flushing, periods of excessive sweating, irritability); weight loss, anorexia, cachexia, and diarrhea; pain, refusal to walk, limping, or refusal to use extremities; symptoms associated with pressure to surrounding organs (e.g., changes in bowel or bladder function); and family history of cancer.
- Perform a complete physical examination to assess for periorbital ecchymosis or proptosis, or both; bluish, movable cutaneous or subcutaneous nodules; abdominal mass that may cross the midline, hepatomegaly, or pelvic mass; enlarged lymph nodes; paralysis, extremity weakness.
- Review laboratory findings.
- Review radiological imaging studies, as indicated.
- Review surgical and pathology reports as indicated.
- Assess the child's degree of pain.

**Interventions:**
- Provide comfort measures.
- Provide pain medication as needed.
- Explain all tests, procedures, and results to the patient and the family.

### Goal

The patient will experience minimal complications related to treatment.

**Assessment:**
- Assess the child for toxicity related to specific chemotherapy agents. (See the discussion of chemotherapy in Section IV, "Childhood Cancer Treatment.")
- Assess the child for toxicity related to radiation therapy, if it is being given. (See the discussion of radiation therapy in Section IV, "Childhood Cancer Treatment.")
- Assess the child for complications related to surgery, if

performed. (See the discussion of surgery in Section IV, "Childhood Cancer Treatment.")
- Assess for signs of infection.
- Assess the child for evidence of fatigue, bleeding, pain, and nutritional deficits.
- Monitor fluids and electrolytes.
- Determine which type of IV access is needed.
- Assess for the possibility of emergency complications.
- Assess for a response to therapy (i.e., a decrease in the size of the mass or enlarged lymph nodes, evaluation of any metastatic disease).

**Interventions:**
- Refer the child for central IV access as needed.
- Provide comfort measures.
- Provide pain medication as needed.
- Provide instruction on proper mouth care, nutrition, and hygiene.
- Educate the family regarding neutropenia, anemia, and thrombocytopenia, as well as the signs and symptoms of infection and fever precautions.
- Obtain cultures and radiological examinations as ordered, when infection is suspected, and initiate antibiotics if indicated.
- Provide alternative methods of nutrition (e.g., oral supplements, nasogastric and parenteral supplements).
- Review all findings of laboratory tests and radiological studies with the patient and the family.

## Goal
The patient and the family will be adequately informed regarding the diagnosis, disease, and treatment.

**Assessment:**
- Assess the level of knowledge of the patient and the family about the diagnosis and disease.
- Assess their level of knowledge about treatment (i.e., surgery, radiation therapy, chemotherapy).
- Assess their learning styles. (See Section VIII, "Patient and Family Education.")
- Assess their understanding of the role of the multidisciplinary team in treating children with neuroblastoma.

**Interventions:**
- Communicate with the patient and the family in an appropriate style.
- Provide them with appropriate educational resources and review the material with them.
- Ensure that the family is aware of when and how to contact the healthcare team.
- Encourage the patient and the family to ask questions related to the diagnosis, disease, and treatment.
- Clarify the information provided by various members of the multidisciplinary team.

## Goal
The patient and the family will cope adequately with the diagnosis.

**Assessment:**
- Assess the family's communication and coping styles in general.
- Assess the family's adjustment to the diagnosis.

**Interventions:**
- Provide the patient and the family with honest answers to their questions.
- Provide emotional support.
- Anticipate the need for referral services (e.g., social work, chaplain, nutritionist, financial assistance, rehabilitation).
- Offer the child age-appropriate "hospital play."
- Offer to introduce a contact family who has dealt with a similar malignancy to talk with the patient and the family.

## Expected Patient and Family Outcomes
The child, the family, or both, can do the following:
- Describe the type of neuroblastoma and the plan of care.
- List the expected and possible toxic side effects of therapy.
- Outline methods to prevent infection.
- Describe the schedule of treatment, procedures, and follow-up care.
- Describe available in-hospital and community resources.
- Demonstrate the skills needed to care for the child at home.
- Explain how and when to contact the healthcare team if problems or questions arise.

# Osteosarcoma

*Judith Ann Holloway*

## Definition
*Osteosarcoma* is a primary malignant tumor of the bone.

## Pathophysiology
Osteosarcoma is distinguished from other bone tumors by the production of osteoid substance. These tumors have varying degrees of osteoblastic, chondroblastic, and fibroblastic differentiation.

## Incidence and Etiology
Osteosarcoma is the most common bone tumor and the sixth most common malignancy in children; in adolescents and young adults, it is the third most frequent neoplasm (after leukemias and lymphomas). There are 5.6 cases per 1 million children of European ancestry younger than 15 years of age, with approximately 400 children and adolescents younger than 20 years old diagnosed in the United States each year. Incidence is slightly lower in children without European ancestry. Peak incidence is in the second decade of life, during the adolescent growth spurt. Osteosarcoma often occurs earlier in girls because of their earlier growth spurt, but it is more common in boys because of their large bone volume. Osteogenic sarcoma occurs in approximately 56% of all malignant bone tumors in children and adolescents.

Three percent of osteosarcomas result from irradiation, but this applies to the older population and occurs between 4 and 40 years (the median is 12–16 years) after receiving radiation. Two percent of patients with Paget's disease, a premalignant condition, will develop osteosarcoma after age 50. Patients with hereditary retinoblastoma or carriers of the mutations of the p53 gene have a genetic predisposition to develop osteosarcoma, but the

| Table 2-10. Causes of Osteosarcoma | |
|---|---|
| **Exposure or Characteristic** | **Comments** |
| **Known risk factors** | |
| Prior treatment for childhood cancer with radiation therapy and/or chemotherapy | There is an increased risk following radiotherapy for childhood cancer. |
| | Independent of radiotherapy, treatment with alkylating agents increases the risk of developing osteosarcoma. |
| Hereditary retinoblastoma, Li-Fraumeni syndrome, and Rothmund-Thomson syndrome | Increased risk is well documented for these genetic conditions. |
| Radium | High doses of the radioisotope radium are known to cause osteosarcoma in adults. Whether the low levels sometimes found in drinking water confer risk to children or adults is unknown. |
| **Factors for which evidence is limited or inconsistent** | |
| Growth and development | There has been some suggestion that taller stature is associated with increased risk, but the results of more recent studies do not support this finding. One study showed an association with earlier age at onset of secondary sex characteristics in females and lower weight gain during pubertal growth spurt in males. |
| Prior trauma to tumor site | One study found a small positive association between damage to the tumor site and increased risk of osteosarcoma. |
| Prenatal exposure and development | Short birth length and fetal X rays were associated with an increased risk in a single study. |
| Parental exposures | An association with chicken farming and another with gardening fertilizer, herbicides, or pesticides have been reported in single studies. |
| Fluoride in drinking water | The few epidemiologic studies as well as ecologic and time-trend analyses suggest that fluoride is unlikely to cause osteosarcoma. |

*Source:* National Cancer Institute SEER data 1975–1995.

majority of cases are of unknown cause. Li-Fraumeni syndrome describes a condition in which mutations of the p53 gene are inherited. Patients have a 50% chance of developing a malignancy (usually bone or breast) by the age of 30 and a 90% chance of developing a cancer by the age of 70 (**Table 2-10**).

## Clinical Presentation

The patient may have pain that is dull, aching, and constant and is often worse at night; the average duration of the pain is 3 months before osteosarcoma is diagnosed. Pain often is attributed to trauma, which is common in active adolescents. Patients may or may not have a soft-tissue mass or swelling. This disease most commonly involves the long bones (e.g., distal femur, proximal tibia, humerus). Patients may have altered gait or function of the extremity because of their reluctance to use the affected limb. Approximately 15%–20% of patients present with visible macrometastatic disease, with the majority of these metastatic lesions found in the lungs. A small portion of patients present with bone metastasis with or without associated pulmonary metastasis. Bone metastasis at presentation carries an extremely poor prognosis.

## Diagnostic

The diagnostic includes an evaluation of the extent of disease before therapy is initiated. An evaluation should include the following:
- A complete history of the current illness, including the location, duration, and intensity of pain; limping or refusal to bear weight; and the presence of mass
- A complete physical examination, including observation for soft-tissue mass, abnormal gait, limited range of motion, circumference of the affected and nonaffected limbs, and warmth and tenderness associated with the affected limb
- Radiographic findings of the extremity, which often may include a sunburst pattern, mixed regions of sclerosis and lytic lesions of bone; Codman's triangle (i.e., an isolated cuff of reactive subperiosteal new bone at the boundary of any benign or malignant mass that rapidly elevates the periosteum); and chest X ray to assess for the possible presence of metastatic disease. Although radiographic findings are highly suggestive of a malignant bone tumor, a biopsy is always required to confirm the diagnosis
- An assessment for a pathological fracture, which can be present with any malignant or benign bone tumor
- A bone scan to assess for an increased uptake of radioisotope at tumor sites or areas of healing bone
- A computed tomography (CT) scan of the chest to reveal the presence and extent of pulmonary lesion(s)
- A magnetic resonance imaging (MRI) scan to assess for soft-tissue, nerve and vessel involvement, and tumor boundaries
- Laboratory studies such as serum alkaline phosphate, which is increased in 40% of patients. (Elevations are not uncommon in adolescents because they are undergoing normal bone growth.) Approximately 30% of patients have an elevated serum lactic dehydrogenase
- Arteriography, which may be helpful for determining the extent of blood or vascular flow to the tumor that is not noted with MRI
- Fine-needle, core, or open incisional biopsy, which is

important for determining histology. An open biopsy is preferred to allow for obtaining an ample bone specimen for testing. The initial biopsy should be done at a pediatric oncology center.

## Prognostic Considerations

The most important prognostic factor is extent of disease at diagnosis. Pulmonary metastasis at diagnosis is an important prognostic variable, has an impact on the management of the disease, and greatly decreases the survival time. The location of the tumor will direct the surgical procedure (i.e., limb salvage or surgical resection). Spinal osteosarcoma has a poor prognosis because it is not possible to completely resect the tumor. Tumor size also has been cited as an important prognostic factor. Large tumors (more than 15 cm) correlate with a dismal prognosis. A poor prognosis is also associated with patients younger than 10 years old, males, and serum and tumor tissue alkaline phosphatase levels. Patients who respond to preoperative chemotherapy (more than a 98% necrosis) have more favorable outcomes.

## Treatment and Prognosis

Successful treatment requires chemotherapy inasmuch as all patients are presumed to have microscopic metastases. More than 80% of patients with osteosarcoma treated with surgery only will develop metastatic disease. Chemotherapy consists of high-dose MTX (Mexate), doxorubicin (Adriamycin), and cisplatin (Platinol), as well as ifosfamide (Ifex) and etoposide (VP-16). After initial chemotherapy is given, surgery for tumor resection and reconstruction of the limb is then performed and is followed by additional chemotherapy. The overall survival rate is 65%–70%.

Although osteosarcoma is a typically radioresistant tumor, radiation may be used for metastatic disease or palliation. Treatment of a lung metastasis includes resection and possible irradiation of the areas. The event-free survival rate for metastatic osteosarcoma is approximately 20%–30% (**Figure 2-4**).

## Surgery

The goal is to obtain a wide margin—a zone of 5 mm or more of normal healthy tissue—around the tumor. The type of surgery is dependent upon the tumor type and location, age of the patient, response to preoperative chemotherapy, surgeon's preference, and the decision of the patient or the family.

Patients undergoing either limb salvage or amputation often achieve similar functional outcomes. However, these two surgical groups of patients are at risk for decreased quality of life, social isolation, poor self-esteem, and limitations in employment and future health insurance coverage.

## Limb Salvage Procedure

An endoprosthetic device, such as a total knee or hip joint, is implanted after the diseased bone is removed. The allograft, bone,

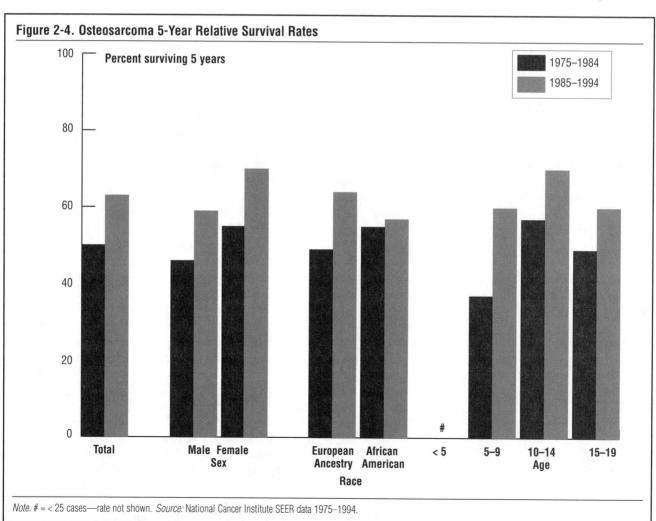

Figure 2-4. Osteosarcoma 5-Year Relative Survival Rates

Note. # = < 25 cases—rate not shown. Source: National Cancer Institute SEER data 1975–1994.

or soft tissue can become infected and result in additional surgeries and even amputation. Ten percent of patients will have mechanical failure of the endoprosthesis that results from routine use and will need to undergo replacement procedures.

### Arthrodesis
Arthrodesis (i.e., fusion of the joint) involves replacement of the joint with allograft or cadaver bone.

### Amputation
This procedure is used especially for expendable bones, such as a fibula, rib, toe, finger, or ulna.

### Rotationplasty
This involves an excision of the femur (and preservation of the lower leg), after which the lower leg is turned 180 degrees. The foot, which is now facing backward, becomes the knee. This procedure improves functional ability, as it is similar to a below-the-knee amputation and the patient can be fitted with a prosthesis.

### New Therapies
Current clinical trials are assessing the use of monoclonal antibodies, such as trastuzumab (Herceptin), used concurrently with the standard front-line chemotherapy in an effort to determine improved efficacy for disease-specific therapy. Inhaled granulocyte-macrophage colony-stimulating factor (GM-CSF) also is being studied for individuals who have recurrent pulmonary metastases.

## Recurrent Disease
A routine chest radiograph and plain films of the affected limb are needed if a recurrence is to be detected early. Recurrent disease most commonly occurs within 3 years of the original diagnosis; 85% of recurrences occur in the lung. There is less possibility of a cure if a recurrence appears within 2 years after therapy is discontinued.

## Nursing Assessment and Interventions
### Goal
The patient will experience minimal complications related to the onset of tumor.
   **Assessment:**
- Review the type of bone cancer and the location and extent of the disease.
- Obtain a complete history, including the incidence and duration of symptoms (e.g., limping, presence of masses), predisposing factors (e.g., exposure to radiation, cytotoxic drugs, genetic abnormalities), and family history.
- Perform a complete physical examination to assess for the presence of a mass, warmth, tenderness, and bilateral limb circumference.
- Review the laboratory findings.
- Review the radiological imaging studies as indicated.
- Review the surgical and pathology reports as indicated.
- Assess the child's degree of pain.
   **Interventions:**
- Provide comfort measures.
- Provide pain medication as needed.
- Explain all tests, procedures, and results to the patient and the family.

### Goal
The patient will experience minimal complications related to the treatment.
   **Assessment:**
- Assess the child for toxicity related to specific chemotherapy agents. (See the discussion of chemotherapy in Section IV, "Childhood Cancer Treatment.")
- Assess the child for toxicity related to radiation therapy, if it has been given. (See the discussion of radiation therapy in Section IV, "Childhood Cancer Treatment.")
- Assess the child for complications related to surgery, if it has been done. (See the discussion of surgery in Section IV, "Childhood Cancer Treatment.")
- Assess the need for rehabilitative therapies.
- Assess the child for signs of infection.
- Assess the child for evidence of fatigue, bleeding, pain, and nutritional deficits.
- Monitor fluid intake and output and electrolytes.
- Determine which type of IV access is needed.
- Assess for the possibility of emergency complications.
- Assess for response to therapy (i.e., a decrease in the size of the mass or enlarged lymph nodes, evaluation of any metastatic disease).
   **Interventions:**
- Refer the child for central IV access, as needed.
- Provide comfort measures.
- Provide pain medication as needed.
- Provide instruction on proper mouth care, nutrition, and hygiene.
- Educate the family regarding neutropenia, anemia, thrombocytopenia, as well as the signs and symptoms of infection and fever precautions.
- Obtain cultures and radiological examinations, as ordered, when infection is suspected, and initiate antibiotics if they are indicated.
- Provide alternative methods of nutrition (e.g., oral supplements, nasogastric and parenteral supplements).
- Review all findings of laboratory tests and radiological studies with the patient and the family.

### Goal
The patient and the family will be adequately informed regarding the patient's diagnosis, disease, and treatment.
   **Assessment:**
- Assess the level of knowledge of the patient and the family about the diagnosis and disease.
- Assess their level of knowledge about treatment (i.e., surgery, radiation therapy, chemotherapy).
- Assess their learning styles. (See Section VIII, "Patient and Family Education.")
- Assess their understanding of the role of the multidisciplinary team in treating children with osteosarcoma.
   **Interventions:**
- Communicate with the patient and the family in an appropriate style.
- Provide them with appropriate educational resources and review the material with them.

- Determine that the family is aware of when and how to contact the healthcare team.
- Encourage the patient, the family, or both, to ask questions related to the diagnosis, disease, and treatment.
- Clarify information provided by various members of the multidisciplinary team.

### Goal
The patient and the family will cope adequately with the diagnosis.
**Assessment:**
- Assess the family's communication and coping styles in general.
- Assess the family's adjustment to the diagnosis.
- Assess the patient and the family for adjustment to limb salvage or amputation.

**Interventions:**
- Provide the patient and the family with honest answers to their questions.
- Provide emotional support.
- Provide counseling resources for patients experiencing amputation or rotationplasty as needed.
- Anticipate the need for referral services (e.g., social work, chaplain, Candlelighters, American Cancer Society, Leukemia Society).
- Offer the child age-appropriate "hospital play"; provide the patient and the family with information on local children's cancer camps.
- Offer to introduce a contact family who has dealt with a similar malignancy to talk with the patient and the family.

## Expected Patient and Family Outcomes
The child, the family, or both can do the following:
- Describe the type of osteosarcoma and the plan of care.
- List the expected and possible toxic side effects of therapy.
- Outline methods to prevent infection.
- Describe the schedule of treatment, procedures, and follow-up care.
- Describe available community resources.
- Demonstrate the skills needed to care for the child at home.
- Explain how and when to contact the healthcare team if problems or questions arise.

# Ewing's Sarcoma of Bone and Soft Tissue and Peripheral Primitive Neuroectodermal Tumors

*Rebecca D'Amore*

## Definition
*Ewing's sarcoma* was first described by James Ewing in 1921 as an undifferentiated bone tumor that differs from osteosarcoma because of its radiosensitivity. It was initially thought to be of endothelial origin and was later found to be of neural crest origin. Classic Ewing's sarcoma most frequently occurs in the bone. Extraosseous Ewing's sarcoma (EES), peripheral primitive neuroectodermal tumor (PNET), and malignant small-cell tumor of the thoracopulmonary region, or Askin's tumor—all of which are now known to be neoplasms of neuroectodermal origin—have similar histologic and immunohistochemical characteristics as well as shared chromosomal translocations; all are considered to be along the same spectrum of tumors as Ewing's sarcoma of bone. Therefore, all of these entities are considered part of the Ewing's sarcoma family of tumors (ESFT). PNET is the most highly differentiated tumor on the spectrum.

## Pathophysiology
Ewing's sarcoma is a tumor composed of small, round cells with blue granules and characteristic chromosomal translocations. EWS-FLI1 t(11;22; q24;q12) occurs in approximately 90% of tumors within the ESFT. In the ESFT that lack the EWS-FLI1 translocation, the EWS-ERG translocation t(21;22;q22;q12) occurs in 5%–10% of these types of tumors. The most commonly occurring cytogenetic alternations in this family of tumors are Trisomy 8 (55%), Trisomy 12 (33%), and 9q21 LOH (p16; INK4; 33%). In addition, p53 mutations are detected in 5%–20% of ESFT cases. Ewing's sarcoma cells require special markers or staining to differentiate them from other small, round cell tumors. The ESFT stain with vimentin and express CD 99.

## Incidence and Etiology
The ESFT are the second most common bone malignancies in childhood and adolescence. In the United States, 200 children and adolescents younger than 20 years of age are diagnosed with Ewing's sarcoma annually. This represents 34% of bone cancer diagnoses, equaling 2.9 cases per 1 million children. They are most common in the second decade of life, with a slight predominance in males. The majority of patients are European American or Hispanic (the tumors are exceedingly rare among children of Asian and African descent), and they are not commonly associated with congenital diseases of childhood (**Table 2-11**).

## Clinical Presentation
Almost all patients present with pain that often is intermittent and often has been present from a few weeks to months prior to diagnosis. The pain will usually be described as *mild that worsened over time,* may be intensified with exercise, and is often worse at night. A distinct soft-tissue mass is sometimes present, depending on the primary site of disease. It may be difficult to determine if the primary tumor is bone with an associated large soft-tissue mass or soft-tissue mass that invades the bone. Pathological fractures are present in 10%–15% of cases. Constitutional symptoms, such as fever, malaise, anorexia, or weight loss are present in 10%–20% of patients at initial presentation.

Distribution of primary sites is split evenly between the extremities (53%) and the central axis (47%; e.g., pelvis, chest wall, spine/paravertebral region, head and neck). Hemorrhage and necrosis often are seen and may be mistaken for infection. Approximately 25% of patients have overt metastatic disease at diagnosis (e.g., lung, bone, bone marrow). However, subclinical metastatic disease is believed to be present in most cases due to the 80%–90% relapse rate associated with the use of local therapy alone.

## Diagnostic
The diagnostic includes an evaluation of the extent of disease before therapy is started. Evaluation should include the following:

- Complete history of the current illness regarding pain (i.e., location, duration, and intensity), limp or limited range of motion, and presence of a mass
- Physical examination to assess for soft-tissue mass, warmth, and tenderness; abnormal gait and limited range of motion; and circumference of the affected and nonaffected limb
- Plain radiograph of the affected area to assess primary site and presence of fracture. The ESFT often appear as a loss of the normal sharp, dense, cortical bone. Due to the presence of finely destructive lesions, the radiographic appearance is often described as "moth-eaten." An "onion-skin" appearance also is present as a result of the periosteal reaction within the layers of reactive bone
- Plain radiograph of the chest to assess for metastatic disease
- Bone scan to assess for increased uptake of radioisotope at the tumor sites or areas of healing bone
- Computed tomography scan of the chest to reveal the presence and extent of pulmonary lesion(s)
- Magnetic resonance imaging scan to reveal soft tissue, nerve and vessel involvement, and tumor boundaries. Scans rarely are normal after treatment
- Laboratory studies, including complete blood count, chemistries, LDH, and erythrocyte sedimentation rate. An elevated sedimentation rate and white blood cell count can be seen with the ESFT and can be confused with osteomyelitis.
- An initial biopsy at a pediatric oncology center. Poorly planned biopsies of bone may lead to pathological fractures or contamination of other tissue.
- Bilateral bone marrow aspirations and biopsies
- Baseline cardiovascular, pulmonary, renal, and hepatic function studies
- Baseline assessment of neurologic, musculoskeletal, and psychological function.

## Prognostic Considerations

The presence of clinically detectable metastatic disease at diagnosis is associated with poor outcomes and is the most significant prognostic indicator. Patients with ESFT with a primary lesion in the pelvis have a poor prognosis; patients with primary lesions in a distal extremity or rib fare best. Tumor size is related significantly to outcome in some studies. Older age has been associated with a poor prognosis. Deletion of the short arm of chromosome 1p, homozygous deletions of CDKN2A and p16/p14ARF, and p53 mutations have all been associated with an inadequate response to chemotherapy, resulting in a poorer prognosis. The serum LDH level may be a prognostic indicator (i.e., a higher level is associated with a poorer prognosis; **Figure 2-5**).

## Treatment and Prognosis

### Chemotherapy

Chemotherapy for ESFT consists of a combination of several agents: ifosfamide (Ifex), cyclophosphamide (Cytoxan), vincristine (Oncovin), etoposide (VP-16), doxorubicin (Adriamycin), and dactinomycin (Actinomycin D).

### Local Control

Surgery or radiation therapy is dependent upon the tumor's location and response to chemotherapy, as noted with disease restaging. ESFT responds well to radiation therapy, with total tumor dose equal to 55–60 Gy. Surgical procedures such as limb salvage or amputation may be necessary to achieve maximal tumor resection. Local control measures should not compromise systemic therapy because of the overall poorer prognosis associated with metastatic disease. If the patient presents with lung metastases, he or she will receive lung irradiation.

### Cure Rates

Cure rates of localized ESFT are 60%–70%. Distal lesions are more easily cured than axial lesions. The cure rate for metastatic ESFT is 18%–30%.

### Recurrent Disease

Recurrent disease is indicative of a poor prognosis. The chance of survival is related to the site and extent of recurrence, biology of

### Table 2-11. Causes of Ewing's Sarcoma (ES)

| Exposure or Characteristic | Comments |
| --- | --- |
| **Known risk factors** | |
| Race | ES is almost exclusively a disease of European ancestry children, with rates approximately 9 times those in African Americans. |
| **Risk factors for which evidence is limited or inconsistent** | |
| Growth | As for osteosarcoma, recent studies have not found a consistent association with increased height or weight or age at pubertal growth. |
| Hernia | An association was found between hernias and increased risk in one study. |
| Paternal occupation | Paternal occupation in agriculture has been associated with increased risk in two studies, although only in one were the results statistically significant. |
| Ingestion of poison or overdose of medication | A prior poisoning episode was more common among cases than controls in a single study. |
| Family history of cancer | ES has been reported in several pairs of siblings. However, more than one family member with ES is rare. In a study of more than 200 cases, none had a relative with ES. Unlike osteosarcoma, ES is not part of the Li-Fraumeni syndrome. |

*Source*: National Cancer Institute SEER data 1975–1995.

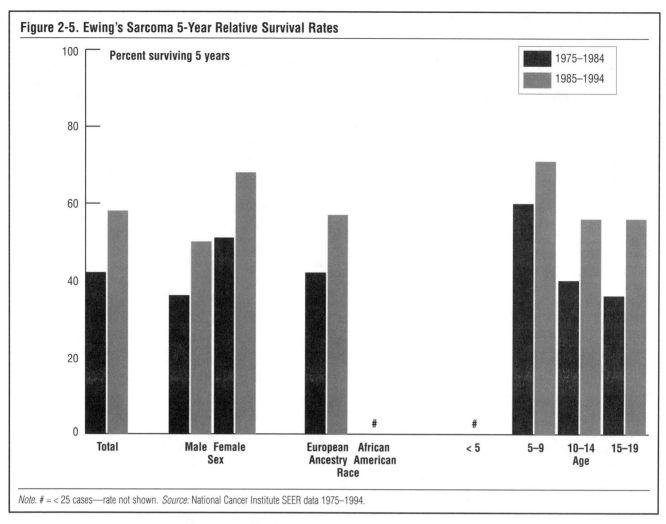

Figure 2-5. Ewing's Sarcoma 5-Year Relative Survival Rates

Note. # = < 25 cases—rate not shown. Source: National Cancer Institute SEER data 1975–1994.

tumor cells, aggressiveness of previous treatment, length of time between treatment, and recurrence and age (patients younger than 11 years old have improved survival rates). Chemotherapy agents not previously used are considered when there is a recurrence. Treatment may include surgery, radiation, or both. In some centers, metastatic, refractory or relapsed disease, or large inoperable tumors are being treated with high-dose therapy followed by autologous stem-cell rescue. There is no conclusive evidence that this type of high-dose therapy is beneficial. The secondary malignancy rate may be as high as 30%. Overall survival rate for recurrent disease is less than 20%.

## Nursing Assessment and Interventions

### Goal
The patient will experience minimal complications related to the onset of ESFT.
  **Assessment:**
- Know the type of malignancy, location and extent of disease, and presenting symptoms.
- Obtain a complete history, including the incidence and duration of symptoms (e.g., the presence of mass, warmth, tenderness, limited range of motion) and family history.
- Perform a complete physical examination to determine the presence of mass, warmth, tenderness, and bilateral limb circumference.
- Review the laboratory findings.
- Review radiological imaging studies as indicated.
- Review surgical and pathology reports as indicated.
- Assess the child's degree of pain.
  **Interventions:**
- Provide comfort measures.
- Provide pain medication as needed.
- Explain all tests, procedures, and results to the patient and the family.

### Goal
The patient will experience minimal complications related to treatment.
  **Assessment:**
- Assess the child for toxicity related to specific chemotherapy agents. (See the discussion of chemotherapy in Section IV, "Childhood Cancer Treatment.")
- Assess the child for toxicity related to radiation therapy if it has been given. (See the discussion of radiation therapy in Section IV, "Childhood Cancer Treatment.")
- Assess the child for complications related to surgery, if performed. (See the discussion of surgery in Section IV, "Childhood Cancer Treatment.")
- Assess the need for rehabilitation therapies after surgery.
- Assess for signs of infection.
- Assess the child for evidence of fatigue, bleeding, pain, and

nutritional deficits.
- Monitor fluid intake and output and electrolytes.
- Determine which type of IV access is needed.
- Assess for the possibility of emergency complications.
- Assess for the child's response to therapy (i.e., decrease in size of the mass or enlarged lymph nodes, evaluation of any metastatic disease).

  **Interventions:**
- Refer the child for central IV access as needed.
- Provide comfort measures.
- Provide pain medication as needed.
- Provide instruction on proper mouth care, nutrition, and hygiene.
- Educate the family regarding neutropenia, anemia, and thrombocytopenia, as well as the signs and symptoms of infection and fever precautions.
- Obtain cultures and radiological examinations as ordered, when infection is suspected, and initiate antibiotics if indicated.
- Provide alternative methods of nutrition (e.g., oral supplements, nasogastric and parenteral supplements).
- Review all findings of laboratory studies and radiological studies with the patient and the family.

### Goal
The patient, the family, or both will be adequately informed regarding the diagnosis, disease, and treatment.

  **Assessment:**
- Assess the level of knowledge of the patient and the family about the diagnosis and disease.
- Assess their level of knowledge regarding treatment (i.e., surgery, radiation therapy, chemotherapy).
- Assess their learning styles. (See Section VIII, "Patient and Family Education.")
- Assess their understanding of the role of the multidisciplinary team in treating children with ESFT.

  **Interventions:**
- Communicate with the patient and the family in an appropriate style.
- Provide them with appropriate educational resources and review the material with them.
- Determine that the family is aware of when and how to contact the healthcare team.
- Encourage both the patient and the family to ask questions related to the diagnosis, disease, and treatment.
- Clarify information provided by various members of the multidisciplinary team.

### Goal
The patient and the family will cope adequately with the diagnosis.

  **Assessment:**
- Assess the family's communication and coping styles in general.
- Assess the family's adjustment to the cancer diagnosis and treatment.

  **Interventions:**
- Provide the patient and the family with honest answers to their questions.
- Provide them with emotional support.
- Anticipate their need for referral services early (e.g., social work, chaplain, Candlelighters, American Cancer Society, Leukemia Society).
- Offer the child age-appropriate "hospital play."
- Offer to introduce a contact family who has dealt with a similar malignancy to talk with the patient and the family.

### Expected Patient and Family Outcomes
The child, the family, or both can do the following:
- Describe ESFT and the plan of care.
- List the expected and possible toxic side effects of therapy.
- Outline methods for preventing infection.
- Describe the schedule of treatment, procedures, and follow-up care.
- Describe available community resources.
- Demonstrate the skills needed to care for the child at home.
- Explain how and when to contact the healthcare team if problems or questions arise.

## Tumors of the Kidney

*Eileen Duffey-Lind*

### Definition
Tumors of the kidney are primary tumors arising from the kidney.

### Pathophysiology

#### Description
Tumors of the kidney are most often Wilms' tumors, which are large, rapidly growing, vascular abdominal tumors. They frequently have a fragile gelatinous capsule. Wilms' tumors are divided into two categories:

#### Favorable Histology
This tumor has an undifferentiated, primitive development. It is composed of stromal, epithelial, and blastemic tissue (precursor of stromal and epithelial cells).

#### Anaplastic
This type of tumor has anaplastic nuclear changes, is present in about 5% of patients with Wilms' tumor, and is more common in older children. It is rarely seen in the first 2 years of life; then it increases in frequency in patients older than 5 years of age, accounting for approximately 13% of patients with Wilms' tumor. It is significantly more frequent in African American than in Caucasian children. Focal anaplasia does not confer a poor prognosis, whereas diffuse anaplasia does. Anaplasia is associated with resistance to chemotherapy.

#### Clear-Cell Sarcoma of the Kidney
This tumor is the second most common pediatric renal neoplasm and is associated with a significantly higher rate of relapse and death than favorable-histology Wilms' tumor. It also is associated with a wider distribution of metastases, including to the brain, bone, and soft tissue, as well as an extended period during which metastases may present.

### Rhabdoid Tumor of the Kidney

This is not Wilms' tumor; it is a rare, highly malignant renal tumor. It may metastasize to the brain and lungs. Rhabdoid tumor of the kidney occurs more frequently in infants, with 85% of cases occurring within the first 2 years of life. Typically, the tumor is widely metastatic at presentation, and in both the National Wilms Tumor Study Group (NWTSG) and International Society of Pediatric Oncology (SIOP) studies more than 80% of children die within 1 year of diagnosis.

### Nephrogenic Rests

These are precursor cells to Wilms' tumor. Nephroblastomatosis refers to multiple nephrogenic rests, which are classified by their position within the kidney—Intralobar (ILNR) or perilobar (PLNR). Only a small number develop a clonal transformation into Wilms' tumor.

### Renal-Cell Carcinoma

The classic form of renal-cell carcinoma is rare in children who do not have a genetic predisposition to it. It is a rare subtype that is seen in adolescence and young adulthood, with a male predominance.

### Renal Medullary Carcinoma

This is a rare, highly lethal tumor that is virtually restricted to patients with sickle-cell hemoglobinopathy, most commonly sickle-cell trait. The median age at which it occurs is 13 years.

### Congenital Mesoblastic Nephroma

This is a distinctive renal neoplasm of infancy. It occurs predominantly in infants, with a median age of 2 months. It comprises about 5% of childhood kidney tumors, with twice as many males diagnosed as females. The poor response to chemotherapy and radiation highlights the importance of surgical resection.

### Incidence and Etiology

Wilms' tumor represents 6% of childhood cancers, and the total incidence in the United States is estimated at 500 cases per year. From 1975 to 1995, the annual incidence was 7.6 cases per 1 million in children younger than 15 years.

Wilms' tumors are seen slightly less frequently in boys (0.92:1.00) than in girls; the median age at diagnosis is slightly younger for boys. The age at diagnosis peaks at 2 to 3 years; these tumors are rare in children older than 5 years of age. For boys the mean age at diagnosis for those with unilateral disease is 41.5 months compared with 46.9 months among girls. The mean age at diagnosis for those who present with bilateral disease is 29.5 months for boys and 32.6 months for girls.

Familial cases account for approximately 1%–2% of all Wilms' tumor cases. These are usually autosomal-dominant with variable penetrance. Tumors of the kidney are associated with aniridia (i.e., congenital absence of iris), hemihypertrophy, genital or renal malformations, Beckwith-Wiedemann syndrome (including macroglossia, omphalocele, hemihypertrophy, and visceromegaly), and other overgrowth syndromes (**Table 2-12**).

Most patients with Wilms' tumor have normal chromosomes, but a gene deletion at 11p13 is noted in the tumor cells of many patients and, frequently, in all cells of patients with aniridia. One hypothesis is that the Wilms' tumor suppressor gene (WT1) located at 11p13 suppresses the activity of the tumor-transforming gene located elsewhere on chromosome 11. A second Wilms' tumor gene (WT2) has been found at 11p15; the same gene deletion is seen in Beckwith-Wiedemann syndrome. Alterations on band 11p15 may predispose a person to the development of Wilms' tumor. The incidence of p53 mutations of sporadic anaplastic-histology Wilms' has been shown to be 75%.

### Clinical Presentation

Tumors of the kidney most often present with an asymptomatic abdominal mass and are frequently found by family members or during a routine physical examination. Pain, malaise, and hematuria are present in 20%–30% of patients with kidney tumors. Twenty-five percent of patients have hypertension, which has been attributed to an increase in renin activity. Rapid abdominal enlargement, anemia, and hypertension occur in a subset of patients who have a sudden subcapsular hemorrhage; eggshell-type calcifications may be visible on plain film. The lungs, liver, and regional lymph nodes are the most common sites of metastatic disease. Seven percent involve both kidneys, either at diagnosis or subsequently; 7% of bilateral lesions are not noted on preoperative imaging studies; and 12% are unilateral with multicentric foci. Neurological signs may indicate brain metastases. The primary tumor may extend to the inferior vena cava or right atrium.

### Diagnostic

The diagnostic includes an evaluation of the extent of the disease before therapy is started. An evaluation should include the following:

- A complete history of the current illness, including information about the location of the pain, its duration, and intensity (bone pain may indicate metastases, often in the long bones); presence of abdominal mass, including location and size; and hematuria
- A complete physical examination to assess for hemihypertrophy (partial or complex), aniridia, Beckwith-Wiedemann syndrome, distended abdominal veins, cryptorchidism, hypospadius, and abdominal mass
- A complete blood count, urinalysis, renal function and liver function tests, and serum chemistries
- An abdominal ultrasound to determine tumor size and shape, vessel involvement, and the presence of thrombus in the inferior vena cava and right atrium
- An abdominal computed tomography (CT) scan is recommended to further evaluate the nature and extent of disease. A magnetic resonance imaging (MRI) of the abdomen may be used in place of CT scans and may be particularly valuable for the assessment of nephrogenic rests
- A chest radiograph to assess for metastases
- A chest CT scan, which may reveal lesions not noted on a chest X ray. A biopsy might have to be obtained to determine whether Stage IV disease is present.
- Bone scan and X ray skeletal survey should be obtained in children with renal-cell carcinoma and clear-cell sarcoma of the kidney
- Brain imaging with MRI or CT scans should be obtained for children with clear-cell sarcoma, renal-cell carcinoma, or rhabdoid of the kidney.

**Other considerations:** Initial Wilms' tumor assessment does not routinely check for liver, bone, and brain metastases unless warranted by presenting signs and symptoms.

**Staging:** Wilms' tumors are classified by stage (**Table 2-13**).

## Prognostic Considerations

Histology (i.e., a favorable histology versus anaplastic) is the most significant prognostic consideration. Lymph node involvement is an adverse prognostic factor. Metastatic disease at the time of diagnosis remains an important prognostic indicator. Children entered in the National Wilms' Tumor Study (NWTS)-1 are younger than 24 months of age and have a significantly better prognosis than do older children. Tumor size, the age of the patient, histology, lymph node metastases, and local features of the tumor, such as capsular or vascular invasion, have in the past been predictive of risk for tumor recurrence or progression. These may change when more effective treatment regimens are developed. This has been seen with previous evaluations of prognostic factors among children on the NWTS.

Associations between tumor-specific loss of heterozygosity (LOH) for both chromosomes 16q and 1p in NWTS-5 have been found in a subset of favorable histology patients to have a significantly increased risk of relapse and death. LOH for these chromosomal regions is now being used as an independent prognostic factor together with disease stage to weigh intensity of treatment against risk of treatment failure.

## Treatment and Prognosis

The NWTS has systematically studied Wilms' tumor since 1969. The overall relative 5-year survival rate for children with Wilms' tumor was approximately 92% for cases diagnosed between 1985 and 1994, an improvement from the 81% survival rate for cases diagnosed between 1975 and 1984. Relative survival rates were slightly higher for females than males and slightly higher for African American children than for Caucasian children.

### Surgery

Surgery, with a transperitoneal approach and nephrectmy, is most frequently used as an initial treatment. The contralateral kidney and sample lymph nodes must also be examined for tumor. Extensive lymph node dissection is not necessary, however. Small amounts of residual tumor are not associated with a major decrease in the survival rate. Preoperative chemotherapy is given to patients with an intravascular spread of disease, for very large invasive tumors, or for patients for whom there is an anesthesia-related risk. Preoperative chemotherapy prevents an adequate assessment of staging. Patients whose tumors are staged on the basis of imaging only should be considered to have a Stage III tumor.

When bilateral disease is present, an initial staging and biopsy of both kidneys are performed, followed by approximately 6 weeks of chemotherapy, a nephrectomy of the more involved side, and a partial nephrectomy of the other kidney. Seventy-

### Table 2-12. Causes of Wilms' Tumor (WT)

| Exposure or Characteristic | Comments |
|---|---|
| **Known risk factors** | |
| Race | Incidence in Asians is about half that in African Americans and European Americans. |
| Aniridia, genitourinary anomalies, WAGR syndrome (Wilms' tumor, aniridia, genitourinary abnormalities, mental retardation), Beckwith-Wiedemann syndrome, Denys-Drash syndrome, Simpson-Golabi-Behmel syndrome | Risk is increased in children with these congenital anomalies and genetic conditions. The study of children with WAGR led to the identification of one of the WT genes. |
| **Factors for which evidence is suggestive but not conclusive** | |
| Paternal occupation | An increased risk for fathers employed as welders or mechanics has been reported in several studies. |
| **Factors for which evidence is inconsistent or limited** | |
| High birth weight | Association with birth weight over 4,000 grams has been reported in some studies. |
| Parental exposure to pesticides | One study found an increased risk for parental occupational exposure to pesticides. Another study found an association with household insect extermination. |
| Ionizing radiation (in utero) | Prenatal diagnostic X ray was associated with increased risk in one study. |
| Maternal consumption of coffee and tea during pregnancy | Three studies reported association with coffee and tea; another did not replicate this finding. |
| Maternal hair dye use during pregnancy | Use was associated with risk in one study, but not in others. |
| Maternal medication use during pregnancy | Studies reported associations with various drugs including hormones, antibiotics, dipyrone, metoclopramide, and pethrane anesthesia during delivery. Most of these results were found in a single study. |
| Maternal occupation | One study found an association with job groupings that included hairdressers, electronic and clothing manufacturing workers, laboratory workers, and dental assistants. |

*Source:* National Cancer Institute SEER data 1975–1995.

**Table 2-13. National Wilms' Tumor Study (NWTS) Group Staging for Renal Tumors**

| Stage | Description/Incidence |
|---|---|
| I | Tumor confined to the kidney and completely resected. No penetration of the renal capsule or involvement of renal sinus vessels—43%. |
| II | Tumor extends beyond the kidney but is completely resected (negative margins and lymph nodes). At least one of the following has occurred: penetration of the renal capsule, invasion of the renal sinus vessels, biopsy of tumor before removal, spillage of tumor locally during removal—23%. |
| III | Gross or microscopic residual tumor remains postoperatively, including inoperable tumor, positive surgical margins, tumor spillage involving peritoneal surfaces, regional lymph node metastases, or transected tumor thrombus—23%. |
| IV | Hematogenous metastases or lymph node metastases outside the abdomen (e.g., lung, liver, bone, brain)—10%. |
| V | Bilateral renal Wilms' tumors at onset—5%. |

*Source:* Data from National Cancer Institute NCI–PDQ.

five percent of patients with bilateral disease will have residual tumor in the remaining kidney after surgery, but the survival rate remains high.

**Chemotherapy**

The following chemotherapy options are based on the National Wilms' Tumor Study V and current studies: AREN0532 *(very-low-, low-, standard-risk FH Wilms')*, AREN0533 *(higher-risk FH Wilms')*, and AREN0321 *(high-risk renal)*.

**Stage 1, favorable or anaplastic (focal or diffuse):** NWTS V-Regimen EE-4A; nephrectomy with lymph node sampling and 18 weeks of chemotherapy with vincristine and actinomycin-D
*Current Studies.*
- *AREN0532.* Patients with LOH at 1p and 16q are upstaged to DD-4A: vincristine, actinomycin, and doxorubicin for 24 weeks. No radiation therapy is used. Other Stage 1 patients are treated on EE-4A after nephrectomy. Patients younger than 2 years of age who have a tumor weighing less than 550 gm and negative microscopic lymph nodes are eligible for observation only.
- *AREN0321.* Anaplasia (focal or diffuse) is treated with DD-4A and radiation therapy.

**Stage II, favorable:** NWTS V—Regimen EE-4A
*Anaplasia (focal).* Regimen DD-4A
*Anaplasia (diffuse).* Regimen I
Nephrectomy with lymph node sampling, abdominal radiation, and 24 weeks of chemotherapy with vincristine, doxorubicin, etoposide, cyclophosphamide, and mesna.
*Current Studies.*
- *AREN0532:* Patients with LOH at chromosomes 1p and 16q will be upstaged to receive treatment with DD-4A. Stage II patients will be treated with EE-4A.
- *Focal anaplasia.* Stage II: DD-4A and radiation therapy
- *AREN0321 (diffuse anaplasia):* UH-1 regimen calls for cyclophosphamide, carboplatin, and etoposide alternating with vincristine, doxorubicin, and cyclophosphamide for 30 weeks and radiation therapy.

**Stage III, favorable:** NWTS V—Regimen DD-4A and abdominal radiation.
*Anaplasia (focal and diffuse).* Regimen I
*Current Studies.*
- *AREN0532:* Patients with LOH at chromosomes 1p and 16q will be moved to AREN0533 with regimen M (dactinomycin, doxorubicin, and vincristine alternating with cyclophosphamide and etoposide) for 24 weeks and radiation therapy.
- *Focal anaplasia:* AREN0321 consists of standard DD-4A and radiation therapy.
- *Diffuse anaplasia:* AREN0321 consists of UH-1 regimen and radiation therapy.

**Stage IV, favorable:** This treatment level includes nephrectomy with lymph node sampling, abdominal radiation according to local stage of renal tumor, bilateral pulmonary radiation for patients with chest X ray evidence of pulmonary metastases, and 24 weeks of chemotherapy with vincristine, doxorubicin, and actinomycin-D.

*Focal anaplasia.* Treatment consists of nephrectomy with lymph node sampling, abdominal radiation according to local stage of renal tumor, bilateral pulmonary radiation for patients with chest X ray evidence of pulmonary metastases, and 24 weeks of chemotherapy with vincristine, doxorubicin, and actinomycin-D.

*Diffuse anaplasia.* Treatment consists of nephrectomy with lymph node sampling, abdominal radiation according to local stage of renal tumor, bilateral pulmonary radiation for patients with chest X ray evidence of pulmonary metastases, and 24 weeks of chemotherapy with vincristine, doxorubicin, etoposide, cyclophosphamide, and mesna.

*Current Studies.*
- *Favorable histology—AREN0533:* Patients with pulmonary metastases will start with DD-4A. Pulmonary metastases will be reevaluated at 6 weeks with CT scan. If complete resolution of pulmonary metastases occurs, the patients will be considered rapid responders and will continue on DD-4A without any pulmonary radiation. Patients who do not have complete response are called slow responders and will be switched to regimen M and radiation therapy to the abdomen and lungs. Patients with LOH at 1p and 16q will be treated with regimen M with radiation therapy to all sites of disease.
- *Focal and diffuse:* No measurable disease
- *Anaplasia:* AREN0321 consists of UH-1 regimen and radiation therapy.
- *Diffuse anaplasia with measurable disease:* AREN0321 consists of window therapy for 12 weeks with irinotecan and vincristine. If patient responds to the window therapy, he or she will receive

UH-2 (cyclophosphamide, carboplatin, and etoposide alternating with vincristine, doxorubicin, and cyclophosphamide; vincristine, irinotecan, and radiation) for 30 weeks. Patients not responsive to the window will receive regimen UH-1 and radiation.

**Stage V, individualized:** Patients should undergo bilateral renal biopsies with staging for each kidney. Initial treatment is with DD-4A if the renal tumors are favorable and if anaplastic histology they should receive regimen I. Following 6 weeks of chemotherapy, the patient should be reassessed. If no further reduction in tumor size is observed, then a second-look surgical procedure should be performed. Chemotherapy or radiation, or both, is dependent on the child's response to initial therapy.

- *AREN0534:* Bilateral and bilaterally predisposed
  **Clear-cell sarcoma, Stages I–IV:** Regimen I and radiation
  *Current Study.*
- *AREN0321:* Patients with lymph node dissection, Stage 1, will be treated with only regimen I. Stages II and III will be treated with regimen I and radiation. Stage IV will be treated with UH-1 and radiation therapy.
  **Malignant rhabdoid, Stages I–IV:** No satisfactory treatment has been developed.
  *Current Studies.*
- *AREN0321:* Regimen UH-1
- *Renal-cell carcinoma, Stages I–IV:* AREN0321 calls for gross total resection and associated lymph nodes. Renal-cell carcinoma has never been studied in a cooperative group setting. It is not responsive to conventional chemotherapy.

## Radiation Therapy

The port is extended to cross the midline to prevent scoliosis. With tumors that have a favorable histology, radiation therapy is needed only for Stage III and Stage IV disease. After lung irradiation, the doses of chemotherapy may have to be decreased. The whole abdomen is treated when patients have had tumor spillage during surgery or when patients have had diffuse peritoneal seeding. On protocol AREN0533, lung radiation has been recommended for patients who do not have complete resolution after 6 weeks of therapy.

## Recurrent Disease

Approximately 15% of patients with favorable-histology Wilms' tumor and 50% of patients with anaplastic Wilms' tumor experience relapse. There is less chance of a cure if a recurrence appears within 12 months of diagnosis. Patients who have an abdominal recurrence after radiation or a recurrence after treatment with doxorubicin (Adriamycin) have a poor prognosis and need aggressive treatment. Patients with Stage II–IV anaplastic-histology at diagnosis have a very poor prognosis upon recurrence. Relapse treatment often consists of etoposide (VP-16), carboplatin and ifosfamide (ICE), cyclophosphamide-etoposide, and carboplatin-etoposide or autologous bone marrow transplantation. The most common sites of disease recurrence with all stages are the lungs and pleura, tumor bed, and liver. Less frequently, recurrences can occur in the bone, brain, and distant lymph nodes. Most recurrences (approximately 90%) occur within the first 2 years after diagnosis, and the remainder occur in the next 2 years. Children in a more favorable group should be treated aggressively with relapse because they generally have a good response to retrieval therapy. Longer follow-up for clear-cell sarcoma patients is needed because relapses are known to occur as long as 5 years after diagnosis.

## Nursing Assessment and Interventions

### Goal

The patient will experience minimal complications related to the onset of tumor.

**Assessment:**
- Know the type of malignancy, location and extent of disease, and presenting symptoms.
- Obtain a complete history, including the incidence and duration of symptoms (e.g., presence of abdominal mass, hematuria), predisposing factors (e.g., hemihypertrophy, aniridia, Beckwith-Wiedemann syndrome), and family history.
- Perform a complete physical examination to assess for the presence of abdominal mass, hypertension, hemihypertrophy, aniridia, distended abdominal veins, genitourinary abnormalities, and neurological changes.
- Review the laboratory findings.
- Review the radiological imaging studies, as indicated.
- Review surgical and pathology reports, as indicated.
- Assess the child's degree of pain.

**Interventions:**
- Provide comfort measures.
- Provide pain medication as needed.
- Explain all tests, procedures, and results to the patient and the family.

### Goal

The patient will experience minimal complications related to treatment.

**Assessment:**
- Assess the child for toxicity related to specific chemotherapy agents. (See the discussion of chemotherapy in Section IV, "Childhood Cancer Treatment.")
- Assess the child for toxicity related to radiation therapy, if it has been given. (See the discussion of radiation therapy in Section IV, "Childhood Cancer Treatment.")
- Assess the child for complications related to surgery, if it has been performed. (See the discussion of surgery in Section IV, "Childhood Cancer Treatment.")
- Assess for signs of infection.
- Assess the child for evidence of fatigue, bleeding, pain, and nutritional deficits.
- Monitor fluid intake and output and electrolytes.
- Determine which type of IV access is needed.
- Assess for the possibility of emergency complications.
- Assess for the child's response to therapy (i.e., a decrease in the size of mass or enlarged lymph nodes, evaluation of any metastatic disease).

**Interventions:**
- Refer the child for central IV access, as needed.
- Provide comfort measures.
- Provide pain medication as needed.
- Provide instruction on proper mouth care, nutrition, and hygiene.

- Educate the family regarding neutropenia, anemia, and thrombocytopenia, as well as about the signs and symptoms of infection.
- Obtain cultures and radiological examinations as ordered, when infection is suspected, and initiate antibiotics if indicated.
- Provide alternative methods of nutrition (e.g., oral supplements, nasogastric and parenteral supplements).
- Review all of the findings of laboratory studies and radiological studies with the patient and the family.

### Goal
The patient, the family, or both, will be adequately informed regarding diagnosis, disease, and treatment.

**Assessment:**
- Assess the level of knowledge of the patient and the family about diagnosis and disease.
- Assess their level of knowledge regarding treatment (i.e., surgery, radiation therapy, chemotherapy).
- Assess their learning styles. (See Section VIII, "Patient and Family Education.")
- Assess the patient's and the family's understanding of the role of the multidisciplinary team in treating children with renal tumors.

**Interventions:**
- Communicate with the patient and the family in an appropriate style.
- Provide them with appropriate educational resources and review the material with them.
- Determine that the family is aware of when and how to contact the healthcare team.
- Encourage both the patient and the family to ask questions related to diagnosis, disease, and treatment.
- Clarify information provided by various members of the multidisciplinary team.

### Goal
The patient and the family will cope adequately with the diagnosis.

**Assessment:**
- Assess the family's communication and coping styles in general.
- Assess the family's adjustment to the diagnosis.

**Interventions:**
- Provide the patient and the family with honest answers.
- Provide them with emotional support.
- Anticipate the need for referral services (e.g., social work, chaplain, Candlelighters, American Cancer Society).
- Offer the child age-appropriate "hospital play."
- Offer to introduce a contact family who has dealt with a similar malignancy to talk with the patient and the family.

### Expected Patient and Family Outcomes
The child, the family, or both are able to do the following:
- Describe the type of kidney tumor and the plan of care.
- List the expected and possible toxic side effects of therapy.
- Outline methods for preventing infection.
- Describe the schedule of treatment, procedures, and follow-up care.
- Describe available community resources.
- Demonstrate the skills needed to care for the child at home.
- Describe how and when to contact the healthcare team if problems or questions arise.

## Rhabdomyosarcoma
*Julie McMahon*

### Definition
*Rhabdomyosarcoma* (RMS) is a malignant tumor of mesenchymal cell origin, most often arising from cells of skeletal muscle lineage. This type of tumor can develop in tissues in which striated muscle cells are not normally found.

### Pathophysiology
RMS is a small, round blue-cell tumor. It is classified as an RMS when muscle cell characteristics (e.g., cross striations on muscle proteins, such as actin, myosin, desmin, myoglobin, Z-band, protein, and myoD) are noted on pathologic review, using both microscopic techniques and molecular genetic techniques.

The histological classifications of RMS are botryoid/spindle-cell, embryonal, alveolar, and undifferentiated. The botryoid and spindle-cell types generally have the best prognosis. The embryonal type has an intermediate prognosis. The undifferentiated sarcoma subtype has a poorer prognosis, as does the alveolar type. Two-thirds of rhabdomyosarcomas are diagnosed as embryonal. Although these tumors may develop almost anywhere in the body, there exist certain clusters of features specific to age at diagnosis, site of primary tumor, and histology that are more common. Children younger than 8 years of age are most commonly diagnosed with head and neck tumors, which are most commonly embryonal if they arise from the orbit. Adolescents are more likely to have extremity tumors of the alveolar variety. RMS is seen almost exclusively in infants, developing from the vagina or the bladder. In older children, botryoid arises from the nasopharynx.

### Incidence and Etiology
There are 350 new cases of RMS in the United States each year, 4.3 cases per 1 million children. After neuroblastoma and Wilms' tumor, RMS is the most common extracranial solid tumor of childhood. The majority of RMS cases are diagnosed before age 9, with another peak incidence during early- to mid-adolescence.

African American girls have just half the incidence rate of Caucasian girls, but no demonstrated difference has been noted among boys in these two racial groups. Lower incidence rates are seen in Asia than in industrialized Western countries. This tumor is slightly more common in males than in females (a 1.3–1.4:1 ratio).

### Genetics and Molecular Biology
The development of RMS occurs sporadically in the majority of cases; however, its development also has been associated with certain familial syndromes. Neurofibromatosis and the Li-Fraumeni syndrome are linked to the p53 tumor suppressor gene, and Beckwith-Wiedemann syndrome, which is marked by abnormalities on 11p15—where the insulin-like growth factor-2 (IGF-2) gene is located—has been associated with RMS. It has been argued that children with these germline mutations should have their therapy altered because of the increased risk of developing

cancer associated with the syndromes. Treatment, including radiation, epipodophyllotoxins, and alkylating agents—which also have potential carcinogenic properties—may need to be adjusted for this patient population in the future.

The two major histologic subtypes of RMS, embryonal and alveolar, have been found to have different genetic alterations, as well. The alveolar subtype is associated with the translocation of chromosome 2 and 13, designated as t(2;13), and the involvement of the *PAX3* gene. This gene is believed to regulate early neuromuscular development, thus interfering with normal growth and contributing to the development of RMS; it is seen as an adverse prognostic factor. The embryonal subtype is associated with loss of heterozygosity at the 11p15 corresponding position (locus). Both alveolar and embryonal RMS have been associated with the overproduction of IGF-2.

## Clinical Presentation

RMS, depending on the site, is detected by the appearance of a mass or a disturbance of normal body function. The head and neck, including the orbit and parameningeal areas, are the sites of 35% of these tumors. The signs and symptoms for orbital tumors include proptosis and ophthalmoplegia; for nonorbital parameningeal tumors, they are nasal, aural, or sinus obstruction, muco-purulent or sanguinous discharge, cranial nerve palsies, or signs of increased intracranial pressure (ICP). For nonparameningeal tumors, the symptoms include painless growth, which often is localized. The genitourinary tract is the site of 25% of RMSs, which are found most often in the bladder or prostate. The signs and symptoms include hematuria, urinary obstruction, extrusion of the tumor, vaginal discharge, painless pelvic or testicular mass, and constipation. Twenty percent are found in the extremities, where the signs and symptoms include swelling of the soft tissue, either with or without tenderness or erythema. Other sites (i.e., trunk, pelvis, retroperitoneal areas, perineum, biliary tract, liver, brain, trachea, heart, breast, ovary) account for 25%, and the signs and symptoms depend upon the location of the tumor. On occasion, no primary tumor is found.

## Diagnostic

The diagnostic includes an evaluation of the extent of disease before therapy is initiated. An evaluation should include the following components:

- a complete history of the current illness, including the incidence and duration of symptoms (e.g., location of the pain as well as its duration and intensity; presence of mass, warmth, tenderness; neurological changes; hematuria), fatigue, and family history (e.g., p53 dilution, neurofibromatosis)
- a complete physical examination to assess for the presence of a mass (warmth, tenderness); proptosis and rhinorrhea; hematuria, pallor; lymphadenopathy; neurological changes; and signs of increased ICP
- a computed tomography (CT) scan or magnetic resonance imaging (MRI) study of the affected area to define the mass
- a technetium-99m bone scan to rule out osseous metastasis
- a CT scan of the chest to rule out metastasis
- a CT scan of the abdomen/pelvis to rule out clinically occult abnormalities of the gut
- an ultrasound as adjuvant to CT scans for tumors of the pelvis to help with localization
- bilateral bone marrow aspirates and biopsies
- a radiograph of the affected part for a baseline evaluation
- a complete blood count with differential, creatinine, liver function tests, blood urea nitrogen (BUN), electrolytes, calcium, phosphorus, magnesium, and uric acid
- a tumor biopsy, which is necessary for diagnosis
- a blood sample for molecular diagnostic tests to determine characteristic abnormalities—polymerase chain reaction techniques (PCR)
- baseline coagulation studies (i.e., prothrombin time, activated partial thromboplastin time, fibrinogen)
- a blood sample for analysis of gene translocation, which is of great value in diagnosis of undifferentiated tumors.

## Prognostic Considerations

The stage, site, age, histology, surgical respectability, and absence or presence of nodal disease or metastatic disease all contribute to the final outcome of patients with RMS. The presence of metastatic disease is the greatest prognostic indicator (**Table 2-14**). Genetics and the molecular biology of tumors are also being considered as prognostic indicators of RMS. The 4-year survival rate is >70% for *PAX7* versus 10% for *PAX3* in cases with metastatic disease. There is a significant increased risk of relapse and death in patients with metastatic disease if their tumors express *PAX3*. Alveolar histology and more than two metastatic sites of disease also indicate a poor prognosis for a child with RMS.

## Treatment and Prognosis

The Intergroup Rhabdomyosarcoma Study (IRS) group was formed in 1972, and today the majority of children with RMS are enrolled in IRS studies. There are three recognized modalities with which to treat children with RMS: surgical removal (if feasible), radiation, and chemotherapy.

### Surgery

A surgical resection should always be performed if it is feasible. A second surgery may be necessary if residual disease is present after the initial surgery.

Resection is often feasible for head and neck tumors. Routine node sampling is not necessary because the incidence of regional node involvement is low.

A radical inguinal orchiectomy and a resection of the spermatic cord are performed to treat paratesticular tumors. Routine node sampling is controversial.

Vulvar and vaginal tumors often respond to induction chemotherapy; thus, initial widespread excision can be avoided.

Uterine and proximal vaginal tumors may require hysterectomy, but oophorectomy often is avoided. Distal vaginal preservation usually is possible. Second-look surgery is performed for patients with gross residual disease.

Previously, radical surgical procedures were performed to excise bladder and prostate tumors, resulting in high morbidity. A total cystectomy and pelvic exenteration are now performed only when patients do not achieve local control by chemotherapy and radiation.

An initial complete resection is recommended for extremity tumors if limb function will not be greatly impaired; amputation

### Table 2-14. Intergroup Rhabdomyosarcoma Studies (IRS) Grouping and Staging Criteria

**IRS Clinical Group**

- **Group I:** Tumors that are completely removed by surgery
- **Group II:** Tumors that are removed, but with tumor at the edge of the surgical margin and/or in regional lymph nodes
- **Group III:** Local tumors that cannot be removed by surgery
- **Group IV:** Distant metastatic disease present at diagnosis

**IRS Modified Tumor, Node, Metastases (TNM) Stage**

- **Stage I:** Localized tumor involving the orbit (the area near the eye), head, and neck area except for parameningeal sites (next to the membranes covering the brain), or genitourinary tract tumors except bladder and prostate.
- **Stage II:** Localized small tumors of any site not in Stage I. The tumor must be less than 5 cm (about 2 inches), and there must not be regional lymph node spread.
- **Stage III:** Localized tumor at any site not included in Stage I. The tumor is greater than 5 cm (2 inches) in diameter and/or has spread to regional lymph nodes.
- **Stage IV:** Distant metastatic tumor is present at diagnosis.

*Source:* Data from National Cancer Institute NCI–PDQ.

is rarely required. Regional node sampling is recommended.

A complete resection is difficult for pelvic, retroperitoneal, and intrathoracic tumors.

With metastatic disease, the value of pulmonary nodule resection is unclear.

### Radiation Therapy

Radiation therapy is used for most patients, except for children with Group I tumors who have undergone a complete resection. It is important for tumor control and survival. The current IRS protocol (IRS-V) recommends postoperative conventional external beam radiation therapy (EBRT) doses of 36–41.4 Gy for treating microscopic residual disease and 50.4 Gy in 1.8-Gy fractions for treating gross disease (Maharaj, Nimako, & Hadley, 2007). Radiation therapy is usually begun after 9–12 weeks of chemotherapy, unless it is needed at diagnosis on an emergency basis to relieve spinal-cord compression or to reduce intracranial meningeal extension. Intraoperative radiation or radiation implants occasionally are used. Radiation therapy in very young children (younger than 6 years old) has shown to lead to significant late effects, and studies monitoring the dose of radiation therapy necessary for local control are ongoing. Although strategies such as intensity-modulated radiation therapy (IMRT) and proton beams may improve outcome without compromising long-term function, continued research is necessary.

### Chemotherapy

Chemotherapy is used for all patients except a small subset of patients with Group I tumors. Vincristine (Oncovin), dactinomycin (actinomycin-D), doxorubicin (Adriamycin), cyclophosphamide (Cytoxan), ifosfamide (Ifex), and etoposide (VP-16) are the most commonly used agents. Topotecan (hycamtin) and irinotecan (CPT-11) are newer agents that are being used in combination with other chemotherapy agents in an attempt to increase cure rates.

### Treatment Results

IRS-III, the third IRS study, found that orbital, nonbladder, and nonprostate genitourinary tumors have the best prognosis. Intermediate results have been obtained for other head and neck sites, as well as for bladder and prostate tumors. The worst prognosis is associated with tumors in these sites: extremity, cranial parameningeal, truncal, pelvic, retroperitoneal, and paravertebral.

The fourth IRS study identified ifosfamide plus doxorubicin as a significant drug pairing for improving outcomes in patients with metastatic RMS. Although certain groups of patients appear to have benefited from the increased alkylator intensity of IRS-IV, this strategy did not improve the outcome for the majority of patients when it was compared with the IRS-III treatment. IRS-V, the currently accruing protocol for treating RMS, has two major objectives: to evaluate the activity of irinotecan in patients with newly diagnosed metastatic RMS and to evaluate the efficacy of adding topotecan to the standard three-drug regimen of vincristine, dactinomycin, cyclophosphamide (VAC) for patients with intermediate-risk tumors.

### Recurrent Disease

Although rare 3 or 4 years after diagnosis, recurrence can take place many years after treatment is completed. Recurrence should always be documented by biopsy or fine needle aspiration with, at minimum, imaging studies to evaluate fully. Treatment for a local recurrence consists of surgical excision and chemotherapy with agents that have not previously been used. Although cure rates are low, cures are possible.

It is almost impossible to cure metastatic recurrence. Current research is examining ways to overcome drug resistance as well as exploring the potential role of bone marrow or peripheral stem-cell transplantation. Tumor vaccines and immune therapy targeted to specific tumor pathogenesis, as well as antiangiogenic therapy, are also currently being investigated.

### Nursing Assessment and Interventions

#### Goal

The patient will experience minimal complications related to the onset of tumor.

**Assessment:**
- Know the type of malignancy, location and extent of disease, and presenting symptoms.
- Obtain a complete history, including incidence and duration of symptoms (e.g., pain, fatigue, presence of mass,

hematuria, neurological changes) and family history (e.g., p53, neurofibromatosis).
- Perform a complete physical examination to establish the presence of mass (location, tenderness), proptosis, rhinorrhea, pallor, petechiae, lymphadenopathy, hepatosplenomegaly, and neurological changes.
- Review laboratory findings.
- Review radiological imaging studies as indicated.
- Review surgical and pathology reports as indicated.
- Assess the child's degree of pain.

**Interventions:**
- Provide comfort measures.
- Provide pain medication as needed.
- Explain all tests, procedures, and results to the patient and the family.

## Goal
The patient will experience minimal complications related to treatment.

**Assessment:**
- Assess the child for toxicity related to specific chemotherapy agents. (See the discussion of chemotherapy in Section IV, "Childhood Cancer Treatment.")
- Assess the child for toxicity related to radiation therapy, if it is given. (See the discussion of radiation therapy in Section IV, "Childhood Cancer Treatment.")
- Assess the child for complications related to surgery, if performed. (See discussion of surgery in Section IV, "Childhood Cancer Treatment.")
- Assess for signs of infection.
- Assess the child for evidence of fatigue, bleeding, pain, and nutritional deficits.
- Monitor fluid intake and output and electrolytes.
- Determine which type of IV access is needed.
- Assess for the possibility of emergency complications.
- Assess the patient's response to therapy (i.e., a decrease in the size of the mass or enlarged lymph nodes, changes in any metastatic disease).

**Interventions:**
- Refer the child for central IV access as needed.
- Provide comfort measures.
- Provide pain medication as needed.
- Provide instruction on proper mouth care, nutrition, and hygiene.
- Educate the family regarding neutropenia, anemia, thrombocytopenia, signs and symptoms of infection, and fever precautions.
- Obtain cultures and radiological examinations as ordered, when infection is suspected, and initiate antibiotics if indicated.
- Provide alternative methods of nutrition (e.g., oral supplements, nasogastric or parenteral supplements).
- Review all findings of laboratory studies and radiological studies with the patient and the family.

## Goal
Both the patient and the family will be adequately informed regarding the diagnosis, disease, and treatment.

**Assessment:**
- Assess the level of knowledge of the patient and the family about the diagnosis and disease.
- Assess their level of knowledge about treatment (i.e., surgery, radiation therapy, chemotherapy).
- Assess their learning styles. (See Section VIII, "Patient and Family Education.")
- Assess their understanding of the role of the multidisciplinary team in treating RMS.

**Interventions:**
- Communicate with the patient and the family in an appropriate style.
- Provide them with appropriate educational resources and review the material with them.
- Ensure that the family is aware of when and how to contact the healthcare team.
- Encourage both the patient and the family to ask questions related to the diagnosis, disease, and treatment.
- Clarify information provided by various members of the multidisciplinary team.

## Goal
The patient and the family will cope adequately with the diagnosis.

**Assessment:**
- Assess the family's communication and coping styles in general.
- Assess the family's adjustment to the diagnosis.

**Interventions:**
- Provide the patient and the family with honest answers to their questions.
- Provide emotional support.
- Anticipate the need for referral services (e.g., social work, chaplain, Candlelighters, American Cancer Society, Leukemia Society).
- Offer the child age-appropriate "hospital play."
- Offer to introduce a contact family who has dealt with a similar malignancy to talk with the patient and the family.

## Expected Patient and Family Outcomes
The child, the family, or both can do the following:
- Describe the type of RMS and the plan of care.
- List the expected and possible toxic side effects of therapy.
- Outline methods for preventing infection.
- Describe the schedule of treatment, procedures, and follow-up care.
- Describe available community resources.
- Demonstrate the skills needed to care for the child at home.
- Explain how and when to contact the healthcare team if problems or questions arise.

## Reference
Maharaj, N. R., Nimako, D., & Hadley, G. P. (2007). Multimodal therapy for the initial management of genital embryonal rhabdomyosarcoma in childhood. *International Journal of Gynecological Cancer, 18*(1), 190–192.

# Retinoblastoma

*Diane Baniewicz*

## Definition
*Retinoblastoma* is the most common primary intraocular cancer seen in children.

## Pathophysiology
Retinoblastoma consists of a chalky white intraocular mass, often containing calcified foci and large areas of necrosis. It most commonly originates in the posterior retina, arising from the inner layers of the retina and growing into the vitreous humor (endophytic), or arising from the outer layers of the retina and growing toward the subretinal space (exophytic). It can originate from one or more foci in one or both eyes, or, in rare cases, it can present as trilateral disease with an additional focus of tumor in the pineal gland.

## Histology
Retinoblastoma is characterized by cells with scant cytoplasm and hyperchromic nuclei of various sizes, arranged in tight bouquet-like clusters called rosettes.

## Metastatic Disease
Metastatic retinoblastoma can occur as the result of local intraocular extension into the vitreous with distal spread through the optic nerve. Extraocular extension can lead to hematogenous and lymphatic dissemination.

## Incidence and Etiology
There are 200 new cases of retinoblastoma in the United States each year; 70%–80% of these are unilateral. No differences in incidence based on race or gender have been noted. Eighty percent of children who present with this disease are younger than 4 years of age. Retinoblastoma can occur as hereditary or familial form (40%), or as nonhereditary or sporadic form (60%).

## Hereditary (Familial Form)
This form presents as either bilateral or multifocal unilateral disease. Bilateral disease, which can present asynchronously, occurs at a younger age (median age of 7 months) than the spontaneous form (median age of 23 months). The hereditary form is associated with deletion, translocation, or errors in transcription affecting chromosome 13, band q14 and is inherited as an autosomal dominant trait. The retinoblastoma gene, RB1, is contained in chromosome 13q14. The RB1 gene is a tumor suppressor gene. The deletion of tumor suppressor genes predisposes individuals to malignancies. Mutations of RB1 are seen in patients with hereditary and nonhereditary retinoblastoma.

The prototype for analysis of inherited cancer syndromes is explained by Knudson's two-hit theory. One chromosomal mutation is inherited from a parent and a second mutation occurs after conception and affects a somatic retinal cell. Errors in transcription occur more often in the paternal allele, suggesting that germline mutations occur more frequently during spermatogenesis than oogenesis. The hereditary form of retinoblastoma predisposes affected patients to secondary malignant neoplasms.

## Clinical Presentation
Leukocoria ("cat's eye reflex"), lack of the normal red reflex of the eye, is the most common presentation. Strabismus, esotropia, exotropia, decreased vision, or inflammatory signs are other symptoms.

## Diagnostic
The diagnostic includes an evaluation of the extent of the disease before therapy is begun. An evaluation should include the following:

- Complete history of the current illness, including information about familial incidence of retinoblastoma, ocular loss of unknown etiology, decreased vision in one eye, and changes in the appearance of the eyes (e.g., strabismus, leukocoria)
- Complete physical examination, including an assessment of the patient's visual acuity or tracking, strabismus, esotropia, exotropia, and leukocoria
- Direct and indirect funduscopic examination under anesthesia by a retinal surgeon
- Ultrasound, computed tomography scan, or magnetic resonance imaging (MRI) study of the brain and orbits are the most common radiologic tests completed to confirm diagnosis, determine the extent of disease, and visualize ectopic disease of the pineal gland
- MRI study of orbits is a superior method of localizing the intraocular extent of the disease
- Lumbar puncture and bone marrow aspirates are performed in patients with signs and symptoms of metastatic disease. Staging is determined by the Reese-Ellsworth classification for the extent of intraocular disease (**Table 2-15**).

---

**Table 2-15. Reese-Ellsworth Classification of Retinoblastoma**

**Reese-Ellsworth Staging for Retinoblastoma**

**Group I: Very Favorable**
A. Solitary tumor; < 4 disc diameters (dd*) in size at or behind the equator
B. Multiple tumors; no tumor > 4 dd in size at or behind the equator

**Group II: Favorable**
A. Solitary tumor; 4–10 dd in size at or behind the equator
B. Multiple tumors; 4–10 dd in size at or behind the equator

**Group III: Doubtful**
A. Any lesion anterior to the equator
B. Solitary tumors > 10 dd in size behind the equator

**Group IV: Unfavorable**
A. Multiple tumors; some > 10 dd in size
B. Any lesion extending anteriorly to the ora serrata

**Group V: Very Unfavorable**
A. Tumors involving more than half of the retina
B. Vitreous seeding

*1 dd = 1.5 mm

From *Nursing Care of Children and Adolescents with Cancer* (3rd ed., p. 593), ed. C. R. Baggott, K. P. Kelly, D. Fochtman, & G. V. Foley, 2007, Glenview, IL: Association of Pediatric Hematology/Oncology Nurses.

## Prognostic Considerations

The overall prognosis is excellent; 96% of patients have a disease-free, 5-year survival rate. The extent to which the tumor invades the optic nerve affects prognosis in metastatic disease. The spread of the disease to the central nervous system (CNS) is associated with a poor outcome. The potential for preservation of useful vision depends on the stage of the disease at diagnosis and the treatment that has been given.

## Treatment and Prognosis

Treatment and diagnosis depend on the form (i.e., hereditary or sporadic) and the stage of the retinoblastoma. The goal is to preserve useful vision without compromising the patient's chances for survival. Bilateral hereditary (i.e., familial) retinoblastoma can occur asynchronously; therefore, conservative management of a neonate with unilateral presentation of retinoblastoma is indicated. Enucleation is indicated when retinal damage is so extensive that useful vision is unlikely. Chemotherapy is being utilized more often as treatment for patients with intraocular retinoblastoma. The major objective of current clinical trials is to decrease tumor size so that surgical options are more likely to be an option than radiotherapy, thereby decreasing the risk of secondary cancers and orbital or facial abnormalities. All patients must be followed with frequent funduscopic examinations to detect recurrent or new disease.

Treatment includes one or more of the following:
- Surgery—Enucleation, which is removal of the affected eye.
- Chemotherapy—Frequently used IV chemotherapy includes carboplatin, etoposide, and vincristine (CEV). Local subconjunctival carboplatin has also been used.
- Radiation therapy—Retinoblastoma is a radiosensitive tumor; external beam radiation is used to treat advanced disease. Plaque radiotherapy is a radioactive implant placed over the base of the tumor.
- Focal therapy—Cryotherapy is the use of cold temperatures to kill cancer cells. *Thermotherapy* is the use of heat to kill cancer cells. Laser photocoagulation uses lasers to destroy blood vessels that nourish cancer cells.

## Recurrent Disease

Recurrent disease portends a poor prognosis. Radiation therapy or systemic chemotherapy provide palliation.

## Nursing Assessment and Interventions

### Goal
The patient will experience minimal complications related to the onset of tumor.

**Assessment:**
- Know the type of malignancy, location, and extent of disease.
- Obtain a complete history, including familial incidence of retinoblastoma or ocular loss of unknown etiology, decreased vision in one eye, and other changes in the appearance of the eye.
- Perform a complete physical examination, including an assessment of visual acuity or tracking in infants, strabismus, esotropia, exotropia, and leukocoria.
- Review laboratory findings.
- Review radiological imaging studies as indicated.
- Review surgical and pathology reports as indicated.
- Assess the child's degree of pain.

**Interventions:**
- Provide comfort measures.
- Provide pain medication as needed.
- Explain all tests, procedures, and results to the patient and the family.

### Goal
The patient will experience minimal complications related to treatment.

**Assessment:**
- Assess the child for toxicity related to specific chemotherapy agents. (See the discussion of chemotherapy in Section IV, "Childhood Cancer Treatment.")
- Assess the child for toxicity related to radiation therapy, if given. (See the discussion of radiation therapy in Section IV, "Childhood Cancer Treatment.")
- Assess the child for complications related to surgery, if performed. (See the discussion of surgery in Section IV, "Childhood Cancer Treatment.")
- Assess for signs of infection.
- Assess the child for evidence of fatigue, bleeding, pain, and nutritional deficits.
- Monitor fluid and electrolytes.
- Determine which type of IV access is needed.
- Assess for the possibility of emergency complications.
- Assess for a response to therapy (i.e., a decrease in the size of the mass or enlarged lymph nodes, evaluation of any metastatic disease).

**Interventions:**
- Refer the child for central IV access, as needed.
- Provide comfort measures.
- Provide pain medication as needed.
- Provide instruction on proper mouth care, nutrition, and hygiene.
- Educate the family about neutropenia, anemia, thrombocytopenia, the signs and symptoms of infection, and fever precautions.
- Obtain cultures and radiological examinations as ordered, when infection is suspected, and initiate antibiotics if indicated.
- Provide alternative methods of nutrition (e.g., oral supplements, nasogastric or parenteral supplements).
- Review all findings of laboratory studies and radiological studies with the patient and the family.

### Goal
Both the patient and the family will be adequately informed regarding the diagnosis, disease, and treatment.

**Assessment:**
- Assess the level of knowledge of the patient and the family about the diagnosis and disease.
- Assess their level of knowledge about treatment (i.e., surgery, radiation therapy, chemotherapy).
- Assess their learning styles. (See Section VIII, "Patient and Family Education.")

- Assess their understanding of the role of the multidisciplinary team in treating children with retinoblastoma.

  **Interventions:**
- Communicate with the patient and the family in an appropriate style.
- Provide them with appropriate educational resources and review the material with them.
- Ensure that the family is aware of when and how to contact the healthcare team.
- Encourage both the patient and the family to ask questions related to the diagnosis, disease, and treatment.

### Goal
The patient and the family will cope adequately with the diagnosis.

  **Assessment:**
- Assess the family's communication and coping styles in general.
- Assess the family's adjustment to the diagnosis.

  **Interventions:**
- Provide the patient and the family with honest answers.
- Provide them with emotional support.
- Anticipate the need for referral services (e.g., social work, chaplain, Candlelighters, American Cancer Society, Leukemia Society, and national resources for the visually impaired such as CureSearch, Eyecancer Network, Helen Keller International World Headquarters, Prevent Blindness America).
- Offer the child age-appropriate "hospital play."
- Offer to introduce a contact family who has dealt with a similar malignancy to talk with the patient and the family.

## Expected Patient and Family Outcomes
The child, the family, or both can do the following:
- Describe the type of retinoblastoma and the plan of care.
- List the expected and possible toxic side effects of therapy.
- Outline methods for preventing infection.
- Describe the schedule of treatment, procedures, and follow-up care.
- Describe available community resources.
- Demonstrate the skills needed to care for the child at home.
- Explain how and when to contact the healthcare team if problems or questions arise.

# Rare Tumors of Childhood

*Elisa S. Frederick*

This chapter will cover a few rare tumors of pediatric oncology. It will not cover the rarest of the rare or all rare tumors in their entirety—just the ones most commonly seen in pediatric oncology. Certain malignancies are classified as rare tumors in pediatric oncology because they originate from epithelial tissues (the source of most adult cancer) rather than embryonal tissues (the origin of most childhood cancers). These rare cancers are diagnosed more commonly in the 15- to 19-year-old age group (**Figure 2–6**).

Children and their families who are affected by the diagnosis of a rare cancer need additional support because there is often little information available about these particular cancers. It is important for a pediatric oncology nurse to identify resources and reduce the isolation felt by these children and their families.

## Nasopharyngeal Carcinoma
### Definition
*Nasopharyngeal carcinoma* is a primary malignancy of the nasopharyngeal epithelium.

### Incidence and Etiology
It is rare in children—only 3% of all nasopharyngeal carcinomas occur in children who are younger than 19 years of age. It is the second-most-common tumor (after rhabdomyosarcoma [RMS]) of the upper respiratory tract in children and is associated with Epstein-Barr virus (EBV). EBV titers may be used as tumor markers. There is a high incidence of EBV-associated tumors in Asia. This strongly suggests that there is an environmental and genetic cause in the tumor's pathology.

### Clinical Presentation
Nasopharyngeal carcinomas develop in the pharyngeal recesses and spread to the cervical lymph nodes. Lymphadenopathy is often the first and only presenting symptom. Other symptoms include epistaxis, nasal obstruction, tribmus, hearing loss, ear pain, headache, and chronic otitis media. Fifty percent of all patients have cranial nerve involvement. Nasopharyngeal carcinomas metastasize locally to lymph nodes and to the lungs, vertebrae, long bones, or liver.

### Treatment and Prognosis
Treatment includes radiation therapy to extended fields (6,000–7,000 cGy) and frequently has long-term effects such as xerostomia and fibrosis of the neck muscles. Low-stage tumors have been successfully treated with radiation alone, whereas more advanced tumors have been treated with adjuvant chemotherapy. Chemotherapy, including cisplatin (Platinol), fluorouracil (5-FU), MTX (Mexate), bleomycin (Blenoxane), vincristine, cyclophosphamide, doxorubicin, and etoposide, is often used. Patients with small tumors have a more favorable prognosis than patients with tumors that extend outside of the nasopharynx. The overall survival is 78%.

## Fibrosarcoma
### Definition
*Fibrosarcoma* is a malignancy of fibrous tissue.

### Incidence and Etiology
Fibrosarcoma is one of the most common soft-tissue sarcomas (non-RMS) in children and adolescents and is the most common soft-tissue sarcoma that occurs in children younger than 1 year of age. Two peak incidences occur: the first is in children younger than 5 years of age, and the second is in children 10–15 years of age. These two types are referred to as congenital, or infant, and adult forms of fibrosarcoma. Tumors in infants usually are benign. The adult form of this disease has been associated in some patients with previous exposure to radiation.

# Section II Pediatric Cancers

## Clinical Presentation
The most common site for fibrosarcoma is an extremity, especially its distal segments. Fibrosarcoma also can occur in the trunk or in the head and neck. Presenting symptoms are variable, depending upon the site of the primary tumor.

## Treatment and Prognosis
The treatment for infant fibrosarcoma is wide surgical excision (conservative surgical approach). Late local recurrences have been noted in 17%–43% of cases; however, this does not appear to affect overall survival for this population.

Older children (10–15 years old) usually require preoperative chemotherapy to reduce tumor size before surgical resection, as well as to prevent metastases. The purpose of surgery is to achieve a wide local excision, or amputation, if necessary. Chemotherapy treatment is similar to that used to treat RMS, including doxorubicin (Adriamycin), ifosfamide (Ifex), etoposide (VP-16), vincristine (Oncovin), dactinomycin, cyclophosphamide (Cytoxan), and dacarbazine in various combinations. Prognosis is dependent on the site of the primary lesion and extent of disease. Congenital fibrosarcoma has a 5-year survival rate of 95%; an older child has a 5-year survival rate of approximately 60%. The prognosis for recurrent or progressive disease, with the exception of infants, is poor, with the most common site of metastasis being the lung.

## Malignant Hepatic Tumors

### Definition
*Malignant hepatic tumors* are malignant tumors of the liver. Most are hepatoblastomas and hepatocellular carcinomas.

### Incidence and Etiology
Approximately 50% of hepatic tumors are malignant, whereas other hepatic lesions may be hemangiomas or hamartomas. The median age of patients with hepatoblastoma is 1 year, and the median age for patients with hepatocellular carcinoma is 12 years. Hepatoblastoma is associated with some constitutional syndromes, such as familial adenomatous polyposis, Beckwith-Wiedemann syndrome, and Li-Fraumeni syndrome. It is also associated with chromosomal abnormalities. Hepatocellular carcinoma in patients younger than 15 years of age is associated with the hepatitis B virus. Hepatocellular carcinoma also is associated with the prolonged use of anabolic steroids and cirrhosis.

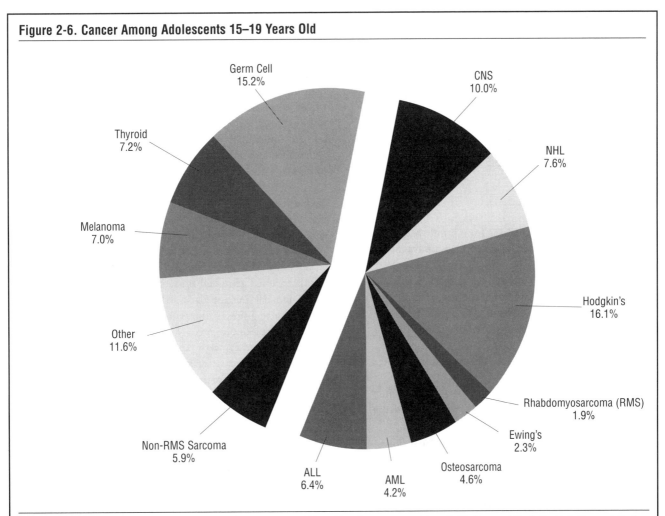

Figure 2-6. Cancer Among Adolescents 15–19 Years Old

Distribution of cancer types, age < 5, all races, both sexes, SEER, 1986–1995. (Adapted from Cancer among adolescents 15–19 years old by Smith, M. A., Gurney, J. G., & Ries, G. In L. A. G. Ries, M. A. Smith, J. G. Gurney, M. Linet, T. Tamra, J. L. Young, et al. [Eds.], *Cancer incidence and survival among children and adolescents: United States SEER Program 1975–1995* [p. 159], 1999. Bethesda, MD: National Cancer Institute, NIH Pub. No. 99–4649.)

## Clinical Presentation

Hepatoblastoma most often presents as an asymptomatic abdominal mass. Pallor, weight loss, and jaundice are rare. Many patients with hepatoblastoma present with osteopenia, which regresses with tumor resection. Hepatocellular carcinoma often presents with abdominal distension and mass in the patient's right upper quadrant. Abdominal pain, nausea, and vomiting are common. The patient may be jaundiced and have associated splenomegaly. The patient's levels of alpha-fetoprotein may be elevated.

## Treatment and Prognosis

A complete resection may be made possible by preoperative chemotherapy in hepatoblastoma and hepatocellular carcinoma. The most common agents used for hepatoblastoma are fluorouracil (5-FU), vincristine (Oncovin), doxorubicin (Adriamycin), and cisplatin (Platinol). The cure rates are high for hepatoblastoma. Overall survival rates for children who have complete resection of their primary tumor exceed 75%. The following characteristics are correlated with a poor prognosis: tumor involvement in both lobes of the liver; multifocal, disseminated liver metastasis; distant metastasis; vascular invasion; embryonal differentiation; and serum alpha-fetoprotein (less than 100,000 ng/ml or more than 100,000 ng/ml). Recurrent disease most often appears in the liver or lungs. Cure is possible for metastatic disease if metastases are surgically resected.

The survival rate for patients with hepatocellular carcinoma is between 10% and 20%. A variant form of hepatocellular carcinoma known as fibrolamellar is associated with a high rate of surgical respectability and improved overall survival, compared with typical hepatocellular carcinoma. Hepatocellular carcinoma is difficult to resect and to cure, even with complete resection. Radiation is of little benefit in treating hepatic tumors. The efficacy of liver transplantation is being investigated.

## Germ-Cell Tumors

### Definition

*Germ-cell tumors* are tumors arising from primitive germ-cells, or embryonal cells, and can occur in the gonads or in sites along the migratory path of the germ-cells from the yolk sac to the gonads. The morphological type varies according to the site and the patient's age. It is not uncommon for one tumor to include more than one cell type. The classifications of these tumors include teratomas, germinomas, endodermal sinus tumors, choriocarcinomas, and embryonal carcinomas.

Types of ovarian tumors include dysgerminoma, teratoma (these are often benign), malignant mixed germ-cell tumor, endodermal sinus tumor (also called yolk sac tumor), gonadoblastoma, choriocarcinoma, embryonal carcinoma, and polyembryoma.

Types of testicular tumors include endodermal sinus tumor, embryonal carcinoma, teratoma (often benign), teratocarcinoma, gonadoblastoma, seminoma, choriocarcinoma, and mixed germ-cell tumor.

Types of extragonadal germ-cell tumors include teratoma, endodermal sinus tumor (also called yolk sac tumor), and embryonal carcinoma.

### Incidence and Etiology

Germ-cell tumors, which account for 1% of all childhood tumors, are associated with abnormal sex chromosomes, central nervous system (CNS) and genitourinary abnormalities, and malformations of the low spine. Most sacrococcygeal teratomas occur in girls; most ovarian tumors occur in postmenarchal girls. The incidence for testicular tumors has two peaks—one in infancy and the other postpubertal—and is higher in males with a history of cryptorchidism.

### Clinical Presentation

The most common sites of metastasis for germ-cell tumors are the lungs, liver, regional nodes, and CNS. They rarely spread to the bone marrow. Alpha-fetoprotein and β-human chorionic gonadotropin levels are often elevated.

The most common germ-cell tumor is teratoma, which in infants often appears with large external masses (often sacrococcygeal). Other primary sites include the cervical neck, upper jaw, nasopharynx, intracranium, retroperitoneum, mediastinum, and gonads. Patients with ovarian tumors often have abdominal pain and swelling, palpable mass, nausea, vomiting, constipation, or genitourinary symptoms. Most testicular tumors present as painless irregular scrotal masses, often with hydroceles or inguinal hernias.

### Treatment and Prognosis

Individualized multimodal treatment is necessary because of the variety of germ-cell tumors. Surgical resection is the treatment of choice for benign germ-cell tumors such as teratoma. In malignant tumors, removal is indicated if it can be done without sacrificing vital structures or organs, or both. Otherwise, debulking or biopsy only is appropriate.

Chemotherapy is given initially in an attempt to debulk the tumor so that a second surgical procedure can be done. It is recommended that malignant lesions with microscopic residual, lymph-node disease or metastatic disease receive platinum-based chemotherapy. Drugs frequently used include cisplatin, bleomycin, vincristine, etoposide, dactinomycin, cyclophosphamide, and doxorubicin. Cisplatin, etoposide, and bleomycin are the standard drugs used in current studies.

Site, stage, and alpha-fetoprotein (AFP) level have prognostic significance for germ-cell tumors. Current survival for Stages I and II gonadal sites approaches 100%, and survival for Stages III and IV gonadal sites is approximately 95%. Survival for extragonadal tumors is approximately 90% for Stages I and II and 75% for Stages III and IV. Retroperitoneal and testicular primary sites of disease have been associated with an improved prognosis. Sacrococcygeal and mediastinal tumors have a poorer prognosis.

## Synovial Sarcoma

### Definition

*Synovial sarcoma* is a tumor of fibrous and epithelial origins.

### Incidence and Etiology

This type of tumor is most commonly seen in older children and young adults, with approximately 31% of cases occurring in patients younger than 20 years of age (median age of 13). Incidence is slightly higher in males than in females (1.2:1.0).

## Clinical Presentation

Synovial sarcoma most often occurs in a lower extremity, especially in the knee and thigh. It also occurs in the upper extremities as well as in the trunk, head, and neck. The lung is the most common site of metastatic disease, and it also can spread to regional lymph nodes.

## Treatment and Prognosis

Because this tumor is rare in children, the guidelines for optimal treatment are not firmly established. Wide local excision is the treatment of choice for the primary tumor. Radiation may be used to control microscopic residual disease. This tumor is chemoresponsive; however, the role of adjuvant chemotherapy is still being investigated. Poor prognosis is related to the presence of metastases; a tumor that is larger than 5 cm; tumor invasiveness; a primary site other than the hand, foot, or knee; older age at diagnosis; bone or neurovascular invasion; and poor histologic differentiation.

# Alveolar Soft-Part Sarcoma

## Definition

*Alveolar soft-part sarcoma* is a soft-tissue sarcoma of unclear histogenesis.

## Incidence and Etiology

This rare type of sarcoma is usually seen in patients who are 15–35 years of age.

## Clinical Presentation

This sarcoma, seen most often in the orbit and in the head and neck in children, is often a slow-growing, asymptomatic mass that does not produce symptoms. In adults, it is most commonly seen in the extremities. The lung is the most common site of metastasis, followed by the brain, bone, and lymph nodes.

## Treatment and Prognosis

Complete local excision is the most common initial therapeutic treatment. Alveolar soft-part sarcoma grows slowly, but recurrent disease is common and difficult to treat. Despite the fact that more than 80% of patients with this type of sarcoma are alive 2 years after diagnosis, most patients die of this disease, sometimes as long as 20 years after diagnosis. Radiation and chemotherapy (anthracycline-based regimen) often are used for recurrent disease and are increasingly being used during initial treatment.

## Nursing Assessment and Interventions

### Goal

The patient will experience minimal complications related to the onset of a rare tumor.

**Assessment:**
- Know the type of rare malignancy, its location, and the extent of the disease.
- Obtain a complete history, including the incidence and duration of symptoms (e.g., fatigue, epistaxis, weight loss, full abdomen, neurological changes), predisposing factors (e.g., exposure to radiation, cytotoxic drugs, anabolic steroids, genetic abnormalities), and family history.
- Perform a complete physical examination that includes an assessment for the presence of mass (warmth, tenderness), pallor, jaundice, ascites, lymphadenopathy, hepatosplenomegaly, and neurological changes.
- Review laboratory findings.
- Review radiological imaging studies as indicated.
- Review surgical and pathology reports as indicated.
- Assess the child's degree of pain.

**Interventions:**
- Provide comfort measures.
- Provide pain medication as needed.
- Explain all tests, procedures, and results to the patient and the family.

### Goal

The patient will experience minimal complications related to the treatment.

**Assessment:**
- Assess the child for toxicity related to specific chemotherapy agents. (See the discussion of chemotherapy in Section IV, "Childhood Cancer Treatment.")
- Assess the child for toxicity related to radiation therapy, if given. (See the discussion of radiation therapy in Section IV, "Childhood Cancer Treatment.")
- Assess the child for complications related to surgery, if performed. (See the discussion of surgery in Section IV, "Childhood Cancer Treatment.")
- Assess for signs of infection.
- Assess the child for evidence of fatigue, bleeding, pain, and nutritional deficits.
- Monitor fluid intake and output and electrolytes.
- Determine whether there is a need for IV access.
- Assess for the possibility of emergency complications.
- Assess for the child's response to therapy (i.e., a decrease in the size of the mass or enlarged lymph nodes, evaluation of any metastatic disease).

**Interventions:**
- Refer the child for central IV access as needed.
- Provide comfort measures.
- Provide pain medication as needed.
- Provide instruction on proper mouth care, nutrition, and hygiene.
- Educate the family regarding neutropenia, anemia, and thrombocytopenia, as well as the signs and symptoms of infection and fever precautions.
- Obtain cultures and radiological examinations as ordered, when infection is suspected, and initiate antibiotics if indicated.
- Provide alternative methods of nutrition (e.g., oral supplements, nasogastric or parenteral supplements).
- Review all findings of laboratory studies and radiological studies with the patient and the family.

### Goal

Both the patient and the family will be adequately informed about the diagnosis, disease, and treatment.

**Assessment:**
- Assess the level of knowledge of the patient and the family about the diagnosis and disease.
- Assess their level of knowledge about treatment (i.e., surgery, radiation therapy, chemotherapy).

- Assess their learning styles. (See Section VIII, "Patient and Family Education.")
- Assess their understanding of the role of the multidisciplinary team in treating children with rare tumors.

**Interventions:**
- Communicate with the patient and the family in an appropriate manner.
- Provide them with appropriate educational resources and review the material with them.
- Ensure that the family is aware of when and how to contact the healthcare team.
- Encourage both the patient and the family to ask questions related to the diagnosis, disease, and treatment.

## Goal
The patient and the family will cope adequately with the diagnosis.

**Assessment:**
- Assess the family's communication and coping styles in general.
- Assess the family's adjustment to the diagnosis.

**Interventions:**
- Provide the patient and the family with honest answers.
- Provide them with emotional support.
- Anticipate the need for referral services (e.g., social work, chaplain, Candlelighters, American Cancer Society, Leukemia Society).
- Offer the child age-appropriate "hospital play."
- Offer to introduce a contact family who has dealt with a similar malignancy to talk with the patient and the family.

## Expected Patient and Family Outcomes
The child, the family, or both can do the following:
- Describe the type of rare malignancy and the plan of care.
- List the expected and possible toxic side effects of therapy.
- Outline methods for preventing infection.
- Describe the schedule of treatment, procedures, and follow-up care.
- Describe available community resources.
- Demonstrate the skills needed to care for the child at home.
- Explain how and when to contact the healthcare team if problems or questions arise.

# Bibliography

### Overview of Childhood Cancer
American Cancer Society. (2007). *Cancer facts and figures 2007.* Retrieved May 26, 2008, from www.cancer.org/downloads/STT/CAFF2007PWSecured.pdf.

Bleyer, A., O'Leary, M., Barr, R., & Ries, L. A. G. (2006). *Cancer epidemiology in older adolescents and young adults 15 to 29 years of age, including SEER INCIDENCE and SURVIVAL: 1975–2000.* Retrieved May 26, 2008, from http://seer.cancer.gov/publications/aya/.

### Epidemiology of Childhood Cancer
American Cancer Society. (2007). *Cancer facts and figures.* Retrieved November 10, 2007, from www.cancer.org/docroot/stt/stt_0.asp.

Birch, J. M., & Bleyer, A. (2007). Epidemiology and etiology of cancer in adolescents and young adults. In W. A. Bleyer & R. D. Barr (Eds.), *Cancer in adolescents and young adults* (pp. 39–59). Berlin: Springer.

Bleyer, A., O'Leary, M., Barr, R., & Ries, L. A. G. (Eds.). (2006). *Cancer epidemiology in older adolescents and young adults 15 to 29 years of age, including SEER incidence and survival: 1975–2000* (NIH Publication No. 06-5767). Bethesda, MD: National Cancer Institute.

CureSearch National Childhood Cancer Foundation (NCCF), Children's Oncology Group (COG). (2007). *Incidence.* Retrieved November 10, 2007, from www.curesearch.org/our_research/index_sub.aspx?id=1475.

CureSearch NCCF, COG. (2007). *Epidemiology Committee.* Retrieved November 10, 2007, from www.curesearch.org/our_research/index_sub.aspx?id=1779.

Gurney, J. G., & Bondy, M. L. (2006). Epidemiology of childhood cancer. In P. A. Pizzo & D. G. Poplack (Eds.), *Principles and practice of pediatric oncology* (5th ed., pp. 1–13). Philadelphia: Lippincott Williams & Wilkins.

Look, A. T., & Aplan, P. D. (2006). Molecular and genetic basis of childhood cancer. In P. A. Pizzo & D. G. Poplack (Eds.), *Principles and practice of pediatric oncology* (5th ed., pp. 38–85). Philadelphia: Lippincott Williams & Wilkins.

Plon, S. E., & Malkin, D. (2006). Childhood cancer and heredity. In P. A. Pizzo & D. G. Poplack (Eds.), *Principles and practice of pediatric oncology* (5th ed., pp. 14–37). Philadelphia: Lippincott, Williams & Wilkins.

Ruccione, K. S. (2002). Biologic basis of cancer in children and adolescents. In C. R. Baggott, K. P. Kelly, D. Fochtman, & G. V. Foley, (Eds.), *Nursing care of children and adolescents with cancer* (pp. 24–63). Philadelphia: W.B. Saunders.

Ruccione, K., Waskerwitz, M., Buckley, J., Perin, G., & Hammond, G. D. (1994). What caused my child's cancer? Parents' responses to an epidemiology study of childhood cancer. *Journal of Pediatric Oncology Nursing, 11*(2), 71–84.

Thiele, C. J., & Khanna, C. (2006). Biology of childhood cancer. In P. A. Pizzo & D. G. Poplack (Eds.), *Principles and practice of pediatric oncology* (5th ed., pp. 86–117). Philadelphia: Lippincott Williams & Wilkins.

### Leukemia
Arber, D., Stein, A., Carter, N., Ikle, D., Forman, S., & Slovak, M. (2003). Prognostic impact of acute myeloid leukemia classification. *American Journal of Clinical Pathology, 119*(5), 672–680.

Feinberg, S. L. (2007). Leukemias. In M. J. Hockenberry & D. Wilson (Eds.), *Wong's nursing care of infants and children* (8th ed., pp. 1583–1587). St. Louis: Mosby.

Golub, T. R., & Arceci, R. J. (2006). Acute myelogenous leukemia. In P. A. Pizzo & D. G. Poplack (Eds.), *Principles and practice of pediatric oncology* (5th ed., pp. 591–644). Philadelphia: Lippincott Williams & Wilkins.

Harris, N. L., Jaffe, E., Diebold, J., Flandrin, G., Muller-Hermelink, H. K., Vardiman, J., et al. (1999). World Health Organization classification of neoplastic diseases of the hematopoietic and lymphoid tissues: Report of the Clinical Advisory Committee meeting–Airlie House, Virginia, November 1997. *Journal of Clinical Oncology, 17,* 3835–3849.

Margolin, J. R., Steuber, C. P., & Poplack, D. G. (2006). Acute lymphoblastic leukemia. In P. A. Pizzo & D. G. Poplack (Eds.), *Principles and practice of pediatric oncology* (5th ed., pp. 538–590). Philadelphia: Lippincott Williams & Wilkins.

Smith, M., Arthur, D., Camitta, B., Carrol, A. J., Crist, W., Gayon, P., et al. (1996). Uniform approach to risk classification and treatment assignment for children with acute lymphoblastic leukemia. *Journal of Clinical Oncology, 14,* 18–24.

Tubergen, D., & Blyer, A. (2007). The leukemias. In R. Kliegman, R. Behrman, H. Jenson, & B. Stanton (Eds.), *Nelson textbook of pediatrics* (18th ed., pp. 2115–2123). Philadelphia: W.B. Saunders.

### Non-Hodgkin's Lymphoma

Link, M. P., & Weinstein, H. J. (2006). Malignant Non-Hodgkin's lymphoma in children. In P. A. Pizzo & D. G. Poplack (Eds.), *Principles and practice of pediatric oncology* (5th ed., pp. 722–747). Philadelphia: Lippincott Williams & Wilkins.

Pinkerton, R. (2005). Continuing challenges in childhood non-Hodgkin's lymphoma. *British Journal of Haematology, 130,* 480–488.

Rademaker, J. (2006). Hodgkin's and Non-Hodgkin's lymphomas. *Radiologic Clinics of North America, 45,* 69–83.

Shukla, N. N., & Trippett, T. M. (2006). Non-Hodgkin's lymphoma in children and adolescents. *Current Oncology Reports, 8,* 387–394.

### Hodgkin's Lymphoma

Hudson, M. M., Donaldson, S. S., & Onciu, M. (2006). Hodgkin lymphoma. In P. A. Pizzo & D. G. Poplack (Eds.), *Principles and practice of pediatric oncology* (5th ed., pp. 695–721). Philadelphia: Lippincott Williams & Wilkins.

Lister, T. A, Crowther, D., Sutcliffe, S. B., Glatstein, E., Canellos, G. P., Young, R. C., et al. (1989). Report of a committee convened to discuss the evaluation and staging of patients with Hodgkin's disease: Cotswolds meeting. *Journal of Clinical Oncology, 7*(11), 1630–1636.

National Cancer Institute. (2007). *Childhood hodgkin lymphoma treatment.* Retrieved October 24, 2007, from www.cancer.gov/cancertopics/pdq/treatment/childhodgkins/healthprofessional.

### Central-Nervous-System Tumors

Blaney, S., Kun, L., Hunter, J., Rorke-Adams, L., Lau, C., Strother, D., & Pollack, I. (2006). Tumors of the central nervous system. In P. A. Pizzo & D. G. Poplack (Eds.), *Principles and practice of pediatric oncology* (5th ed., pp. 786–864). Philadelphia: Lippincott Williams & Wilkins.

Central Brain Tumor Registry of the United States (CBTRUS). (2007). *Fact sheet.* Retrieved October 12, 2007, from www.cbtrus.org/factsheet/factsheet.html.

Kun, L. (2005). Tumors of the posterior fossa and spinal-cord. In E. Halperin, E. Constine, N. Tarbell, & L. Kun (Eds.), *Pediatric radiation oncology* (4th ed., pp. 89–133). Philadelphia: Lippincott Williams & Wilkins.

Louis, D., Ohgaki, H., Wiester, O., Cavenee, W., Berger, P., Jouvet, A., et al. (2007). The 2007 WHO classification of tumours of the central nervous system. *Acta Neuropathology, 114,* 97–109.

Packer, R. (1999). Brain tumors in children. *Archives of Neurology, 56,* 421–425.

Quinones-Hinojosa, A., Gullati, M., & Schmidt, M. (2004). Intramedullary spinal-cord tumors. In N. Gupta, A. Banjerjee, & D. Hass-Kogan (Eds.), *Pediatric CNS tumors* (pp. 167–182). Berlin: Springer.

Ryan-Murray, J., & Petriccione, M. (2007). Central nervous system tumors. In C. R. Baggott, K. P. Kelly, D. Fochtman, & G. V. Foley (Eds.), *Nursing care of children and adolescents with cancer* (3rd ed., pp. 503–523). Glenview, IL: Association of Pediatric Hematology/Oncology Nurses.

Shiminski-Maher, T., Cullen, P., & Sansalone, M. (2002). Posterior fossa syndrome. In *Childhood brain & spinal-cord tumors: A guide for families, friends and caregivers* (pp. 157–158). Sebastopol, CA: O'Reilly.

### Neuroblastoma

Brodeur, G. M., & Maris, J. M. (2006). Neuroblastoma. In P. A. Pizzo & D. G. Poplack (Eds.), *Principles and practice of pediatric oncology* (5th ed., pp. 933–970). Philadelphia: Lippincott Williams & Wilkins.

Brodeur, G. M., Pritchard, J., Berthold, F., Carlsen, N. L. T., Castel, V., Castleberry, R. P., et al. (1993). Revision of the international criteria for neuroblastoma diagnosis, staging, and response to treatment. *Journal of Clinical Oncology, 11,* 1466–1477.

Cheung, N. K., & Cohn, S. L. (Eds.). (2005). *Neuroblastoma.* Berlin: Springer.

Dadd, G. (2007). Neuroblastoma. In C. R. Baggott, K. P. Kelly, D. Fochtman, & G. V. Foley (Eds.), *Nursing care of children and adolescents with cancer* (3rd ed., pp. 545–554). Glenview, IL: Association of Pediatric Hematology/Oncology Nurses.

Matthay, K. K., Villablanca, J. G., Seeger, R. C., Stram, D. O., Harris, R. E., Ramsay, N. K., et al. (1999). Treatment of high-risk neuroblastoma with intensive chemotherapy, radiotherapy, autologous bone marrow transplantation and 13-cis-retinoic acid. Children's Cancer Group. *The New England Journal of Medicine, 341,* 1165–1173.

### Osteosarcoma

Ferrari, S., Briccoli, A., Mercuri, M., Bertoni, F., Picci, P., Tienghi, A., et al. (2003). Postrelapse survival in osteosarcoma of the extremities: Prognostic factors for long-term survival. *Journal of Clinical Oncology, 21,* 710–715.

Lane, J. M., Christ, G. H., Khan, S. N., & Backus, S. I. (2001). Rehabilitation for limb salvage patients: Kinesiological parameters and psychological assessment. *Cancer, 92,* 1013–1019.

Link, M. P., Gebhardt, M. C., & Meyers, P. A. (2006). Osteosarcoma. In P. A. Pizzo & D. G. Poplack (Eds.), *Principles and practice of pediatric oncology* (5th ed., pp. 1074–1109). Philadelphia: Lippincott Williams & Wilkins.

### Ewing's Sarcoma of Bone and Soft Tissue and Peripheral Primitive Neuroectodermal Tumors

Carvajal, R., & Meyers, P. (2005). Ewing's sarcoma and primitive neuroectodermal family of tumors. *Hematology/Oncology Clinics of America, 19,* 501–525.

Ginsberg, J. P., Woo, S. Y., Johnson, M. E., Hicks, M. J., & Horowitz, M. E. (2002). Ewing's sarcoma family of tumors: Ewing's sarcoma of bone and soft tissue and the peripheral primitive neuroectodermal tumors. In P. A. Pizzo & D. G. Poplack (Eds.), *Principles and practice of pediatric oncology* (4th ed., pp. 973–1016). Philadelphia: Lippincott Williams and Wilkins.

Grier, H. E., Krailo, M. D., Tarbell, N. J., Link, M. P., Fryer, C. J., Pritchard, D. J., et al. (2003). Addition of ifosfamide and etoposide to standard chemotherapy for Ewing's sarcoma and primitive neuroectodermal tumor of bone. *New England Journal of Medicine, 348,* 694–701.

### Tumors of the Kidney

Argani, P., Perlman, E. J., Breslow, N. E., Browning, N. G., Green, D. M., D'Angio, G. J., et al. (2000). Clear cell sarcoma of the kidney: A review of 351 cases from the National Wilms' Tumor Study Group Pathology Center. *American Journal of Surgical Pathology, 24,* 4–18.

Bardessy, N., Falkoff, D., Petruzzi, M. J., Nowak, N., Zabel, B., Adam, M., et al. (1994). Anaplastic Wilms' tumour, a subtype displaying poor prognosis, harbours p53 gene mutations. *Nature Genetics, 7,* 91–97.

Beckwith, J. B., & Larson, E. (1989). Clear cell sarcoma of kidney. *Pediatric Pathology, 9,* 211–218.

Beniers, A. J., Efferth, T., Füzesi, L., Granzen, B., Mertens, R., & Jakse, G. (2001). p53 expression in Wilms' tumors: A possible role as a prognostic factor. *International Journal of Oncology, 18,* 133–139.

Breslow, N., Olshan, A., Beckwith, J. B., & Green, D. M. (1993). Epidemiology of Wilms' tumor. *Medical and Pediatric Oncology, 21,* 172–181.

Breslow, N., Olshan, A., Beckwith, J. B., Moksness, J., Feigl, P., & Green, D. (1994). Ethnic variation in the incidence, diagnosis, prognosis and follow-up of children with Wilms' tumor. *Journal of the National Cancer Institute, 86,* 49–51.

Crist, W. M., & Kun, L. E. (1991). Common solid tumors of childhood. *New England Journal of Medicine, 324,* 461–471.

Dome, J. S., Cotton, C. A., Perlman, E. J., Breslow, N. E., Kalapurakal, J. A., Ritchey, M. L., et al. (2006). Treatment of anaplastic histology Wilms' tumor: Results from the fifth National Wilms' Tumor Study. *Journal of Clinical Oncology, 24,* 2352–2358.

Dome, J. S., Ritchey, M. L., Kalapurakal, J., Perlman, E. J., Coppes, M. J., & Grundy, P. E. (2006). Renal tumors. In P. A. Pizzo & D. G. Poplack (Eds.), *Principles and practice of pediatric oncology* (5th ed., pp. 907–932). Philadelphia: Lippincott Williams & Wilkins.

Drigan, R., & Androkites, A. L. (2007). Wilms' tumor. In C. R. Baggott, K. P. Kelly, D. Fochtman, & G. V. Foley (Eds.), *Nursing care of children and adolescents with cancer* (3rd ed., pp. 568–574), Glenview, IL: Association of Pediatric Hematology/Oncology Nurses.

Faria, P., Beckwith, J. B., Mishra, K., Zuppan, C., Weeks, D. A., Breslow, N., et al. (1996). Focal versus diffuse anaplasia in Wilms tumor—new definitions with prognostic significance: A report from the National Wilms Tumor Study Group. *American Journal of Surgical Pathology, 20,* 909–920.

Furtwaengler, R., Reinhard, H., Leuschner, I., Schenk, J. P., Goebel, U., Claviez, A., et al. (2006). Mesoblastic nephroma—A report from the Gesellschaft fur Pädiatrische Onkologie und Hämatologie (GPOH). *Cancer, 106,* 2275–2283.

Grundy, P. E., Breslow, N. E., Beckwith, J. B., Moksness, J., Finklestein, J. Z., & D'Angio, G. J. (1994). Treatment of children with clear-cell sarcoma of the kidney: A report from the National Wilms Tumor Study Group. *Journal of Clinical Oncology, 12,* 2132–2137.

Grundy, P. E., Breslow, N. E., Li, S., Perlman, E., Beckwith, J. B., Ritchey, M. L., et al. (2005). Loss of heterozygosity for chromosomes 1p and 16q is an adverse prognostic factor in favorable-histology Wilms tumor: A report from the National Wilms Tumor Study Group. *Journal of Clinical Oncology, 23,* 7312–7321.

Malkin, D., Sexsmith, E., Yeger, H., Williams, B. R. G., & Coppes, M. J. (1994). Mutations of the p53 tumor suppressor gene occur infrequently in Wilms' tumor. *Cancer Research, 54,* 2077–2079.

Petruzzi, M. J., & Green, D. M. (1997). Wilms' tumor. *Pediatric Clinics of North America, 44,* 939–952.

Vujanić G. M., Harms, D., Sandstedt, B., Weirich, A., de Kraker, J., & Delemarre, J. F. (1999). New definitions of focal and diffuse anaplasia in Wilms tumor: The International Society of Paediatric Oncology (SIOP) experience. *Medical and Pediatric Oncology, 32*(5), 317–323.

**Rhabdomyosarcoma**

Kotsubo, C. S. (2007). Rhabdomyosarcoma. In C. R. Baggott, K. P. Kelly, D. Fochtman, & G. V. Foley (Eds.), *Nursing care of the child with cancer* (3rd ed., pp. 555–567). Glenview, IL: Association of Pediatric Hematology/Oncology Nurses.

Leaphart, C., & Rodeberg, D. (2007). Pediatric surgical oncology: Management of rhabdomyosarcoma. *Surgical Oncology, 16*(3), 173–185.

Wexler, L. H., Meyer, W. H., & Helman, L. J. (2006). Rhabdomyosarcoma and the undifferentiated sarcomas. In P. A. Pizzo & D. G. Poplack (Eds.), *Principles and practice of pediatric oncology* (5th ed., pp. 972–1001). Philadelphia: Lippincott Williams & Wilkins.

**Retinoblastoma**

Dulczak, S., & Frothingham, B. (2007). Retinoblastoma. In C. R. Baggott, K. P. Kelly, D. Fochtman, & G. V. Foley (Eds.), *Nursing care of children and adolescents with cancer* (3rd ed., pp. 589–597). Glenview, IL: Association of Pediatric Hematology/Oncology Nurses.

Hurwitz, R. L., Shields, C. L., Shields, J. A., Chevez-Burrios, P., Hurwitz, M. Y., & Chintagumpala, M. M. (2002). Retinoblastoma. In P. A. Pizzo & D. G. Poplack (Eds.), *Principles and practice of pediatric oncology* (4th ed., pp. 825–841). Philadelphia: Lippincott Williams & Wilkins.

Knudson, A. G. (1971). Mutation and cancer: Statistical study of retinoblastoma. *Proceedings of the National Academy of Sciences USA, 68,* 820–823.

Shields, C. L., Mashayekhi, M., Au, A. K., Czyz, C., Leahey, A., Meadows, A., et al. (2006). The international classification of retinoblastoma predicts chemoreduction success. *Opthalmology, 113,* 2276–2280.

Shields, C. L., & Shields, J. A. (2004). Diagnosis and management of retinoblastoma. *CancerControl: Journal of the Moffitt Cancer Center. 11,* 2–11.

Zhu, X. P., Dunn, J. M., Phillips, R. A., Goddard, A. D., Paton, K. E., Becker, A., et al. (1989). Preferential germline mutation of the parental allele in retinoblastoma. *Nature, 340,* 312–313.

**Rare Tumors of Childhood**

Albritton, K., Goldberg, J., & Pappo, A. S. (in press). Rare tumors. In S. H. Orkin, D. Ginsburg, D. G. Nathan, A. T. Look, D. E. Fisher, & S. E. Lux (Eds.), *Nathan and Oski's hematology of infancy and childhood* (7th ed.). Philadelphia: W.B. Saunders.

Hockenberry, M. J., & Kline, N. E. (2002). Nursing support of the child with cancer. In P. A. Pizzo & D. G. Poplack (Eds.), *Principles and practice of pediatric oncology* (4th ed., pp. 1333–1349). Philadelphia: Lippincott Williams & Wilkins.

Muller, B. U., Lopez-Terrada, D., & Finegold, M. J. (2006). Tumors of the liver. In P. A. Pizzo & D. G. Poplack (Eds.), *Principles and practice of pediatric oncology* (5th ed., pp. 888–904). Philadelphia: Lippincott Williams & Wilkins.

Okcu, M. F., Hicks, J., Merchant, T. E., Andrassy, R. J., Pappo, A. S., & Horowitz, M. E. (2006). Nonrhabdomyosarcomatous soft tissue sarcomas. In P. A. Pizzo & D. G. Poplack (Eds.), *Principles and practice of pediatric oncology* (5th ed., pp. 1033–1073). Philadelphia: Lippincott Williams & Wilkins.

O'Neill, J. B. (2007). Rare tumors. In C. R. Baggott, K. P. Kelly, D. Fotchman, & G. V. Foley (Eds.), *Nursing care of children and adolescents with cancer* (3rd ed., pp. 598–617). Glenview, IL: Association of Pediatric Hematology/Oncology Nurses.

Pappo, A. S., & Furman, W. L. (2006). Management of infrequent cancers of childhood. In P. A. Pizzo & D. G. Poplack (Eds.), *Principles and practice of pediatric oncology* (5th ed., pp. 1172–1201). Philadelphia: Lippincott Williams & Wilkins.

Soule, E. H., & Pritchard D. J. (1977). Fibrosarcoma in infants and children: A review of 110 cases. *Cancer, 40,* 1711–1721.

# Section III  Overview of Hematology

Nancy E. Kline

## Section Outline

**Origin of Blood Cells**

**Anemia**

**Neutropenia**

**Thrombocytopenia**

**Bibliography**

# Origin of Blood Cells

*Jane Hennessy and Tamara E. Scott*

## Definition

There are two major components of whole blood: plasma (the fluid portion) and formed elements (the cellular portion). Plasma is approximately 90% water and 10% solutes. Albumin, electrolytes, and proteins are the main solutes. Clotting factors, globulins, circulating antibodies, and fibrinogen are the proteins in the plasma. White blood cells (WBCs), red blood cells (RBCs), and platelets are the cellular elements of blood.

The major blood-forming organs (hematopoietic organs) of the body are bone marrow (myeloid tissue) and the lymphatic system. The lymphatic system consists of lymph (fluid), lymphatic vessels, and lymphoid structures (lymph nodes, spleen, thymus, and tonsils). After birth, the bone marrow, spleen, and liver are the primary organs for hematopoiesis and cell removal.

## Pathophysiology

All formed elements of blood are formed in bone marrow and are believed to originate from a primitive cell called a pluripotent stem cell (**Figure 3-1**).

Recent research suggests that bone marrow stem cells also may be useful in the repair of other organs. Experiments in animals and people suggest possible applications in cardiac repair after myocardial infarction, spinal cord and central nervous system repair after injuries or strokes, and even liver cell replacement (Krause, 2002).

RBCs (erythrocytes) survive approximately 120 days in the peripheral circulation. As they age, their membranes become fragile and eventually rupture. Hemoglobin is broken down into hemosiderin (iron) and bilirubin. Most of the iron (hemosiderin) is reused by the bone marrow for production of new RBCs or stored in the liver and other tissues for future use. The bilirubin is excreted by the liver in the bile.

Normally there is a homeostatic balance between RBC production and destruction. The production of erythropoietin by the kidneys in response to tissue hypoxia is the basic regulator of erythrocyte production. When erythropoietin is released into the bloodstream, the bone marrow is stimulated to make new RBCs. During this time, there is a rapid increase in red cell production; therefore, not all of the circulating erythrocytes will be totally mature, which accounts for an increase in the reticulocyte count. If a rise in the reticulocyte count does not occur at times of tissue hypoxia or with increased destruction of red cells, bone marrow failure could be the cause.

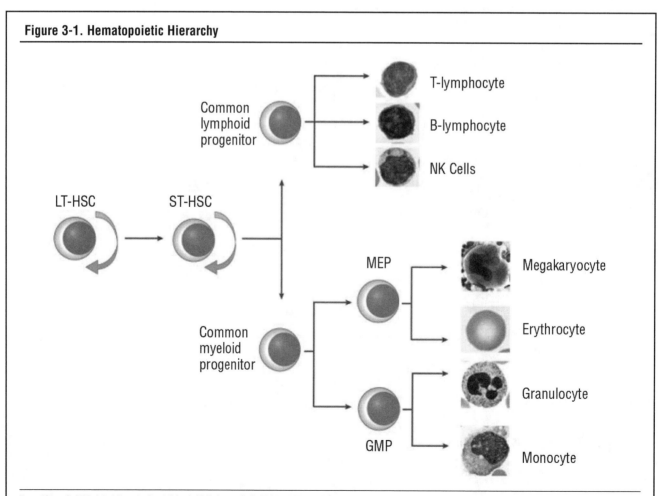

Figure 3-1. Hematopoietic Hierarchy

From "Stem Cell Model of Hematopioesis" by A. Y. H. Leung & C. M. Verafaillie, 2004, in *Hematology: Basic Principles and Practice (4th ed.)*, ed. E. Benz, S. Shattil, B. Furie, H. Cohen, L. Silberstein, et al., Oxford, United Kingdom: Elsevier. Copyright 2004 by Elsevier. Reprinted with permission.

# Section III Overview of Hematology

When tissues are adequately oxygenated, erythropoietin production ceases. The RBCs transport oxygen to tissues in response to their needs, not in response to the circulating numbers of erythrocytes. Oxygen transport depends on the number of circulating RBCs and the amount of normal hemoglobin in the cell. (See the subsection "Anemia" for a discussion of hemoglobin, hematocrit, and RBC indices.)

WBCs (leukocytes) are produced in both the bone marrow and the lymph tissue. They are categorized as granulocytes and agranulocytes. The granulocytes (neutrophils, basophils, and eosinophils) survive 12–14 hours in blood and about 5 days in tissues. Agranulocytes (monocytes and lymphocytes) can survive for years in tissues. Platelets (thrombocytes) have an average life span of 7–10 days in the blood.

## Normal Blood Cell Parameters

Normal blood values vary during infancy, childhood, and adolescence. **Table 3-1** indicates mean normal blood values from infancy through adulthood.

## Function of Red Blood Cells

The major function of RBCs is to transport hemoglobin, which, in turn, carries oxygen to all cells of the body. RBCs catalyze the reaction between carbon dioxide and water, allowing large quantities of carbon dioxide to react with blood that is transported to the lungs. The hemoglobin serves as an acid-base buffer, which, when combined with carbon dioxide, maintains the blood pH at a constant level.

## Function of White Blood Cells

**Neutrophils:** Neutrophils are the primary defense in bacterial infection. Neutrophils are able to phagocytize and kill bacteria.

**Monocytes:** Monocytes are large phagocytic cells that are involved in the early stage of inflammatory reaction.

**Lymphocytes:** Lymphocytes are involved in the development of antibodies and delayed hypersensitivity and are of two types: B cells, which synthesize and secrete an antibody, and T cells, which are lymphocytes that have circulated through the thymus gland. When exposed to an antigen, the T cells rapidly divide and produce large numbers of new T cells that are sensitized to the antigen. Some are called "killer cells" because they secrete certain compounds and assist B cells in destroying foreign proteins. T cells also play a significant role in the body's resistance to the proliferation of cancer cells.

**Eosinophils:** Eosinophils seem to have parasiticidal properties and can selectively destroy parasites, but their function is not completely known. They may also function in immediate allergic or anaphylactic hypersensitivity reactions. They are also thought to release a substance called profibrinolysin, which, when activated to form fibrinolysin, digests fibrin, thereby helping to dissolve a clot.

**Basophils:** Basophils are seen in increased amounts during the healing phase of inflammation and during prolonged inflammation, but their function is not completely understood. They exit the blood vessels and become mast cells in the tissue. They are responsible for histamine release, which results in increased permeability of the vessels to allow WBCs to exit the vessels at the site of injury.

## Function of Platelets

Platelets adhere to the endothelium to form a plug to stop bleeding. The first platelets to arrive at an injury site release substances that attract other platelets to the site. They release serotonin at the injury site, which causes vasoconstriction.

### Reference

Krause, D. S. (2002). Plasticity of marrow-derived stem cells. *Gene Therapy, 9*, 754–758.

### Table 3-1. Estimated Normal Mean Values and Lower Limits of Normal (95% Range) for Hemoglobin, Hematocrit, and MCV and MCH

| Age (years) | Hemoglobin (gm/dL) Mean | Lower Limit | Packed Cell Volume (%) Mean | Lower Limit | MCV (fL) Mean | Lower Limit | MCH (pg) Mean | Lower Limit |
|---|---|---|---|---|---|---|---|---|
| 0.5–4 | 125 | 110 | 36 | 32 | 80 | 72 | 28 | 24 |
| 5–10 | 130 | 115 | 38 | 33 | 83 | 75 | 29 | 25 |
| 11–14F | 135 | 120 | 39 | 34 | 85 | 77 | 29 | 26 |
| 11–14M | 140 | 120 | 41 | 35 | 85 | 77 | 29 | 26 |
| 15–19F | 135 | 120 | 40 | 34 | 88 | 79 | 30 | 27 |
| 15–19M | 150 | 130 | 43 | 37 | 88 | 79 | 30 | 27 |
| 20–44F | 135 | 120 | 40 | 35 | 90 | 80 | 31 | 27 |
| 20–44M | 155 | 135 | 45 | 39 | 90 | 80 | 31 | 27 |

*Note.* Hemoglobin and MCH were obtained by Coulter counter, packed cell volume was obtained by centrifugation, and MCV was obtained from packed cell volume divided by the Coulter red-cell count. All data are based on venous blood in whites after excluding individuals with laboratory evidence of iron deficiency or inflammatory disease. Hemoglobin values are rounded out to the nearest 5 gm/dL. Red-cell indices are calculated from combined data for both sexes because of the relatively minor difference in values.

MCV= mean corpuscular volume; MCH= mean corpuscular hemoglobin.

From *Rudolph's Pediatrics* (21st ed.) by A. M. Rudolph & C. D. Rudolph, 2003, The McGraw-Hill Companies, New York. Copyright 2003 by The McGraw-Hill Companies. Reprinted with permission.

# Anemia

*Jane Hennessy*

## Definition

*Anemia* is a reduction of circulating hemoglobin, resulting in a decrease in the oxygen-carrying capacity of the red blood cells (RBCs).

## Pathophysiology

The hemoglobin within RBCs carries nearly all of the oxygen to the tissues throughout the body. When the hemoglobin concentration is decreased, tissues, muscles, and organs receive less oxygen. Anemia can be caused by an impaired or decreased production of RBCs, nutritional deficiencies, metabolic disturbances, or increased erythrocyte destruction. Any of these four causes can also occur in combination.

## Clinical Presentation

A review of systems should include the following:
- General—change in behavior, fatigability, inactivity, malaise
- Skin—onset of pallor, jaundice, petechiae, ecchymoses, rashes, ulcerations
- Head—headaches, dizziness, trauma
- Eyes—scleral jaundice, diplopia, blurring, spots, cataracts
- Ears—tinnitus, vertigo
- Nose—epistaxis
- Mouth and throat—stomatitis, swelling, bleeding gums, ulceration of buccal mucosa, change in the texture of the tongue
- Neck—adenopathy
- Cardiopulmonary—palpitations, dyspnea, edema, dizziness
- Gastrointestinal—bleeding, diarrhea, melena, vomiting, anorexia
- Genitourinary—hematuria, menstrual irregularities, urinary frequency
- Musculoskeletal—muscle pain or cramps, joint pain, swelling, stiffness, weakness, numbness, coldness, discoloration of extremities
- Nervous system—loss of consciousness, syncope, paresthesia, seizures, decreased mental concentration
- Endocrine—temperature intolerance, polyuria, polydipsia, polyphagia.

The physical examination should be carefully assessed for the following:
- General—performance status, mental acuity and concentration, general appearance, height and weight for age, rate of growth
- Skin—color of skin or pallor, jaundice, pigmentation, pinkness of the palmar creases, nailbeds, conjunctiva, mucous membranes and lips, petechiae, ecchymoses, leg ulcers
- Head and neck—circumference, shape of skull, ecchymoses, bumps, hair texture and pattern
- Eyes—scleral jaundice
- Ears—abnormal hearing screen
- Nose—bleeding
- Mouth—pallor of the mucosa, ulcerations, bleeding, hematoma
- Tongue—texture and color, swelling
- Neck—adenopathy, thyroid enlargement
- Heart—tachycardia, increased pulsations, heart murmur
- Lungs—increased rate and depth of respirations
- Abdomen—splenomegaly, hepatomegaly
- Genitalia—inflammation, ulcerations, bleeding, edema
- Rectum—ulcerations, bleeding, hemorrhoids
- Musculoskeletal—painful swollen joints, stiffness, discoloration of extremities, spoon nails, triphalangeal thumbs
- Lymph nodes—swelling, tenderness
- Nervous system—paresthesia, decreased mental concentration.

## Diagnostic Workup

An evaluation of anemia in a child includes a comprehensive history and physical examination as outlined above. Children with anemia should have a complete blood cell count, RBC indices, reticulocyte counts, and a review of the peripheral smear. All values must be compared with age-matched normal values.

**Hemoglobin and hematocrit:** Hemoglobin is a true indicator of the physiological potential of blood to transport oxygen to tissue. Hematocrit indicates the percentage of the volume of circulating packed red cells of the total blood and is approximately three times the concentration of hemoglobin in gm/dL.

**Reticulocyte count:** The reticulocyte count is a direct measurement of production of RBCs by the bone marrow and indicates the activity of the bone marrow.

**RBC indices:** RBC indices (mean corpuscular volume [MCV], mean corpuscular hemoglobin [MCH], and mean corpuscular hemoglobin concentration [MCHC]) are based on ratios of RBC volume, RBC count, and hemoglobin concentration.

**ABO and Rh type:** Prior to transfusion, the patient's blood type must be cross-matched for ABO and Rh type against the donor's red cells to determine the presence or absence of agglutination. Antibody screening, using Coombs' tests, also must take place. The direct Coombs' test identifies antibodies on the surface of the red cell, whereas the indirect Coombs' test identifies antibodies in serum.

## Treatment

Because children often tolerate a decreased hemoglobin concentration, they may not develop symptoms of anemia. However, when they are symptomatic, scheduled for surgery or radiation therapy, or entering a myelosuppressive period, treatment is indicated. The standard treatment for anemia is a leukocyte-reduced, irradiated, packed RBC transfusion of 10 ml/kg. Although criteria for transfusion vary widely, most institutions recommend transfusion when hemoglobin values reach at least 6–7 gm/dL, if the child is symptomatic. Children receiving radiation therapy need to maintain hemoglobin levels of 10 gm/dL or higher to get the maximum benefit from the therapy.

The U.S. Food and Drug Administration (FDA) has approved the use of recombinant human erythropoietin (rHuEPO, epoetin alfa) in children. Buyukpamukcu, Varan, Kutluk, and Akyuz (2002) found that epoetin alfa is effective during myelosuppression for boosting hemoglobin levels or in place of transfusion and is safe in pediatric cancer patients. Razzouk and colleagues (2006) also found that weekly erythropoietin is tolerated in children with cancer, results in increased hemoglobin, and may decrease the need for transfusions. Epoetin alfa could be particularly helpful for families with objections to blood transfusions based on religious beliefs.

## Nursing Assessment and Interventions

The nurse must be knowledgeable about the signs and symptoms of anemia and be able to perform a comprehensive history and assessment (see "Clinical Presentation," which is presented earlier in this subsection). Nursing interventions for a child with anemia include the following:
- Observe laboratory data for evidence of a decrease in hemoglobin and notify the healthcare team.
- Monitor for complications related to anemia.
  - Assess skin for pallor, decreased capillary refill, or prolonged redness.
  - Assess for decreased energy, fatigue, lethargy, or irritability.
  - Assess for tachycardia, tachypnea, and dyspnea.
  - Assess for headache, hypotension, or syncope.
  - Assess level of consciousness.
- Monitor patient for transfusion reactions.
- Monitor patient for signs and symptoms of volume overload.
- Maximize the child's physical tolerance.
  - Provide oxygen, as ordered, when decreased oxygen creates difficulty breathing.
  - Provide quiet play activities that promote physical and intellectual development.
  - Promote times for rest and sleep.
- Teach the family about anemia.
  - Discuss anemia as the cause of the child's irritability, short attention span, and changing moods.
  - Review ways to save energy and decrease fatigue.
  - Describe signs and symptoms for parents to observe, including a change in color, increased heart rate and respirations, dyspnea, and diaphoresis.
- Administer erythropoietin if needed.

## Expected Patient and Family Outcomes

- Family members report the signs, symptoms, and complications of anemia or treatment for anemia to the healthcare team.
- The healthcare team's interventions minimize physical activity and promote oxygenation.
- The child has minimal complications related to anemia.

### References
Buyukpamukcu, M., Varan, A., Kutluk, T., & Akyuz, C. (2002). Is erythropoietin alfa a treatment option for chemotherapy-related anemia in children? *Medical and Pediatric Oncology, 39,* 455–458.

Razzouk, B. I., Hord, J. D., Hockenberry, M., Hinds, P. S., Feusner, J., Williams, D., et al. (2006). Double-blind, placebo-controlled study of quality of life, hematologic end points, and safety of weekly epoetin alfa in children with cancer receiving myelosuppressive chemotherapy. *Journal of Clinical Oncology, 24*(22), 3583–3589.

# Neutropenia

*Jane Hennessy and Tamara E. Scott*

## Definition

*Neutropenia* is usually defined as a reduction in circulating neutrophils of less than 1,000 absolute neutrophil count (ANC) in infants 2 weeks to 1 year of age or less than 1,500 ANC in children older than 1 year. The risk of serious bacterial infection is increased when ANC is below 500. ANC is calculated by multiplying the total white blood cell (WBC) count by the percentage of neutrophils and bands in the differential.

Some institutions use the absolute granulocyte count, which is calculated by multiplying the total WBC count by the percentage of monocytes, neutrophils, and bands in the differential.

## Pathophysiology

There are many types of neutropenia seen in children. Neutropenia may be a presenting sign of malignancy involving the bone marrow. It occurs most commonly in children with acute lymphoblastic leukemia or acute nonlymphocytic leukemia. It also can be seen as a presenting sign in patients with neuroblastoma and lymphoma. Neutropenia also can be a sign of relapse in patients with leukemia if it persists for longer than expected after chemotherapy.

This discussion will focus on neutropenia secondary to chemotherapy or radiation therapy, or both, for treatment of a childhood malignancy. The administration of chemotherapy results in suppression of the bone marrow and circulating WBCs. This immunosuppression results from an interruption of the normal replication of the bone marrow cells. Cytotoxic drugs that commonly cause neutropenia are listed in **Table 3-2**.

Irradiation also results in suppression of the bone marrow. Its effects, like those of chemotherapy, are transient; however, ablating doses are given when preparing patients for hematopoietic stem cell transplantation. Bactrim and dapsone, two of the drugs used for pneumocystis prophylaxis, are also known to cause neutropenia in some children.

## Clinical Presentation

A child with neutropenia often is asymptomatic. If a child with cancer presents with an ANC below 1,000, a complete review of systems, with attention to the following, should be done:
- Skin—erythema, edema, ulcerations
- Lungs—cough, tachypnea
- Ears, nose, and throat—rhinorrhea, ear pain, throat pain, sinus tenderness
- Mouth—stomatitis, erythema of gums, ulceration of buccal mucosa, difficulty swallowing
- Gastrointestinal—perirectal pain, diarrhea.

The physical examination should meticulously assess for the following:
- Skin—integrity of the area of central venous access (if present), any venipuncture or fingerstick site, any open lesion
- Lungs—tachypnea, presence of cough, presence of adventitious sounds in the lung fields

- Ears, nose, and throat—rhinorrhea (color and consistency), sinus tenderness, erythematous tympanic membranes, erythema of the pharynx
- Mouth—ulcerations, stomatitis, erythema of the gums
- Gastrointestinal—perirectal erythema or tenderness, or both, perirectal laceration.

## Diagnostic Workup

An evaluation of neutropenia is dependent upon several factors, such as time since the patient's last chemotherapy, presence of fever, and signs of infection, among others. (See Section V, "Side Effects of Treatment," for a more complete discussion of children with fever and neutropenia.) All febrile (38.3 °C or 101 °F) neutropenic patients should have the following:

- a history and physical examination (as outlined earlier in "Clinical Presentation")
- blood cultures from all lumens of indwelling venous catheters (peripheral cultures may be obtained with a new temperature spike)
- urinalysis and urine culture
- stool culture (if diarrhea is present)
- chest X ray (at the discretion of the patient's healthcare provider).

Nonfebrile neutropenic patients do not need to have any special studies or diagnostic workup unless some other sign of infection is present.

### Table 3-2. Chemotherapy Agents that Cause Neutropenia

| Drug | Nadir (Days) | Recovery (Days) |
|---|---|---|
| **Severe** | | |
| Carboplatin | 21–24 | 28–35 |
| Cytarabine | 14–18 | 21–28 |
| Daunomycin | 10–14 | 21–28 |
| Etoposide | 7–10 | 21–28 |
| Nitrogen mustard | 14 | 28 |
| Teniposide | 5–15 | 24–28 |
| Topotecan | 8–11 | 14–21 |
| **Mild** | | |
| BCNU | 21–35 | 42–50 |
| Busulfan | 14–21 | 28 |
| CCNU | 40–50 | 60 |
| Cisplatin | 14–23 | 21–39 |
| Cyclophosphamide | 10–14 | 21 |
| Dactinomycin | 14–21 | 21–28 |
| Doxorubicin | 10–14 | 21–28 |
| Hydroxyurea | 10 | 21 |
| Melphalan | 10–14 | 42–50 |
| Mercaptopurine | 14 | 21 |
| Methotrexate | 7–14 | 14–21 |
| Thiotepa | 14 | 21 |
| Vinblastine | 5–9 | 14–21 |

## Treatment

Many childhood cancer treatment regimens, especially those expected to cause a high degree of myelosuppression, now use granulocyte colony-stimulating factor (G-CSF) starting 1–5 days after chemotherapy and before the onset of neutropenia. The recommended dosage is 5–10 μg/kg administered subcutaneously once a day for 10–14 days.

## Nursing Assessment and Interventions

### Assessment

The nurse must be knowledgeable about the signs and symptoms of neutropenia and be able to perform a comprehensive history and assessment (see the earlier discussion in "Clinical Presentation"). The nurse should assess for signs of infection (fever; oral lesions; erythema at central venous access site; open skin lesion; perirectal irritation or laceration; cough; rhinorrhea; tachypnea; complaints of ear or throat pain, or both; and diarrhea).

### Interventions

Nursing interventions for a child with neutropenia depend upon the severity of the condition and can include the following actions:

- Observe laboratory data for evidence of a decrease in ANC and notify the physician or responsible healthcare provider.
- Monitor for complications related to neutropenia (watching for signs and symptoms of septic shock).
- Protect the child from exposure to infection by advising the child and the family to take the following measures:
  - Wash hands well.
  - Decrease the child's exposure to crowds when ANC is less than 500.
  - Keep the child away from individuals known to have infections.
  - Do not use rectal thermometers or suppositories.
  - Avoid exposure to molds (e.g., digging in soil).
  - Practice good mouth care.
- Teach families about neutropenia.
  - Instruct family members on how to protect the child from infection (as previously listed).
  - Teach family members to monitor for signs and symptoms of infection.
- Instruct parents to notify their physician or a responsible healthcare provider immediately if the child develops a fever higher than 101 °F (38.3 °C) or any signs of infection.

## Expected Patient and Family Outcomes

- There is an early identification of complications related to neutropenia.
- The family and the child are knowledgeable about neutropenia, the signs and symptoms of infection, and the ways to avoid exposure to infection.
- The child has minimal complications related to the neutropenia.

# Thrombocytopenia

*Jane Hennessy*

## Definition
*Thrombocytopenia* is a quantitative decrease in the number of circulating platelets in the peripheral blood and is defined as a platelet count of less than 100,000/mm$^3$.

## Pathophysiology
There are many causes of thrombocytopenia in a child with a malignancy. Bone marrow replacement of malignant cells or bone marrow suppression induced by intense chemotherapy or radiation therapy can cause thrombocytopenia. Chemotherapy causes destruction of rapidly dividing normal hematopoetic cells and malignant cells, which results in a decrease in the number of platelet precursors. This decrease usually occurs within 7 days or as late as 21 days after administration of chemotherapy agents. Radiation therapy causes the destruction of rapidly dividing normal hematopoetic cells in radiation treatment fields such as the pelvis, sternum, and proximal ends of long bones.

In addition to chemotherapy agents as a cause of a decrease in platelets, other pharmacological agents may be associated with platelet dysfunction. For example, aspirin inhibits platelet aggregation. Penicillin G, ampicillin, carbenicillin, and ticarcillin can also cause transient dysfunction. Amphotericin B has also been implicated as a cause of platelet dysfunction.

## Clinical Presentation
Approximately 75% of all children with leukemia are symptomatic with thrombocytopenia at the initial diagnosis. These symptoms include the following:
- Skin—bruising, petechiae, purpura
- Nose and mouth—bleeding from the gums, nose, or both
- Genitourinary and gastrointestinal—blood (whether microscopic or obvious) in urine, stool, or emesis
- Eyes—scleral bleeding
- Neurological—intracranial bleeding (This may be seen especially if the WBC count is > 300,000/mm$^3$ and is a result of ruptured intracerebral vessels damaged by leukocyte sludging or by nodules or leukemic cells). The patient's physical examination should assess for the signs and symptoms previously listed.

## Diagnostic Workup
An evaluation of thrombocytopenia is initiated by obtaining a complete blood count with platelets. In addition to the platelet count, a complete history and physical are conducted to assess for symptoms of thrombocytopenia (e.g., bruising, bleeding, petechiae, ecchymoses). The severity of the thrombocytopenia dictates the type of treatment or even whether treatment is warranted.

## Treatment
When the platelet count drops below 20,000/mm$^3$, minor bleeding episodes generally occur; spontaneous internal hemorrhage does not occur until the platelet count is 10,000/mm$^3$ or less. Treatment is indicated if there is active bleeding. The standard treatment for thrombocytopenia is a random-donor, leukocyte-reduced platelet transfusion of 1 unit of platelets per 10 kg of body weight. Matched ABO and Rh platelet transfusions are usually preferred. Although A and B antigens are only slightly expressed on platelets, the transfusion of incompatible platelets could result in low-grade hemolysis due to plasma antibodies or erythrocyte contamination.

Policy regarding the use of prophylactic platelet transfusion, including the specific platelet values used as criteria for transfusion before procedures, varies. The American Society of Clinical Oncology (ASCO) adopted guidelines based on a study by Schiffer and colleagues (2001), which recommended that the threshold for platelet transfusions in children be set at a platelet count of 10,000/mm$^3$. Higher thresholds may be considered for certain comorbidity factors and invasive procedures. Howard and colleagues (2000) demonstrated that there was no evidence of serious complications from lumbar punctures when the platelet count was between 11,000/mm$^3$ and 20,000/mm$^3$. Platelet transfusion should be avoided to decrease the likelihood of alloimmunization.

## Nursing Assessment and Interventions
### Assessment
The nurse must be knowledgeable about the signs and symptoms of thrombocytopenia and be able to perform a comprehensive history and assessment (see "Clinical Presentation," which is presented earlier in this subsection).

### Interventions
Nursing interventions for a child with thrombocytopenia include the following:
- Review laboratory reports for the platelet count and alert the healthcare team.
- Monitor for complications related to thrombocytopenia, and assess skin, stools, urine, gums, emesis, sputum, and nasal secretions for blood.
- Monitor for transfusion reactions.
- Prevent and decrease the risk of bleeding by
  - applying pressure directly to all needle puncture sites for 5 minutes
  - reducing the risk of constipation by administering a prescribed stool softener
  - encouraging the use of a soft-bristle toothbrush and avoiding dental floss and sharp food items, such as chips and ice, to decrease gum irritation
  - encouraging the patient to avoid contact sports or activities that might cause injury
  - advising sexually active adolescent patients to take precautions to avoid trauma during sexual relations
  - providing safe environments (e.g., using helmets, knee pads, and padded cribs)
  - administering hormonal therapy to inhibit menses if necessary
  - keeping invasive procedures to a minimum
  - instructing the patient and the family about how to treat epistaxis (The child's nostril should be pinched against the nasal septum by applying constant pressure for at least 10 minutes. The child should not lie down while

the nose is bleeding because excess blood can drip into the nasopharynx and cause nausea and vomiting.)
- ensuring that no rectal temperatures are taken and no other manipulations (e.g., enemas and suppositories) are done
- advising that adolescents use electric razors.
• Teach the child and the family about thrombocytopenia. They should be instructed on how to decrease the risk of complications of thrombocytopenia and to report the signs and symptoms to the healthcare team.

## Expected Patient and Family Outcomes
• The patient is protected from bleeding.
• The patient and the family verbalize an understanding of how to reduce the risk and complications of thrombocytopenia.
• The patient and the family identify the signs and symptoms of thrombocytopenia to report to medical staff.

### References
Howard, S. C., Gajjar, A., Ribeiro, R. C., Rivera, G. K., Rubnitz, J. E., Sunderland, J. T., et al. (2000). Safety of lumbar puncture for children with acute lymphocytic leukemia and thrombocytopenia. *JAMA: The Journal of the American Medical Association, 284,* 2222–2224.

Schiffer, C. A., Anderson, K. C., Bennett, C. L., Bernstein, S., Elting, L. S., Goldsmith, M., et al. (2001). Platelet transfusion for patients with cancer: Clinical practice guidelines of the American Society of Clinical Oncology. *Journal of Clinical Oncology, 19,* 1519–1538.

## Bibliography

### Origin of Blood Cells
Abshire, T. C. (2001). Sense and sensibility: Approaching anemia in children. *Contemporary Pediatrics, 18*(9), 104–113.

Norville, R., & Bryant, R. (2007). Blood component deficiencies. In C. R. Baggott, K. P. Kelly, D. Fochtman, & G. V. Foley (Eds.), *Nursing care of children and adolescents with cancer* (3rd ed., pp. 347–364). Glenview, IL: Association of Pediatric Hematology/Oncology Nurses.

Sieff, C. A., Nathan, D. G., & Clark, S. C. (2003). The anatomy and physiology of hematopoiesis. In D. G. Nathan & S. H. Orkin (Eds.), *Nathan and Oski's hematology of infancy and childhood* (pp. 171–255). Philadelphia: W.B. Saunders.

### Anemia
Norville, R., & Bryant, R. (2007). Blood component deficiencies. In C. R. Baggott, K. P. Kelly, D. Fochtman, & G. V. Foley (Eds.), *Nursing care of children and adolescents with cancer* (3rd ed., pp. 347–364). Glenview, IL: Association of Pediatric Hematology/Oncology Nurses.

Panzarella, C., Baggott, C. R., Comeau, M., Duncan, J. M., Groben, V., Woods, D. A., et al. (2007). Management of disease and treatment-related complications. In C. R. Baggott, K. P. Kelly, D. Fochtman, & G. V. Foley (Eds.), *Nursing care of children and adolescents with cancer* (3rd ed., pp. 279–318). Glenview, IL: Association of Pediatric Hematology/Oncology Nurses.

### Neutropenia
Alexander, S. W., Walsh, T. J., Freifeld, A. F., & Pizzo, P. A. (2002). Infectious complications in the pediatric cancer patient. In P. A. Pizzo & D. G. Poplack (Eds.), *Principles and practice of pediatric oncology* (pp. 1239–1283). Philadelphia: Lippincott Williams & Wilkins.

Kline, N. E. (2007). Prevention and treatment of infections. In C. R. Baggott, K. P. Kelly, D. Fochtman, & G. V. Foley (Eds.), *Nursing care of children and adolescents with cancer* (3rd ed., pp. 266–278). Glenview, IL: Association of Pediatric Hematology/Oncology Nurses.

Norville, R., & Bryant, R. (2007). Blood component deficiencies. In C. R. Baggott, K. P. Kelly, D. Fochtman, & G. V. Foley (Eds.), *Nursing care of children and adolescents with cancer* (3rd ed., pp. 347–364). Glenview, IL: Association of Pediatric Hematology/Oncology Nurses.

Taketomo, C. K., Hodding, J. H., & Kraus, D. M. (2008). *Pediatric dosage handbook* (14th ed.). Hudson, OH: Lexi-Comp, Inc.

### Thrombocytopenia
Demetri, G. D. (2001). Targeted approaches for the treatment of thrombocytopenia. *The Oncologist, 6,* 15–23.

Norville, R., & Bryant, R. (2007). Blood component deficiencies. In C. R. Baggott, K. P. Kelly, D. Fochtman, & G. V. Foley (Eds.), *Nursing care of children and adolescents with cancer* (3rd ed., pp. 347–364). Glenview, IL: Association of Pediatric Hematology/Oncology Nurses.

Panzarella, C., Baggott, C. R., Comeau, M., Duncan, J. M., Groben, V., Woods, D. A., et al. (2007). Management of disease and treatment-related complications. In C. R. Baggott, K. P. Kelly, D. Fochtman, & G. V. Foley (Eds.), *Nursing care of children and adolescents with cancer* (3rd ed., pp. 279–318). Glenview, IL: Association of Pediatric Hematology/Oncology Nurses.

# Section IV  Childhood Cancer Treatment

Nancy E. Kline

## Section Outline

**Diagnostic and Staging Procedures**

**History of Chemotherapy**

**Clinical Trials**

**Chemotherapy**

**Guidelines for Safe Handling of Chemotherapy**

**Administration of Vesicants**

**Surgery**

**Radiation Therapy**

**Hematopoietic Stem-Cell Transplantation**

**Biologic Response Modifiers**

**Cell and Gene Therapy**

**Complementary and Alternative Treatments**

**Bibliography**

# Diagnostic and Staging Procedures

*Nancy E. Kline*

## Principles of Treatment

Diagnostic and staging procedures provide the tools for an accurate diagnosis of childhood cancer. Prompt and accurate diagnosis of a malignancy is essential to begin appropriate treatment, achieve remission, and optimize long-term survival.

## Role in Childhood Cancer

Diagnostic procedures enable a healthcare team to determine the type and location of a malignancy as well as the extent of metastasis. Accurate diagnosis allows for the planning and initiation of treatment.

## Diagnostic Procedures

### History and Physical Assessment

A history and physical assessment are the most basic and inexpensive diagnostic tools, yet they are highly important. Parents often are the first to detect physical changes in their child. Symptoms such as fatigue, malaise, anorexia, recurrent infections or fevers, lymphadenopathy, bone or joint pain, enlarged abdomen, headache, and bleeding are suggestive of childhood cancers (**Table 4-1**). A detailed physical history that includes information on the child's growth and development, a family history, and a physical assessment help to determine how to proceed with a diagnostic evaluation.

### Laboratory Tests

A child with a suspected cancer will have routine blood work and urinalysis done upon arrival at a clinic or admission to a hospital. A complete blood count (CBC) with a differential and serum chemistries is commonly performed. If a patient is evaluated for a particular malignancy, additional tests will be ordered.

**CBC with a differential:** A significantly elevated white blood cell count with the presence of lymphoblasts can be indicative of leukemia. Malignancies that have bone-marrow involvement (e.g., neuroblastoma) may cause the hemoglobin, hematocrit, and platelets to be low.

**Serum chemistries:** This routine study helps to evaluate the body's response to the cancer process. It reflects metabolic compensation and organ function and usually includes an assessment of electrolytes as well as liver and renal functions.

**Urinalysis:** A routine urinalysis provides general information regarding renal function.

**Tumor markers:** A tumor marker is a characteristic or substance that can indicate the presence of a specific tumor. Testing for tumor markers can be useful at diagnosis and in follow-up treatment. For example, alpha-fetoprotein is elevated (i.e., >20 ng/ml) in patients with hepatoblastoma, teratoma, and germ-cell tumors; and beta human chorionic gonadotropin (β-hCG) is elevated in patients with hepatoblastoma and germ-cell tumors.

**Immunophenotyping and cytogenetics:** Tumor cells can be identified, classified, and described using immunophenotyping of monoclonal antibodies. Cytogenetic studies can determine whether any chromosomal abnormalities exist within the tumor.

### Nursing Assessment and Interventions

**Assessment:**
- Determine whether the patient has had prior experience with phlebotomy procedures.
- Assess the patient's and the family's knowledge of the blood test to be performed.

**Interventions:**
- Prepare the patient and the family for the blood test by explaining it in developmentally appropriate terminology.
- Position the child for phlebotomy work.
- Use comforting strategies (e.g., performing a venipuncture "on the count of three" to help a child feel ready for the discomfort and serve as a distraction).
- Tell the family when the test results will be ready.

### Expected Patient and Family Outcomes

- The family understands which laboratory tests are being performed.
- Trauma to the patient is minimized.

## Invasive Diagnostic Procedures

### Bone-Marrow Aspiration (BMA) and Biopsy

A BMA is performed when leukemia is suspected, the tumor has possibly spread to the bone marrow, or a CBC suggests malfunctioning bone marrow. This procedure is done using an aseptic technique. A topical anesthetic is used to anesthetize the skin, and an injectable anesthetic is used to anesthetize the bone.

The sites most frequently chosen for aspiration are the posterior or anterior iliac crest; the sternum generally is not used because of its close proximity to the vital organs. For the procedure, a needle with a stylet is inserted though the bony cortex into the bone-marrow cavity. The stylet is removed, a syringe is connected to the needle, and bone marrow is aspirated. The collected specimen is used to prepare slides for a microscopic examination to determine the cell type and morphology. If leukemia is suspected, the following tests are performed: flow cytometry and immunophenotyping, karyotyping, and cytogenic analysis. Bone marrow that is packed with leukemic cells may be difficult to aspirate, causing increased discomfort to and anxiety in the patient and the family (more than one site may have to be used).

A bone-marrow biopsy is performed if leukemia or metastasis to the bone marrow from a solid tumor is likely. It is done using an aseptic technique. A local anesthetic usually is used to anesthetize the skin and bone. The biopsy is similar to a BMA, except that a large Jamshidi needle is used to remove an actual core of bone and bone marrow. The Jamshidi needle is turned and rocked as it is inserted into the bone. The needle is then removed with the core of bone marrow inside.

### Lumbar Puncture (LP)

An LP is performed to determine whether cancer (e.g., leukemia, lymphoma, or brain tumor) is present in the cerebral spinal fluid (CSF). A patient who has symptoms indicative of increased intracranial pressure at diagnosis also may have CSF pressure measured. For this aseptic procedure, the patient is placed in a position that exposes the vertebrae. The two most common positions are lying on the side with knees pulled up and back arched or sitting cross-legged with back arched. A topical anesthetic is administered; a

### Table 4-1. Symptoms Suggestive of Childhood Cancers

| Symptoms | Possible Malignancy | Possible Nonmalignant Condition |
|---|---|---|
| Pallor, fatigue, or malaise | Leukemia, lymphoma, neuroblastoma | Iron-deficiency anemia |
| Bleeding, bruising, petechiae | Leukemia, neuroblastoma | Coagulopathy, ideopathic thrombocytic purpura |
| Weight loss, night sweats | Hodgkin's lymphoma | Viral illness, tuberculosis |
| Edematous face and neck | Non-Hodgkin's lymphoma, leukemia | Thrombus in superior vena cava |
| Pancytopenia | Leukemia, neuroblastoma | Infection, aplastic anemia |
| Lymphadenopathy | Hodgkin's or Non-Hodgkin's lymphoma | Infection |
| Bone pain and fevers | Leukemia, Ewing's sarcoma | Osteomyelitis, trauma |
| Limping | Bone tumors, leukemia, neuroblastoma | Osteomyelitis, trauma |
| Vaginal bleeding | Yolk sac tumor, rhabdomyosarcoma | Trauma, menses |
| Chronic drainage from the ear | Rhabdomyosarcoma, histiocytosis | Otitis media, otitis externa |
| Cat's eye reflex | Retinoblastoma | Coats's disease, severe uveitis |
| Abdominal mass | Wilms' tumor, neuroblastoma, hepatoblastoma | Renal or ovarian cyst |
| Headache, morning vomiting | Brain tumor | Migraine or tension headache |

local anesthetic also may be used if necessary. A needle with a stylet is inserted between the lumbar vertebrae at the level of the iliac crest. The stylet is removed, and the CSF is collected in tubes to be tested for glucose, protein, cell differential, and cytology. Additional tests may be ordered if necessary. This procedure can be done quickly if the patient is kept calm and positioned properly. A moving child can lead to a traumatic LP, resulting in a bloody specimen or harm to the patient.

### Nursing Assessment and Interventions

**Assessment:**
- Assess the patient's and the family's knowledge of LP and BMA or biopsy.
- Assess the patient's platelet count if an LP is necessary; consult the physician or nurse practitioner if the platelet count is less than 50,000; if the patient is symptomatic, consider a platelet transfusion.
- Assess the child's and the family's level of fear and anxiety.

**Interventions:**
- Prepare the child and the family for the procedure by explaining it to them beforehand in a developmentally appropriate manner (see preparation for procedures in Section VI, "Supportive Care").
- Assure the patient and the family that the patient will be kept as comfortable as possible and may even fall asleep if sedation is used.
- Apply topical anesthetic to the BMA and/or LP sites at least 60–90 minutes prior to the procedure.
- Administer conscious sedation as ordered (see conscious sedation in Section VI, "Supportive Care").
- Position the patient properly.
  – Bone marrow aspiration and biopsy—Place the patient in a prone or supine position (depending on the site) with the patient's face turned away from the practitioner (the sight of large needles is frightening, even to a sleepy child).
  – Lumbar puncture—Place the patient so that his or her vertebrae are exposed and draw the knees up toward the chest (as described in the discussion of LP in the subsection "Invasive Diagnostic Procedures") to separate the vertebrae for easy entry into the subarachnoid space. Maintain the patient's shoulder alignment perpendicular to the examination table and do not allow the shoulders to fall forward, as doing so could restrict access to the lumbar spaces. It may work best if the patient is in a sitting position and leaning over a pillow or rolled towel toward the assisting nurse, with the patient's back to the practitioner.
- Follow the guidelines for distracting and preparing patients for procedures (see Section VI, "Supportive Care," for information on preparing patients prior to procedures).
- Use universal precautions when handling specimens.
- Apply pressure to the LP or BMA site after the procedure.
- Apply a sterile bandage to the LP site. (A pressure dressing may be required for a BMA site.)
- Remove the dressing during the first 24 hours after the procedure to examine the site for bleeding and signs of infection. A saturated dressing is a medium for bacterial growth and can lead to infection of the site.

### Expected Patient and Family Outcomes
- The patient and the family are prepared for a BMA, biopsy, or LP.
- Trauma to the patient is minimized.
- The BMA, biopsy, or LP site remains free of infection.
- The patient is able to better cope with procedures that may need to be done in the future.

### Imaging Studies

Imaging tests are used to locate tumors and metastases and to stage malignancies. Advances in technology have decreased the need for more invasive procedures.

## Radiological Studies

Various structures of the body have different densities. X rays allow for visualization of the skeleton and internal organs. The patient is required to remain still to allow for a clear picture. Sedation is not necessary because it is painless and quick. The most common X rays performed for diagnostic purposes are a chest X ray, which is used to look for tumors in the lungs, mediastinum, or chest wall, and a skeletal survey, which is an X ray of the entire skeleton that allows for visualization of metastases to bone. X rays of specific areas of the body can be done to determine whether further imaging is needed.

## Computerized Tomography (CT) Scan

CT, sometimes called computerized axial tomography, provides images of planes of the body. A CT scan takes serial X rays of each plane of the area studied, stores this information, and then completes a three-dimensional view. The scanner does this by rotating the X-ray beam completely around the patient. The patient is required to remain still throughout the test, which usually takes 30 minutes.

Either intravenous (IV) or oral contrast dye may be ordered. An IV contrast may be used to help illuminate malignancies. Oral contrast is used for abdominal CT scans to help visualize all aspects of the gastrointestinal tract. The patient usually drinks contrast dye the night before the test and again 2 hours before the test. The dye usually is mixed in clear fluids, and the patient is given nothing to eat or drink until the test is completed. If the patient is not willing to drink the dye mixture, a nasogastric tube may be placed to administer the contrast dye.

## Magnetic Resonance Imaging (MRI)

This scan uses radio waves and magnets to produce a highly defined, computerized image of the body. Radio waves are emitted toward the body and various tissue types absorb the energy. The magnets then pick up the signals produced from the body tissue, and a computer scan is done. All metal items, including IV poles and pumps, must be detached from the patient's body. If it is suspected that a patient has a metastatic brain tumor or spinal masses, a gadolinium contrast dye may be administered. The patient must remain still for up to 1 hour while the scan is being performed; therefore, sedation may be required.

## Bone Scan

A bone scan detects the presence, size, and location of a malignancy or metastases in the bone. A radioisotope dye is injected intravenously 2–4 hours before the scan. Although the dye is radioactive, it emits about the same amount of radiation as an X ray. Any areas of disease will have an increased uptake of the dye. During the scan, the patient must remain still and may have to be secured to the table. Sedation may be necessary.

## Positron Emission Tomography (PET) Scan

PET uses isotopes of 18 fluorodeoxyglucose (FDG) to obtain images of physiologic and metabolic activity. A PET scan is an extremely effective, efficient technique for the diagnosis and evaluation of neuroblastoma, Hodgkin's disease, Non-Hodgkin's lymphoma, bone tumors, lung and colon cancer, and brain tumors. Viable tumors can be distinguished from necrotic tissue neoplasm and scar tissue on a PET scan (Kushner, Yeung, & Larson, 2000). The patient must fast prior to the scan to allow for maximum tissue uptake of FDG, which is administered intravenously, and IV fluids with dextrose should be avoided 6 hours before the test to prevent a false-positive result.

## Ultrasound

An ultrasound examines the body structures with the use of sound waves. A transducing gel is placed on the patient's skin, and then an ultrasound transducer is placed on and moved over the skin. Sound waves are emitted to the body tissues, which produce echoes. The returned echoes are then processed and recorded on film, which provides an image on a monitor. This image can be used to visualize an abdominal mass. The patient may be required to ingest fluids orally before the test is conducted, because a full bladder enables visualization of certain organs. The length of the procedure is approximately 30 minutes. The child must remain still for an ultrasound; however, sedation usually is not needed.

## Echocardiogram

An echocardiogram, which is an ultrasound of the heart, displays the chambers of the heart, and its contractility, septa integrity, and valve function. It also measures cardiac blood flow and the ejection fraction. It can detect a tumor, vegetation, thrombus, or pericardial effusions. An echocardiogram may be done at the time of diagnosis if the patient has abnormal heart sounds. It is performed routinely on patients who receive anthracyclines to evaluate for cardiotoxicity. The patient must remain still for this procedure, which lasts 15–30 minutes.

## Nursing Assessment and Interventions

**Assessment:**
- Assess the patient's developmental level and ability to follow instructions (i.e., ability to remain still).
- Assess the need for sedation and for IV access.
- Assess the patient's and the family's understanding of the test to be done.

**Interventions:**
- Explain the radiological study to be performed, including what it will be like, the length of time required for the test, and the results; explain that the test does not hurt but that the patient has to remain still.
- Remain supportive of the patient and the family, because awaiting the diagnosis of a malignancy is a stressful and life-changing time.
- Do not give the patient anything to eat or drink before sedation, and follow institutional guidelines.
- If the patient is scheduled to have an abdominal CT, administer an oral contrast dye as ordered (usually mixed with a clear fluid of the patient's choice). Do not give the patient anything to eat or drink, and explain the reason for this to the patient and the family.
- If the patient is to be given an IV contrast dye, explain to the patient and the family why this is required, what it feels like (i.e., the patient may experience a sensation of warmth or flushing), and establish IV access.
- Use a heparin (Liquaemin) flush to prepare the venous access device if the patient is to have an MRI; remove the IV tubing, pump, and pole; remove any metal objects from the patient's body.
- Assist the patient with positioning during the test as needed.

### Expected Patient and Family Outcomes
- The patient and the family feel adequately prepared for the diagnostic studies.
- Trauma to the patient is minimized.
- Optimal studies are obtained.

### Reference
Kushner, B. H., Yeung, H. W., & Larson, S. M. (2000). Extending positron emission tomography scan utility to high-risk neuroblastoma: Fluorine-18 fluorodoxyglucose positron emission tomography as sole imaging modality in follow-up of patients. *Journal of Clinical Oncology, 19,* 3397–3405.

# History of Chemotherapy

*Christine Sullivan*

The modern age of chemotherapy began in the 1940s when the first effective chemotherapy agent, mechlorethamine (nitrogen mustard), an alkylating agent derived from a chemical weapon, was found to benefit patients with advanced-stage lymphoma. The majority of the agents in use today were discovered by the late 1960s. With rare exceptions, chemotherapeutic agents were developed based on empirical observations rather than systematic scientific efforts. The complex biology of cancer cells, as well as the supporting cells that allow malignant cells to thrive, continues to hinder research efforts. Yet, as of 2007, the field of pediatric oncology can still boast an overall cure rate for childhood cancer of well above 75%. The scientific milestones and evolution of the research environment detailed here serve to illustrate not only the hard-won victories of the past, but also the immense challenges ahead.

## The 1940s and 1950s
Several important discoveries in the field of cancer chemotherapy were made during the 1940s, including the discovery of antitumor antibiotics and the use of folic-acid antagonists to treat leukemia. Dr. Sydney Farber noted that children with leukemia often were deficient in folic acid; paradoxically, he found that supplementation of folic acid resulted in an acceleration of the disease. Dr. Farber began to study folic-acid antagonists, and in 1947, he treated a child with leukemia with aminopterin, a predecessor to methotrexate. The child achieved a complete remission, the first remission ever induced in childhood leukemia.

During the 1950s, significant progress was made in the development of new chemotherapeutic drugs. These drugs included fluorouracil (5-FU), 6-thioguanine (6-TG), mercaptopurine (Purinethol), dactinomycin (Actinomycin-D), methotrexate (Mexate), cyclophosphamide (Cytoxan), melphalan (Alkeran), and busulfan (Mylaran). In 1954, the Cancer and Leukemia Group B and the Children's Cancer Group were formed. In 1955, the first randomized clinical trial began, and Congress provided funding for the National Chemotherapy Program. All chemotherapy-related research efforts in the United States during this time were government funded.

## The 1960s and 1970s
Single-agents therapies of the 1940s and 1950s were rarely curative because of drug resistance and/or the inability to administer the drugs in adequate doses without devastating toxicities. In the early 1960s, a significant advance in combination chemotherapy was made with the initiation of the vincristine (Oncovin)/doxorubicin (Adriamycin)/methotrexate (Mexate)/prednisone (Deltasone) program for acute leukemia initiated by Dr. Emil Freireich. For the first time, a combination of four drugs, each with different mechanisms of action, were administered as intensive intermittent therapy. This design allowed dosing that produced maximum effectiveness and time for recovery of normal cells after each course. The success of this regimen set a precedent for the intermittent, intensive, combination-chemotherapy regimens used today. The 1960s and 1970s also saw the first use of platinum agents and MOPP (mechlorethamine, Oncovin, prednisone, and procarbazine) as a successful treatment for Hodgkin's disease. Phase I trials for Adriamycin began in the 1970s.

In the 1970s, it also was determined that methotrexate could be injected intrathecally into the cerebrospinal fluid to control the spread of leukemia to the meninges. This discovery was based on the sanctuary theory that leukemic blasts could survive in the cerebral spinal fluid and seed the bone marrow if not halted. In the early 1970s, St. Jude Children's Research Hospital added central-nervous-system prophylaxis to all leukemia protocols, which dramatically improved cure rates. Drug development slowed in the 1970s, yet important cancer biology discoveries had an impact on treatment approaches. Cancer researchers had believed that a tumor first developed locally, spread to regional lymph nodes, and then metastasized widely. Adjuvant chemotherapy following less radical surgery was introduced, and the resulting improved survival rates validated systemic treatment of metastatic tumors.

Between 1969 and 1980, several pediatric cooperative groups evolved from Acute Leukemia and Cancer Cooperative Groups A and B to include the Children's Cancer Study Group, established in 1974, and the Pediatric Oncology Group (POG), formed in 1980. In addition, two other groups were established: the National Wilms Tumor Study Group (formed in 1969) and the Intergroup Rhabdomyosarcoma Study Group (formed in 1972).

## The 1980s and 1990s
The 1980s introduced a new series of chemotherapeutic agents. The topoisomerase inhibitors (i.e., tenoposide and etoposide, the first stable camptothecin analog, irinotecan and taxane, and paclitaxel [Taxol]) were introduced. Taxol was found to be active against ovarian cancer. The National Cancer Institute signed a collaborative research agreement with Bristol-Myers Squibb in 1991, and Taxol became the first commercially profitable chemotherapeutic agent.

During the 1990s, therapies that more effectively addressed side effects such as nausea and vomiting began to emerge. The antiemetic Ondansetron, derived from a new class of serotonin antagonists, addressed even the most highly emetic agents. Growth factors (neupogen) shortened postchemotherapy bone-marrow nadirs, thereby decreasing treatment delays. In addition, cardiac and bladder toxicities were ameliorated with the use of the protectant agents dexrazoxane and mesna.

Ongoing efforts to increase chemotherapy doses were finally accomplished with the advent of bone-marrow and cord-blood transplantation, stem-cell rescue, and growth factors. In pediatric oncology, prognostic indicators were used to tailor therapies to a patient's specific needs. The goal was to promote continued improvement in survival rates while delivering the smallest amount of drug possible. This strategy sought to prevent unnecessary late effects of chemotherapy as childhood cancer survivors lived into adulthood. Survivorship programs flourished throughout this period.

## 2000 and Beyond

In December 2004, Clofarabine became the first chemotherapy agent approved by the U.S. Food and Drug Administration (FDA) for refractory pediatric acute lymphoblastic leukemia without prior approval for an adult indication. This was the outcome of legislation enacted to entice pharmaceutical companies to develop pediatric chemotherapeutic agents. Specifically, in 1998, the FDA's Pediatric Rule advocated for the development of pediatric agents. In 2002, the Best Pharmaceuticals for Children Act, which encompassed the Pediatric Exclusivity Provision, offered pharmaceutical companies the ability to extend by 6 months their exclusive rights to a new agent in exchange for their commitment to the development of pediatric agents (FDA, 2002). The legislation was extended in 2007.

In 2003, the United Kingdom's Children's Cancer Study Group, the Pediatric Oncology Group, the National Wilms Tumor Study Group, and the Intergroup Rhabdomyosarcoma Study Group merged to form the Children's Oncology Group in an effort to streamline research efforts.

Pharmacogenetics, the study of genetic variations in drug-processing genes and, ultimately, a child's ability to process drugs, has led to thiopurine-S-metyltransferase gene testing in leukemia patients experiencing myelosuppression out of proportion for treatment with mercaptopurine and thioguanine.

The age of molecularly targeted agents is upon us. A pediatric agent as targeted as Gleevec for chronic myelogenous leukemia would be a welcome addition to the traditional chemotherapy. However, cancer is a highly diverse group of diseases with a vast array of resistance mechanisms, and many believe that the basic principles of cancer treatment and drug resistance still apply. Combination chemotherapy in the future likely will combine targeted drugs and traditional cytotoxic agents.

**Reference**

U.S. Food and Drug Administration (FDA) (2002). *Best Pharmaceuticals for Children Act.* Retrieved May 26, 2008, from www.fda.gov/opacom/laws/pharmkids/contents.html.

# Clinical Trials

*Elizabeth A. Gilger*

## Principles of Treatment

A *clinical trial* is a scientific experiment designed to answer a specific medical question, usually about the therapeutic effect of a specific treatment. A well-designed clinical trial should answer the medical question with certainty and provide information that is reliable and easy to analyze and interpret. The procedure for conducting a clinical trial, as well as all pertinent background information, is compiled into a protocol. The protocol serves as the comprehensive document that guides treatment management. This allows for a systematic and consistent treatment plan among participating investigators.

## Phases of Clinical Trials

Clinical trials are divided into four phases of research. Each phase has a unique purpose as well as some general characteristics that are common to protocols in that phase.

### Phase I

Phase I determines the maximally tolerated dose (MTD) of an investigational agent or combination of agents using a strict administration schedule that is then recommended for use in efficacy studies. The starting dose in children is usually 80% of the MTD for adults. The toxicities related to the therapy and the pharmacokinetic profile of the agent also are described from Phase I data. Phase I studies usually involve a small trial that includes 15–25 patients with refractory cancer for which no other effective therapies are known. Patients must have adequate organ function as well as a reasonable life expectancy and ability to function. In addition, all standard therapeutic options for curative treatment must have been exhausted. Patients and families choose Phase I trials hoping for a possible cure, disease response, or control of symptoms, or to help other patients by contributing to scientific knowledge.

### Phase II

Phase II is designed to determine the efficacy of a new agent in treating specific types of cancer. Studies are disease specific and based on biochemical data, pharmacological data, or both; preclinical screening in human tumor cell lines; or a suggestion of the agent's antitumor activity in Phase I trials.

All patients must have measurable disease and normal major organ function as well as a reasonable life expectancy and functional status. Patients who have not already received intensive treatment are the best candidates for Phase II trials. The number of patients varies and is based on the number of patients needed to allow meaningful statistical conclusions to be drawn about the treatment; the sample size should minimize the chance that a potentially ineffective drug will be accepted or that a potentially effective drug will be rejected. When clinical trials are used to evaluate a treatment regimen rather than a specific agent, Phase I and Phase II trials can be combined; they then are referred to as a pilot study.

### Phase III

Phase III is used to assess the role of a new treatment in terms of overall response, survival, and quality of life of newly diagnosed patients with a specific diagnosis. The goal of the trial is to determine whether the treatment is equivalent with or superior to the current or standard treatment. Randomization between the experimental group and the control group to avoid systematic bias as well as stratification by specific prognostic factors is a key element. Phase III trials require large numbers of patients; therefore, protocols usually must be implemented at a number of institutions or through cooperative groups.

## Phase IV

Phase IV is meant to further investigate the long-term safety and efficacy of a treatment and takes place after the new treatment is approved for standard use. These trials are less common in pediatric oncology than trials in other phases, but their goal is to decrease side effects, toxicities, and late effects of treatment while continuing to provide acceptable cure rates.

## Regulatory Requirements

To conduct clinical research, investigators must comply with federal guidelines compiled by the U.S. Food and Drug Administration (FDA). The guidelines are as follows:

- All research with human subjects must be approved by an institutional review board, which serves to protect the rights of research subjects. Institutional review-board approval must be obtained before the protocol may be implemented, the approval must be renewed at least annually, all changes (i.e., amendments) to the protocol also must be approved, and all unexpected serious toxicities (termed adverse drug reactions or serious adverse events) and the deaths of any subjects in the study must be reported.
- Before treatment can begin, all patients or their parents or legal guardians must sign an informed-consent document that has been approved by an institutional review board. Although it is not legally necessary to obtain consent from the child, children of an appropriate age should be informed about their participation in the trial and their assent must be obtained. Assent indicates that the child agrees with participation in a research study. In a clinical trial, the informed-consent document must describe in lay terms the research; the purpose of the research; and the risks, benefits, duration of, and alternatives to the research. The document should also describe any compensation that will be offered, explain how confidentiality will be ensured, note the responsibilities of the researcher in the event of adverse effects, and the financial implications and voluntary nature of the treatment. In a randomized study, because the patient, the parent, or both must give informed consent before the randomized assignment is made, they thereby agree to all of the treatment methodologies in the protocol.
- The participants' medical records should contain complete documentation of their eligibility; the treatment and any modifications, outcome, and toxicities; and the results of the studies required by the protocol. These records must be kept for at least 7 years after the new drug application is filed with the FDA.
- All investigational drugs require strict record keeping. Drug-accountability logs, which detail the disposition of every dose of drug, must be maintained. These logs are subject to audits and must match the available supply of the drug in the study.

## Nursing Assessment and Interventions

Nurses play a vital role in treating patients in clinical trials.

### Assessment

- Ensure that a patient is eligible for a protocol before beginning investigational therapy, all required studies are completed, consents are signed, and compliance with the protocol is maintained.
- Ensure that investigational drugs or therapies are given safely; pay special attention to checking doses, as they may vary throughout the study or be considerably different from a standard dosing regimen; ensure that all laboratory work and follow-up evaluations are done as stated; assess the patient carefully for adverse side effects; and thoroughly document in the medical record any side effects.

### Interventions

- Serve as an advocate for the patient and the family (this is the role of a nurse who has rapport with the patient and the family and is able to assess their concerns about an investigational therapy), help the patient and the family ask questions of the treating physician, and ensure that issues are addressed and the patient and the family are comfortable and proceeding with the investigational therapy. (Patients and families who do not wish to participate in clinical trials may require support and assurance that their care will not be compromised if they choose not to participate.)
- Provide support for the family. Be respectful of choices that families make and support their decisions regardless of the patient's outcome. The families, not the healthcare providers, are the ones who must live with the consequences of the decisions they make.
- Provide education for the patient. This is an important responsibility of nurses who are involved in clinical research. In addition to giving the patient and the family initial information concerning the treatment plan, the investigator should also explain the risks and benefits associated with and alternatives to the investigational therapy. After this initial discussion, the nurse can reinforce education regarding all aspects of the treatment plan; for example, how drugs will be delivered, how many injections will be required, and methods that will be used to control side effects. The nurse also should be prepared to discuss clinical research in general and direct patients and families to clinical-trial Web sites and registries, thus allowing them to make an informed decision about participation.

## Expected Patient and Family Outcome

The patient or the family or both are able to make an informed decision regarding treatment for cancer.

# Chemotherapy

*Christine Sullivan*

## Principles of Treatment

The purpose of using chemotherapy to treat cancer is to prevent the cancer cell from dividing, metastasizing, and ultimately resulting in the death of the patient. Chemotherapeutic agents are designed to treat cancer by preventing the proliferation of cancer cells; however, their cytotoxic effects also indiscriminately interfere with the proliferation of normal cells. To fully understand how chemotherapy works, it is important to examine the way in which a normal cell reproduces and to compare this with cancer-cell growth.

## Normal Cellular Division—The Cell Cycle

The cell cycle consists of four periods, or phases, of cellular growth and a resting phase (G0). For cellular proliferation to occur, there must be duplication of the cellular genetic material, deoxyribonucleic acid (DNA), followed by mitosis (M phase), or the phase of the cell cycle that results in the division of the cell into two identical daughter cells. The following are the phases of the cell cycle (**Figure 4-1**):

- *G1*, the first gap, is the first phase that a cell enters when it leaves the resting phase. This is the phase during which ribonucleic acid (RNA) synthesis and protein synthesis occur. The time span of G1 is widely varied; during this period, cells spend the largest portion of their dividing lives.
- *S* is the synthesis phase during which the DNA is replicated.
- *G2*, the second gap, is the premitotic phase in which RNA synthesis is completed.
- *M* is the phase in which mitosis occurs.

Normal cells proceed through the cell cycle in a consistent manner in response to feedback mechanisms and are protected by tumor-suppressor genes. They have a defined number of cell divisions and are programmed for cell death, or apoptosis, as they age or are damaged.

## Malignant Cellular Division

A primary characteristic of a cancer cell is that it has lost the usual mechanisms to control growth that a normal cell exhibits. A cancer cell experiences unchecked growth due to the following deviations from normal cellular behavior:

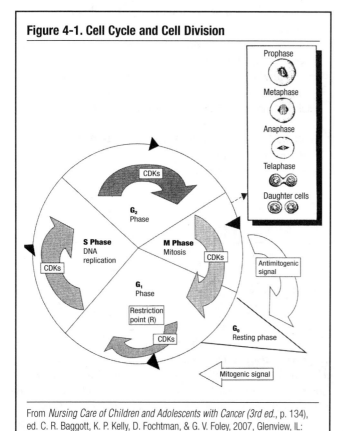

**Figure 4-1. Cell Cycle and Cell Division**

From *Nursing Care of Children and Adolescents with Cancer* (3rd ed., p. 134), ed. C. R. Baggott, K. P. Kelly, D. Fochtman, & G. V. Foley, 2007, Glenview, IL: Association of Pediatric Hematology/Oncology Nurses.

- Cancer cells do not seem to have a preset number of divisions before death; thus, apoptosis is avoided.
- Cancer cells do not appear to be inhibited by contact, but rather, they continue to divide into an unorganized mass.
- Cancer cells do not require the usual amount of growth factors, and some cancer cells even produce their own growth factor.

## Role in Childhood Cancer

Since the introduction of chemotherapy, survival statistics for childhood cancers have improved dramatically. Prior to the advent of chemotherapy, treatment consisted of surgery and radiation that primarily addressed local disease. Chemotherapy offers a means of controlling systemic disease and provides a more comprehensive approach to cancer treatment. Chemotherapeutic agents are now included in disease-specific treatment protocols based on their synergy and improved treatment responses when used in combination.

Chemotherapy is used in several different ways to achieve total destruction of the cells of a given malignancy:

- *Multimodal therapy* involves the use of chemotherapy in combination with another type of therapy, such as radiation, surgery, or both.
- *Adjuvant chemotherapy* is the use of chemotherapy as well as surgery and/or radiation to address residual disease or suspected metastases.
- *Combination chemotherapy* is a multidrug regimen that employs several agents found to be effective against a specific tumor and has varied toxicities and mechanisms of action.
- *Neoadjuvant chemotherapy* refers to the use of chemotherapy preoperatively to debulk a tumor prior to its surgical excision.
- *Sanctuary therapy*, or *regional chemotherapy*, is chemotherapy that is delivered directly to an area where malignant cells may not be fully eradicated by systemic chemotherapy alone (e.g., intrathecal chemotherapy for central nervous system [CNS] prophylaxis in the treatment of leukemia). Sanctuary and regional chemotherapy also may refer to high-dose chemotherapy administered intra-arterially to decrease systemic effects.

## Classification of Chemotherapy Agents

Chemotherapeutics typically are divided into several different classes, each of which has several types of agents. A class of drugs can be defined according to the mechanism of action, the molecular structure, or the physiological action of the agent. An agent's mechanism of action determines whether it is classified as cell-cycle specific or nonspecific. Cell-cycle-specific agents (**Table 4-2**) are most effective during active phases of the cell-cycle, whereas cell-cycle-nonspecific agents are effective during all phases of the cell cycle (**Table 4-3**). Agents are selected for use in combination to achieve maximum cell kill. Chemotherapeutic agents can be classified as follows (specific agents are described in more detail in **Table 4-4**):

### Alkylating Agents

These drugs contribute their alkyl group to sites on DNA or other macromolecules, causing DNA disruptions that interfere with replication and transcription.

### Antibiotics

Antitumor antibiotics are natural agents synthesized by a variety of bacteria and fungi. They interfere with cellular metabolism through numerous mechanisms. In general, they form stable complexes with DNA, interfering with the synthesis of DNA and RNA.

## Antimetabolites
These drugs appear to be similar to naturally occurring metabolites that are used by cells to make nucleic acids; they act by inhibiting essential enzymes or by causing the nucleic acids to produce nonfunctional end products.

## Plant Products
These drugs are derived from natural sources or manufactured from compounds extracted from plants. The natural products include mitotic inhibitors known as vinca alkaloids.

**Additional plant products include the epipodophyllotoxins and camptothecins:** These agents inhibit topoisomerase II and I, respectively, causing DNA breaks.

## Hormones (corticosteroids)
These steroidal drugs enter the cell and bind with macromolecules in the cytoplasm. Ultimately, they enter the cell nucleus, bind with DNA, and interfere with transcription.

## Miscellaneous
Included in this category are drugs whose mechanisms of action are not understood or do not fit into any other category. Examples include enzymes such as L-asparaginase (Elspar).

Delivering the most effective chemotherapy with the least amount of damage to normal cells, and ultimately to the patient, remains the primary challenge of chemotherapy treatment for cancer. **Table 4-5** provides a list of methods used to overcome chemotherapy resistance and normal cell damage.

## Method of Delivery
Chemotherapeutic agents are delivered by oral, subcutaneous, intramuscular, intravenous, intrathecal, and intraarterial routes. The administration route is selected based on the chemical properties of the agent and the desired effect.

## Potential Side Effects
Most chemotherapeutic agents have a variety of side effects related to their mechanism of action. A goal of combination chemotherapy is to use agents that have either different types of toxicities or different timing of toxicities (see Section V, "Side Effects of Treatment").

The following are among the general toxicities of chemotherapy:
- Gastrointestinal: nausea, vomiting, diarrhea, constipation, impaired liver function, pancreatitis, anorexia, and electrolyte imbalances
- Skin/mucosal: mucositis, stomatitis, rashes, discoloration, increased sensitivity to sunlight, and alopecia
- Hematologic: anemia, neutropenia, and thrombocytopenia
- Immunosuppression
- Other: pulmonary, renal, neurological, or cardiac damage; possible sterility.

## Nursing Assessment and Interventions
The responsibilities of a pediatric hematology/oncology nurse regarding the safe administration of chemotherapy are daunting. Few other nursing responsibilities are associated with such a small margin for error. In light of this fact, institutions that provide chemotherapy to children should have a well-educated team that includes pediatric oncologists, pharmacists, and registered nurses responsible for ordering, dispensing, and administering these agents.

### Assessment
The nurse should have a thorough understanding of the drug that is administered and should be able to discuss with the patient and the family the drug's mechanism of action and its potential side effects. The following factors also should be included in a baseline assessment before administering a chemotherapeutic agent to a patient:

*(continued on page 88)*

### Table 4-2. Cell-Cycle-Specific Agents

| Plant Alkaloids | Antimetabolites |
|---|---|
| Etoposide (VP 16) | Mercaptopurine |
| Tenoposide (VM 26) | Thioguanine |
| Paclitaxel | 5 Fluorouracil |
| Docetaxel | Gemcitabine |
| Topotecan | Fludarabine |
| Irinotecan | Cladribine |
| Vincristine | Nelarabine |
| Vinblastine | Clofarabine |
| Vinorelbine | Cytarabine |
| | Hydroxyurea |
| | Methotrexate |

### Table 4-3. Cell-Cycle-Nonspecific Agents

| Alkylating Agents | Antitumor Antibiotics | Hormones | Miscellaneous |
|---|---|---|---|
| Mechlorethamine | Dactinomycin | Dexamethasone | Asparaginase |
| Cytoxan | Bleomycin | Prednisone | Retinoids |
| Ifosfamide | Daunorubicin | Hydrocortisone | Imatinib (Gleevac) |
| Melphalan | Doxorubicin | | |
| Lomustine (CCNU) | Idarubicin | | |
| Carmustine (BCNU) | Mitoxantrone | | |
| Busulfan | | | |
| Procarbazine | | | |
| Thiotepa | | | |
| Temozolimide | | | |
| Dacarbazine (DTIC) | | | |
| Cisplatin | | | |
| Carboplatin | | | |

## Table 4-4. Chemotherapeutic Agents

| Drug | Classification | Route | Side Effects | Special Considerations |
|---|---|---|---|---|
| Arsenic trioxide | Differentiating agent | IV | Common: fatigue, fever, rigors, reactions at injection site, nausea, vomiting, diarrhea, increased LFTs, myelosuppression | Safety and efficacy have not been studied in children younger than 5 years of age. |
| Asparaginase (Elspar) | Miscellaneous Cell-cycle nonspecific | Intramuscular (IM), IV | Common: local allergic reaction, hyperammonemia, low fibrinogen<br><br>Occasional: rash, hyperglycemia, abnormal liver function tests, coagulation abnormalities<br><br>Rare: hypersensitivity with anaphylaxis, nausea, vomiting, anorexia, somnolence, lethargy, pancreatitis, convulsions, thrombosis, edema, CNS ischemic attack, renal compromise | IV administration returning to favor, PEG-asparaginase has provided excellent asparagine depletion, use of *E. coli* asparaginase or erwinia asparaginase requires meticulous dosing schedules.<br><br>Have emergency equipment and drugs available.<br><br>Observe patient for at least 1/2 hr after dose.<br><br>Coagulation abnormalities place child at risk for thrombus formation or bleeding. |
| Bleomycin sulfate (Blenoxane) | Antibiotic Cell-cycle nonspecific | IV, IM, subcutaneous (SQ) | Common: none<br><br>Occasional: hyperpigmentation, pneumonitis, high fever 2–6 hr after administration<br><br>Rare: anaphylaxis, fever, hypotension, nausea, vomiting, anorexia, skin rash, mucositis, pulmonary fibrosis, renal failure | High fevers may occur without anaphylaxis; give earlier in the day so it does not occur at night. Rare, lethal anaphylactoid reactions with severe fever and hypotension can occur—have emergency equipment available.<br><br>If test dose is required, administer 1–2 Units IM; wait 1 hr and give remaining dose. Lower dose may need to be given when pulmonary radiotherapy is used.<br><br>Pulmonary function tests are done as baseline, throughout course of therapy and for a period of time after therapy. Patients can develop fibrosis with decreased diffusion capacity. |
| Busulfan (Myleran) | Alkylating agent (alkane sulfonate) Cell-cycle nonspecific | By mouth (PO) | Common: myelosuppression, mild nausea, vomiting, "bronzing" of the skin<br><br>Occasional: seizures with a high dose, oral mucositis, skin breakdown, decreased adrenal function<br><br>Rare: skin rashes, veno-occlusive disease (VOD), amenorrhea, testicular atrophy, gynecomastia, myasthenia symptoms, cataract, atrophic bronchitis | Prophylactic anticonvulsant therapy may be useful in patients receiving high doses of the drug. |
| Carboplatin (Paraplatin) | Alkylating agent (heavy metal) Cell-cycle nonspecific | IV | Common: nausea, vomiting, myelosuppression<br><br>Occasional: electrolyte disturbances, anaphylaxis<br><br>Rare: metallic taste, peripheral neuropathy, hepatotoxicity, renal toxicity, ototoxicity, secondary leukemia | IV infusion over 15 min or longer.<br><br>Aluminum reacts with carboplatin, causing precipitate formation and loss of potency; therefore, do not allow needles or IV sets containing aluminum parts to come in contact with this drug.<br><br>Elimination dependent upon glomerular filtration rate (GFR) and may be prescribed based on GFR and area under the curve (AUC) desired. Premedicate, or consider desensitization if previous hypersensitivity reaction has occurred. |

*continued*

## Table 4-4. Chemotherapeutic Agents *continued*

| Drug | Classification | Route | Side Effects | Special Considerations |
|---|---|---|---|---|
| Carmustine (BCNU, BiCNU) | Alkylating agent (nitrosourea)<br><br>Cell-cycle non-specific | IV | Common: burning with peripheral administration, nausea, vomiting, myelosuppression, alopecia, late pulmonary dysfunction<br><br>Occasional: marked facial flushing, liver dysfunction, thrombophlebitis at injection site<br><br>Rare: brownish discoloration of skin, renal dysfunction, pulmonary fibrosis, secondary malignancy | Avoid extravasation or local contact with skin or conjunctiva.<br><br>Avoid rapid infusion, which is associated with burning or hypotension.<br><br>Use glass containers and polyethylene-lined administration sets for stability. |
| Cisplatin (Platinol) | Alkylating agent (heavy metal)<br><br>Cell-cycle non-specific | IV | Common: nausea, vomiting, anorexia, myelosupression, hypomagnesemia, high-frequency hearing loss, nephrotoxicity<br><br>Occasional: metallic taste, electrolyte disturbances, hearing loss in the normal hearing range<br><br>Rare: peripheral neuropathy, tinnitus, seizure, liver toxicity, secondary malignancy | Synergistic with radiation therapy.<br><br>Aluminum reacts with cisplatin, causing precipitate formation and loss of potency; therefore, do not allow needles or IV sets containing aluminum parts to come in contact with this drug.<br><br>Premedicate with antiemetics; continue throughout and beyond course of therapy, because cisplatin causes delayed nausea and vomiting.<br><br>During course of therapy carefully monitor input and output (I&O).<br><br>Maintain urinary output at least at 2 ml/kg/hr.<br><br>Administer mannitol as ordered to ensure adequate urinary output.<br><br>Intensifies aminoglycoside toxicity and should be used with caution when administered concurrently.<br><br>To decrease risk of hypomagnesemia, supplement with magnesium. |
| Cladribine | Antimetabolite<br><br>Cell-cycle specific | IV | Common: myelosuppression, fever, fatigue, nausea, vomiting<br><br>Occasional: elevated bilirubin and LFTs, diarrhea, paralysis of extremities at high doses<br><br>Rare: acute nephrotoxicity | Visually inspect solution. Precipitate may form at low temperatures but will dissipate at warmer temperatures or by shaking the solution. |
| Clofarabine | Antimetabolite<br><br>Cell-cycle specific | IV | Common: profound bone-marrow suppression with associated infection risk<br><br>Occasional: abnormal hepatic and renal functions<br><br>Rare: tumor lysis and capillary leak syndrome | 0.4 mg/ml dilution, monitor for fever and signs of infection, abnormal liver and kidney functions, metabolic abnormalities, and signs of capillary leak syndrome. |

*continued*

### Table 4-4. Chemotherapeutic Agents continued

| Drug | Classification | Route | Side Effects | Special Considerations |
|---|---|---|---|---|
| Corticosteroid (prednisone, dexamethasone, hydrocortisone, methylprednisolone) | Hormones<br>Cell-cycle non-specific | IV, PO<br>Intrathecal (IT)<br>Equivalent potency:<br>• Cortisone 5·<br>• Hydrocortisone 4<br>• Methylprednisolone 0.8<br>• Dexamethasone 0.15 | Common: hyperphagia, immunosuppression, personality changes, Cushing's syndrome, pituitary-adrenal axis suppression, acne<br>Occasional: poor wound healing, stomach upset, hyperglycemia, gastritis, muscle weakness, osteonecrosis<br>Rare: pancreatitis, electrolyte imbalance, gastrointestinal (GI) bleeding, increased intraocular pressure, hypertension, aseptic necrosis of femoral head, growth retardation, striae, osteopenia, peptic ulcer, cataracts | Decrease salt intake; protect from infection; observe for hyperglycemia. To decrease or prevent GI upset, take with meals or snacks; may need to take with histamine $H_2$-receptor antagonist such as cimetidine, ranitidine. |
| Cyclophosphamide (Cytoxan) | Alkylating agent<br>Cell-cycle non-specific | IV, PO | Common: anorexia, nausea, vomiting, myelosuppression, alopecia, gonadal dysfunction/sterility<br>Occasional: metallic taste, hemorrhagic cystitis, syndrome of inappropriate antidiuretic hormone (SIADH)<br>Rare: transient blurred vision, cardiac toxicity with arrhythmias (in higher doses), myocardial necrosis, pulmonary fibrosis, secondary malignancy, bladder fibrosis | Maintain adequate hydration, urinary output.<br>Check urine for blood frequently.<br>Outpatient therapy should be given early in the day when possible so that toxic metabolites do not accumulate in bladder overnight.<br>Encourage patient to urinate before going to bed at night to empty bladder completely.<br>Administration of high doses of cyclophosphamide should be preceded and followed by IV fluids and mesna. |
| Cytarabine (ara-C, cytosine arabinoside, Cytosar-U) | Antimetabolite<br>Cell-cycle specific | IV, IM, SQ, IT | Common: nausea, vomiting, anorexia, conjunctivitis with higher doses, myelosuppression, stomatitis, alopecia<br>Occasional: flu-like symptoms with fever, diarrhea<br>Rare: encephalopathy, cerebellar dysfunction, or pulmonary capillary leak with higher doses; rash, hepatotoxicity, VOD, pneumonitis, gonadal dysfunction<br>With intrathecal administration: nausea, vomiting, headache, pleocytosis, fever, learning disability, rash, somnolence, meningismus, convulsions, paresis, myelosuppression, ataxia | Administer steroid eyedrops to prevent conjunctivitis with high dose. |
| Dacarbazine (DTIC) | Alkylating agent<br>Cell-cycle non-specific | IV | Common: moderate to severe nausea and vomiting, mild myelosuppression<br>Occasional: flu-like syndrome with malaise, fever, myalgias<br>Rare: veno-occlusive disease and hepatic vein thrombosis | Provide adequate antiemetic coverage. |
| Dactinomycin (actinomycin D, Cosmegen) | Antibiotic<br>Cell-cycle non-specific | IV | Common: nausea, vomiting, local ulceration if extravasated, myelosuppression, alopecia, skin photosensitivity or hyperpigmentation<br>Occasional: diarrhea, mucositis, immune thrombocytopenia, radiation recall<br>Rare: hepatotoxicity | Vesicant—severe tissue damage if extravasation occurs.<br>Protect from light.<br>Avoid preservatives.<br>Do not filter.<br>Radiation recall may occur in an area of previous radiotherapy. |

*continued*

### Table 4-4. Chemotherapeutic Agents *continued*

| Drug | Classification | Route | Side Effects | Special Considerations |
|---|---|---|---|---|
| Daunorubicin (daunomycin, Cerbidine) and Doxorubicin (Adriamycin) | Antibiotic  Cell-cycle non-specific | IV | Common: subclinical cardiac arrhythmias, nausea, local ulceration if extravasated, pink or red color to urine, myelosuppression, alopecia  Occasional: stomatitis, hepatotoxicity, mucositis, cardiomyopathy (cumulative and dose dependent)  Rare: anaphylaxis, allergic reaction, rash, secondary malignancy | Vesicant—severe tissue damage if extravasation occurs.  Warn patient and family about urine discoloration.  Cardiac studies with echocardiogram or multigated angiography (MUGA) scan should be done periodically to monitor cardiac function—must have acceptable cardiac ejection/monitor cumulative dose. |
| Docetaxel (Taxotere) | Plant product (taxane)  Cell-cycle specific | IV | Common: myelosuppression, nausea, vomiting, weakness  Occasional: elevated LFTs, hypersensitivity, epiphora  Rare: hypotension, severe pulmonary toxicity | Premedication with corticosteroids is recommended to decrease hypersensitivity reactions and fluid retention. |
| Etoposide (VP-16, VePesid) | Plant product (epipodophyllotoxin)  Cell-cycle specific | IV, PO | Common: nausea, vomiting, myelosuppression  Occasional: alopecia, enhanced damage due to radiation, diarrhea  Rare: hypotension, anaphylaxis, skin rash, peripheral neuropathy, stomatitis, secondary malignancy | Severe hypotension can occur with rapid infusion.  Concentrations above 0.4 mg/ml have unpredictable stability in solution.  Do not refrigerate IV solution, PO capsules must be refrigerated. |
| 5-Fluorouracil (5-FU, fluorouracil, Adrucil) | Antimetabolite  Cell-cycle specific | IV, PO | Common: nausea, vomiting, metallic taste, immunosuppression, myelosuppression  Occasional: diarrhea, stomatitis, sun sensitivity, hyperpigmentation, dry skin, palmar-plantarery throdysesthesia (red painful skin irritation)  Rare: hypotension, angina, electrocardiogram (ECG) changes, tearing, conjunctivitis and blurred vision, partial loss of nails, headache, visual disturbances, cerebellar ataxia, proctitis | Take on empty stomach (at least 1 hr before or 2 hr after food).  For oral administration mix parenteral solution of 5-FU with flavored water or carbonated beverage; avoid acidic fruit juice. |
| Fludarabine | Antimetabolite  Cell-cycle specific | IV | Common: myelosuppression, nausea, vomiting, mucositis  Occasional: elevated LFTs, peripheral neuropathy, tumor lysis syndrome, fatigue  Rare: respiratory distress and failure | Prophylactic allopurinol, adequate hydration, and urinary alkalinization are used for patients with large initial tumor burdens to avoid tumor lysis syndrome. Avoid exposure by inhalation or by direct contact of the skin or mucous membranes. |
| Gemcitabine | Antimetabolite  Cell-cycle specific | IV | Common: myelosuppression, nausea, vomiting  Occasional: elevated LFTs, flu-like symptoms  Rare: somnolence, hypotension, severe pulmonary toxicity, thrombosis | Maintain adequate hydration. Avoid exposure by inhalation or by direct contact of the skin or mucous membranes. |
| Hydroxyurea (Hydrea) | Antimetabolite  Cell-cycle specific | PO | Common: myelosuppression with rapid drop in WBC count  Occasional: nausea, vomiting, stomatitis, anemia  Rare: rash, facial erythema, dysuria, renal tubular damage, headache, dizziness, jaundice, radiation recall, hallucination, convulsions, nail changes | Take on empty stomach (1 hr before or 2 hr after meals).  Dose often titrated to WBC count.  Do not add to solutions that are acidic or carbonated; alkaline solutions preferred. |

*continued*

## Table 4-4. Chemotherapeutic Agents *continued*

| Drug | Classification | Route | Side Effects | Special Considerations |
|---|---|---|---|---|
| Idarubicin (Idamycin) | Antibiotic (anthracycline) Cell-cycle non-specific | IV | Analogue of daunorubicin with similar activity and side effects | Vesicant—severe tissue damage if extravasation occurs. Protect from light. See daunorubicin. Perhaps less cardiotoxicity than doxorubicin and daunorubicin. |
| Ifosfamide (isophosphamide, Ifex) | Alkylating agent | IV | Analog of cyclophosphamide. Common: nausea, vomiting, anorexia, myelosuppression, alopecia. Occasional: somnolence, confusion, weakness, seizure, SIADH, hemorrhagic cystitis, cardiac toxicities with arrhythmias at high dosages, myocardial necrosis, Fanconi's renal failure. Rare: encephalopathy, peripheral neuropathy, acute renal failure, pulmonary fibrosis, secondary malignancy, bladder fibrosis | Risk of severe hemorrhagic cystitis if given without uroprotection from mesna. Can be mixed with mesna. More severe symptoms may occur at higher doses and after rapid injection. Must receive PO or IV hydration beginning 3–6 hr before and 24 hr after dose. Must monitor I&O and urinary specific gravity. Fanconi's renal failure more common with history of cisplatin use, prior kidney damage, and greater than 70–100 g/m$^2$ cumulative dose. May require electrolyte supplementation with magnesium (Mg), potassium (K+), and phosphorous (PO$^4$). |
| Imatinib (Gleevec) | Miscellaneous | PO | Edema, fluid retention, nausea and vomiting, neutropenia, thrombocytopenia, hepatotoxicity | Take at bedtime to avoid nausea and vomiting; observe for signs of fluid retention; drug metabolism may be altered by some antibiotics, antifungals, and steroids. |
| Interferon (Intron A, Roferon-A) | Protein produced by recombinant DNA technology | IV, IM, SQ | Common: none. Occasional: fever, headache, fatigue, anorexia, nausea, myalgia, arthralgia, diarrhea, depression, confusion. Rare: vomiting, chills, stomatitis, somnolence, psychosis, elevated transaminases, myelosuppression, peripheral neuropathy, sinus tachyarrhythmias, hypocalcemia, hyperkalemia, anaphylaxis, dyspnea, hypotension, rash, dizziness, impotence, alopecia, menstrual disorder | Premedication with magnesium choline salicylate, acetaminophen, or, if not contraindicated, nonsteroidal anti-inflammatory drugs (NSAIDS), may reduce fever and myalgias. |
| Irinotecan (CPT-11, Camptosar) | Plant product Cell-cycle specific | IV | Common: transient early diarrhea, nausea, vomiting, abdominal pain, anorexia, fever, dehydration, alopecia, asthenia, myelosuppression, later onset diarrhea. Occasional: elevation in transaminases, alkaline phosphatase, bilirubin, creatinine, constipation, pain at infusion site. Rare: dermatitis, tremor, hematuria, hypoproteinemia, glucosuria, mucositis, headache, dizziness, disorientation/confusion, facial hot flushes, colitis, pulmonary infiltrates, pneumonitis | May require antidiarrheal for control of diarrhea: atropine for early diarrhea, loperamide for delayed diarrhea. |

*continued*

### Table 4-4. Chemotherapeutic Agents continued

| Drug | Classification | Route | Side Effects | Special Considerations |
|---|---|---|---|---|
| Lomustine (CCNU, CeeNU) | Alkalating agent (nitrosourea) Cell-cycle non-specific | PO | Common: nausea, vomiting, myelosuppression Occasional: anorexia Rare: elevation of liver enzymes, pulmonary toxicity, renal toxicity, cumulative myelosuppression | PO in one dose on an empty stomach, 1 hr before meals or 2 hr after meals. |
| Mechlorethamine (nitrogen mustard, Mustargen, HN2) | Alklylating agent Cell-cycle non-specific | IV | Common: nausea, vomiting, anorexia, metallic taste, phlebitis, alopecia, diarrhea, myelosuppression, gonadal dysfunction/sterility, necrosis if extravasated | Vesicant—can also cause skin irritation with local contact (use sodium thiosulfate and ice). Use within 1 hr after reconstitution. May cause thrombosis, phlebitis, and discoloration of vein. |
| Melphalan (Alkeran, L-PAM, L-sarcolysin) | Alkylating agent Cell-cycle non-specific | PO, IV | Common: anorexia, ulceration if extravasated, nausea, vomiting, myelosuppression, mucositis, diarrhea, alopecia Occasional: lethargy Rare: hypotension, diaphoresis, hypersensitivity reaction, pulmonary fibrosis, sterility, secondary malignancy | Infusion over 15–30 min. Good hydration for 24 hr after IV dose. Furosemide may be given to maintain urinary output after IV dose. Take daily dose at one time. Take on empty stomach. |
| Mercaptopurine (Purinethol, 6-MP) | Antimetabolite Cell-cycle specific | PO | Common: myelosuppression Occasional: anorexia, nausea, vomiting, diarrhea, mucositis Rare: anaphylactic reaction, urticaria, hepatic fibrosis, hyperbilirubinemia | Reduce oral dose 75% if given with allopurinol. Take daily dose at one time, preferably at bedtime on an empty stomach (2 hr after meals). |
| Methotrexate (amethopterin, MTX) | Antimetabolite Cell-cycle specific | IV, IM, PO, IT | Common: transaminase and bilirubin elevations Occasional: nausea, vomiting, anorexia, diarrhea, myelosuppression, stomatitis, photosensitivity, learning disability Rare: dizziness, malaise, blurred vision, allergic reaction, peeling, redness and tenderness of skin—especially soles and palms, alopecia, folliculitis, renal toxicity, leukoencephalopathy, seizures, acute neurotoxicity, lung damage, liver damage, hyperpigmentation, osteoporosis, osteonecrosis and soft tissue necrosis, progressive CNS deterioration Intrathecal administration: nausea, vomiting, headache, pleocytosis, fever, convulsion, learning disability, rash, somnolence, meningismus, convulsions, paresis, myelosuppression, somnolence, ataxia, leukoencephalopathy, progressive DNS deterioration | Renal impairment will enhance toxicity. Advise patients to use sunscreen; severe sunburn can occur even with low weekly doses. When intermediate or high-dose methotrexate is given, leucovorin is administered as a rescue agent. Avoid vitamins containing folic acid to avoid the metabolic block caused by methotrexate. Hydration and urine alkalinization are used with higher dose infusions. Methotrexate readily enters body fluids; patients with effusions may have delayed clearance. Do not give concomitant trimethoprim and sulfamethaxozole, NSAIDs, and aspirin because delayed clearance and increased toxicities may occur. |

continued

### Table 4-4. Chemotherapeutic Agents *continued*

| Drug | Classification | Route | Side Effects | Special Considerations |
|---|---|---|---|---|
| Mitoxantrone (Novantrone, DHAD) | Antibiotic<br>Cell-cycle non-specific | IV | Common: cardiac arrhythmias, nausea, vomiting, worsening side effects due to radiation, local ulceration if extravasated, bluish-green color to urine, myelosuppression, immunosuppression, alopecia<br><br>Occasional: stomatitis, hepatotoxicity, mucositis, cardiomyopathy (dose dependent)<br><br>Rare: anaphylaxis, allergic reactions, rash, secondary malignancy | Vesicant—severe tissue damage if extravasation occurs.<br><br>Not recommended for patients who have received full doses of anthracycline.<br><br>Do not give IV push.<br><br>May discolor urine. |
| Nelarabine (ara-G) | Antimetabolite<br>Cell-cycle specific | IV | Common: peripheral neuropathy is primary toxicity<br><br>Rare: central nervous system toxicity to include somnolence and Guillain-Barre-like ascending paralysis | Prophylactic allopurinol, adequate hydration, and urinary alkalinization are used for patients with large initial tumor burdens to avoid tumor lysis syndrome. |
| Paclitaxel (Taxol) | Plant product (taxane)<br>Cell-cycle specific | IV | Common: pain, swelling, erythema if extravasated, myelosuppression, diminished or absent deep tendon reflexes, alopecia, fatigue<br><br>Occasional: acute anaphylactic reaction, nausea, vomiting, headache, skin rash, mucositis, diarrhea, fever, glove and stocking numbness, hyperesthesia with burning sensation, mild to severe myalgias, increased triglyceride levels | Irritant—avoid extravasation.<br><br>Premedicate with diphenhydramine, dexamethasone, and an $H^2$ receptor blocker.<br><br>Do not administer in any bag or tubing containing polyvinyl chloride (PVC).<br><br>Use filters because small fibers can appear after dilution. |
| Procarbazine (Matulane) | Aklylating agent<br>Cell-cycle non-specific | IV, PO | Common: nausea, vomiting, diarrhea, anorexia, inhibits monoamine oxidase (MAO) activity, myelosuppression, alopecia<br><br>Occasional: headache, flu-like syndrome, gonadal dysfunction/sterility<br><br>Rare: nightmares, hallucinations, hemolytic anemia, pruritus, rash, depression, insomnia, convulsions, coma, stomatitis, pulmonary reaction, hypertension, secondary malignancy | Hypotension and/or CNS depression may occur in the presence of alcohol, narcotics, antihistamines, phenothiazines, phenytoin (Dilantin), tricyclic antidepressants, barbiturates, sympathomimetic drugs, and tyramine-rich foods, such as aged cheese, wine, bananas, yogurt.<br><br>Take 1 hr before or 2 hr after meals. |
| Retinoic acids | Differentiating agents | IV, PO | Common: dry skin, dry mucosa, inflammation of the lips<br><br>Occasional: nausea, vomiting, rash, conjunctivitis, musculoskeletal pains, fatigue, headache, triglyceride elevation, cholesterol elevations, transaminase elevations, retinoic acid syndrome with hyperleukocytosis<br><br>Rare: changes in skin pigmentation, nonspecific GI complaints, dizziness, pseudotumor cerebri, anemia, leukopenia, respiratory distress, fever, hypotension, skeletal hyperostosis | Take with food or meals to enhance absorption.<br><br>Monitor lipid levels.<br><br>Avoid sun exposure, use good lubricant for skin and lips.<br><br>Monitor nutritional status.<br><br>Use saline eye drops as needed. |
| Temozolomide | Alkylating agent<br>Cell-cycle non-specific | PO | Common: mild nausea and vomiting, delayed myelosuppression<br><br>Occasional: fatigue, elevated LFTs | Avoid opening capsules to prevent inhalation or contact with skin or mucous membranes. |

*continued*

## Table 4-4. Chemotherapeutic Agents *continued*

| Drug | Classification | Route | Side Effects | Special Considerations |
|---|---|---|---|---|
| Teniposide (VM-26, Vumon) | Plant product (epipodophyllotoxin) Cell-cycle specific | IV | Common: nausea, vomiting, myelosuppression<br>Occasional: alopecia, enhanced damage due to radiation, diarrhea<br>Rare: hypotension, anaphylaxis, skin rash, peripheral neuropathy, stomatitis, secondary malignancy | Irritant—avoid extravasation.<br>Do not use PVC-containing bags or tubing to administer.<br>Do not refrigerate diluted solutions.<br>Heparin can precipitate; must be flushed from lines.<br>Anaphylaxis or hypotensive reaction with rapid infusion.<br>Flush vein before and after administration. |
| Thioguanine (6-thioguanine, 6-TG) | Antimetabolite Cell-cycle specific | PO | Common: myelosuppression<br>Occasional: anorexia, nausea, vomiting, diarrhea, mucositis<br>Rare: anaphylactic reaction, urticaria, hematuria, crystalluria, hepatic fibrosis, hyperbilirubinemia | Take oral dose at one time, preferably at bedtime on empty stomach (2 hr after meals). |
| Thiotepa (Triethylenethiophosphoramide, Thioplex) | Alkylating agent Cell-cycle non-specific | IV, IM, SQ, IT Intracavitary Intratumor | Common: nausea, vomiting, anorexia, myelosuppression, mucositis and esophagitis at higher doses in conditioning regimens for bone marrow transplant (BMT), gonadal dysfunction/infertility<br>Occasional: pain at injection site, dizziness, headache, inappropriate behavior, confusion, somnolence, increased liver transaminase, increased bilirubin, hyperpigmentation of the skin at higher dose in conditioning regimens for BMT<br>Rare: hives, skin rash, febrile reaction | Use 0.22-micron filter to eliminate haze with IV infusions; solutions that are grossly opaque or contain obvious precipitation should not be used.<br>Dilute reconstituted solutions with NS before use.<br>Should be used within 8 hr of reconstitution. |
| Topotecan (Hycamtin) | Plant product Cell-cycle specific | IV, IT | Common: myelosuppression, alopecia<br>Occasional: nausea, vomiting, diarrhea, mucositis, flu-like symptoms, headache, rash, elevated transaminases, elevated alkaline phosphatase, elevated bilirubin, asthenia<br>Rare: abdominal pain, rigors, microscopic hematuria<br>Intrathecal: Nausea, vomiting, headache, fever, back pain, possible leukoencephalopathy, seizures, or paralysis | Administer IT doses over 5 min to avoid potential adverse reactions. |
| Vinblastine (VLB, vincaleukoblastine, Velban) | Plant product Cell-cycle specific | IV | Common: myelosuppression, alopecia<br>Occasional: constipation, loss of deep-tendon reflexes, paresthesias<br>Rare: nausea, vomiting, anorexia, bone pain, allergic reaction, stomatitis, peripheral neuropathy, hoarseness, ptosis, double vision | Vesicant—severe tissue damage if extravasation occurs.<br>Administer stool softeners; increase bulk and fiber in diet. |

*continued*

### Table 4-4. Chemotherapeutic Agents *continued*

| Drug | Classification | Route | Side Effects | Special Considerations |
|---|---|---|---|---|
| Vincristine (VCR, Oncovin) | Plant product<br>Cell-cycle specific | IV | Common: local ulceration if extravasated, hair loss, loss of deep tendon reflexes<br>Occasional: jaw pain, weakness, constipation, numbness, tingling, clumsiness<br>Rare: paralytic ileus, ptosis, vocal cord paralysis, myelosuppression, CNS depression, seizures, SIADH | Vesicant—severe tissue damage if extravasation occurs.<br>Refrigerate and protect from light.<br>Stool softeners may be given prophylactically or for constipation.<br>Liver dysfunction or concomitant radiation therapy to the liver may enhance toxicity.<br>Must have special overwrap label that bears the statement, "Do not remove covering until moment of injection. Fatal if given intrathecally. For intravenous injection only."<br>Infants may have difficulty feeding because of jaw pain.<br>Maximum single dose: 2 mg regardless of BSA or weight. |
| Vinorelbine | Plant product<br>Cell-cycle specific | IV | Common: constipation, myelosuppression is the dose-limiting toxicity<br>Rare: neurotoxicity, paralytic ileus | Assess bowel habits. Infusion site must be monitored closely to prevent extravasation. |

#### *Supportive Medications*

| Drug | Classification | Route | Side Effects | Special Considerations |
|---|---|---|---|---|
| Allopurinol (Zyloprim) | Enzyme inhibitor; blocks uric acid production by inhibiting xanthine oxidase | IV, PO | Common: rash, fever<br>Occasional: granulomatous hepatitis, ocular lesions, alopecia, slight bone marrow suppression, drowsiness, peripheral neuropathy, GI complaints<br>Rare: agranulocytosis, toxic epidermal necrolysis, severe systemic vasculitis, exfoliative dermatitis | Dose reduction is required in moderate to severe renal impairment.<br>Increased toxicities may occur when used with 6-MP or azathioprine—use with great caution. With cyclophosphamide, warfarin, oral antidiabetic drugs, ampicillin, amoxicillin, or thiazide diuretics, use with caution.<br>Maintain adequate hydration.<br>Physically incompatible with methotrexate—do not give in same IV fluid. |
| Amifostine (Ethyol) | Organic thiophosphate cytoprotective agent | IV | Common: nausea, vomiting, flushing, hypotension, hypocalcemia (with multiple daily or multiple day dosing)<br>Occasional: sleepiness, dizziness, sneezing<br>Rare: hiccups, chills | If multiple doses are administered within a 24-hr period, monitor serum calcium levels and supplement, as needed.<br>Administer with patient lying down.<br>Have normal saline bolus available.<br>Monitor blood pressure frequently during infusion (every 3–5 min).<br>Hypotension often occurs toward the end of the infusion. If hypotension develops, place patient in Trendelenberg's position and administer NS bolus (20 ml/kg over 20 min). If blood pressure normalizes, resume infusion.<br>Doses are given immediately before radiation therapy or chemotherapy.<br>Inspect parenteral solutions for particulate matter or discoloration. Do not use if cloudiness or precipitate is observed.<br>Use with NS solutions only. Compatibility with other solutions has not been examined. |

*continued*

### Table 4-4. Chemotherapeutic Agents continued

| Drug | Classification | Route | Side Effects | Special Considerations |
|---|---|---|---|---|
| Dexrazoxane (Zinecard) | Iron chelator that interferes with iron-mediated free-radical generation | IV | Common: Pain on injection, phlebitis, myelosuppression<br><br>Occasional: transient increases in triglycerides, amylase, and alanine transaminase (ALT), mild nausea, vomiting, and diarrhea<br><br>Rare: neurotoxicity (headache, constipation) | Recommended dose ratio of dexrazoxane:doxorubicin is 10:1.<br><br>Doxorubicin must be given before elapsed time of 30 min from beginning of dexrazoxane infusion.<br><br>Used as cellular rescue when intermediate- or high dose methotrexate is given. |
| Leucovorin calcium (Wellcovorin, citrovorum factor, folinic acid) | Antidote<br><br>Bypasses the inhibitor action of folic acid antagonist (methotrexate) | IV, IM, PO | Rare: allergic sensitization, rash | May be given as a single dose after IT methotrexate.<br><br>Must be given exactly at the times ordered.<br><br>False positive test for urinary ketones.<br><br>Not compatible with cisplatin. |
| Mesna (Mesnex) | Uroprotective agent | IV, PO | Common: bad taste with oral use<br><br>Occasional: nausea, vomiting, stomach pain<br><br>Rare: headache; pain in arms, legs and joints; fatigue; rash; transient hypotension; allergy; diarrhea | May be mixed with cyclophosphamide or ifosfamide.<br><br>Must be given exactly at the times ordered.<br><br>IV dose may be given orally at a higher dose, orally has a foul taste.<br><br>Do not use the multidose vial in young infants or neonates because preservative benzyl alcohol is used. |
| Trimethoprim and sulfamethoxazole (Bactrim, Septrax, Co-Trimoxizole) | Antibiotic used prophylactically to prevent *Pneumocystis carinii* pneumonia | IV, PO | Occasional: neutropenia, anorexia, nausea, vomiting, diarrhea, GI upset, hepatic dysfunction, rash<br><br>Rare: Stevens-Johnson syndrome, toxic epidermal necrolysis | May be given as a prophylaxis for *P. carinii* on a schedule of 3 consecutive days weekly.<br><br>If allergic to Bactrim, may use intravenous or aerosolized pentamidine or PO dapsone.<br><br>Must be diluted in 5% dextrose in water ($D_5W$) solution for IV administration; infuse parenteral solution over 60–90 min; monitor for hyponatremia.<br><br>Not compatible with other drugs in IV solution.<br><br>Avoid use during methotrexate infusion; delays methotrexate clearance and increases risk of toxicities.<br><br>Use sunscreen during use because Trimethoprim increases sensitivity to sun. |

Adapted from material in "2000 Guide for the administration and use of cancer chemotherapeutic agents," by V. Almuete, J. Brisby, B. Delman, et al., 2000, *Oncology Special Edition, 3*, 51–55; "General principles of chemotherapy," by F. Balis, J. Hocenberg, & D. G. Poplack, 2006, in *Principles and practice of pediatric oncology*, ed. P. A. Pizzo & D. G. Poplack, (3rd ed., pp. 215–272), Philadelphia: Lippincott-Raven; *Children's Oncology Group pharmacology manual*, by D. Henry, J. Cartwright, & D. Sinsabaugh, 2000, Arcadia, CA: Children's Oncology Group Operations Center; "Chemotherapy," by A. Renick-Ettinger, 2007, in *Nursing care of the child with cancer*, ed. G. V. Foley, D. Fochtman, & K. H. Mooney (3rd ed., pp. 81–116), Glenview, IL: Association of Pediatric Hematology/Oncology Nurses.

### Table 4-5. Overcoming Chemotherapy Resistance

**Methods to Overcome Chemotherapy Resistance**

1. Development of multidrug resistance (MDR) modulators
2. Administration of chemotherapy at maximum dose intensity (maximum tolerated dose and shortest possible interval between doses)
3. Development of combination chemotherapy regimens (multiple alternating agents used to prevent the development of resistance)

    Characteristics of agents selected for combination chemotherapy regimens:
    – differing side effect profiles
    – action at different phases of cell cycle
    – show synergy with other agents—nonoverlapping toxicities
    – conform to dose intensity principles
4. Utilization of pharmacokinetics, pharmacodynamics, and pharmacogenomics in the development of therapeutic protocols

**Advances to Offset Normal Cell Damage**

1. Investigation of drugs that have shown the ability to modulate MDR by inhibiting P-glycoprotein
2. Normal cell return is improved with supportive care measures, such as the use of growth factors, aggressive antibiotic regimens for infection, safer transportation practices, and early symptom management
3. Dose adjustments are made to offset toxicities, and biochemical modulators are used to improve chemotherapy tolerance
    – Use of leucovorin calcium with high-dose methotrexate to rescue normal cells
    – Use of cryoprotective agents (mesna to prevent bladder toxicity, amifostine to prevent ototoxicity, and dexrazoxane to prevent cardiac toxicity)
    – Use of asparaginase as a rescue drug after methotrexate and cytarabine
4. Children's physiological differences may provide an advantage in terms of drug absorption, distribution, metabolism, excretion, and, ultimately, drug tolerance
5. Better understanding of constitutional genetic abnormalities that affect drug tolerance (e.g., inherited genetic defect in thiopurine methyltransferase)

---

- Ensure that the patient and the family understand the treatment protocol.
- Review the patient's history relative to receiving a particular drug (e.g., determine side effects the patient experienced in the past and the presence of relevant allergies).
- Determine the premedication the patient usually receives to control nausea and vomiting and its effectiveness.
- Be aware of any drug-specific concerns. For example, is it necessary to check when the patient had his or her last bowel movement? Must the patient have any tests done before taking the drug? Is the drug likely to cause an allergic or anaphylactic reaction?
- Know the "five rights" of the drug (i.e., right patient, right schedule, right dose, right drug, and right rate) as well as the right sequence of the drug in the protocol.
- Determine the patient's ability to take the drug as ordered. For instance, can or will the patient take medicine by mouth? Is the patient's platelet count high enough for an injection or lumbar puncture? Is the intravenous (IV) line adequate for chemotherapy, particularly a vesicant?
- Assess the patient's complete blood count (CBC) with a differential and other required laboratory tests to determine, among other concerns, whether the results are within the protocol's parameters.
- Ensure that the chemotherapy doses and drugs are correct by following the institution's policies for double-checking the orders and doses, identifying the correct patient by looking at the arm band, and reviewing the patient's allergy profile.
- Prepare IV chemotherapy according to Occupational Safety and Health Administration (OSHA) guidelines for handling cytotoxic or hazardous drugs, or both. (It is important to remember that oral chemotherapy tablets should be crushed in the pharmacy under a hood to prevent inhalation of the dust.)
- Prepare the appropriate and necessary protective equipment based on the potential for exposure before entering the patient's room (refer to the subsection "Guidelines for Safe Handling of Chemotherapy" for the OSHA guidelines on handling chemotherapeutic agents).
- Monitor the IV site during and after administration of the chemotherapy.
- Teach the family and the patient about drug-specific side effects that may be immediate (e.g., doxorubicin [Adriamycin] can change urine to an orange-to-red color).
- Teach the family about side effects that the patient will experience after administration of the drug (e.g., bone-marrow suppression and alopecia).

### Interventions

Nursing interventions should be specific to the type of chemotherapy that is administered. Care must be taken to accurately assess and document the occurrence of any side effects, particularly if the patient is a participant in a research study. The following are some general considerations:

- Administer appropriate premedications based on the assessment.
- Monitor and document the effectiveness of the antiemetic regimen and any expected side effects.
- Ensure that the chemotherapy is administered as ordered and that if the patient is given a drug intravenously, the site is carefully monitored for evidence of local irritation or reaction.
- Discuss the potential and expected side effects of the drug, and ensure that the caregiver understands any home care that is necessary after administration of the drug.
- Teach the family to anticipate side effects that may occur days or weeks after administration of chemotherapy.
- Follow the institution's policy for handling chemotherapy wastes, including the patient's body fluids, to protect people and the environment from exposure to the cytotoxic drugs.

### Expected Patient and Family Outcomes

- The patient successfully completes the course of chemotherapy with effective management of side effects.
- The patient, the family, or both understand the home care that is necessary after the chemotherapy.

- The patient, the family, or both are aware of the concerns about bone-marrow suppression after chemotherapy and are able to verbalize the proper steps to take to deal with episodes of fever, bleeding, or excessive fatigue.
- The patient and the family are aware of the resources available to help the patient transition back into the school system, if applicable.
- The patient and the family know when the patient's next follow-up visit is scheduled.

# Guidelines for Safe Handling of Chemotherapy

*Susanne B. Conley*

Nurses who administer chemotherapy should be knowledgeable about the risks associated with repeated exposure to these agents. In 1986 the Occupational Safety and Health Administration (OSHA) published its first set of guidelines for the preparation, administration, and disposal of chemotherapeutic agents. OSHA grouped antineoplastic agents into a category labeled "cytotoxic drugs." However, as drug research increased, OSHA revised its guidelines in 1995 and added a new category of drugs, which it labeled "hazardous." *Hazardous drugs* are drugs that require special precautions because of their potential risk to health (OSHA, 2006). The National Institute for Occupational Safety and Health (2004) reports that health risk is evidenced in studies and that safe levels of exposure to cytotoxic agents have not been determined by a reliable method. A list of drugs that should be handled as hazardous can be found in Appendix A of the Centers for Disease Control electronic document (CDC, 2007). The purpose of these guidelines is to provide recommendations consistent with current scientific knowledge. The recommendations apply to all care settings, such as hospitals, outpatient clinics, physicians' offices, and home-care companies. Research indicates that compliance with current safety guidelines offers adequate protection to healthcare workers who are involved in handling and administering chemotherapy agents or caring for the patients who receive them. However, surface contamination studies demonstrate that engineering controls and handling practices do not prevent release of hazardous drugs into the environment, a finding that has led to the development of closed-system devices (Polovitz, 2004).

With today's rapid expansion of chemotherapy services and new agent development, the need for specialized instruction in the safe handling of cytotoxic drugs has become increasingly apparent. Training new personnel in safe work practices, maintaining up-to-date procedure manuals, and evaluating staff exposure to cytotoxic drugs should be an ongoing standard of practice in all settings where hazardous drugs are handled and administered.

## Classification

Hospitals and clinics use OSHA guidelines as a basis for developing their own policies for administration and disposal of cytotoxic and hazardous drugs. Chemotherapy preparation and administration guidelines must also provide optimal protection for the small oncology office and home-care settings.

The following is a summary of the OSHA recommendations (the policies of individual institutions may differ slightly):
- Staff should wear gowns with back closures, disposable, powder-free gloves that have been tested for use with hazardous drugs, and eye protection during drug preparation and administration. Double gloves are recommended for the handling of all hazardous drugs. The inner glove cuff should be under the gown cuff and the outer glove cuff should cover the gown cuff. Use of a closed-system device is recommended to prevent aerosolization during preparation and administration (NIOSH, 2004).
- Intravenous (IV) tubing should have Luer-lock connections and fittings.
- All IV tubing should be primed under a biological safety cabinet (BSC) hood with fluid that does not contain medication before adding cytotoxic drugs, or a closed-system device should be used to decrease exposure risk.
- It is important to remember that oral agents also can cause exposures. The precautions taken with oral drugs should be based on the potential for exposure that exists. For example, a young child may spit out a pill that has been crushed and mixed with liquids. Also, tablets should be crushed only under a BSC hood to prevent inhalation of the dust.
- Potential health risks are associated with biotherapeutic agents.
- Staff should wear appropriate protection to shield them from blood and body fluids for up to 48 hours after chemotherapy has been completed, because patients excrete the drugs in their urine and feces.
- Any unused drugs should be returned to the pharmacy for disposal.
- IV tubing should be disposed of intact as a single unit. Do not remove the spike from the bag and reuse the tubing.
- Gloves and gowns should be disposed of before leaving the room. If either of these items becomes soiled before administration or preparation of a drug is complete, they must be removed and replaced with clean items.
- Soiled tubing, gloves, and gowns should be disposed of in designated containers. These containers must be labeled in accordance with the *Hazard Communication Standard,* as directed by OSHA guidelines.
- Patients' soiled linens, diapers, or emesis basins should be disposed of in the same manner as other equipment and materials if the patient has received chemotherapy within the previous 48 hours.
  - Wash hands thoroughly before and after handling or administering hazardous drugs.
  - Use detergent and water to clean surfaces that have been in contact with hazardous drugs (Polovich, 2004).

## Nursing Assessment and Interventions

### Assessment
- Review the institution's policies before handling or administering cytotoxic or hazardous drugs.

### Interventions
- Prepare protective equipment before entering the patient's room and be aware of cleanup procedures and the location of spill kits.

- Prepare patients and their families for precautions that staff will take before entering their room, such as wearing protective equipment. It can be frightening for them to see staff enter wearing a gown, gloves, and eye gear.
- Prepare patients and their families for home administration of chemotherapy. Caregivers in the home should be given written instructions and personal protective equipment whenever there is a risk that cytotoxic drugs could be released into the environment. Prescriptions for chemotherapy gloves, masks, and spill kits should be given to patients and parents as appropriate.
- Home-care providers and caretakers should be instructed to do the following:
  - Dispose of unused agents in designated containers labeled *hazardous*.
  - Use a designated workplace for handling cytotoxic agents.
  - Work below eye level.
  - Use detergent and water to wash surfaces that come into contact with cytotoxic drugs.
  - Institute universal precautions when handling the blood, vomitus, or excreta of a patient who has received chemotherapy within the previous 48 hours.

## Expected Patient and Family Outcome
Chemotherapy is administered safely and in accordance with OSHA and NIOSH guidelines.

### References
Centers for Disease Control and Prevention (CDC). (2007). *Preventing Hazardous Exposure to Antineoplastic and Other Drugs in Healthcare Settings.* Retrieved May 26, 2008, from www.cdc.gov/niosh/docs/2004-165.

National Institute for Occupational Safety and Health. (2004). *Preventing occupational exposure to antineoplastic and other hazardous drugs in health care settings.* Retrieved September 5, 2007, from www.cdc.gov/niosh/docs/2004-165.

Occupational Safety and Health Administration (OSHA). (2006). *Safety and Health Topics: Hazardous Drugs.* Retrieved May 26, 2008, from www.osha.gov/SLTC/hazardousdrugs/index.html.

Polovich, M. (2004). *Safe handling of hazardous drugs.* Retrieved September 5, 2007, from www.nursingworld.org/ojin/topic25/tpc25_5.htm.

# Administration of Vesicants

*Linda Madsen*

## Definitions
*Vesicants* are agents that have the potential to cause significant tissue injury, including necrosis, if they leak outside of the vascular space. An irritant drug can cause an inflammatory reaction with aching, burning, tightness, pain, and phlebitis at the insertion site or along the vein, but it does not have the potential to cause tissue destruction. Extravasation is the inadvertent administration of a fluid into the tissue surrounding the vascular space.

Extravasation of a vesicant can result in reactions that vary from mild redness and burning to pain, inflammation, tissue necrosis, and cellulitis. The degree of damage depends on the type, dilution, and amount of the agent extravasated. The risk of extravasation is minimized by the proper use of central and peripheral access devices.

Vesicants are categorized as either deoxyribonucleic acid (DNA)-binding or non-DNA-binding.

### DNA-Binding Agents
DNA-binding agents (e.g., anthracyclines), cause ongoing damage by producing free radicals that bind to cellular DNA, causing the drug to be taken up by additional healthy cells. Minimizing dilution and applying a cold compress to the extravasation site can help contain the damage. The full extent of the injury may not be known for days or weeks. Anthracyclines are the most potent vesicants and tend to cause the most significant injuries.

### Non-DNA-Binding Agents
The non-DNA-binding agents (e.g., vinca alkaloids, taxanes) cause much less damage than DNA-binding agents because the injury is confined to the tissues directly affected at the time of the extravasation. Ideally, when these agents extravasate, diluting and diffusing the drug by administering heat and the appropriate antidote is best.

Although a list of agent-specific antidotes has been developed for use in the event of extravasation, well-controlled research on the effectiveness of such antidotes has been marginal at best.

## Role in Childhood Cancer
Vesicants are an integral part of most systemic-therapy protocols because of their effectiveness against a wide variety of malignancies. Careful administration is key to their safe use.

## Classifications and Method of Delivery
Prevention is the best way to avoid extravasation of these agents. Preventive measures include the following:

- Chemotherapy should be administered only by nurses specifically trained to do so.
- Central venous lines are the preferred route for administering vesicants. It is highly recommended, and in some institutions required, that all infusions of vesicants be done using a central venous catheter. Extravasation can still occur because of catheter migration, a break in the line, malposition of the needle, or backflow caused by formation of a fibrin sheath or thrombosis.
- When peripheral access is used, careful site selection is key. Ideally, the vessel chosen has adequate blood flow, and a plastic catheter type of IV has been newly placed and is in an area that allows stabilization of the catheter during administration. Vessels overlying joints and ligaments should be avoided. Vessels with sclerosis, thrombosis, or scar formation should be avoided, as should limbs with impaired circulation or sensation.
- The ability to view the site during administration is key, so transparent dressings are essential for allowing complete visualization of the site.

# Section IV Childhood Cancer Treatment

## Two-Syringe Technique
This technique involves choosing and accessing the appropriate site, flushing with 3–5 ml of normal saline (NS), and assessing blood return and signs of infiltration. After adequate access has been established, the NS syringe is removed and the chemotherapy syringe is attached. The drug is injected slowly while checking for blood return after each 1–2 cc of injected drug, then an additional 3–5 cc of the drug is injected and flushed with saline. A continuous push-pull technique can be used throughout the administration.

## Side-Arm Technique
IV access is obtained as described above. Free-flowing IV fluids are connected to the catheter, and assessment for blood return is made by pinching off the tubing. While the IV fluids are being infused, the drug is injected into the IV line via a side port and then flushed with saline. Assessment for blood return is made throughout administration by pinching the tubing.

If extravasation is suspected, infusion should be stopped immediately. Generally the patient will complain of pain and burning, and slight infiltration close to the site might be seen. The antidote that is chosen is based on the drug classification. **Table 4-6** provides a summary of the available antidotes and a description of how to administer them.

## Nursing Assessment and Interventions
### Assessment
- Assess IV access for patency just before administration. (For a peripheral IV, establishment of a new IV should be strongly considered.) Patency is checked by assessing blood return throughout the administration of the vesicant. If there is no blood return but the IV flushes well, a vesicant should not be given. The institution's policy for assessing a blocked catheter should be followed.
- Ask the patient, to communicate any pain, burning, or other discomfort experienced during or after administration of the drug. Encourage quiet activity during the administration of vesicants.

### Table 4-6. Vesicant and Irritant Agents and Interventions for Extravasation

**Vesicants**

| Drug Name | Temperature | Intervention |
|---|---|---|
| Cisplatin  If more than 20 mL extravasated or concentration greater than 0.5 mg/mL | Cold | Sodium thiosulfate |
| Carboplatin  If concentration greater than 0.5 mg/mL | Cold | Sodium thiosulfate |
| Dactinomycin | Cold | |
| Daunorubicin (anthracycline*) | Cold | Dexrazoxane |
| Doxorubicin | | |
| Epirubicin | | |
| Idarubicin | | |
| Mitoxantrone | | |
| *Liposomal anthracyclines require only cold applications. No antidote is needed. | | |
| Mitomycin | Cold | DMSO |
| Mechlorethamine (Nitrogen Mustard) | Cold | Sodium thiosulfate |
| Oxaplatin | Warm | Sodium thiosulfate |
| Paclitaxel | Cold | Hyaluronidase |
| Vinblastine | Warm | Hyaluronidase |
| Vincristine | | |
| Vinorelbine | | |

**Irritants**

| Drug name | Temperature | Intervention |
|---|---|---|
| Cisplatin  If less than 20 mL extravasated or concentration less than 0.5 mg/mL | Cold | Increasing the diluent and slowing the infusion rate can decrease the pain of irritant agents. |
| Carboplatin  If concentration is less than 0.5 mg/mL | Cold | Same as Cisplatin |
| Dacarbazine | Cold | Same as Cisplatin |
| Etoposide | Warm | Same as Cisplatin |
| Ifosfamide | Cold | Same as Cisplatin |

- Constantly observe the site for redness, swelling, or loss of blood return during IV-push administration. For continuous infusions, assess the site at least hourly and check blood return every 4 hours.
- Be especially aware of patients who are unable to communicate pain, those who have a decreased level of consciousness, or those who are sedated.
- Assess the patient for late signs of extravasation, such as blistering, erythema, ulceration, or sloughing.

### Interventions
- Stop the administration of a vesicant immediately if any burning, swelling, tenderness, loss of blood return, or local redness develops. Do not remove the needle and do not flush the line.
- Notify a provider immediately if extravasation is suspected or occurs.
- Obtain needed supplies for extravasation and follow the institution's policy on extravasation.
- Attempt to withdraw 3–5 mL of fluid from site.
- Apply heat or a cold compress and appropriate antidote as indicated. A separate IV may be needed to administer the antidote.
- Elevate the involved extremity if appropriate.
- Assess anthracycline extravasation using a Wood's lamp initially and throughout the next few days. Illumination with a Wood's lamp identifies the extent of spread of the anthracycline. Document the extravasation per institution policy.
- Early evaluation by a plastic surgeon should be strongly considered in the event of an anthracycline extravasation.

### Expected Patient and Family Outcomes
- The patient has minimal complications related to extravasation.
- The family understands the home interventions needed after extravasation and the importance of follow-up.
- The family reports any changes to the site after vesicant administration.

## Surgery

*Carol Rossetto*

Surgery in combination with chemotherapy or radiation is an important component of a multidisciplinary treatment approach to childhood cancer.

### Principles of Treatment
Surgical treatment of childhood cancer is indicated for the following reasons:
- Diagnostic biopsy
- Staging and "second-look" procedures
- Complete resection of tumor
- Debulking of tumors that are not fully resectable
- Debridement of necrotic tissue
- Many surgical procedures can be done with minimally invasive techniques.
- Complications (e.g., obstruction, infection, bleeding)
- Palliation of symptoms
- Supportive care, such as long-term venous access or gastrostomy tubes for nutritional support.

### Types and Classification of Surgeries

#### Biopsies
Biopsies include fine-needle aspirations, Tru-Cut needle biopsies for larger tissue specimens, and open procedures to remove entire lymph nodes and sections of tumor tissue, especially when material is required for molecular studies.

#### Staging
Staging is indicated when treatment depends on the location of the cancer and the extent of disease involvement. Second-look procedures are used to assess a patient's response to nonsurgical treatment.

#### Complete Resection
A resection is indicated for tumors that can be fully removed without compromising vital structures. This may be done before chemotherapy, radiation, or both, or during the course of these therapies. Tumors such as rhabdomyosarcomas have higher cure rates when resection includes "clean" margins that are free of tumor. Resection in a limb may be done to salvage the limb or to amputate it; although in pediatrics, amputation is avoided whenever possible.

#### Debulking
Debulking involves removing a portion of the tumor mass when it is not possible to remove more than 90% of the mass. This may be done as a first-line therapy or after several courses of chemotherapy or radiation.

#### Minimally Invasive Surgery
Minimally invasive surgery allows for good visualization of the tumor without the need for open surgery. Several small incisions (less than 1 inch in diameter) are made, and an endoscope is passed through these incisions, along with instruments that are manipulated to achieve resection or debulking of smaller wounds. There is a quicker recovery time, which allows for an earlier initiation of therapy in selected cases. Thorascopic and laparoscopic techniques are examples of minimally invasive surgeries.

#### Surgery for Complications
This type of surgery may be done to decompress structures such as the bowel, bladder, or spinal cord. Surgery also may be needed to stop bleeding or to treat pericardial tamponade.

#### Debridement
*Debridement* is the removal of necrotic tissue that impairs wound healing.

#### Palliation
Palliative surgery is performed to relieve the symptoms caused by tumors that have been unresponsive to medical therapy. It also may be done to relieve pain and bleeding.

#### Placement of Venous Access Devices
Surgery may be performed to place tunneled external catheters or implanted venous access devices.

### Upper Gastrointestinal (GI) Endoscopy/Colonoscopy

Used for evaluating the gastrointestinal tract, obtaining a biopsy for diagnosis, or screening to evaluate those at risk for early-onset colorectal cancer following total body irradiation or radiation.

### Robotics

Integration of mechanical engineering and computers has allowed the development of robotic surgery. This type of surgery has enabled the performance of complex minimally invasive surgeries. The application of robotics to minimally invasive surgery may be part of the future of surgical practice.

## Method of Delivery

Surgery in children is almost always performed under general anesthesia to ensure the safety and comfort of the child during the procedure. Exceptions include a mediastinal mass with compression of the trachea or a vena cava, for which general anesthesia would be dangerous. In cases such as these, a combination of local anesthesia, sedation, and positioning are used instead to maintain and protect the airway and venous return while promoting comfort. In older patients, local anesthesia may suffice for line placement or superficial biopsies. Outpatient anesthesia is increasingly used for some procedures.

## Preoperative Management

Children should be in the best possible condition for surgery. Their hydration, nutritional status, and electrolyte balance should be as close to normal levels as possible. Hemodynamically, there should be adequate platelets (>50,000 mm$^3$, depending on type of surgery), clotting factors, hemoglobin (>8 g/dl for adequate oxygenation), and white blood cells (absolute neutrophil count >1,000 mm$^3$). Children may receive either intravenous hydration fluids with electrolyte supplementation, if indicated, or total parenteral nutrition. Transfusions of blood products and antibiotics should be given preoperatively if indicated. Additional laboratory and radiologic studies may need to be ordered on the basis of the patient's specific diagnosis. Preoperative planning may include measures such as vaccinations. In the case of splenectomy, vaccines against *Haemophilus influenza* and pneumococcal and meningococcal infections should precede the surgery (by 4–6 weeks, if possible). Patients with pheochromocytoma should be alpha blocked.

Difficult airway problems or a serious condition merits a preoperative anesthesia consultation.

Parental preparation should include obtaining their informed consent, providing an opportunity for them to ask questions, and relieving any anxiety they may have about the scheduled surgery. Children should be given age-appropriate explanations, as well as an opportunity to handle medical equipment and to tour the operating room, if time permits.

## Postoperative Management

### Airway/Breathing

After anesthesia, it is important to protect against postoperative atelectasis. Atelectasis may be evidenced by fever, labored breathing, or decreased breath sounds.

### Fluid Shifts

Patients will experience fluid shifts for the first few days. These are evidenced by facial edema, general puffiness, weight gain, and decreased urine output.

### Fever

Fevers during the first 3 days after surgery are almost always related to atelectasis. Wound infections usually do not occur for at least 5 days after surgery.

### Tube Management

Drainage tubes that function properly promote healing by evacuating fluids that accumulate in operative sites. These fluids can stress suture lines and compress blood vessels that carry nutrients to the surgical site. Tubes are usually removed when the drainage output is less than 20–30 ml per day.

### Antibiotic

Almost all surgical patients have "on call" antibiotics for the operating room. Antibiotics may or may not be ordered postoperatively, usually depending upon the surgery and the structures involved.

### Pain Management

Intravenous or epidural medications are indicated for the first 2–5 days after surgery. Oral medications should be given as needed after intravenous or epidural medications are discontinued.

## Nursing Assessment and Interventions

### Airway/Breathing

**Assessment:**

- Monitor vital signs with close attention to increases in respiratory rate or fever.
- Auscultate breath sounds for rhonchi, rales, or diminished air movement.
- Monitor oxygen saturation.

**Interventions:**

- Use incentive spirometry or bubble-blowing, depending on the age of the child.
- Encourage position changes, early ambulation, and deep breathing and cough.
- Perform chest physiotherapy, as indicated, to help reexpand the patient's lungs and decrease atelectasis.

### Fluid Status

**Assessment:**

- Assess skin turgor, mucous membranes, and perfusion.
- Monitor blood chemistries when large volume of drainage occurs.

**Interventions:**

- Keep accurate measures of intake and output.
- Replace any drainage (i.e., nasogastric tube) as necessary.

### Fever

**Assessment:**

- Auscultate breath sounds for rhonchi, rales, or diminished breath sounds.

- Monitor patients who have compromised immune systems and who also may require blood cultures, a chest X ray, and antibiotics.
- Assess incision for redness, swelling, drainage, or increased tenderness.
  
  **Interventions:**
  - Administer antipyretics as indicated to promote comfort.
  - Administer antibiotics as ordered.

### Tube Management
**Assessment:**
- Assess tubes for patency and irrigate them as ordered.
  
  **Interventions:**
  - Document the amount and characteristics of drainage.
  - Make sure the tubes are well secured.

### Antibiotics
**Assessment:**
- Monitor the serum level of aminoglycosides.
- Watch for evidence of side effects and drug reactions.
  
  **Intervention:**
  - Administer postoperative antibiotics as ordered.

### Pain Management
**Assessment:**
- Monitor pain, judging manifestations according to patient's age.
- Monitor changes in vital signs, especially increases in heart rate, respiratory rate, or blood pressure.
- Monitor the patient for side effects of the administered medications.
  
  **Interventions:**
  - Use an age-appropriate, objective pain-rating system for evaluating postoperative pain and the effectiveness of analgesic and behavioral interventions.
  - Administer pain medication, as indicated, for discomfort.
  - Consider administering pain medication prior to ambulation, a dressing change, or other potentially uncomfortable activities.

### Wound Care
Some surgeries require extensive wound care and management.

**Assessment:**
- Monitor the dressing for drainage and circle the drainage on the dressing.
- Assess the appearance of the wound and document it in the medical record.
- Monitor wound size and granulation of tissue and monitor for any drainage.
  
  **Intervention:**
  - Change the dressing as ordered.

### Education
**Assessment:**
- Assess the learning needs of the patient and the family and adjust the teaching plan accordingly.
  
  **Intervention:**
  - Instruct the patient and the family to report any symptoms of infection.

### Follow-Up
**Assessment:**
- Decide with the family whether home care will be required for home management.
- Ensure that the family knows whom to call in the event of complications or questions.
- Ensure that the patient keeps appointments for follow-up visits.
  
  **Intervention:**
  - Make the appropriate referrals.

### Expected Patient and Family Outcomes
- The patient, the family, or both are confident and can demonstrate the skills required for caring for the child at home.
- The patient, the family, or both demonstrate competence in any required, specialized skills (e.g., for stoma care) related to the child's surgery.
- The patient, the family, or both know the signs and symptoms of fever as well as wound infections and complications and what to do if these should occur.
- The patient's family is able to provide emotional support to help the child deal with fears and anxieties about the surgery.
- The patient's wound heals properly, thus enabling him or her to resume chemotherapy and radiation.
- The patient views the surgery in either a neutral or a positive way.

## Radiation Therapy

*Joy Hesselgrave and Christine Chordas*

### Principles of Treatment
Radiation therapy (RT) uses high-energy particles or waves to destroy cancer cells. Damage is caused by breaking strands of DNA that prevent cell replication. Methods of delivery focus on minimizing injury to normal tissue, but normal cells around the area may be affected. RT is most effective when cells are in the M and G2 phases, are rapidly dividing, and are well oxygenated. Oxygen is essential to the production of the free radicals that lead to the chemical changes resulting in cell destruction. The rate at which a given dose is administered (i.e., the dose rate) and the administration of daily radiation in divided fractions (i.e., fractionation) also influence the response of cells to RT. A fractionated dose of RT is less toxic to healthy surrounding tissue.

### Role in Childhood Cancer
RT is a treatment modality used for many different types of pediatric cancers. It may be used in combination with chemotherapy, biotherapy, and surgery, or alone. Many solid tumors and lymphomas are radiosensitive. RT can be used to prevent central nervous system disease in children with leukemia or lymphoma. RT also may be used emergently to treat tumors that cause superior

vena cava syndrome, spinal-cord compression, or airway compromise, or those that interfere with other vital organ functions. Palliative RT may be helpful for managing pain and other symptoms that are not responsive to medications.

## Radiation-Therapy Planning Process

The RT planning process includes a consultation with a radiation oncologist who evaluates the patient, discusses the side effects of RT, obtains informed consent, and develops a treatment plan. As part of the treatment-planning process, most patients undergo radiation simulation so that the radiation field can be determined. This is done by using computed tomography or magnetic resonance imaging. During the simulation the exact areas to be irradiated are identified and the necessary markings, immobilization devices, and blocks are created. This helps to ensure that the radiation is consistently delivered to the same location at each RT session.

RT requires that children be immobilized for extended periods of time. Intervention from a child-life specialist, a psychologist, or a social worker to provide education, relaxation, and distraction is invaluable for children receiving RT (see Section VI, "Supportive Care"). Young children and children with increased behavioral distress may require sedation or anesthesia and, therefore, may also require central venous access and airway monitoring.

## Methods of RT Delivery

### External Beam
A well-defined, two-dimensional beam of radiation is aimed toward a specific anatomic site or tumor volume. X rays, gamma rays, or electrons are the most common types of external-beam radiation.

### Brachytherapy
*Brachytherapy* is the temporary or permanent implantation of radioactive "seeds" or "pellets" directly into a body cavity, tissue, or skin surface. Brachytherapy provides a prescribed dose of radiation to a localized area. Pediatric applications primarily have been in children who have soft-tissue tumors, retinoblastoma, and central-nervous-system tumors. Brachytherapy may be done alone or in conjunction with external-beam RT as a boost to the tumor bed.

### Conformal
*Conformal RT* is three dimensional, delivering radiation to the contours of the tumor and area to be treated, as identified in the planning process. Radiation is delivered precisely to conform to the affected area, sparing healthy tissue.

### Intensity Modulated Radiation Therapy (IMRT)
IMRT delivers varying intensities of radiation beams by modulating for high and low doses within the same field. The maximum dose is delivered to the target area, while the surrounding healthy tissue is spared. IMRT also can be used to treat multiple sites at the same time with varying doses of radiation.

### Intraoperative Radiation Therapy (IORT)
IORT is delivered as a single dose to the exposed tumor, tumor bed, and surrounding area while the patient is in surgery. This ensures that the patient receives radiation only at the affected site, preserving healthy tissue. The delivery of this single dose has the biologic effect of several daily fractions.

### Proton
Proton RT is a type of external-beam therapy, which uses proton-charged particles that deliver energy over a short distance known as the Bragg peak (Tarbell, Yock, & Kooy, 2006). A low dose is delivered in front of the tumor, and a high dose is delivered to the entire tumor, with minimal exit radiation. The advantage of this type of radiation is that it can be directed to conform to the tumor, minimizing radiation to normal tissue.

### Stereotactic Radiosurgery
Stereotactic radiosurgery delivers a high dose of radiation via a focused beam to a small, well-circumscribed area of tumor. Stereotactic radiotherapy is similar to stereotactic radiosurgery but is carried out over multiple fractions and can treat larger tumor volumes.

## Potential Side Effects

A dose of radiation to an organ may be associated with a relative probability of a radiation-induced complication. This refers to the concept of minimum tissue tolerance dose (TTD). Different organs have variable TTD values. The risk of side effects is also related to the location of the radiation field, the age of the child (younger children are more vulnerable) and adjuvant chemotherapy. In general, acute early and late effects of radiation are limited to the area of the body that is irradiated, can vary with each patient, and resolve after completion of treatment.

The following discusses some of the acute toxicities associated with RT. (For information on chronic toxicities related to RT, see Section X, "Late Effects of Childhood Cancer.")

### General
Some patients experience fatigue regardless of the location of the radiation. Fatigue usually begins several weeks into a course of treatment and can persist for several months after treatment. Myelosuppression can occur, particularly with RT to the pelvis, sternum, and long bones, or when chemotherapy is given with RT.

### Central Nervous System
In general, RT is not recommended for children under 3 years of age because myelination is incomplete at this age, and RT could cause significant neurocognitive and functional impairment.

**Brain:** Headache, nausea, and vomiting may occur. Somnolence syndrome, which can occur a few weeks to 3 months after cranial irradiation, is characterized by a prolonged period of fatigue and slowed mentation. It generally is resolved completely without intervention within 4–6 weeks.

**Spinal cord:** Transient radiation myelopathy can occur 2–4 months after spinal RT. Symptoms are characterized as an electrical, shocklike sensation after neck flexion. The syndrome is usually self-limiting and frequently is resolved without treatment; corticosteroids are rarely used to manage symptoms.

### Digestive Tract
**Salivary glands:** The salivary glands may swell and become painful after the first RT treatment or two. Increased viscosity of the saliva and a decrease in its volume often occur, causing a dry mouth and throat (i.e., xerostomia). A loss of taste or change in taste may occur and can last for months or years. RT to the parotid gland may be accompanied by an elevated serum amylase. Radiation parotitis usually is resolved quickly.

**Dental disturbances:** Decreased saliva and oral bacteria can result in dental caries. RT can also cause small-teeth (i.e., microdontia) and other dental disturbances. The most severe changes are seen in developing teeth.

**Oral mucosa:** Erythema of the oral mucosa occurs at doses of approximately 20 Gy. At doses greater than 40 Gy, desquamation may develop. Regeneration of the oral mucosa occurs about 2–3 weeks after completion of RT. Children who receive head and neck irradiation may experience dental problems, including abnormal tooth formation and early loss of their permanent teeth.

**Esophagus:** Dysphagia and odynophagia occur at doses of 20 Gy. Symptoms usually are resolved 2–3 weeks after RT is completed.

**Stomach:** Acute nausea and vomiting may occur. Ulceration of the stomach can occur with doses of 45 Gy, but this would be an unusual complication of pediatric RT, because a dose this high is rarely, if ever, given.

**Liver:** Hepatic enlargement, tenderness, and elevation of serum liver function can occur. Radiosensitivity of the liver is increased by combination chemotherapy that includes doxorubicin (Adriamycin), dactinomycin (Actinomycin-D), cyclophosphamide (Cytoxan), and vincristine (Oncovin).

**Small intestine:** Nausea and vomiting can occur after RT. Diarrhea and cramping occur after administration of 20–30 Gy of RT. Obstruction of the small bowel, malabsorption, and fistula formation can occur but are usually late side effects (see Section X, "Late Effects of Childhood Cancer").

**Large intestine:** Frequent diarrhea and tenesmus can occur after administration of 25–50 Gy of RT. Persistent proctitis, rectal ulceration, or stenosis are seen with RT doses greater than 60 Gy.

## Pulmonary

Doses of more than 20 Gy delivered to both lungs can produce radiation pneumonitis. This is characterized by dyspnea, dry cough, tachypnea, tachycardia, and radiographic pulmonary infiltrates. The TTD for RT of the whole lung is 20 Gy. The incidence of radiation pneumonitis increases if some types of chemotherapeutic agents are used (e.g., bleomycin [Blenoxane] and dactinomycin [Actinomycin-D]).

## Cardiac

Incidence of radiation-induced heart disease is higher in patients who are given high doses of radiation or concurrent doxorubicin. RT can cause fibrous thickening of the pericardium. Presentation can include pericardial effusion or pericarditis. Onset of symptoms occurs 2 months to years after RT.

## Urinary Tract

**Kidney:** Acute radiation nephritis can occur 6–12 months after RT, and symptoms are similar to nephrotic syndrome (e.g., hypertension, proteinuria). Medical management usually prevents significant complications. Late symptoms can occur and include hypertension, edema, proteinuria, and azotemia (see Section X, "Late Effects of Childhood Cancer").

**Bladder:** Acute radiation cystitis can occur as a result of pelvic RT. This condition is characterized by urinary frequency and pain on urination. With RT doses higher than 60 Gy, urinary abnormalities may be permanent. Because hemorrhagic cystitis is a common complication of cyclophosphamide (Cytoxan) therapy, RT to the bladder is not given concurrently with cyclophosphamide therapy.

## Reproductive Organs

(See Section X, "Late Effects of Childhood Cancer.")

**Testes:** At doses of 1 Gy, patients may temporarily experience low sperm count, and with RT of 4–6 Gy, azoospermia can persist for 5 years.

**Ovaries:** Administered doses greater than 6 Gy may result in sterilization.

## Hematopoietic

Circulating lymphocytes are acutely sensitive to the effects of RT. Even when little or no bone marrow is included in the RT field, the peripheral lymphocyte count can fall. White blood cells other than lymphocytes and platelets are less sensitive; however, the bone-marrow precursors of these cells are quite sensitive. RT to a large area of bone marrow produces significant declines in the circulating blood count.

## Bones

An RT dose of 6–10 Gy results in slow bone growth at the epiphyseal plate. A dose greater than 20 Gy will arrest growth, and hypoplastic changes in muscle and tissue are often more apparent than the alterations in the bone (see Section X, "Late Effects of Childhood Cancer," for a further discussion of this effect).

## Skin

An RT dose greater than 20 Gy produces erythema. Desquamation of the skin is seen at doses of approximately 40 Gy and moist desquamation occurs at 50 Gy. These reactions are resolved within a few weeks after completion of RT. Temporary alopecia develops after doses of 25–30 Gy. Hair regrowth occurs within 3–4 months after RT. Permanent hair loss may occur with high doses of RT.

## Endocrine glands

Changes in endocrine glands are delayed effects (see Section X, "Late Effects of Childhood Cancer," for a discussion).

## Nursing Assessment and Interventions

RT is usually given in daily fractions, Monday through Friday, for consecutive weeks until the entire dose has been delivered. Most RT is delivered on an outpatient basis. Some side effects, such as stomatitis, nausea, vomiting, diarrhea, neutropenic fever, and increased intracranial pressure, may require hospitalization. During hospitalization, the radiation oncologist and the primary oncologist determine whether the patient should continue with RT or should discontinue therapy until the symptoms improve.

When radiation therapy and chemotherapy are administered together, it is the nurse's responsibility to be aware of the interaction between the two treatment modalities and to monitor for side effects. Acute side effects occur within the first 2–3 weeks, whereas late effects occur at least 3 months after the completion of RT.

### Assessment

Side effects experienced as a result of RT are generally related to the site that was irradiated. Assessment should include the following:

- General—coping, mood, tolerance to RT, fatigue, vital signs, weight, pain
- Central nervous system—headache, nausea and vomiting, somnolence syndrome, malaise, fatigue
- Head and neck—mucositis, pain, xerostomia, dysphagia, esophagitis
- Abdomen—liver tenderness, nausea and vomiting, diarrhea, cramping, tenesmus
- Lungs—dyspnea, chest pain, dry cough
- Heart—chest pain, dyspnea, fever
- Genitourinary—urinary frequency, pain on urination, hematuria
- Hematologic—myelosuppression, fatigue, bruising, and bleeding
- Skin—redness, desquamation, alopecia, pruritus, and pigment changes. Hair loss usually occurs at about the third week of RT, and regrowth begins within 3 months of completion of therapy. Radiation recall is a phenomenon that may be seen when chemotherapy follows radiation. The affected skin may have a painless erythematous area where the patient previously received radiation. This effect also can occur when radiation follows chemotherapy.

## Interventions

Interventions are implemented to decrease the specific side effects caused by RT.

**General:**
- Encourage the child to take rest breaks throughout the day.
- Educate the child and the family about well-balanced nutrition during RT.
- Provide psychosocial support throughout treatment.
- Listen to and support the child and the family as they express their feelings about treatment and side effects.
- Treat pain with supportive measures and appropriate pain medications.

**Central Nervous System:**
- Educate the patient and the family regarding somnolence syndrome.
- Encourage the child to rest during the day.
- Recommend earlier bedtimes.
- Assess and treat headaches, nausea, and vomiting with supportive care, appropriate medications, or both.

**Head and Neck:**
- Offer pain medications as necessary.
- Treat mucositis with appropriate oral hygiene, dietary modifications, and mucosal protectants. Antiplaque rinses and antimicrobial agents may be helpful. (See Section V, "Side Effects of Treatment.") For severe mucositis, hospitalization for parenteral narcotics, hydration, and nutrition may be required.
- Offer nutritional supplements with appropriate oral hygiene, dietary modifications, and mucosal protectants. Antiplaque rinses and antimicrobial agents may be helpful.
- Relieve salivary-gland discomfort with moistening agents and saliva substitutes.

**Abdomen:**
- Provide antiemetics for nausea and vomiting.
- Prevent dehydration and reinforce the importance of oral intake of liquids.
- Treat diarrhea by administering fluids and antidiarrheal agents if indicated. Encourage eating small, frequent meals rich in protein and soluble fibers.
- Monitor intake and weight changes closely.
- Provide sitz baths to keep perirectal area clean.
- Instruct patients and families not to use enemas, rectal suppositories, or thermometers.

**Lungs and Heart:**
- Monitor for dyspnea, hacking cough, and low-grade fever, which may indicate pulmonary changes.
- Monitor for pneumonitis, which may require oxygen, systemic corticosteroids, and cough suppressants.
- Teach deep-breathing exercises.
- Report symptoms to the physician.

**Genitourinary:**
- Monitor for urinary frequency, pain on urination, and hematuria.
- Encourage the patient's oral-liquid intake.
- Report symptoms to the physician.

**Hematologic:**
- Monitor blood counts during RT. Monitoring frequency depends on the site being irradiated and whether there is any concurrent chemotherapy. Some patients may require packed red blood cell transfusions during RT to keep hemoglobin above 10 gm/dL.
- Report to the physician symptoms of fever or increased bruising.

**Skin:**
- Observe skin changes closely.
- Prevent infections.
- Emphasize the importance of keeping skin clean and dry.
- Emphasize gentle bathing or showering and patting dry or drip drying.
- All skin-care products should be completely washed off before RT. During RT, use only skin products recommended by the radiation staff, which may include water-soluble moisturizers and aloe vera and lanolin products. After the course of RT is completed, use moisturizers liberally.
- Recommend using sunscreens with a sun-protection factor of 30 and avoiding prolonged sun exposure and tanning beds.
- Address hair loss and use of head covering or wig. After hair loss, recommend protecting the scalp with a hat or scarf.

## Expected Patient and Family Outcomes

- The patient and the family are knowledgeable about RT.
- The patient and the family understand what to expect during RT treatments.
- The patient experiences minimal side effects during RT.
- The patient and the family understand the specific short-term and late effects that may be experienced after RT.

## Reference

Tarbell, J. J., Yock, T., & Kooy, H. (2006). Principles of radiation oncology. In P. A. Pizzo & D. G. Poplack (Eds.), *Principles and practice of pediatric oncology* (5th ed., pp. 421–432). Philadelphia: Lippincott Williams & Wilkins.

# Hematopoietic Stem-Cell Transplantation

*Robbie Norville*

## Principles of Treatment

The purpose of hematopoietic stem-cell transplantation (HSCT) is to replace diseased, damaged, or absent hematopoietic stem cells with healthy stem cells. In general, allogeneic transplants are used if the patient's bone marrow is diseased. The new immune system from the donor also may be effective in preventing a recurrence of disease by providing a graft-versus-tumor effect. Allogeneic transplants also are used to replace damaged or absent cells for a number of hematologic and immunodeficiency disorders. An autologous transplant is used to provide a stem-cell rescue after high doses of chemotherapy or radiation therapy. In some circumstances, autologous stem cells may be used, even if there is a history of disease in the bone marrow. These stem cells are usually treated or purged to remove residual tumor cells before the infusion.

## Role in Childhood Cancer

Children with malignancies may not always be cured with conventional chemotherapy, surgery, and radiation therapy. Increased doses of chemotherapy and radiation therapy, which might prove to be curative, can cause myelosuppression as a dose-limiting toxicity. Infusion of stem cells previously collected from the patient or stem cells from a healthy donor allows the bone marrow to recover after intensive therapy. In addition, patients who have tumor invasion of the bone marrow benefit from the transplantation of healthy cells from a donor. HSCT plays an important role in treating children who have aggressive malignancies in first remission or who have recurrent disease.

## Types of Hematopoietic Stem-Cell Transplantation

- Allogeneic—The stem cells are collected from someone other than the recipient:
  - Matched related—This type involves a 6/6 antigen match (usually a sibling).
  - Mismatched related—This type involves a 3/6–5/6 antigen match (usually a sibling or a parent).
  - Matched unrelated—This type involves a 5/6 or a 6/6 antigen match from an unrelated donor.
  - Cord blood (related or unrelated)—This type involves a 3/6–6/6 antigen match from cord blood.
- Autologous—The stem cells are collected from the recipient.
- Syngeneic—Stem cells are collected from an identical twin (**Table 4-7** for an overview of the advantages and disadvantages for each type of stem-cell source).

## HLA Typing

Human leukocyte antigen (HLA) refers to a complex series of proteins on the surface of human cells. These proteins, called antigens, make up the major histocompatibility complex, which helps the body recognize cells that are foreign. The HLA class I antigens of primary concern for typing include A, B, and C; the class II antigens include DR, DQ, and DP. The DR antigens are among the predictors for the risk of graft-versus-host disease (GVHD). Each individual inherits one set of antigens from each parent. A biological parent is always at least a 3/6 match for the child (see **Figure 4-2** for an example of HLA typing). Historically, approximately 30% of patients have an HLA-matched sibling donor, so the remaining 70% must consider alternative donors. Through the growth and diversity of national and international donor registries, more patients are receiving stem cells from matched-unrelated donors.

### Table 4-7. A Comparison of the Advantages and Disadvantages of Donor Sources

| Type of Stem-Cell Transplant | Advantages | Disadvantages |
| --- | --- | --- |
| **Allogeneic** | | |
| Matched related | Healthy source of cells<br>Easy access to the donor | Some graft-versus-host disease (GVHD)<br>30% likelihood of a sibling match |
| Mismatched related | Healthy source of cells<br>Easy access to the donor<br>Availability of a donor for most patients | Greater risk of GVHD<br>Risk of graft failure |
| Matched unrelated | Healthy source of cells | Risk of GVHD<br>3–6 month waiting time for donor procurement<br>Few ethnic minority donors<br>Expensive donor charges |
| Cord blood | Healthy source of cells<br>Easy procurement of cells<br>No risk to the donor<br>Decreased chance of viral transmission<br>More diverse human leukocyte antigen types | Limited number of cells per unit<br>Increased time to platelet engraftment<br>Potential transmission of genetic diseases |
| **Autologous** | Easy access to the donor<br>No GVHD | No graft-versus-leukemia effect (increased risk of relapse)<br>Possible tumor contamination |
| **Syngeneic** | Healthy source of cells | Some risk of GVHD |

# Section IV Childhood Cancer Treatment

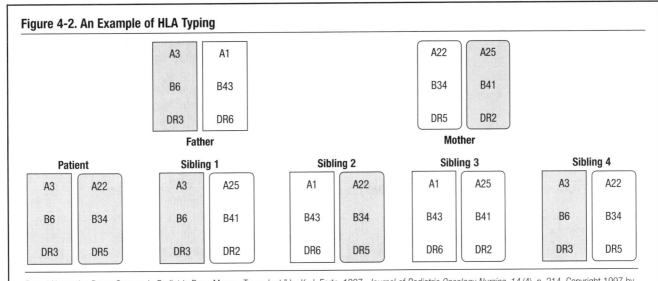

Figure 4-2. An Example of HLA Typing

From "Alternative Donor Sources in Pediatric Bone Marrow Transplant," by K. J. Forte, 1997, *Journal of Pediatric Oncology Nursing, 14* (4), p. 214. Copyright 1997 by W. B. Saunders. All rights reserved. Reprinted with permission.

## Diseases Treated with Hematopoietic Stem-Cell Transplantation

See **Table 4-8** for a list of diseases treated using HSCT and the rationales for treatment.

## Collection of Stem Cells

Stem cells are the immature progenitor cells that mature in the bone marrow. Upon maturation, they are released into the circulation as white cells, red cells, or platelets. Stem cells can be collected from the bone marrow or from peripheral blood or blood from the placenta and umbilical cord that is obtained postpartum.

## Bone-Marrow Harvest

Stem cells are removed from the donor's posterior and, possibly, the anterior iliac crest. This procedure is performed under general anesthesia at most medical centers. Cells are mixed with heparin (Liquaemin) and filtered to remove bone chips, spicules, fat cells, and blood clots. One advantage is that this is a relatively quick and well-tested method of collection. The risks to the donor are associated with general anesthesia, infection, and mild-to-moderate pain at the harvest site.

## Peripheral Stem-Cell Collection

Stem cells are collected through a large catheter by an apheresis machine, which selects the stem cells from the circulating blood on the basis of weight. The remaining cells are reinfused into the patient. Stem cells are mobilized into the peripheral blood circulation through the use of granulocyte colony-stimulating factors, granulocyte-macrophage colony-stimulating factors, or high-dose priming chemotherapy, such as cyclophosphamide (Cytoxan) (for autologous patients only). The stem cells are then mixed with heparin (Liquaemin) and a preservative before being frozen (cryopreservation).

The advantages of this collection method are that there is no need for general anesthesia for the donor, engraftment is faster, and there is presumed to be a decreased risk of tumor contamination compared with autologous marrow harvest. The risks to

## Table 4-8. Diseases for Which Hematopoietic Stem-Cell Transplantation (HSCT) Is a Treatment Option

| Disease | Rationale for HSCT |
|---|---|
| Leukemias, lymphomas | Chemotherapy, with or without total body irradiation, is used to eradicate tumor cells and to make room for engraftment of healthy cells. Irradiation is often used in mismatched and unrelated transplants. |
| Solid tumors: neuroblastoma, sarcoma, brain tumor | High doses of chemotherapy or radiation therapy are given to kill tumor cells. An autologous "rescue" is given to prevent prolonged myelosuppression. |
| Hematologic diseases: thalassemia, sickle-cell disease, severe aplastic anemia, Fanconi anemia | Chemotherapy is given to eradicate cells in the bone marrow and to make space for engraftment of healthy allogeneic cells. The new donor cells will produce normal white cells, red cells, and platelets. |
| Immunodeficiency diseases: Wiskott-Aldrich syndrome, severe combined immunodeficiency syndrome (SCIDS) | Chemotherapy is given to eradicate cells in the bone marrow and to make space for engraftment of healthy allogeneic cells. In the case of SCIDS, chemotherapy may not always be used. |
| Genetic diseases: adrenoleukodystrophy, metachromatic leukodystrophy, Hurler's syndrome | Chemotherapy is given to eradicate cells in the bone marrow. Donor cells, which will eventually produce the deficient enzyme, are infused. |

the donor are associated with bone pain as a consequence of growth-factor administration, reaction to citrate (i.e., numbness and tingling in the fingers and lips or hypotension) during collection, and catheter placement.

## Cord-Blood Collection
Stem cells are collected from a newborn's cord and placenta immediately after birth. The advantages of this practice are quick and easy collection, decreased chance of transmission of viral disease, and less GVHD; however, engraftment may be slower. There is no risk to the donor.

## Stem-Cell-Product Purging and T-Cell Depletion

### Purpose
The purpose of stem-cell purging is to remove any remaining tumor cells before autologous stem-cell transplantation. The purpose of T-cell depletion is to decrease the number of T lymphocytes to help lower the risk of GVHD before allogeneic stem-cell transplantation. The purpose of CD34+ (very young stem cells that are not lymphocytes) selection is to collect specific progenitor cells for infusion in either autologous or allogeneic stem-cell transplantation.

### Methods
**Immunologic technique:** A monoclonal antibody specific for a type of tumor or T lymphocytes is added to the stem-cell product.

**Pharmacological technique:** A chemotherapeutic analog is added to the stem-cell product to kill any remaining tumor cells. An example is 4HC, a derivative of cyclophosphamide.

**Lymphocyte depletion:** Lymphocytes are removed through several different techniques. Elutriation is a method that uses a centrifuge to select cells based on size, and anti-T-cell monoclonal antibody induced systemic T-cell depletion is a method in which antibodies bind with and remove lymphocytes. E-rosetting is a technique in which red blood cells from sheep are added to marrow to bind with T lymphocytes. CD34+ stem-cell selection, a method that involves the addition of a monoclonal antibody that is specific for CD34+ stem cells, results in significant T-cell reduction in the final product.

## Evaluation of a Donor and a Recipient

### Evaluation of a Donor
A donor must have healthy stem cells and be able to tolerate the harvest procedure. The usual age range is 4 months to 65 years. Volunteer donor banks may be more restrictive regarding age requirements. The evaluation should include a physical examination, a complete health history to rule out genetic diseases, and serological testing that includes a complete blood count (CBC) with differential, in addition to a chemistry profile, coagulation screen, infectious-disease testing (e.g., hepatitis profile, HIV, cytomegalovirus [CMV], herpes simplex virus [HSV], Epstein-Barr virus, West Nile virus), cross-matching (to determine whether the donor is ABO compatible with the patient), confirmation of HLA typing, and pregnancy test if appropriate. Donors may be asked to donate an autologous unit of blood prior to harvesting. Issues, such as testing procedures, health risks, and psychological sequelae, should be discussed with donors, especially child donors. Consultation with child-life specialists, social workers, and clergy may be beneficial.

### Evaluation of a Patient
The patient should have a more extensive evaluation than the donor. In addition to the items listed for the donor, the patient's work-up should include organ function tests, such as a chest X ray, echocardiogram, pulmonary function test (if the patient's age is appropriate), creatinine clearance/glomerular filtration rate, audiogram (if the patient has a history of hearing loss or has previously received ototoxic agents), an eye exam (if the patient is to receive total body irradiation), and a dental exam. Other serological tests are thyroid function tests and serum immunoglobulins. Disease-staging evaluations depend on the type of disease and previous areas of involvement and include scans, bone-marrow aspiration, and lumbar puncture. Neuropsychological testing may be performed as a baseline for monitoring of late effects. Information regarding sperm banking and egg harvesting should be provided to age-appropriate patients.

## Conditioning (Preparative) Regimens
The conditioning regimen serves the following purposes:
- eradicates tumor cells (malignancies only)
- immunosuppresses the patient to prevent rejection of the graft and decrease risk of GVHD
- prepares the bone marrow space to allow for the growth of healthy cells.

In general, the duration of the conditioning regimen is 4–9 days. The type and timing of therapy offered depends on the patient's disease and the type of stem cells to be infused. Historically, patients transplanted with malignancies have received fully ablative conditioning regimens in which hematopoietic reconstitution would not occur without hematopoietic stem-cell support. Less intensive (submyeloablative) conditioning regimens given with the aim of facilitating allogeneic engraftment have been used in older patients, those who have been heavily pretreated, and patients with significant comorbidities prior to HSCT. The submyeloablative approach relies on the graft-versus-tumor effect to eradicate the malignancy, uses a variety of regimens based on low-dose total body irradiation and fludarabine, and is associated with an increased rate of graft failure compared with fully ablative regimens.

### Chemotherapy
Chemotherapeutic agents are the mainstay of therapy and are used for most HSCT. Commonly used agents include
- alkylating agents such as cyclophosphamide (Cytoxan), busulfan (Myleran), melphalan (Alkeran), and thiotepa (Thiotepa)
- antimetabolites such as cytarabine (cytosine arabinoside)
- nitrosoureas (carmustine [BCNU])
- heavy metals (carboplatin [CBDCA], cisplatin [Platinol])
- plant alkaloids (etoposide [VP-16]).

### Radiation Therapy (RT)
RT is used to eradicate tumor cells in the central nervous system and sanctuary sites, which may not be responsive to treatment by chemotherapy alone. It is also used to provide increased immunosuppression for patients receiving an unrelated or mismatched transplant and to decrease the risk of graft failure and GVHD.

**Total-body irradiation:** This type of RT is usually given in fractionated doses twice a day for 4–5 days.

**Local-control irradiation:** This type of RT may be given before or after a transplant to patients with solid tumors or to patients who have a history of central nervous system disease.

## Immunotherapy

Immunosuppressive agents such as antithymocyte globulin are used to bind with and destroy the patient's circulating T lymphocytes in an attempt to decrease the incidence of graft rejection. Antithymocyte globulin usually is given once a day for 3 days during the preparative regimen. Newer monoclonal antibodies, such as alemtuzumab (Campath) and CD45, are used to deplete the patient's circulating lymphocytes and to try to decrease the incidence of graft rejection and GVHD.

## Infusion of Stem-Cells

Stem cells harvested from bone marrow, peripheral blood, and cord blood can be frozen and infused at a later time.

## Types of Infusion

**Frozen:** Frozen stem cells most often are used in autologous transplants (i.e., transplants in which cells are collected from the patient). Stem cells are frozen or cryopreserved, most commonly with a preservative called dimethyl sulfoxide (DMSO). DMSO has a garliclike odor that is excreted through the lungs of the patient for 1–2 days after the transplant. DMSO can cause transient cardiac arrhythmias, most commonly bradycardia. Many centers require some form of cardiac monitoring during and immediately after the infusion. Rapid intravenous (IV) infusion is recommended. Stem cells should not be irradiated or filtered.

**Fresh:** Stem cells used for allogeneic transplants usually are fresh when infused, generally within 48 hours of collection. However, frozen peripheral blood and cord-blood stem-cell products are becoming more common in the allogeneic setting. The ABO (i.e., blood-group) status and volume of donor cells dictate the need for red-cell or volume depletion. The method of infusion is slow IV infusion over 2–4 hours. Stem cells should not be irradiated or filtered.

## Nursing Assessment and Interventions

**Assessment:**
- Know the potential side effects and adverse reactions associated with each type of HSCT.
  - For infusion of frozen stem cells, the side effects include a bad taste in the mouth, nausea, vomiting, arrhythmia (bradycardia), hypertension, hemoglobinuria, flushing, allergic reaction (anaphylaxis), renal failure, micropulmonary emboli, fluid overload, and infection.
  - For infusion of fresh stem cells, the side effects include anaphylaxis, hemolytic transfusion reactions, fluid overload, micropulmonary emboli, and infection.
- Assess the patient's and the family's understanding of the infusion and monitoring procedures.
- Assess the patient's vital signs before, during, and after the infusion (an electrocardiogram and pulse-oximetry monitoring may be required).

**Interventions:**
Base nursing interventions on the type of stem-cell infusion that is done.
- For infusion of frozen stem cells, patients are premedicated with an antihistamine, an antiemetic, a corticosteroid and/or antipyretic, and diuretic. Prehydration fluids with an added alkaline base are administered 4–12 hours before the infusion. During the infusion, which is administered through a central venous access device, the patient should be monitored for evidence of adverse reactions. After infusion, the patient should be monitored for adverse reactions according to the institution's policy. Postinfusion fluids (12–24 hours after stem-cell infusion) may be infused, diuretics may be administered to ensure renal perfusion, adequate urine output should be maintained, and alkaline urine should be maintained for 12–24 hours.
- For infusion of fresh stem cells, the premedications include an antihistamine, a corticosteroid, and an antipyretic and/or a diuretic, which may be given if there is an ABO incompatibility or if the patient has a history of transfusion reactions. Prehydration fluids are indicated when there is an ABO incompatibility (administer 12–24 hours before the infusion). During the infusion, the patient should be monitored for evidence of adverse reactions, and stem cells should be infused through a central venous access device. After the infusion, the patient should be monitored for adverse reactions according to the institution's policy. Postinfusion fluids should be administered if there is an ABO incompatibility, and brisk urine output should be maintained for 12 hours.

## Expected Patient and Family Outcomes
- The patient, the family, or both can verbalize the infusion and monitoring procedures.
- The patient tolerates an infusion without adverse reactions.

## Complications of Hematopoietic Stem-Cell Transplantation

Complications related to HSCT primarily are due to alloreactivity (e.g., GVHD, graft failure after allogeneic transplant); risk of infections during hematopoietic and immune reconstitution; and toxicities from the conditioning regimen. **Table 4-9** provides a review of the time sequence of complications with HSCT.

### Bone-Marrow Suppression

All cell lines in the bone marrow are eradicated, causing low levels of hemoglobin, platelets, and white blood cells and an absolute neutrophil count (ANC) of or near 0. It occurs 7–10 days after the conditioning regimen is started.

*Engraftment* is the term used to indicate that the new stem cells have taken hold and are starting to reproduce. The timing of engraftment depends on the stem-cell source, the patient's history of prior therapy, and the patient's condition. An ANC of 500 and a platelet count of 20,000/mm$^3$ without transfusions indicate engraftment. In general, white blood cells engraft before platelets. As red cells engraft, the recipient's blood type changes to that of the donor's. The average number of days after a transplant for WBC and platelet engraftment is listed in **Table 4-10**.

### Table 4-9. Timing of Potential Complications Associated with HSCT

| Early<br>(conditioning to engraftment) | Intermediate<br>(engraftment to first 100 days) | Late<br>(after 100 days) |
|---|---|---|
| Bone marrow suppression | Infections | Immunosuppression |
| Nausea, vomiting, diarrhea, anorexia, mucositis | Acute GVHD | Chronic GVHD |
| Parotitis | Graft failure | Infections |
| Infections | Interstitial pneumonitis | Endocrine dysfunction |
| Skin erythema | | Cataracts |
| Capillary leak syndrome | | Disease recurrence |
| Acute renal insufficiency | | Secondary malignancies |
| Hemorrhagic cystitis | | |
| Veno-occlusive disease | | |
| Seizures | | |

From "Hematopoietic Stem Cell Transplant" by R. Norville, 2005, in *Pediatric Oncology Nursing: Advanced Clinical Handbook*, ed. D. Tomlinson & N. E. Kline (p. 207), Heidelberg, Germany: Springer Science and Business Media. Reprinted with kind permission of Springer Science and Business Media.

Note: GVHD = graft-versus-host disease

### Table 4-10. Average Number of Days After HSCT for Engraftment to Occur

| | Average Number of Days | |
|---|---|---|
| Type of HSCT | ANC >500 | Platelets >20,000 |
| Autologous: peripheral blood stem cells | +12 | +21 |
| Autologous: purged marrow | +28 | +35 |
| Allogeneic: matched sibling | +16 | +28 |
| Allogeneic: matched unrelated | +23 | +28 |
| Allogeneic: unrelated cord blood | +28 | +65 |
| Allogeneic: peripheral blood stem cells | +12 | +16 |

*Note.* ANC = absolute neutrophil count; HSCT = hematopoietic stem-cell transplant.

## Neutropenia

The risk of infection is significantly increased when ANC is lower than 500. Measures for preventing infection include air filtration, hand washing, and screening visitors. Isolation policies vary from institution to institution. Prophylactic antimicrobials may be used to prevent herpes, cytomegalovirus, and fungal and bacterial infections.

## Anemia

Transfusions often are given when hemoglobin levels fall below 8 gm/dL. There is a potential for cardiac and respiratory compromise when hemoglobin levels fall below 7 gm/dL.

## Thrombocytopenia

The risk of bleeding is increased when the platelet count is lower than 200,000 mm$^3$.

**Nursing Assessment and Interventions:**
*Assessment.*
- Inspect the patient's mouth, rectum, IV sites, and all wounds for infection.
- Assess for signs and symptoms of infection: dysuria, sore throat, rectal pain, and cough.
- Check the patient's vital signs every 4 hours.
- Assess the patient for signs and symptoms of anemia, including pallor, fatigue, tachycardia, shortness of breath, and dizziness.
- Test the urine, emesis, and stool for blood.
- Assess for bruising, petechiae, epitaxis, or oozing from the patient's gums or the central venous line.
- Assess the patient for signs and symptoms of bleeding or blood loss.
- Check the WBC, ANC, hemoglobin and hematocrit, and platelet count daily.

*Interventions.*
- Initiate precautions against bleeding.
- Call a physician if the patient is febrile or has other signs and symptoms of infection, anemia, or bleeding.
- Administer antimicrobial therapy and monitor the patient's response to treatment.
- Teach the patient, the family, or both how to provide meticulous oral and perineal hygiene.
- Administer red blood cell transfusions and platelet transfusions as needed (Maintain an Hgb ≥8.0 and a platelet count ≥20,000/mm$^3$. All blood products except stem cells should be irradiated and leukocyte depleted).
- Administer oxygen if needed to prevent tissue hypoxia.
- Teach the patient, the family, or both the signs and symptoms of infection, anemia, and thrombocytopenia.

**Expected Patient and Family Outcomes:**
- The patient experiences minimal complications related to infection or blood loss.
- The patient, the family, or both understand the signs and symptoms of infections, anemia, and bleeding.
- The patient, the family, or both are able to perform self-care activities to prevent infection and bleeding.

## Infectious Complications

Infections occur because of the absence of WBCs after the preparative regimen, the use of immunosuppressive therapy to prevent or treat GVHD, and the prolonged absence of donor immunoglobins after initial engraftment. All of the infections listed in **Table 4-11** can occur later, particularly if the patient is treated with immunosuppressive therapy, such as steroids.

**Prevention:** If the patient or the donor is HSV positive, acyclovir (Zovirax) should be administered. If the patient or the donor is CMV positive, a higher dose of acyclovir or valacyclovir should be administered starting the day before stem-cell transfusion; after engraftment of the stem cells occurs, ganciclovir (Cytovene) or foscarnet (Foscavir) should be administered. Controversy exists about the efficacy of immunoglobin (IgG) therapy. Some centers infuse IgG every 2–4 weeks; other centers treat only patients with low IgG levels. Many centers use fluconazole (Diflucan) or low-dose amphotericin B (Fungizone) as prophylaxes for fungal infections.

**Assessment and Interventions:**
*Assessment.*
- Check the patient's temperature every 4 hours and as needed.
- Assess the patient for signs and symptoms of infection every 8 hours.

*Interventions.*
Treatment varies according to institutional policies and sensitivity data.
- Draw blood cultures and start broad-spectrum antibiotics as soon as possible for a first fever; obtain a chest X ray and take a throat or urine culture if applicable.
- Draw blood cultures once a day for subsequent fevers; if the patient appears ill, alter the therapy to provide the broadest coverage. (Patients who continue to be febrile for more than 5 days should be placed on a treatment dose of amphotericin B [Fungizone]. Computerized tomography scanning to assess for areas of infection should be considered.)

**Table 4-11. Infectious Complications of HSCT**

| Types of Possible Infection | Time of Occurrence |
| --- | --- |
| Bacterial (gram-positive and gram-negative) | 2–3 weeks after HSCT |
| Viral: herpes simplex virus | 2 weeks after HSCT |
| Viral: cytomegalovirus | 2–4 months after HSCT |
| Fungal: *Candida, Aspergillus* | 1–2 months after HSCT |
| Protozoa: *Pneumocystis* | 2–4 months after HSCT |
| Viral: varicella zoster | 1–6 months after HSCT |

*Note.* HSCT = hematopoietic stem-cell transplant.

**Expected Patient and Family Outcomes:**
- The patient experiences minimal infectious complications.
- The patient, the family, or both understand the signs and symptoms of infection.

## Gastrointestinal (GI) Toxicity

Nausea or vomiting can begin within the first 24 hours of starting the conditioning regimen and continue through the first week after the transplantation. Vomiting can recur after a transplantation because of antibiotics, infections, GVHD, or slow mucosal healing.

Diarrhea can begin at any time during the preparative regimen and can continue for as long as 2 weeks after HSCT. Causes of delayed diarrhea include infection, refeeding syndrome, or GVHD.

Anorexia can start during the preparative regimen and can continue for several months after HSCT. Causes include a change in taste sensation, dry mouth, damaged mucosa, nausea and vomiting due to the preparative regimen, and GVHD.

Mucositis usually starts by the 3rd day after the HSCT, peaks by the 7th through the 10th day and starts to heal by the 12th day (healing often occurs with engraftment of WBCs).

**Nursing Assessment and Interventions:**
*Assessment.*
- Assess the patient for nausea, vomiting, diarrhea, oral lesions, and pain.
- Check the patient's weight on a daily basis.
- Assess the patient's intake and output during every shift.

*Interventions.*
- Give scheduled antiemetic agents (serotonin antagonists), such as ondansetron (Zofran) or granisetron (Kytril), during the preparative regimen; add steroids for breakthrough vomiting.
- Serotonin antagonists may be discontinued 1–2 days after transplant. Continue other agents, such as benzodiazepenes, as long as needed for nausea and vomiting.
- Administer fluids or total parenteral nutrition as needed.
- Discontinue total parenteral nutrition and start nasogastric feedings if the gut has healed and the patient remains unable to eat by mouth.
- Offer nutritional counseling and supplements.
- Send a specimen for a stool culture if the patient develops diarrhea.
- Promote good oral hygiene, perirectal hygiene, and skin care.
- Administer opioid IV for pain associated with mucositis.

**Expected Patient and Family Outcomes:**
- The patient experiences minimal discomfort due to nausea, vomiting, diarrhea, and mucositis.
- The patient receives adequate fluids and caloric intake.

## Capillary-Leak Syndrome

Tissue damage from the conditioning regimen causes the release of cytokines (e.g., IL-2 and tumor necrosis factor). This, in turn, causes increased capillary permeability, which can lead to weight gain, fluid retention, ascites, or pulmonary edema. The highest risk for its occurrence is 7–14 days after HSCT.

**Nursing Assessment and Interventions:**
*Assessment.*
- Assess the patient for signs and symptoms of fluid overload (e.g., intake greater than output, weight gain, high blood pressure, "wet lungs").

*Interventions.*
- Notify a physician if the patient has signs and symptoms of fluid overload.
- Administer diuretics as needed.
- Administer a renal dose of dopamine (Intropin) to increase renal perfusion.

**Expected Patient and Family Outcome:**
- The patient experiences minimal complications associated with capillary leak syndrome.

## Veno-Occlusive Disease

The conditioning regimen and previous liver damage may cause the veins of the liver to become narrow and fibrotic, which can lead to obstruction of blood flow, liver enlargement, and ascites. Risk factors include preexisting liver disease, intensity of conditioning regimen, use of RT, and pretransplant fever. The classic presentation of veno-occlusive disease includes elevated bilirubin, 5% weight gain, and painful hepatomegaly, which can progress to ascites and encephalopathy. It occurs 7–21 days after HSCT. Management is supportive with careful fluid management. Debibrotide with fibrinolytic, antithrombotic, and anti-ischemic properties has shown promising results in investigational studies. It has been suggested that this syndrome be renamed *sinusoidal syndrome*.

**Nursing Assessment and Interventions:**
*Assessment.*
- Measure strictly the patient's intake and output.
- Assess the patient's weight and abdominal girth twice each day.
- Check the patient's liver- and kidney-function studies.
- Assess the patient for evidence of ascites, pain in the right-upper quadrant, and jaundice.
- Check the platelet count and other coagulation studies (e.g., coagulation profile, antithrombin III [ATIII] level) as needed. (The use of anticoagulants is controversial. Some centers advocate the replacement of ATIII if the serum level is low.)

*Intervention:*
Administer diuretics and pain medications as needed.

**Expected Patient and Family Outcomes:**
- The patient has minimal complications associated with veno-occlusive disease.
- The patient has adequate pain control.
- The patient and family understand the signs and symptoms and the management of veno-occlusive disease.

## Graft Failure

Primary graft failure can occur if the stem-cell dose is too low or if the patient's immune system has not been completely ablated, thereby allowing the body to recognize the donor cells as foreign. Other causes of graft failure include myelosuppressive medications, viral or fungal infections, or recurrence of tumor.

Primary graft failure occurs within the first 100 days after HSCT. Secondary graft failure can occur within 1 year of HSCT. The purpose of administration of immunosuppressants prior to HSCT is to prevent graft failure. To treat graft failure, another infusion of donor cells can be administered with or without additional immunosuppression.

**Nursing Assessment and Interventions:**
*Assessment.*
Check the CBC with a differential on a daily basis.

*Interventions.*
- Provide supportive care measures to prevent or treat infection.
- Help the patient and the family identify coping strategies if engraftment does not occur.

**Expected Patient and Family Outcome:**
The patient experiences minimal complications throughout the period of pancytopenia.

## Acute Graft-Versus-Host Disease

*Acute graft-versus-host disease* (AGVHD) is an immune-mediated response in which the immunocompetent donor T-cells recognize the recipient antigens as foreign and mount an attack. This results from the alloreactivity between the donor and recipient as the donor T-lymphocytes recognize antigen disparities. The onset of AGVHD occurs within the first 100 days after HSCT; it usually coincides with engraftment. The donor cells recognize the patient's body as foreign and mount an attack. The target organs include the skin, liver, and gut. A red maculopapular rash typically starts on the palms and soles and spreads down from the head to the trunk and, lastly, down the lower extremities. A severe rash includes blister formation and desquamation. An elevated bilirubin count indicates liver involvement. Watery, green diarrhea that contains pieces of bowel tissue is most characteristic of gut involvement (see **Table 4-12** for staging and grading).

Preventive measures include administration of agents such as cyclosporine (Sandimmune), tacrolimus (Prograf), methotrexate (Mexate), steroids, or monclonal antibodies. T-cell depletion prior to stem-cell infusion may also prevent or limit AGVHD.

**Nursing Assessment and Interventions:**
*Assessment.*
- Assess the patient for clinical signs and symptoms of AGVHD (e.g., skin rash, diarrhea, abdominal pain, and elevated bilirubin).
- Measure strictly the patient's intake and output and assess the patient's fluid and electrolyte status if he or she has diarrhea.
- Assess the patient for right-upper quadrant pain, diffuse abdominal pain, and generalized skin pain.

*Interventions.*
- Prepare the patient and the family for the patient's skin or rectal biopsy (the patient may also need an endoscopy).
- Administer immunosuppressive therapy. First-line therapy is usually administration of high-dose steroids. Second-line therapy varies according to institutional priorities. (See **Table 4-13** for the mechanisms of action and the toxicities of immunosuppressive agents used to prevent and treat AGVHD.)
- Provide symptom management for skin AGVHD, including the use of hypoallergenic skin moisturizers, gel dressings, or porcine dressings for severe desquamation.
- Provide adequate pain control.
- Teach the patient and the family about the signs, symptoms, and treatment associated with AGVHD.
- Teach the patient and the family self-care measures for controlling symptoms.

### Table 4-12. Graft-Versus-Host Disease (GVHD) Stage and Grading Systems

**Staging of Individual Organ System(s)**

| Organ | Stage | Description |
| --- | --- | --- |
| Skin | +1 | Maculopapular (M-P) eruption over <25% of body area |
|  | +2 | Maculopapular eruption over 25%–50% of body area |
|  | +3 | Generalized erythrodema |
|  | +4 | Generalized erythrodema with bullous formation and often with desquamation |
| Liver | +1 | Bilirubin 2.0–3.0 mg/dl; SGOT 150–750 IU |
|  | +2 | Bilirubin 3.1–6.0 mg/dl |
|  | +3 | Bilirubin 6.1–15.0 mg/dl |
|  | +4 | Bilirubin >15.0 mg/dl |
| Gut | +1 | Diarrhea >30 ml/kg or >500 ml/day |
|  | +2 | Diarrhea >60 ml/kg or >1,000 ml/day |
|  | +3 | Diarrhea >90 ml/kg or >1,500 ml/day |
|  | +4 | Diarrhea >90 ml/kg or >2,000 ml/day; or severe abdominal pain and bleeding with or without ileus |

**Overall Grading of Acute GVHD**

| Grade | Skin Staging | Liver Staging | | Gut Staging |
| --- | --- | --- | --- | --- |
| I | +1 to +2 | 0 | | 0 |
| II | +1 to +3 | +1 | and/or | +1 |
| III | +2 to +3 | +2 to +4 | and/or | +2 to +3 |
| IV | +2 to +4 | +2 to +4 | and/or | +2 to +4 |

Adapted from material in *Graft-versus-host disease* (2nd ed.), by N. J. Chao, 1999, Austin, TX: R. G. Landes.

**Expected Patient and Family Outcomes:**
- The patient experiences minimal complications associated with AGVHD.
- The patient and the family can identify the signs and symptoms associated with AGVHD and its treatment.
- The patient and the family can describe self-care measures for symptom control.

## Chronic Graft-Versus-Host Disease

*Chronic graft-versus-host disease* (CGVHD) is a chronic autoimmune syndrome that resembles collagen vascular disease. Like AGVHD, it targets the skin, liver, and GI tract. The symptoms include dry eyes and mouth, oral ulcerations, hair loss, brittle nails, thin skin with lichenoid and sclerodermatous changes, weight loss, malabsorption of food, elevated liver enzymes and bilirubin, obstructive lung disease, contractures, immunosuppression, and thrombocytopenia. CGVHD can occur from 100 days to 2 years after BMT. Although CGVHD can occur de novo, it often occurs in patients with previous AGVHD. Risk factors for development of CGVHD include prior AGVHD, donor-recipient HLA disparity, and increased patient age.

Treatment consists of immunosuppressant therapy that includes many of the same agents used to treat AGVHD. Most patients are treated with cyclosporine (Sandimmune) or tacrolimus (Prograf) and steroids that are tapered slowly over several months. Several new agents are now available for the treatment of CGVHD (**Table 4-13**).

**Nursing Assessment and Interventions:**
*Assessment.*
- Assess the patient for clinical manifestations of CGVHD.
- Assess the patient's nutritional status.
- Assess for evidence of infection or bleeding (particularly if the patient is taking steroids).
- Check the patient's CBC and electrolytes as needed.

*Interventions.*
- Administer immunosuppressive therapy and monitor the side effects.
- Maintain measures to prevent infection.
- Use products to lubricate the patient's eyes and mouth as needed.
- Teach the patient and the family to apply skin moisturizers and protect the patient's skin from sunlight; emphasize the need to use sunscreen.
- Teach the patient and the family the signs and symptoms, therapeutic agents, and symptom-management strategies associated with CGVHD.

**Expected Patient and Family Outcomes:**
- The patient experiences minimal complications associated with CGVHD.
- The patient and the family can identify the signs and symptoms and self-care measures associated with CGVHD.

### Table 4-13. Immunosuppressive Agents Used in Graft-Versus-Host Disease Prevention and Treatment

| Agent/Treatment | Mechanism of Action | Possible Side Effects |
| --- | --- | --- |
| Antithymocyte globulin (Atgam) | Eliminates antigen reactive T lymphocytes | Fever, chills, hypotension, rash, anaphylaxis, serum sickness |
| Azathioprim (Imuran) | Inhibits synthesis of DNA and RNA | Fever, chills, rash, vomiting, myelosuppression, hepatotoxicity |
| Corticosteroids | Suppresses immune system and inflammation | Myelosuppression, mood swings, hypertension, hyperglycemia, gastrointestinal bleeding, osteoporosis, acne, cushingoid syndrome, muscle wasting |
| Cyclosporine (Sandimmune, Neoral) | Inhibits production and release of IL-2; inhibits IL-2-induced activation of T lymphocytes | Renal toxicity, hypertension, magnesium wasting, hyperkalemia, tremors, seizures, gingival hypertrophy, hirsutism, cortical blindness |
| Daclizubab (Zenapax) | Inhibits IL-2-mediated activation of lymphocytes | Hypertension, headache, diarrhea, vomiting, edema |
| Hydroxychloroquine (Plaquenil) | Impairs complement-dependent antigen-antibody reaction | Ocular toxicity, nausea, diarrhea, rash, headache, myelosuppression, photosensitivity |
| Infliximab (Remicade) | Binds with TNFα | Fever, chills, rash, hypotension, headache, nausea |
| Methotrexate (Mexate) | Inhibits DNA synthesis by competitively binding with dihydrofolate reductase | Renal toxicity, hepatotoxicity, mucositis |
| Muromonab-CD3 (Orthoclone, OKT3) | Modulates T lymphocyte antigen CD3 complex, inactivating T lymphocytes | Reaction to first dose: (cytokine release) fever, chills, diarrhea, dizziness, chest pain, wheezing, tremor |
| Mycophenolate Mofetil (Cellcept) | Inhibits T- and B-cell proliferation, cytotoxic T-cell generation, and antibody secretion | Myelosuppression, abdominal pain, vomiting, headaches, hypertension, renal toxicity |
| Pentostatin (Nipent) | Inhibits DNA synthesis | Fever, chills, rash, vomiting, myelosuppression |
| Psoralen and ultraviolet radiation (PUVA) | Causes apoptosis of T lymphocytes | Tanning or darkening of skin, itching, stinging sensation |
| Sirolimus (Rapamune) | Inhibits T lymphocyte activation and proliferation | Hypertension, diarrhea, peripheral edema, rash |
| Rituximab (Rituxan) | Binds with CD20 antigen on B lymphocytes | Fever, chills, rash, headache, nausea |
| Tacrolimus (Prograf, Protopic) | Inhibits T-cell activation | Renal toxicity, hypertension, magnesium wasting, hyperkalemia, tremors, seizures, gingival hypertrophy, hirsutism, cortical blindness |
| Thalidomide | Decreases the number of helper T cells; increases the number of suppressor T cells | Peripheral neuropathies, constipation, sedation, rash, birth defects |

## Pulmonary Complications

**Cytomegalovirus (CMV) Pneumonitis:** *CMV pneumonitis* is bilateral-interstitial pneumonia caused by cytomegalovirus. The signs and symptoms include tachypnea, cough, and low-grade fever. It can occur 2–4 months after HSCT. Some form of prophylaxis is offered when the recipient or donor is CMV seropositive pretransplant. The prophylaxis may be either ganciclovir IV-form engraftment through 100 days posttransplant or CMV antigenemia monitoring with ganciclovir treatment when virus is detected. Treatment consists of ganciclovir (Cytovene), high-dose immunoglobulin therapy, foscarnet (Foscavir), or cidofovir (Vistide).

**Pulmonary Hemorrhage:** Pulmonary hemorrhage is diffuse bleeding in the lungs that is thought to be caused by the release of cytokines at the time of engraftment. It occurs at the time of engraftment. Treatment consists of platelet transfusions, ventilation, and high-dose steroid therapy.

**Pulmonary Edema:** Pulmonary edema is increased capillary permeability that causes fluid to leak into the lungs. Clinical features include weight gain, fluid retention, ascites, cough, and shortness of breath. It occurs 1–2 weeks after HSCT. Treatment consists of the aggressive use of diuretics; intubation may be necessary.

**Nursing Assessment and Interventions:**
*Assessment.*
- Assess the patient's vital signs and respiratory status every 4–8 hours.
- Send surveillance blood cultures or other studies to the laboratory to test for CMV.

- Check pulse oximetry or a blood gas if the patient is in respiratory distress.
  *Interventions.*
- Administer antiviral therapy, monoclonal antibodies, diuretics, or steroids as needed.
- Administer blood products as needed.
- Administer supplemental oxygen or ventilation as needed.
- Provide anticipatory guidance to the patient, the family, or both, if the patient requires intensive respiratory support.
  **Expected Patient and Family Outcomes:**
- The patient experiences minimal pulmonary complications.
- The patient, the family, or both understand the signs, symptoms, and treatment associated with CMV pneumonitis, pulmonary hemorrhage, or edema.

## Renal Toxicity

**Acute Renal Failure:** Acute renal failure is due to damage of the epithelial cells of the lining of the renal tubules caused by medications that are toxic to the kidneys or by decreased blood flow. RT, immunosuppressive agents, and viruses can cause nephritis. The creatinine and blood urea nitrogen increase, and there is decreased ability to excrete fluid and metabolic waste. Dialysis may be required if the toxicity is severe. Increased incidence is associated with medications that are toxic to the kidneys.

  **Nursing Assessment and Interventions:**
  *Assessment.*
- Monitor the patient's blood chemistries on a daily basis.
- Monitor the levels of medications that are toxic to the kidneys (e.g., cyclosporine [Sandimmune], tacrolimus [Prograf], vancomycin [Vancocin], and amphotericin B [Fungizone]).
- Assess the patient's intake and output during every shift.
- Check the patient's weight every day.
  *Interventions.*
- Adjust the dose and frequency of medications that are toxic to the kidneys, as ordered.
- Administer a renal dose of dopamine (Intropin) to promote renal perfusion.
- Use dialysis if the renal failure is severe.

## Hemorrhagic Cystitis

The primary causes include a metabolite of cyclophosphamide (Cytoxan) that irritates the bladder mucosa and causes bleeding, viruses such as adenovirus and BK virus, and RT. Hemorrhagic cystitis can occur within 24 hours of administration of chemotherapy and as late as several months after HSCT. Signs and symptoms include hematuria (microscopic or gross), urinary frequency, dysuria, suprapubic pain, and bladder spasms.

  **Nursing Assessment and Interventions:**
  *Assessment.*
- Measure the patient's intake and output.
- Test the patient's urine for blood at least once a day.
- Culture the urine for viruses if hematuria occurs.
- Assess the patient frequently to determine whether he or she has pain with urination.
  *Interventions.*
- Administer vigorous hydration (i.e., 1.5 times the maintenance level), and encourage the patient to empty the bladder frequently.
- Administer mesna (Mesenex) in conjunction with cyclophosphamide (Cytoxan).
- Provide continuous bladder irrigation if the cystitis is severe.
- Administer pain medications as needed.
  Expected Patient and Family Outcomes:
- The patient experiences minimal renal toxicity and complications associated with hemorrhagic cystitis.
- The patient, the family, or both understand the supportive care measures used to prevent or treat renal toxicity or cystitis.

## Discharge Planning

General discharge criteria can include the following:
- The patient has an ANC of 500.
- The patient is afebrile and preferably is off IV antibiotics.
- The patient is able to take oral medications (especially immunosuppressant therapy).
- The patient's oral intake of calories and fluids is 50% of his or her caloric need (or the patient is on total parenteral nutrition or nasogastric feedings).
- The family is able to care for the central venous line and any nutritional support that is needed.
- Any transplant complication is resolved or controlled.
- The family understands the discharge instructions, including the purposes of medications and infection precautions.

Parents should receive education about the following issues prior to discharge:
- the importance of calling a member of the transplant team immediately when the child has signs or symptoms of fever, bleeding that does not stop within a few minutes, severe vomiting or diarrhea, change in level of consciousness, breathing difficulty, skin rash, or exudate at the central venous line site
- the importance of communicating the signs or symptoms related to decreased appetite or weight loss; intermittent nausea, vomiting, or diarrhea; mild headache; mild cough; or fatigue at the next clinic visit
- how to take a temperature accurately
- how to care for the central venous line at home
- the importance of protecting the skin from sunlight
- the importance of checking with the stem-cell transplant team before taking medications or immunizations
- swimming, pets, and the child's reentry to school.

## Outpatient Follow-Up

Outpatient follow-up appointments are tailored to meet the needs of the patient. The frequency of clinic visits is based on the type of transplant, engraftment status, and unresolved complications. In general, it is necessary to check the blood counts, serum chemistries, and medication levels (cyclosporine [Sandimmune] or tacrolimus [Prograf]) frequently for the first 3 months after HSCT. Patients who receive an autologous transplant usually do not have to be followed as closely as patients who receive allogeneic transplants, and care may be transferred to the referring oncologist when engraftment has occurred and HSCT complications have been resolved. Patients who receive an allogeneic transplant are followed closely by the HSCT team for the first 100 days, are seen regularly for the first year after transplant, and are seen annually thereafter.

### Significant Tests to Be Done 1 Year After HSCT
- CBC with differential
- chemistry panel
- immunoglobulin levels
- immune-function tests
- thyroid-function tests
- follicle-stimulating hormone, lutenizing hormone, estradiol for girls, and testosterone for boys
- pulmonary function tests
- cardiac function tests
- ophthalmologic examination
- bone-marrow aspiration (if indicated by the protocol or clinical scenario)
- creatinine clearance/glomerular filtration rate
- neuropsychological evaluation.

### Readmission to the Hospital
Readmission to the hospital can occur for any of the following reasons:
- fever
- infection that requires intravenous antibiotics
- new onset or flare-up of GVHD
- active bleeding
- respiratory distress
- uncontrolled hypertension
- uncontrolled vomiting, diarrhea, or dehydration
- alteration in mental status or seizures.

### Late Effects

#### CGVHD
CGVHD is a chronic immune disorder that occurs between 100 days and 2 years after HSCT. Organs that can be involved include the skin, mouth, gastrointestinal tract, liver, lungs, eyes, and vaginal mucosa. It is most common for patients to present with sicca syndrome (i.e., dry, burning, itching eyes), a dry mouth with ulcerations and changes in taste, and skin changes (e.g., dyspigmentation, desquamation, and lichenoid-type changes).

#### Immunosuppression
Patients who have had an autologous or allogeneic HSCT without chronic GVHD have few infectious complications 100 days after the HSCT. Patients who experience chronic GVHD are profoundly immunosuppressed from the disease itself as well as from the therapy used to treat it. Infectious complications can include varicella zoster, CMV, pneumocystic pneumonia, and other latent viruses such as adenovirus and parainfluenza virus.

#### Cataracts
Posterior cataracts, which are usually bilateral, occur in 20% of patients who receive total body irradiation; the average peak onset of formation is 3 years after HSCT. Glucocorticosteroids also can increase the risk of cataract formation. The treatment is surgical removal of the cataracts.

#### Endocrine Dysfunction
Endocrine dysfunction is manifested in the following complications (in general, none of the complications listed occur in children who are treated with cyclophosphamide [Cytoxan] alone):
- thyroid dysfunction—due to increased thyroid-stimulating hormone and decreased thyroxine levels caused by total body irradiation; treatment is thyroid replacement therapy
- growth and developmental delays—occur in most children who receive total body irradiation or steroid therapy or who have GVHD; treatment may include growth-hormone therapy
- ovarian dysfunction—involves more permanent infertility and menopausal symptoms in females who receive chemotherapy after puberty than in those who receive chemotherapy before puberty; total body irradiation may result in primary gonadal failure in females regardless of their age
- testicular dysfunction—includes sterility, azoospermia, and premature ejaculation in males who are treated with total body irradiation; treatment can include hormone-replacement therapy; total body irradiation results in primary gonadal failure in males regardless of their age.

#### Pulmonary Complications
Pulmonary complications can include interstitial pneumonitis, restrictive disease, and, less commonly, obstructive disease. Possible causes include total body irradiation, cytotoxic agents, chronic GVHD, and infectious pathogens (pneumonitis only).

#### Secondary Malignancies
Secondary malignancies are reported to occur at rates up to seven times higher than normal. Possible causes include cytotoxic chemotherapy, total body irradiation, viral infection, high-dose steroid therapy, and genetic predisposition.

#### Recurrence of Disease
Relapse is seen more often in patients who have had more aggressive disease before HSCT. In general, patients with acute myeloblastic leukemia or acute lymphocytic leukemia who receive transplants while they are in remission are reported to have relapse rates of 5%–30%. Those who receive transplants during a more advanced stage of disease have relapse rates of 40%–80%. Unfortunately, the prognosis is quite poor for patients who have relapses, especially those that recur within 1–2 years after HSCT.

## Biologic Response Modifiers

*Robin McCune*

### Principles of Treatment
*Biologic response modifiers* (BRMs) are agents or therapeutic approaches that stimulate the body's immune system to eliminate tumor cells. BRMs include monoclonal antibodies, cytokines, tyrosine kinase inhibitors, and vaccines. BRMs, also referred to as "target therapy," have been added to the three standard approaches to cancer treatment (i.e., surgery, radiation, and chemotherapy) and are recognized as the fourth modality in cancer treatment.

### Role in Childhood Cancer
BRMs are used for the treatment and diagnosis of various pediatric diseases, including cancer. Understanding the characteristics of malignant cells has enabled researchers to develop specific agents that interfere with those unique characteristics. Because

these agents selectively attack targeted pathways and tumor-receptor sites, normal cells and processes are not affected. The end result is fewer associated organ toxicities. However, BRMs have their own set of side effects.

The three major ways that BRMs affect the host-tumor response include modifying the immune response to the tumor, acting directly against the tumor by suppressing tumor growth or killing the tumor cell, and altering other biological activities that can directly or indirectly influence the viability of the tumor. Targeted therapy focuses on cell-membrane receptors, signaling pathways, enzymatic activity, and regulatory cell-growth controls. Many BRMs target the signaling pathway of cells. These pathways are a means of communication within the cell to perform the necessary functions of cell activity, which include survival, proliferation, metastasis, and angiogenesis. When these pathways and receptor sites are blocked or intercepted, communication within the cell is halted and tumor cellular activity ceases.

## Types and Classification

### Monoclonal Antibodies

Monoclonal antibodies (MABs) are immunoglobulin molecules produced for a single clone of cells that bind to a unique target site on a specific antigen. The identification of tumor antigens has provided a new method for diagnosis and treatment of malignancies. More than 20 MABs are available commercially, and many more are in development (**Table 4-14**). Those that have demonstrated some utility in pediatric malignancies include Mylotarg for acute myelogeneous leukemia and rituximab for Non-Hodgkin's lymphoma and Epstein-Barr virus-lymphoproliferative disease. Others (e.g., daclizumab, infliximab, etanercept) have been found useful in the treatment of AGVHD but require further study, and still others (e.g., palivizumab) may prove useful in the treatment of respiratory syncytial virus in immunocompromised patients.

**Use as diagnostic indicators:** Radioactive isotopes can be attached to MABs that aid in the detection of cancer cells. MABs are used to confirm the diagnosis of gliomas and lung, kidney, prostate, and breast cancers. Examples include bectumomab (ImmuRaid-LL2, LymphoScan) for imaging Non-Hodgkin's lymphoma; ibritumomab tiuxetan bound to In-111 (Zevalin) for imaging B-cell Non-Hodgkin's lymphoma; capromab pendetine (ProstaScint) for imaging prostate cancer; Tc-99 oregovomab (OvaRex) for imaging ovarian cancer; and In-111 satumomab (OncoScint) and Tc-99 votumumab (HumaSPECT) for imaging colorectal cancer.

**Use as therapeutic treatment modalities:** MABs can be used alone or with drugs, toxins, or radionuclides. When MABs are combined with radionuclides, they are referred to as radiopharmaceuticals. Radiopharmaceuticals are MABs that have a radioactive source attached to them. Cancer cells have specific and unique antigens on the cell surface that the radiopharmaceutical targets. The patient is given the MAB intravenously, the MAB recognizes the specific protein on the cancer cell and attaches to it, and then the radioactive substance on the MAB delivers radiation to the cancer cell and destroys it. This method of delivery allows treatment to be administered directly to the malignant cells and spares normal cells from the side effects usually seen with chemotherapy.

### Cytokines

Cytokines are nonantibody proteins that regulate the immune response. The cells of the immune system are their primary source, and immunoregulation is their primary function. Classes of cytokines include interferons, interleukins, and the hematopoietic growth factors.

**Interferons:** Interferons are cytokines that are recognized for their direct antiproliferative effects on tumor cells and for their ability to activate natural killer cells. Three classes of interferons exist: alpha interferon (IFN[alpha]) and beta interferon (IFN[beta]) play a more important role as antiviral and antiproliferative proteins, whereas gamma interferon (IFN[gamma]) has more potent immunoregulatory properties. Interferons have subcutaneous, intramuscular, and intravenous (IV) routes of administration.

**Interleukins:** Interleukins are natural proteins produced by macrophages or activated T cells that function as messengers between the cells of the immune system. Interleukins are labeled IL, followed by a number based on the order of their discovery (e.g., IL-1, IL-2, IL-3). IL-2, which has shown clinical activity in patients with renal-cell cancer and melanoma, is under investigation for use in combination with other cancer-treatment modalities. Interleukins have subcutaneous and intravenous (IV) routes of administration.

**Hematopoietic growth factor:** Hematopoietic growth factors are responsible for the differentiation and maturation of blood cells. Hematopoietic growth factors shorten the myelosuppression associated with disease or chemotherapy regimens, can facilitate an increase in the dose and/or the intensity of the chemotherapy regimen, reduce the risk of infections, serve as an adjunct to peripheral stem-cell harvest, and accelerate bone-marrow transplant recovery. They are classified according to the major cell line they affect.

- Epoetin (Epogen, Procrit)—Erythropoietin, which is normally produced by the kidneys, regulates and controls the production and maturation of red blood cells. Epoetin, the synthetic version of erythropoietin, is used primarily to treat chemotherapy-related anemia and anemia related to chronic renal failure. It is administered subcutaneously.
- Darbepoetin alfa (Aranesp)—Darbepoetin alfa is a long-acting form of epoetin used to treat chemotherapy-related anemia and anemia related to chronic renal therapy. A major advantage of darbepoetin alfa is that it has a longer half-life than epoetin and requires less frequent dosing. One disadvantage is that darbepoetin alfa has a higher incidence of subcutaneous pain than epoetin.
- Granulocyte-macrophage colony-stimulating factor (GM-CSF)(Leukine)—GM-CSF is produced by a variety of immune cells and affects multiple cell lineages, including early myeloid, erythroid, and megakaryocytic progenitors. It is also capable of activating mature granulocytes, eosinophils, and monocytes and macrophages. It has subcutaneous and IV routes of administration.
- Granulocyte colony-stimulating factor (G-CSF; Neupogen)—G-CSF is produced primarily by monocytes and macrophages. It increases the number of granulocytes (mainly neutrophils) and also may increase phagocytic activity and antibody-dependent killing. It has subcutaneous, IV, and oral routes of administration.

### Table 4-14. Biotherapeutic Agents Used in Pediatric Malignancies and Hematopoietic Stem-Cell Transplantation

| Biotherapeutic Agent | Classification | Route | Clinical Application |
| --- | --- | --- | --- |
| Alemtuzumab (Campath) | Monoclonal antibody | IV | B-cell chronic lymphocytic leukemia, T-cell prolymphocytic leukemia; investigational for prevention of GVHD in patients receiving hematopoietic stem-cell transplantation |
| Arsenic trioxide (Trisenox) | Differentiating agent | IV | APL in patients with refractory or relapsed APL; investigational for treating AML and CML in patients who have not responded to other regimens |
| Bevacizumab (Avastin) | Monoclonal antibody | IV | Refractory solid tumors; future investigational for Ewing's sarcoma and neuroblastoma |
| Bortezomib (Velcade) | Tyrosine kinase inhibitor | IV | Multiple myeloma, investigational for relapsed lymphoma |
| CH 14.18 Chimeric MoAb Anti-GD2 | Monoclonal antibody | IV | Neuroblastoma |
| Daclizumab (Zenapax) | Monoclonal antibody | IV | Investigational for GVHD |
| Dasatinib (Sprycel) | Tyrosine kinase inhibitor | PO | ALL Ph+ resistance, CML, melanoma |
| Erlotinib (Tarceva) | Tyrosine kinase inhibitor | PO | Investigational for pediatric glioma, AML, and MDS |
| Epratuzumab | Monoclonal antibody | IV | Investigational for leukemia, Non-Hodgkins lymphoma |
| Gentuzumab Ozogamicin (Mylotarg) | Monoclonal antibody | IV | CD+ AML; investigational for MDS and CML |
| Ibritumomab Tiuxetan (Zevalin) | Radiopharmaceutical | IV | Relapsed or refractory B-cell Non-Hodgkins lymphoma |
| Imatinib mesylate (Gleevac) | Tyrosine kinase inhibitor | PO | Ph chromosome + CML; investigational for newly diagnosed CML, Ph+ ALL, recurrent glioblastoma multiforme and peripheral nerve sheath tumors |
| Infliximab Rituximab (Rituxan) | Monoclonal antibody | IV | B-cell Non-Hodgkins lymphoma, B-cell ALL; investigational for GVHD, post-transplant LPD, and immune mediated thrombocytopenia |
| Nilotinib | Tyrosine kinase inhibitor | PO | Investigational for Ph+ ALL and glioma |
| Tositumomab and iodine 131 tositumomab (Bexxar) | Radiopharmaceutical | IV | CD20 positive Non-Hodgkins lymphoma |
| Trastuzumab (Herceptin) | Monoclonal antibody | IV, IM | Osteosarcoma |
| Vizilizumab (Nuvion) | Monoclonal antibody | IV | Investigational for acute GVHD prophylaxis |

*Note:* AML = acute myelogenous leukemia; APL= acute promyelocytic leukemia; CML = chronic myeloid leukemia; GVHD = graft-versus-host disease; IM = intramuscular; IV = intravenous; LPD = lymphoproliferative disorders; MDS = myelodysplastic syndrome; PO = orally.

- Pegfilgrastim (Neulasta)—Pegfilgrastim is the long-acting form of filgrastim. Filgrastim is administered in daily injections, and pegfilgrastim is administered via subcutaneous injection every 3 weeks.

### Protein Tyrosine Kinase Inhibitors

Tyrosine kinases are enzymes that function to catalyze the phosphorylation of tyrosine. Phosphorylation occurs when a phosphate group is transferred from adenosine triphosphate (ATP) to the amino acid tyrosine and is important in signal transduction. Several protein kinases are overexpressed in a variety of cancers. Protein tyrosine kinases (PTKs) provide a molecular on-off switch in cellular signal transduction pathways, as well as a connector that binds proteins to one another. Cellular signal transduction pathways regulate key cell functions including proliferation, metabolism, differentiation, and apoptosis by transferring information from outside the cell into the nucleus of the cell.

PTKs are divided into two main groups, receptor PTKs and cellular PTKs. Receptor PTKs have three domains: (a) a transmembrane domain, (b) an intracellular catalytic domain, and (c) an extracellular ligand-binding domain. The transmembrane domain holds the receptor in the plasma and the extracellular domain binds growth factors. The intracellular catalytic domain functions to induce dimerization (receptor pairing), which enables autophosphorylation of tyrosine residues outside the catalytic domain. This process creates phosphotyrosine docking sites for proteins to transfer signals within the cell. Cellular PTKs are found in the cytoplasm, nucleus, or plasma membrane. Many cellular PTKs focus on cell growth, whereas others are involved in growth inhibition, differentiation, and cell adhesion.

Bcr-abl is a type of tyrosine kinase created by the Philadelphia chromosome, which is overexpressed in CML. Bcr-abl decreases the response to stimuli for apoptosis. Imatinib mesylate (Gleevec) blocks proliferation and induces apoptosis in cancer cells with Bcr-abl genes. Gefitinib (Iressa) is an epidermal growth factor receptor (EGFR) that inhibits signal transduction within the cancer cells and prevents the cells from growing and dividing. EGFR tyrosine kinase is pivotal in the invasion, metastasis, growth, and angiogenesis of nonsmall-cell lung cancer.

Malignant cells are extremely self-sufficient in growth signals. Two important growth factors are the focus of many targeted therapy agents: EGFR and the vascular endothelial growth factor (VEGF). The EGFR is a transmembrane tyrosine kinase receptor that is frequently expressed in many tumors. The signaling pathways of EGFR are involved in cancer-cell proliferation, apoptosis, angiogenesis, invasions, and metastasis. VEGF is an important protein that stimulates angiogenesis and cell migration. When tumors reach 2 mm, they must form their own blood supply to continue to proliferate. They do this through a process called angiogenesis, whereby new blood vessels are formed. Examples of agents that target these growth factors include cetuximab, an anti-EGFR monoclonal antibody; gefitinib and erlotinib, EGFR-specific tyrosine kinase inhibitors; trastuzumab, an antihuman EGFR type 2 (HER2)-related monoclonal antibody; lapatinib, a dual inhibitor of both EGFR- and HER2-associated tyrosine kinases; and bevacizumab, an anti-VEGF monoclonal antibody. Both EGFR and HER2 are targets found on cancer cells, whereas VEGF is a target that acts in the tumor microenvironment. Clinical studies are focusing on how best to incorporate targeted therapy into current treatment regimens that use combination therapy.

## Vaccines

Vaccines are being developed to treat cancer as well as to prevent cancer development. A vaccine's function is to initiate an immune response to foreign antigens. Researchers are looking at multiple strategies for inducing an immune response to cancerous tumors using vaccines. The U.S. Food and Drug Administration has approved only two preventive cancer vaccines, Hepatitis B vaccine and Gardasil. The Hepatitis B virus is associated with some liver cancers. Gardasil has been approved for the prevention of cervical cancer that is caused by a type of human papillomavirus (HPV). Gardasil also protects against infection from a specific HPV type that causes genital warts. There are currently no approved therapeutic vaccines; however, several vaccines are in the investigative stage for follicular B-cell Non-Hodgkin's lymphoma, kidney cancer, cutaneous melanoma, prostate cancer, and multiple myeloma.

## Other (investigational)

Mifamurtide (L-MTP-PE) is a BRM that recently completed a phase III study for the treatment of newly diagnosed osteosarcoma. L-MTP-PE is a synthetic lipophilic molecule derived from a component of the bacterial cell wall that is capable of stimulating an immune response. Once ingested by phagocytosis, L-MTP-PE activates the cell that then seeks out and destroys tumor cells without harming normal cells. It has an IV route of administration.

## Potential Side Effects

### Monoclonal Antibodies
MABs have a high incidence of infusion-related toxicities, including allergic reactions, fever, chills, rigors, malaise, nausea, vomiting, and hypotension. Severe, potentially fatal infusion reactions can occur.

### Cytokines
**Interferons:** The incidence and severity of side effects increase with dosage. They include flu-like syndrome (e.g., fever, chills, myalgias, arthralgias, headache), fatigue and malaise, anorexia, diarrhea, changes in mental status (e.g., poor concentration, somnolence, depression, forgetfulness, irritability), abnormal liver-function tests, neutropenia, thrombocytopenia, skin irritation, and bone pain.

**Interleukins:** The side effects of interleukins are flu-like syndrome (e.g., fever, chills, myalgias, arthralgias, and headache), vascular leak syndrome that involves shifts from intravascular or intracellular areas to extravascular or extracellular areas, skin and mucosal changes, nausea, vomiting, central nervous system changes, and altered laboratory values.

**Hematopoietic growth factors:** The side effects of erythropoietin (Epogen) are hypertension, headaches, fever, myalgia, and rashes. The side effects of GM-CSF are flu-like symptoms (e.g., fever, fatigue, bone pain, myalgias, arthralgias, headache, pain, or erythema at the injection site) and "first-dose" phenomena (e.g., flushing, hypoxia, tachycardia, and oxygen desaturation). The side effects of G-CSF are bone pain, joint pain, fever, rashes, and pain at the injection site.

### Tyrosine Kinase Inhibitors
The incidence and severity of side effects and toxicities vary among patients, doses, and particular agents. Side effects include diarrhea, cardiac dysfunction, skin rash, pruritus, folliculitis, hair changes, paronychial inflammation of nails, hand-foot syndrome, skin discoloration, and hypertension.

### Vaccines
Currently, the only known side effect is soreness at the injection site.

## Nursing Assessment and Interventions

### Assessment
- Know the risks associated with the use of each BRM to assess for side effects.
- Assess the patient's and the family's understanding of the drug to be given and their readiness to learn.
- Assess patient's compliance with orally administered medications.
- Assess patient's knowledge of dosing instructions (e.g., with/without food).
- Assess patient's knowledge of food-drug interactions (e.g., grapefruit juice with warfarin, antidepressants, or antibiotics) and importance of not repeating the dose if vomiting occurs.

### Interventions
- Maximize the safety of the administration of BRMs in patients by taking the following measures:
  - Ensure aseptic preparation and administration.
  - Identify the location of emergency supplies and be prepared to manage a hypersensitivity reaction.
  - Obtain the patient's baseline pulse, respiration, blood pressure, and temperature prior to administration of BRMs and monitor during infusion per protocol.
  - Administer premedications (e.g., acetaminophen [Tylenol], diphenhydramine [Benadryl], and hydrocortisone) when they are warranted.
  - Teach patients and their families about the signs and symptoms of adverse reactions to BRMs (e.g., fever of more than 103°F, shortness of breath) and to report them immediately so that appropriate interventions can be taken.
- Monitor for and know when to anticipate the following complications of BRM therapy:
  - increased pulse rate, orthostatic blood-pressure changes, fever patterns, and critical changes in laboratory values
  - excessive fatigue, weight gain or loss of more than 10% in 1 week, changes in mental status (e.g., confusion, somnolence,

psychosis), chest pain, arrhythmias, hypotension, dyspnea, edema)
  – local inflammation or severe allergic reactions.
- Intervene to decrease the incidence and severity of complications associated with BRM therapy.
  – Encourage measures to maintain skin integrity (e.g., caution when getting out of bed or changing position, application of lubricants after bathing, avoidance of any scrubbing of the skin).
  – Assess changes in mental status at regular intervals, teach the family to monitor for behavioral changes, and evaluate the impact of changes in mental status on the patient's functional status.
  – Administer supportive medical therapy (e.g., albumin, diuretics, fluids, vasopressors) as needed for capillary leak syndrome; instruct the patient to change positions slowly to avoid dizziness; and report decreased urinary output, hypotension, dyspnea, and weight gain of more than 10% in 1 week.
  – Teach the patient and the family essential self-care skills for continuing BRMs after discharge and provide literature on BRMs.
  – Teach strategies for managing any chronic side effects of therapy (e.g., fatigue, anorexia, diarrhea, changes in mental status).

### Expected Patient and Family Outcomes
- The patient and the family can describe the type of treatment with BRMs and the rationale for therapy.
- The patient and the family know the immediate and long-term complications associated with the type of biotherapy and self-care measures to decrease the incidence and severity of the complications of biotherapy.
- The patient and the family demonstrate the self-care skills required for administration of biotherapy.
- The patient and the family can list changes in the patient's condition that should be reported to the healthcare team.

## Cell and Gene Therapy

*Robbie Norville*

### Principles of Treatment
Cell and gene therapies are additions to the current multidisciplinary approach of chemotherapy, radiation, surgery, and hematopoietic stem-cell transplantation (HSCT) for the treatment of pediatric malignancies. *Gene therapy* can be defined as a therapeutic approach to disease treatment that involves replacing, removing, or introducing genetic material into cells. Therapeutic applications include gene transfer (repair), prodrug metabolizing enzyme gene therapy, drug-resistance gene therapy, gene marking, and immunotherapy. Cell therapy involves the administration of autologous or allogeneic cells for a therapeutic effect. These therapies include stem-cell transplantation and strategies for manipulating or modulating the patients' immune status, such as vaccines and adoptive transfer of modified T cells. Even though more than 1,000 clinical protocols for gene therapy have been approved, it remains an experimental approach to cancer that is still in its infancy (Gottschalk, Rooney, & Brenner, 2006).

There are four major approaches to incorporating gene therapy into the treatment of childhood cancers (High & Brenner, 2005):
- The tumor itself can be modified by repairing the genetic defects associated with the malignant process, by introducing a gene that triggers an antitumor immune response, or by delivering a prodrug-metabolizing enzyme that renders the tumor sensitive to the corresponding cytotoxic agent.
- The immune system response to the tumor can be modified by altering the specificity of immune-system cells.
- The drug sensitivity of normal host tissues can be decreased by delivering cytotoxic drug-resistance genes to marrow precursor cells.
- The efficacy of therapies can be monitored closely by "marking" normal or malignant cells to help distinguish the targeted cells.

Successful gene therapy requires the following:
- identification of the responsible gene and successful replications (i.e., manufacturing) of normal copies of the gene
- development of effective methods for inserting the normal gene into a sufficient number of the patient's appropriate cells
- the expression of the inserted gene's normal gene product at a level adequate for treatment of the disease without toxicity or interference with normal cell functioning.

The duration of the therapeutic response to gene therapy depends upon the cell population targeted for gene transfer. Dividing cell populations (e.g., hematopoietic cells, skin fibroblasts) allows modified genes to pass to successive cell generations, thereby producing a long-term therapeutic effect. In nondividing mature-cell populations (e.g., kidney, brain), the effect of modified genes is limited to the life span of the target cells, producing a temporary response that requires repeated applications of gene therapy to maintain a long-term therapeutic effect.

If gene therapy is to become a viable option, it must be accomplished in a manner that is both cost efficient and that yields acceptable risk-benefit ratios.

### Role in Childhood Cancer
The ultimate role of gene therapy in treating childhood cancer remains unclear, though the results of early clinical trials using this approach have shown promise. Future options for cancer treatment likely will involve some form of gene therapy. This therapy should be useful in the treatment of cancer because cancers are the result of genetic mutations or the loss of genetic material. However, like chemotherapy, gene therapy is unlikely to become a cure-all for childhood cancer. Limitations to the widespread application of gene therapy for cancer treatment include limited technical ability to transfer and express new genes in target cells, lack of vector (i.e., carrier) specificity, limited antitumor effect of the transgene (i.e., the gene transferred from one cell to another), and the inability to target every tumor cell.

## Types and Classifications

### Gene Transfer

Gene transfer is the process of inserting one or more genes into a cell. All approaches to gene therapy depend on techniques for gene transfer. There are two gene-transfer techniques:

- *Ex vivo*, or indirect gene transfer, involves a transfer of genetic material to target cells that have been removed from the host and manipulated in the laboratory. After the transfer of the genetic material, the modified cells are reimplanted into the host.
- *In vivo*, or direct gene transfer, is the transfer of genetic material directly to target cells located within the host.

Both gene transfer techniques require a vector that can be used to transfer the required genes into the target cells of the host (see the discussion in "Method of Delivery").

### Somatic-Cell Gene Transfer

Somatic-cell gene transfer is the insertion of corrected or altered genes into nonreproductive human cells. It is the only form of gene therapy approved for clinical trials.

### Germ-Cell Gene Transfer

Germ-cell gene transfer involves the insertion of genetic material into reproductive cells (either sperm or egg cells). Germ-cell gene therapy has controversial ethical and societal implications.

## Method of Delivery

A gene-transfer vector is the mechanism by which the gene is transferred into the cell. The process of introducing a transgene into a cell is called transduction. There are two types of vectors: viral vectors and nonviral vectors.

### Viral Vectors

Viral vectors use the inherent ability of viruses to carry foreign genetic material into cells. The virus to be used as the vector, modified so that it will not replicate, infects the desired cell by introducing the new genetic material into its cytoplasm or genome. If the vector also enters the deoxyribonucleic acid (DNA) of the transduced cell, this information is passed to its daughter cells through mitosis. Otherwise, the new gene (i.e., the transgene) exists as an extra chromosomal episome and is diluted out during cell division.

**Retroviral vectors:** Retroviral vectors are ribonucleic acid (RNA) viruses that convert their RNA to DNA in the cells they infect and then insert their DNA directly into the cell genome (i.e., chromosomes), which contains all of the genetic material of the cell. They require dividing cell populations so that the genetic material can be inserted into the genome of the host cell. The limitations of the use of retroviral vectors are the risk of random insertion of the genetic material into any of the chromosomes of the target cell (i.e., lack of specificity), the risk of insertional mutagenesis (mutation of the chromosome), and the risk that the virus could retain the ability to replicate itself, which could result in viremia, which is rare but possible.

**Adenoviral vectors:** Adenoviral vectors are DNA viruses that are carried into the cytoplasm of the host cell but do not integrate their DNA into the genome of the cell. Because they do not require cell division to introduce DNA into the host cell, adenoviral vectors can enter a wide variety of dividing and nondividing cell populations. Limitations related to the use of adenoviral vectors include their ability to stimulate a host-immune response and their lack of long-term persistence in the host cell, requiring repeated applications of the vector to maintain a consistent therapeutic response.

### Nonviral Vectors

Nonviral vectors rely on the transfer of genetic material into host cells through chemical or physical methods. This genetic material does not become integrated into the host genome.

**Liposomes:** Liposomes are the most common nonviral vectors in use. DNA is contained within the lipid structure of their biodegradable fatty droplets and is delivered directly to the cell when the liposome fuses with the cell membrane. Cell division is not required to introduce the DNA. Liposomes can enter into a wide variety of dividing and nondividing cell populations.

The advantages of liposomes are that they are nontoxic, the extensive safety testing necessary for viral vectors is not required, and they have the potential to insert multiple copies of the transferred gene into the host target cells. Limitations include their restricted targeting ability and short-term persistence in the host cell, thus requiring repeated applications of the vector to maintain the therapeutic response in the host target cells.

## Application to Cancer Therapy

Current gene-transfer techniques applied to cancer therapy include modification of the tumor by inserting genetic material into the tumor to correct the specific genetic defects causing the malignancy, inserting genes that encode enzymes able to convert harmless prodrugs into lethal cytotoxins, or enhancing the immune recognition of tumors. The polyclonal nature of most pediatric malignancies makes tumor correction especially problematic; it is hoped that certain individual genetic abnormalities that are amenable to correction will prove to be key to the malignant process. In addition, this approach requires the majority of tumor cells to be transduced, which is not feasible with the vectors that are currently available.

Transfer of prodrug-metabolizing enzyme therapy involves the insertion of genes into cancer cells that encode enzymes able to convert harmless prodrugs into lethal cytotoxins. This approach has been explored in phase I treatments of retinoblastoma and supratentorial brain tumors and is now used for the treatment of several localized or recurrent adult malignancies (High & Brenner, 2005). In this strategy, the tumor is injected directly with a vector carrying the herpes simplex virus-1 thymidine kinase gene, which converts ganciclovir into a metabolite that acts as a "suicide gene" by killing dividing cells (tumor cells). In some tumors, neighboring cancer cells that have not taken up the transgene also are killed by what is known as the "bystander effect." It is believed that this effect occurs when channels between cells, known as gap junctions, allow the toxic metabolite to spread from the transduced cell in which it was produced to neighboring nontransduced cells.

Modification of the sensitivity of normal host cells to cytotoxic drugs, thus increasing the therapeutic index of these agents, is another therapy. The multidrug-resistant-1 gene is the most widely studied drug-resistant gene to date. This gene, once inserted, acts as a drug-efflux pump and prevents the accumulation of small toxic molecules, including a range of cytotoxic drugs. The transfer of drug-resistant genes into hematopoietic stem cells would exert a protective effect, attenuating drug-induced myelosuppression. Researchers are studying other drug-resistant genes, including dihydrofolate reductase, which protects against methotrexate, and the bacterial nitroreductase, which protects against thiotepa (Abernathy & Wilson, 2000; Biagi, Bollard, Rousseau, & Brenner, 2003).

Although not directly therapeutic, gene marking of hematopoietic progenitor cells provides information that can be used to improve therapies that incorporate autologous stem-cell transplantation. Gene marking has been used to address questions regarding cancer biology and clinical issues, specifically for determining the source of relapse after autologous stem-cell transplant, learning more about normal marrow reconstitution, and evaluating ways to accelerate the reconstitution process.

*Immunotherapy* refers to any approach aimed at enhancing the immune system to treat diseases. Strategies for generating immune responses to inadequately presented tumor-associated antigens or for boosting existing immune responses to eradicate malignancies include vaccines and adoptive immunotherapy. Tumor-vaccine studies are being evaluated to enhance the immune recognition of tumors with poor immunogenicity. Transduced tumor cells are being used as vaccines in adjuvant therapy to prevent relapse in patients with presumed minimal-residual disease. Tumor vaccines in patients have been well tolerated, producing little systemic toxicity with only local inflammation at the injection site. Tumor vaccines are undergoing evaluation in more than 300 different clinical trials. The vaccine trials for neuroblastoma have used both autologous and allogeneic transduced cells. The autologous vaccine trials have demonstrated an increased frequency of tumor-specific cytotoxic T lymphocytes (CTLs) in responders, which provided a mixed response of disease stabilization in patients with advanced disease. Subsequent allogeneic vaccine studies for neuroblastoma demonstrated that a combination of two stimulating agents at different phases of the immune response may be superior to a single-agent approach. This process of combining two agents that act at different phases of T-cell activation is undergoing evaluation in pediatric and adult high-risk acute leukemias (High & Brenner, 2005).

A donor lymphocyte infusion (DLI) after HSCT to augment the graft-versus-leukemia effect is an example of adoptive immunotherapy. Although DLIs are successful at eliminating minimal residual disease, graft-versus-host disease (GVHD) is a potentially life-threatening complication. Adoptive transfer of CTLs directed at viral or tumor antigens is an example of adoptive immunotherapy. Clinical studies have demonstrated the feasibility and safety of administering Epstein-Barr virus (EBV) CTLs to prevent and treat Epstein-Barr virus-lymphoproliferative disease (EBV-LPD) in postallogeneic transplant patients. The use of EBV-specific CTLs has been evaluated in pediatric patients with EBV-associated lymphoproliferative disease after HSCT and solid-organ transplant, EBV-positive Hodgkin's disease, and nasopharyngeal carcinoma (Gottschalk et al., 2006). Clinical trials using adoptive immunotherapy for the treatment of EBV-positive Hodgkin's disease are evaluating CTLs that recognize multiple antigens expressed on the tumor cells. This strategy could improve the effectiveness of CTL therapy and minimize tumor-cell evasion.

## Potential Side Effects

Because of the experimental status of gene therapy, the risks associated with patient safety and toxicity are not well defined. The ratio of relative risk to the potential benefit to the patient must be carefully evaluated. All gene-therapy protocols require stringent review by institutional review boards, the U.S. Food and Drug Administration, and the National Institutes of Health Recombinant DNA Advisory Committee prior to their implementation in humans. Long-term monitoring strategies must be ongoing for all clinical trials with gene therapy.

### Risk of Retroviral-Viremia Infection of Healthcare Providers and Patients

Viral vectors are modified to make them incompetent for replication. Rigorous safety testing and quality control in the manufacturing of retroviral vectors is ongoing to ensure the safety of the vectors. Healthcare providers should follow standard precautions in direct-care situations. Patients should be monitored over the long term for the possibility of developing retroviral viremia.

### Risk of Insertional Oncogenesis for Patients Receiving Retroviral Gene Therapy

Random insertion of genetic material by retroviral vectors could alter normal cellular function and lead to malignant transformation. Ongoing patient monitoring and safety testing to define this risk should continue.

### Side Effects of Overall Gene-Transfer Protocols

Gene-transfer protocols are well tolerated with minimal short-term toxicity. Specific side effects include the following:

**Viral therapy:** The constitutional symptoms experienced by patients participating in studies of retroviruses are fever, chills, fatigue, nausea, vomiting, and anorexia. Localized symptoms related to retrovirus studies are cutaneous reactions, induration, erythema, pruritus, pain, and skin irritation; central nervous system symptoms are meningeal inflammation, headache, and seizure. The symptoms experienced by patients participating in adenovirus studies include fatigue, fever, hypoxemia, pulmonary infiltrates, and abnormalities in lung function (transient).

**Nonviral therapy:** The symptoms associated with liposome studies are pain at the time of injection and transient pneumothorax.

## Nursing Assessment and Interventions

### Assessment

The nurse's role in gene-therapy trials parallels that of the nurse in traditional phase I and phase II clinical drug trials. Gene therapy can be a component of a larger therapeutic trial with a documented toxicity profile. Patients can receive gene therapy in a variety of patient-care settings. The direct caregiver is required to provide careful planning of patient care as well as to monitor and document expected and unexpected short- and long-term toxicities.

- Be knowledgeable about the clinical trial, treatment schema, known and potential toxicities, and symptom management.
- Establish safe parameters for administration of treatments.
- Identify, through an assessment of the patient, past treatment or symptom-management problems and current medical problems that could affect the patient's tolerance to therapy.

- Identify, monitor, and record the patient's subjective and objective responses to the investigational therapy and symptom management.
- Assist with long-term monitoring of the patient's response to therapy and identification of trends related to toxicities, benefits of the therapy, or both.
- Be fully informed in order to be viewed as an essential member of the research team and to function effectively in the role of patient advocate and educator.
- Have a basic understanding of genetics and its relationship to cancer and the concepts of gene therapy (i.e., the unique nature of genetic information).
- Understand the goals and limitations of the clinical-trial process as it applies to gene therapy and the participants in gene therapy.
- Appreciate the ethical, societal, and cultural concerns aroused by the implications of the molecular genetic revolution and the concept of gene therapy, and be aware of the specific implications these have for participating patients and healthcare providers.

### Interventions
- Provide accurate, understandable information that allows for meaningful participation by the patient and the family during the informed-consent process and for future care.
- Provide ongoing clarification of the procedures, toxicities, and expectations related to the patient's participation in the clinical trial to the patient and the family.
- Uphold and advocate for patients' rights during the clinical-trial process.
- Maintain ongoing communication and dialogue with the research team regarding the patient's and the family's concerns.
- Discuss the financial considerations, including third-party funding, of the patient's participation in the clinical-research trials.
- Protect and uphold the patient's and the family's rights to privacy and confidentiality.

### Expected Patient and Family Outcomes
- The patient and the family are able to explain their understanding of the purpose, procedures, limitations, and risks of the treatment plan and their decision about participating.
- The patient and the family recognize the importance of unusual symptoms and their potential relationship to the experimental treatment and are able to establish ongoing communication with the healthcare team.
- The patient and the family express satisfaction that their needs are being met and that their basic rights are respected and supported by the healthcare team.

### References
Abernathy, E., & Wilson, H. B. (2000). Gene therapy: Overview and implications for peripheral stem cell transplantation. In P. C. Buchsell & P. M. Kapustay (Eds.), *Stem cell transplantation: A clinical textbook* (pp. 11.3–11.17). Pittsburgh, PA: Oncology Nursing Press.

Biagi, E., Bollard, C., Rousseau, R., & Brenner, M. (2003). Gene therapy for pediatric cancer: State of the art and future perspectives. *Journal of Biomedicine and Biotechnology, 1,* 13–24.

Gottschalk, S., Rooney, C. M., & Brenner, M. K. (2006). Cell and gene therapies. In P. A. Pizzo & D. G. Poplack (Eds.), *Principles and practice of pediatric oncology* (pp. 433–451). Philadelphia: Lippincott Williams & Wilkins.

High, K. A., & Brenner, M. K. (2005). Gene transfer for hematologic disorders. In R. A. Hoffman, E. J. Benz, S. J. Shattil, B. Furie, H. J. Cohen, L. E. Silverstein, et al. (Eds.), *Hematology: Basic principles and practice* (pp. 1829–1841). Philadelphia: Elsevier Inc.

## Complementary and Alternative Treatments

*Janice Post-White*

### Principles of Treatment
Also referred to as integrative therapies or integrated health care, complementary and alternative medicine (CAM) encompasses practices and therapies outside of conventional medicine. CAM is recommended as an adjunct to standard treatment (complementary) and not as a replacement for (alternative) conventional care. The focus of CAM research in childhood cancer is to evaluate the safety and efficacy of therapies in children, provide evidence-based therapies that improve supportive care, and promote the patient's participation in the care of his or her body, mind, and spirit.

### Types of Complementary and Alternative Therapies
The National Center for Complementary and Alternative Medicine of the National Institutes of Health designates four major domains of CAM (NCCAM, 2007):

#### Mind-Body Medicine
These interventions use the mind to influence symptoms or physical responses and are considered the most mainstream CAM techniques. Evidence exists for effectiveness of cognitive-behavioral therapies, biofeedback, and imagery.

#### Biologically Based Practices
These practices encompass substances found in nature, such as herbs, foods, vitamins, and unproven alternative substances such as antineoplastons and shark cartilage. Vitamins and herbs are among the most frequently used CAM therapies in cancer; they also have the greatest potential to interact with conventional treatment (Richardson & Strauss, 2002).

#### Manipulative and Body-Based Practices
These methods encompass chiropractic, massage, and osteopathy to reduce fatigue and pain and restore the structure and function of the musculoskeletal and nervous systems. Several Cochrane databases and meta-analyses support the use of massage in adults and children with cancer for the management of anxiety, pain, fatigue, and distress (Ezzo, 2007).

#### Energy Medicine
These therapies channel spiritual or healing energy to manipulate or interrupt energy fields either within the body (biofields) or external to the body (electromagnetic fields). Qi gong, reiki,

therapeutic touch, and healing touch involve identifying and correcting energy imbalances and promoting energy flow. There is limited evidence for efficacy and no scientific evidence for the mechanism of action.

In addition, the National Institutes of Health acknowledges whole medical systems that have philosophies and practices independent from conventional Western medicine and use a combination of therapies from the four domains. Traditional Chinese medicine relies on acupuncture, herbs, asian massage (i.e., shiatsu), qi gong, and tai chi to maintain or restore the proper balance of qi, or vital life energy. Ayurvedic medicine, which originated in India, emphasizes restoring the innate harmony of the body, mind, and spirit through diet, exercise, meditation, yoga, herbs, massage, and controlled breathing. Naturopathic medicine also relies on innate healing and emphasizes health restoration through diet, acupuncture, herbs, chiropractic care, ultrasound, light therapy, counseling, and homeopathy. Homeopathy seeks to stimulate the body's ability to heal itself through the administration of very small doses of highly diluted substances that if taken in larger doses would produce illness or symptoms (an approach referred to as "like cures like").

## Role in Childhood Cancer

Thirty-one percent to 84% of children and adolescents with cancer use CAM (Sencer & Kelly, 2006); herbal therapies, supplements, and massage are most commonly used. CAM is most often used to manage side effects, to cope with the emotional aspects of illness, or to boost the immune system, although there is little evidence to support biological effects.

Although few scientifically rigorous studies have been conducted to determine whether CAM therapies in children are effective, mind-body therapies, massage, aromatherapy, and acupuncture are considered safe and feasible in children with cancer and may help reduce symptoms (Ladas, Post-White, Hawks, & Taromina, 2006). No known published research exists on energy therapies or whole medical systems for children with cancer.

## Potential Side Effects

Herbs and supplements carry a greater risk of side effects and potential for interactions than other CAM therapies (Weiger et al., 2002). Currently, there are no standards for recommended pediatric dosages and there is little oversight of the herbal or nutritional industries, which has resulted in products with uneven quality and purity. It is important to help parents weigh the risks against the potential benefits, evaluate interactions with treatment and medications, determine recommended doses and frequency, and find qualified licensed or certified practitioners who are experienced in working with children (American Academy of Pediatrics, 2001).

## Nursing Assessment and Interventions

### Assessment

It is especially important to keep communication open by assuming a nonjudgmental approach and asking patients and families what CAM they use; documenting its use, including dosages, frequency, and reasons for use; and evaluating its effects. Use of CAM and potential interactions with treatment should be assessed at diagnosis, during each hospitalization, and at every phase of medical treatment. Parents should be asked to bring in the bottles of vitamins or supplements that their child uses. Determining the therapies used and the reasons that families use CAM can give insight into which therapies work for individual patients and symptoms and provide an understanding of patients' emotional or resource needs.

### Interventions

The Oncology Nursing Society's position on the use of CAM requires that nurses assess for CAM use; rely on credible sources and providers when giving information to patients; evaluate CAM for safety, efficacy, cost, third-party-payer coverage, ethics, and liability; and evaluate their own beliefs regarding CAM (Oncology Nursing Society, 2000). Misrepresentation of facts or expectations voids informed consent and triggers legal liability (Monaco & Smith, 2002). The bibliography provides resources and Web sites for identifying CAM clinical trials and evidence-based research.

- Assess objectively the therapies that parents or adolescents are using or considering using.
- Document what is being used and why, including dosages and frequency.
- Ascertain all known and suspected potential side effects and interactions with treatment.
- Explore how the child, adolescent, or parent expects the therapy to help.
- Offer supportive therapies that can be used at home at any time, such as acupressure, aromatherapy, massage by a parent or friend, music, relaxation, yoga, and meditation.
- Provide a list of local resources, including practitioners who have pediatric experience.
- Provide reliable resources for information on specific therapies, including where to obtain them.
- Ask questions to ensure that the family has considered the risks, benefits, and cost.
- Discuss options for insurance reimbursement. Reimbursement typically requires a medical order and inpatient service; however, state laws and insurance policies vary.
- Monitor the patient's response to any CAM therapies used. At each visit, ask whether CAM therapies are still being used and whether they have been helpful.
- Assess for negative responses, including allergic reactions, side effects, emotional distress, or financial hardship.
- Periodically assist the family to evaluate the need and value of the therapy.

## Expected Patient and Family Outcomes

- The family makes informed decisions regarding choice of CAM therapies for their child.
- Families work with trained providers who have experience with pediatric patients.
- Resources consulted by families are current, reputable, and reliable.
- Families report to their providers their use of CAM, any side effects, and perceived benefits attributable to CAM therapies.

## References

American Academy of Pediatrics. (2001). Counseling families who choose complementary and alternative medicine for their child with chronic illness or disability: Committee on Children with Disabilities. *Pediatrics, 107,* 598–601.

Ezzo, J. (2007). What can be learned from Cochrane systematic reviews of massage that can guide future research? *Journal of Alternative and Complementary Medicine, 13*(2), 291–295.

Ladas, E. J., Post-White, J., Hawks, R., & Taromina, K. (2006). Evidence for symptom management in the child with cancer. *Journal of Pediatric Hematology/Oncology, 28*(9), 601–615.

Monaco, G. P., & Smith, G. (2002). Informed consent in complementary and alternative medicine: Current status and future needs. *Seminars in Oncology, 29,* 601–608.

National Center for Complementary and Alternative Medicine. (2007, February). *CAM basics: What is CAM?* (NCCAM Publication No. D347). Retrieved October 15, 2007, from http://nccam.nih.gov/health/whatiscam.

Oncology Nursing Society. (2000). Oncology Nursing Society position on the use of complementary and alternative therapies in cancer care. *Oncology Nursing Forum, 27,* 749.

Richardson, M. A., & Strauss, S. E. (2002). Complementary and alternative medicine: Opportunities and challenges for cancer management and research. *Seminars in Oncology, 29,* 531–545.

Sencer, S., & Kelly, K. M. (2006) Bringing evidence to complementary and alternative medicine for children with cancer. *Journal of Pediatric Hematology/Oncology, 28,* 186–189.

Weiger, W. A., Smith, M., Boon, H., Richardson, M. A., Kaptchuk, T. J., & Eisenberg, D. M. (2002). Advising patients who seek complementary and alternative medical therapies for cancer. *Annals of Internal Medicine, 137,* 889–903.

## Bibliography

### Diagnostic and Staging Procedures

Guillerman, R. P., Braverman, R. M., & Parker, B. R. (2006). Imaging studies in the diagnosis and management of pediatric malignancies. In P. A. Pizzo & D. G. Poplack (Eds.), *Principles and practice of pediatric oncology* (5th ed., pp. 236–289). Philadelphia: Lippincott Williams & Wilkins.

Leonard, M. (2007). Diagnostic evaluations and staging procedures. In C. R. Baggott, K. P. Kelly, D. Fochtman, & G. V. Foley (Eds.), *Nursing care of children and adolescents with cancer* 3rd ed., (pp. 66–89). Glenview, IL: Association of Pediatric Hematology/Oncology Nurses.

Wirth, A., Seymour, J. F., Hicks, R. J. (2002). Fluorine-18 fluorodeoxyglucose positron emission tomography, gallium-67 scintigraphy, and conventional staging for Hodgkin's disease and non-Hodgkin's lymphoma. *American Journal of Medicine, 112,* 262–268.

### History of Chemotherapy

Aplenc, R. (2004). Phamacogenetic determinants of outcome in acute lymphoblastic leukemia. *British Journal of Hematology, 125,* 421–434.

Adamson, P. C., Balis, F. M., Berg, S., & Blaney, S. M. (2006). General principles of chemotherapy. In P. A. Pizzo & D. G. Poplack (Eds.), *Principles and practice of pediatric oncology* (5th ed., pp. 290–365). Philadelphia: Lippincott Williams & Wilkins.

Kardinal, C. G. (1993). Cancer chemotherapy in historical perspective. *Journal of the Louisiana State Medical Society, 14,* 175–177.

Ratain, M. J. (2006). The Cancer and Leukemia Group B Pharmacology and Experimental Therapeutics Committee: A historical perspective. *Clinical Cancer Research, 12,* 3612s–3616s.

Smith, M. A. (2006). Molecularly targeted therapies and biotherapeutics. In P. A. Pizzo & D. G. Poplack (Eds.), *Principles and practice of pediatric oncology* (5th ed., pp. 366–404). Philadelphia: Lippincott Williams & Wilkins.

### Clinical Trials

Berg, S. L., Sather, H., & Ellenberg, S. S. (2006). Cancer clinical trials: Design, conduct, analysis, & reporting. In P. A. Pizzo & D. G. Poplack (Eds.), *Principles and practice of pediatric oncology* (5th ed., pp. 501–524). Philadelphia: Lippincott Williams & Wilkins.

Chang, A. (2004). Nurses' perceptions of phase I clinical trials in pediatric oncology: A review of the literature. *Journal of Pediatric Oncology Nursing, 21,* 343–349.

Hinds, P. S., Gilger, E. A., Eder, M., & Kodish, E. (2002). The nurse as witness in the research consent/assent process: An inherently problematic role or an ethical obligation? *Journal of Pediatric Oncology Nursing, 19,* 35–40.

Joffe, S., Fernandez, C. V., Pentz, R. D., Ungar, D. R., Mathew, N. A., Turner, C. W., et al. (2006). Involving children with cancer in decision-making about research participation. *Journal of Pediatrics, 149*(6), 862–868.

Levi, R. B., Marsick, R., Drotar, D., & Kodish, E. (2000). Diagnosis, disclosure, and informed consent: Learning from parents of children with cancer. *Journal of Pediatric Hematology/Oncology, 22,* 3–12.

McCray, A. T. (2000). Better access to information about clinical trials. *Annals of Internal Medicine, 133,* 609–614.

National Cancer Institute. (n.d.). *Understanding clinical trials.* Retrieved May 26, 2008, from www.nci.nih.gov/clinicaltrials/understanding.

National Library of Medicine. (n.d.). *Understanding clinical trials.* Retrieved May 26, 2008, from http://clinicaltrials.gov.

Simon, C. M., Siminoff, L. A., Kodish, E. D., & Burant, C. (2004). Comparison of the informed consent process for randomized clinical trials in pediatric and adult oncology. *Journal of Clinical Oncology, 22,* 2708–2717.

Simon, R. (2004). Design and analysis of clinical trials. In V. T. DeVita Jr., S. Hellman, & S. A. Rosenberg (Eds.), *Cancer: Principles and practice of oncology* (pp. 471–489). Philadelphia: Lippincott Williams & Wilkins.

U.S. Food and Drug Administration. (n.d.) *Clinical trials.* Retrieved May 26, 2008, from www.fda.gov/oashi/clinicaltrials/default.htm.

U.S. Department of Health and Human Services. (2005). *Code of federal regulations* (Title 45, Part 46). Washington, DC: Author.

### Chemotherapy

Adamson, P. C., Balis, F. M., Berg, S., & Blaney, S. M. (2006). General principles of chemotherapy. In P. A. Pizzo & D. G. Poplack (Eds.), *Principles and practice of pediatric oncology* (5th ed., pp. 290–365). Philadelphia: Lippincott Williams & Wilkins.

Ettinger, A. G., Bond, D. M., & Sievers, D. (2007). Chemotherapy. In C. R. Baggott, K. P. Kelly, D. Fochtman, & G. V. Foley (Eds.), *Nursing care of children and adolescents with cancer* (3rd ed., pp. 133–176). Glenview, IL: Association of Pediatric Hematology/Oncology Nurses.

Kline, N. E. (Ed.). (2004). *The pediatric chemotherapy and biotherapy curriculum* (1st ed.). Glenview, IL: Association of Pediatric Oncology Nurses.

Reid, D., & Wilson, K. (2003). Principles of chemotherapy. In K. Wilson, W. Landier, & J. D. Wallace (Eds.), *APON's foundations of pediatric hematology/oncology nursing: A comprehensive orientation and review course.* Glenview, IL: Association of Pediatric Oncology Nurses.

Wittes, R. E. (2003). Therapies for cancer in children—past successes, future challenges. *New England Journal of Medicine, 348,* 747–749.

**Guidelines for Safe Handling of Chemotherapy**

Occupational Safety and Health Administration. (2004). Code of federal regulations. (Title 29, Chapter VII, CFR 1910.21, pp. 111–115). Retrieved May 4, 2007, from Office of the Federal Register via GPO Access: www.access.gpo.gov/nara/cfr/waisidx_04/29cfr1910_04.html.

Occupational Safety and Health Administration. (1999). *OSHA Technical manual* (TED 1-0.15A, Section VI, Chapter 2). Retrieved May 6, 2007, from U.S. Department of Labor Web site: www.osha.gov/dts/osta/otm/otm_vi/otm_vi_2.html.

Polovich, M., White, J. M., & Kelleher, L. O. (Eds.). (2005). *Chemotherapy and biotherapy: Guidelines and recommendations for practice.* Pittsburgh, PA: Oncology Nursing Society Publishing Division.

**Administration of Vesicants**

Bertelli, G., Gozza, A., Forno, G. B., Vidili, M. G., Silvestro, S., Venturini, M., et al. (1995). Topical dimethylsulfoxide for the prevention of soft tissue injury after extravasation of vesicant cytotoxic drugs: A prospective clinical study. *Journal of Clinical Oncology, 13,* 2851–2855.

Langstein, H. N., Duman, H., Seelig, D., Butler, C. E., & Evans, G. R. (2002). Retrospective study of the management of chemotherapeutic extravasation injury. *Annals of Plastic Surgery, 49,* 369–374.

Mouridsen, H. T., Langer, S. W., Buter, J., Eidtmann, H., Rosti, G., de Wit, M., et al. (2007). Treatment of anthracycline extravasation with Savene (dexrazoxane): Results from two prospective clinical multicentre studies. *Annals of Oncology, 18*(3), 546–550.

Wickham, R., Engelking, C., Sauerland, C., & Corbi, D. (2006). Vesicant extravasation. Part II: Evidence-based management and continuing controversies. *Oncology Nursing Forum, 33*(6), 1143–1150.

**Surgery**

Bhatia, S., Blatt, J., & Meadows, A. T. (2006). Late effects of childhood cancer and its treatment. In P. A. Pizzo & D. G. Poplack (Eds.), *Principles and practice of pediatric oncology* (5th ed., pp. 1490–1514). Philadelphia: Lippincott Williams & Wilkins.

Pappo, A. S., & Furman, W. L. (2006). Management of infrequent cancers of childhood. In P. A. Pizzo & D. G. Poplack (Eds.), *Principles and practice of pediatric oncology* (5th ed., pp. 1172–1201). Philadelphia: Lippincott Williams & Wilkins.

Woo, R. K., & Krummel, T. M. (2006). Advanced and emerging surgical technologies and the process of innovation. In J. L. Grosfeld, J. A. O'Neill Jr., E. W. Fonkalsrud, & A. G. Coran (Eds.), *Pediatric surgery.* (6th ed., pp. 31–76). Philadelphia: Mosby Elsevier.

**Radiation Therapy**

Bolderston, A., Lloyd, N. S., Wong, R. K. S., Holden, L., & Robb-Blenderman, L. (2006). The prevention and management of acute skin reactions related to radiation therapy: A systematic review and practice guideline. *Supportive Cancer Care, 14,* 802–817.

Hogle, W. P. (2006). The state of the art in radiation therapy. *Seminars in Oncology Nursing, 22,* 212–220.

Klosky, J. L., Tyc, V. L., Tong, X., Srivastava, D. K., Kronenberg, M., de Armendi, A. J., et al. (2007). Predicting pediatric distress during radiation therapy procedures: The role of medical, psychosocial, and demographic factors. *Journal of the American Academy of Pediatrics, 119,* 1159–1166.

Otmani, N. (2007). Oral and maxillofacial side effects of radiation therapy on children. *Journal of the Canadian Dental Association, 73,* 257–260.

Stern, J., & Ippoliti, C. (2003). Management of acute cancer treatment induced diarrhea. *Seminars in Oncology Nursing, 19,* 11–16.

**Hematopoietic Stem-Cell Transplantation**

Andrykowski, M. A., Bishop, M. M., Hahn, E. A., Cella, D. F., Beaumont, J. L., Brady, M. J., et al. (2005). Long-term health-related quality of life, growth, and spiritual well-being after hematopoietic stem-cell transplantation. *Journal of Clinical Oncology, 23,* 599–608.

Bollard, C. M., Krance, R. A., & Heslop, H. E. (2006). Hematopoietic stem cell transplantation in pediatric oncology. In P. A. Pizzo & D. G. Poplack (Eds.), *Principles and practice of pediatric oncology* (5th ed., pp. 476–500). Philadelphia: Lippincott Williams & Wilkins.

Centers for Disease Control and Prevention. (2000). *Guidelines for preventing opportunistic infections among hematopoietic stem cell transplant recipients.* Retrieved November 20, 2007, from www.cdc.gov/mmwr/pdf/rr/rr4910.pdf.

Fisher, V. L., & Abramovitz, L. Z. (2006). A brief overview of hematopoietic stem-cell transplantation. In R. M. Kline (Ed.), *Pediatric hematopoietic stem cell transplantation* (pp. 601–624). New York: Informa Healthcare.

Foss, F. M., Gorgun, G., & Miller, K. B. (2002). Extracorporeal photopheresis in chronic graft-versus-host disease. *Bone Marrow Transplantation, 20,* 719–725.

Heiney, S. P., Bryant, L. H., Godder, K., & Michaels, J. (2002). Preparing children to be bone marrow donors. *Oncology Nursing Forum, 29,* 1485–1489.

Jacobsohn, D. A., & Vogelsang, G. B. (2002). Novel pharmacotherapeutic approaches to prevention and treatment of GVHD. *Drugs, 62,* 879–889.

Kemp, J., & Dickerson, J. (2002). Interdisciplinary modular teaching for patients undergoing progenitor cell transplantation. *Clinical Journal of Oncology Nursing, 6,* 157–160.

Laffan, A., & Biedrzychi, B. (2006). Immune reconstitution: The foundation for safe living after an allogeneic hematopoietic stem cell transplantation. *Clinical Journal of Oncology Nursing, 10,* 787–794.

Norville, R. (2005). Hematopoietic stem cell transplantation. In D. Tomlinson & N. E. Kline (Eds.), *Pediatric oncology nursing: Advanced clinical handbook* (pp. 201–217). New York: Springer.

Rizzo, J. D., Wingard, J. R., Tichevi, A., Lee, S. J., Van Lint, M. T., Burns, L. J., et al. (2006). Recommended screening and preventive practices for long-term survivors after hematopoietic stem cell transplantation: Joint recommendations of the European Group for Blood and Marrow Transplantation, the Center for International Blood and Marrow Transplant Research, and the American Society of Blood and Marrow Transplantation. *Biology of Blood and Marrow Transplantation, 12,* 138–151.

Ryan, L. G., Kristovich, K. M., Haugen, M. S., Coyne, K. D., & Hubbell, M. M. (2007). Hematopoietic stem cell transplantation. In C. R. Baggott, K. P. Kelly, D. Fochtman, & G. V. Foley (Eds.), *Nursing care of children and adolescents with cancer* (3rd ed., pp. 212–255). Glenview, IL: Association of Pediatric Hematology/Oncology Nurses.

Weisdorf, D. J. (2005). Complications after hematopoietic stem cell transplantation. In R. Hoffman, E. J. Benz, S. J. Shattie, B. Furie, H. J. Cohen, L. E. Silverstein, et al. (Eds.), *Hematology: Basic principles and practice* (pp. 1855–1870). Philadelphia: Elsevier.

Zaia, J. A. (2002). Prevention and management of CMV-related problems after hematopoietic stem cell transplantation. *Bone Marrow Transplantation, 29,* 633–638.

**Biologic Response Modifiers**

Arceci, R. J., & Cripe, T. P. (2002). Emerging cancer-targeted therapies. *Pediatric Clinics of North America, 49,* 1339–1368.

Cheung, N. V., Kushner, B. H., & Kramer, K. (2001). Monoclonal antibody-based therapy of neuroblastoma. *Hematology/Oncology Clinics of North America, 15,* 853–866.

Gemmill, R., & Idell, C. (2003). Biological advances for new treatment approaches. *Seminars in Oncology Nursing, 19*(3), 162–168.

Gobel, B. (2007). Hypersensitivity reactions to biological drugs. *Seminars in Oncology Nursing, 23*(3), 191–200.

Kaplow, R. (2005). Innovations in antineoplastic therapy. *Nursing Clinics of North America, 40,* 77–94.

Mocellin, S., Wang, E., & Marincola, F. M. (2001). Cytokines and immune response in the tumor microenvironment. *Journal of Immunotherapy, 24,* 392–407.

National Cancer Institute. *Cancer vaccine fact sheet.* Retrieved August 14, 2007, from www.cancer.gov/cancertopics/factsheet/cancervaccine.

Rosenberg, S. A. (2001). Progress in the development of immunotherapy for the treatment of patients with cancer. *Journal of Internal Medicine, 250,* 462–475.

National Institutes of Health. (n.d.). *Tyrosine kinase inhibitors: Molecules with an important mission.* Retrieved October 4, 2007, from www.nih.org/pages/tyrosine_kinase_inhibitors.html.

National Institutes of Health. (2007). *Tyrosine kinase overview: Enzyme explorer.* Retrieved October 4, 2007, from www.sigmaaldrich.com/area_of_interest/biochemicals/enzyme_explorer/key_resources/proteinkinase_explorer/tyrosine_kinase_overview.html.

Van Esser, J. W., Niesters, H. G., van der Holt, B., Meijer, E., Osterhaus, A. D., Gratama, J. W., et al. (2002). Prevention of Epstein-Barr virus-lymphoproliferative disease by molecular monitoring and preemptive rituximab in high-risk patients after allogeneic stem cell transplantation. *Blood, 99,* 4364–4369.

Woolery-Antill, M. (2007). Biotherapy. In C. R. Baggott, K. P. Kelly, D. Fochtman, & G. V. Foley (Eds.), *Nursing care of children and adolescents with cancer* (3rd ed., pp. 177–211). Glenview, IL: Association of Pediatric Hematology/Oncology Nurses.

**Cell and Gene Therapy**

Liu, K. (2003). Breakthroughs in cancer gene therapy. *Seminars in Oncology Nursing, 19,* 217–226.

Loud, J. T., Peters, J. A., Fraser, M., & Jenkins, J. (2002). Applications of advances in molecular biology and genomics to clinical cancer care. *Cancer Nursing, 25*(2), 110–122.

**Complementary and Alternative Treatments**

American Botanical Council. (2007). *Herbal medicine: Expanded Commission E online* (2007). Retrieved October 15, 2007, from http://content.herbalgram.org/abc/herbalmedicine.

National Cancer Institute, National Institutes of Health. *Complementary and alternative medicine in cancer treatment: Questions and answers fact sheet.* (2006, January). Retrieved October 15, 2007, from www.cancer.gov/cancertopics/factsheet/therapy/CAM.

The National Center for Complementary and Alternative Medicine, National Institutes of Health. (2008, May 14). *Clinical trials.* Retrieved October 15, 2007, from http://nccam.nih.gov/clinicaltrials.

Office of Dietary Supplements, National Institutes of Health. (2005, August). *Vitamin and Mineral Supplement Fact Sheets.* Retrieved October 15, 2007, from http://ods.od.nih.gov/Health_Information/Vitamin_and_Mineral_Supplement_Fact_sheets.aspx.

U.S. Food and Drug Administration. *The FDA Safety Information and Adverse Event Reporting Program* (2007, October). Retrieved October 15, 2007, from www.fda.gov/medwatch/.

# Section V  Side Effects of Treatment

Cheryl Rodgers

## Section Outline

**Bone-Marrow Suppression**

**Impairment of the Immune System**

**Central-Nervous-System Complications**

**Ototoxicity**

**Endocrine Abnormalities**

**Cardiac and Pulmonary Complications**

**Gastrointestinal Complications**

**Renal and Bladder Complications**

**Skin Changes**

**Musculoskeletal Complications**

**Nutritional Complications**

**Growth and Developmental Complications**

**Pain**

**Oncologic Emergencies**

**Bibliography**

# Bone-Marrow Suppression

*Pat Wills Alcoser*

Bone marrow provides an environment for the formation of red blood cells (RBCs), white blood cells (WBCs), and platelets. Because the hematopoietic system has a rapid turnover, cells are constantly being regenerated. Hematologic and oncologic diseases and their related treatments can have a direct impact on this regeneration process. Bone-marrow suppression is the most common dose-limiting component of cancer therapy. During the nadir, infection and bleeding can occur and require blood-product support and the use of biologic response modifiers to stimulate bone-marrow activity. Biologic response modifiers can include one or more of the following: erythropoietin (Epogen) or darbepoietin alfa (Aranesp) to stimulate red-cell production; granulocyte-colony stimulating factor (GCSF; Neupogen), granulocyte macrophage-colony stimulating factor (GM-CSF; Leukine) or pegfilgrastim (Neulasta) to stimulate granulocyte production; and interleukin 11 (IL-11[oprelvekin or Neumega]) to stimulate platelet production.

## Conditions Related to Bone-Marrow Suppression

The following conditions are related to bone-marrow suppression.

### Anemia

**Definition:** *Anemia* is a deficiency in the number of circulating RBCs required for normal tissue and organ oxygenation (see Section III, "Overview of Hematology").

**Clinical presentation:** The symptoms are fatigue, pallor, tachycardia or gallop heart rhythm, hemoglobin less than or equal to 7.5 gm/dL, and hematocrit of 20% or less.

### Thrombocytopenia

**Definition:** Thrombocytopenia is a decrease in the total number of circulating platelets required for blood clotting (see Section III, "Overview of Hematology"). The severity of thrombocytopenia is defined by the following parameters:

- Mild: Platelet count = 75,000/mm$^3$ to within normal limits
- Moderate: Platelet count = 50,000–74,900/mm$^3$
- Moderately severe: Platelet count = 20,000–49,900/mm$^3$
- Severe: Platelet count <20,000/mm$^3$.

**Clinical presentation:** The symptoms can include oozing of the gums, epistaxis, petechiae, ecchymosis, hematuria, and hematochezia.

### Neutropenia

**Definition:** *Neutropenia* is a reduction in circulating neutrophils determined by the percentage of segmented neutrophils and band neutrophils that constitute the total WBC (see Section III, "Overview of Hematology"). The absolute neutrophil count (ANC) is calculated as follows:

(% bands + % segmented neutrophils) × total WBC = ANC.

The severity of neutropenia is defined by the following parameters:

- Mild: ANC = 1,500–1,900/mm$^3$
- Moderate: ANC = 1,000–1,499/mm$^3$
- Moderately severe: ANC = 500–999/mm$^3$
- Severe: ANC <500/mm$^3$.

**Clinical presentation:** Neutropenia can be asymptomatic. If there are signs or symptoms of anemia or thrombocytopenia, a patient is also frequently neutropenic. The symptoms of neutropenia can be fever and infection (i.e., bacteremia or viral, fungal, opportunistic [e.g., *Pneumocystis carinii* pneumonia] infection) (see Section VI, "Supportive Care").

**Disease-related risk factors:** The disease-related risk factors are acute lymphoblastic leukemia (ALL), acute nonlymphoblastic leukemia, metastatic bone-marrow involvement caused by solid tumors, or aplastic anemia.

**Treatment-related risk factors:** The treatment-related risk factors are myelosuppressive chemotherapy and radiation, including cranial or spinal radiation; radiation involving flat bones such as the ribs, sternum, and pelvis; and total body irradiation. Supportive care measures, such as hyperhydration, can have a dilutional effect on the complete blood count (CBC), and medications such as trimethoprim-sulfamethoxazole (Bactrim) can cause myelosuppression.

## Medical Management

### Anemia

Packed RBC transfusions at 10–15 mL/kg of body weight can be given if clinical symptoms are present. A synthetic preparation of erythropoietin (Epogen) may be given to some patients to stimulate RBC production. The dose is 150–300 units/kg subcutaneously or intravenously every other day. Aranesp is a long-acting, synthetically made erythropoietin that is given on a weekly basis. Dosing begins at 0.45 mcg/kg and should be carefully titrated for effect. Studies in adults have shown occurrences of dose-related cardiomyopathy.

### Thrombocytopenia

Platelet transfusions are administered at a dose of 6 units/m$^2$; single-donor units should be given whenever possible. Depending on the disease, a medically stable patient who has shown no evidence of bleeding may be transfused when the platelet count is less than 10,000–20,000/mm$^3$ (or according to institutional practice). A patient who is bleeding, has significant infection, has residual intracranial tumor, or requires surgical intervention may need transfusions to keep the platelet count greater than 50,000/mm$^3$. Irradiated, leukocyte-depleted blood products can be given to children receiving cancer treatment; cytomegalovirus-negative blood products should be administered to patients who are potential or actual bone-marrow-transplant candidates, according to institutional practice.

Interleukin-11 is a thrombopoietic growth factor that stimulates proliferation and maturation of megakaryocytes in the bone marrow, resulting in increased circulating platelets. It is administered subcutaneously at 75–100 mcg/kg/day for 10–21 days.

### Neutropenia

GCSF, GM-CSF, or pegfilgrastim may be used selectively in some patients, depending upon the treatment protocol or institutional practice. Administration of colony-stimulating factors (CSFs) results in an early release of neutrophils from the bone marrow, decreasing the duration of the neutrophil nadir. The dose of GCSF is 5–10 mcg/kg/day, while the dose of GM-CSF is 250 mcg/m$^2$/day. Pegfilgrastim dosage is 0.1 mg/kg once per chemotherapy cycle. Pegfilgrastim is given by subcutaneous injection. GCSF and GM-CSF may be given subcutaneously or intravenously, though both are thought to have better efficacy if given via the subcutaneous route. CSF therapy is discontinued when the ANC reaches the value indicated by either the treatment protocol or the institutional recommendation.

## Complications

Potential complications associated with blood-product support for anemia and thrombocytopenia include transfusion reactions, as well as hypersensitivity, alloimmunization, or both. Symptoms can include urticaria, fever, chills, rigors, hemolytic reactions, and volume overload. Although the blood supply in the United States is extremely safe, there is still a small risk for the following infections from a contaminated product: hepatitis B, hepatitis C, cytomegalovirus, human immunodeficiency virus, and bacteremia. Graft-versus-host disease is a complication that can occur in severely immunocompromised patients who have received numerous transfusions (see the subsection "Blood Product Support" in Section VI, "Supportive Care").

Potential complications associated with CSFs, GCSF, GM-CSF or pegfilgastrim are fever, bone pain, and allergic reactions manifested by rash, urticaria, dyspnea, tachycardia, and/or hypertension. In particular, GCSF and GM-CSF are contraindicated in patients who have a history of allergy to *E. coli* or L-asparaginase.

The complications that are associated with erythropoietin and darbepoietin alfa are hypertension, seizures, thrombotic events, and cardiomyopathy. A rapid increase in hemoglobin is associated with increased risk of complications; avoid hemoglobin increases >1 gm/dL during any 2-week period.

Side effects of treatment with oprelvekin (IL-11; Neumega) include fever, headaches, and flu-like symptoms.

Fungal infections are a potential complication of prolonged neutropenia, extended antibiotic treatment, or both.

## Nursing Assessment and Interventions

### Assessment
- Know the timing of the nadir associated with various types of therapies.
- Review the patient's response to previous therapy.
- Review the patient's CBC and differential results.

### Interventions
- Teach the patient and the family about the importance of knowing the patient's blood counts and how blood counts are affected by treatment.
- Teach the patient and the family about neutropenic precautions. The patient should avoid large crowds or ill persons, limit participation in contact sports, and engage in quiet activities when his or her blood-cell count is low. Fever greater than 101°F (38.4°C) is a major concern when the child is neutropenic. Strict handwashing should be done before and after eating, after going to the bathroom, touching dirty items or body fluids, or after touching pets.
- Teach the patient and the family about the signs and symptoms of anemia: pallor, fatigue, tachycardia, and shortness of breath.
- Teach the patient and the family about the signs and symptoms of thrombocytopenia: ecchymosis, epistaxis, petechiae, hematuria, and hematochezia.
- Discuss the pros and cons of directed donor transfusions. Transfusion of a blood product from a potential bone-marrow donor to the patient may impair engraftment in the patient at the time of bone-marrow transplantation.

## Expected Patient and Family Outcomes
- The patient and the family understand the implications of bone-marrow suppression and can identify the signs and symptoms of anemia, thrombocytopenia, and infection to seek early medical intervention as needed.
- The patient and the family comply with prophylactic and supportive-care measures.

# Impairment of the Immune System

*Pat Wills Alcoser*

Both the cellular and the humoral components of the immune system are altered when a child has cancer. Innate immunity that allows for nonspecific phagocytosis of invading microorganisms is diminished in states of neutropenia. Lymphocyte function can be affected by either the disease process or the associated treatment. Impairment of T and B lymphocytes results in a deficient production of antibodies and decreased ability to process antigens, thereby altering a patient's ability to resist infection. In a state of immunosuppression, children are susceptible to bacterial, fungal, and viral infections.

## Common Infections Associated with an Impaired Immune System

### Pneumocystis Carinii Pneumonia
**Definition:** *Pneumocystis carinii* pneumonia (PCP) is the most common protozoal infection in immunosuppressed children. It is manifested by pneumonitis or pneumonia or both and frequently is fatal. Almost all PCP cases occur in cancer patients who are not compliant with PCP prophylaxis or who have not been placed on prophylaxis by their healthcare provider. However, children who are immunocompromised because of human immunodeficiency virus (HIV) infection or acquired immune deficiency syndrome (AIDS) have been infected with PCP despite documented evidence that they have complied with the prophylactic regimen.

**Clinical presentation:** PCP symptoms can include fever, cough, tachypnea, nasal flaring, intercostal retractions, decreased oxygen saturation, increased respiratory effort, and diffuse bilateral alveolar disease with or without hyperinflation as revealed by chest radiograph. Definitive diagnosis is made through finding *Pneumocystis carinii* organisms in the lung tissue or respiratory secretions obtained by open-lung or transbronchial biopsy or by bronchoalveolar lavage.

**Risk factors:** The risk factors include immunosuppression, neutropenia, malignancy, and HIV infection or AIDS.

**Medical management:** The prophylactic treatment of choice is trimethoprim-sulfamethoxazole (TMP-SMZ; trade names

Bactrim, Septra) given by mouth at a dose of 5 mg/kg/day, divided twice daily for 3 days a week. If a child does not tolerate TMP-SMZ, other prophylactic regimens are available. These include (in order of preference): Dapsone given orally at a dose of 2 mg/kg/day (maximum dose is 100 mg/day) once daily or 4 mg/kg (maximum dose is 400 mg/week); aerosolized pentamidine isoethionate (Pentam-300) 300 mg via Respirgard II inhaler, given monthly; or atovaquone 30 mg/kg given orally daily in children 1–3 months of age and 45 mg/kg given orally daily in children older than 2 years. Treatment for active infection includes therapy with either TMP-SMZ, pentamidine, or atovaquone, and supportive measures include corticosteroids, oxygen, and mechanical ventilation as needed.

**Potential complications:** Complications can include chronic pulmonary disease, prolonged interruption of cancer treatment, or death.

**Nursing Assessment and Interventions:**
*Assessment.*
- Review the prophylaxis regimen for PCP with the patient and the family.
- Assess for symptoms of PCP.

*Interventions.*
- Tell the patient and the family that PCP can be prevented with prophylactic treatment.
- Inform the patient and the family that prophylaxis must continue for approximately 6 months after treatment ends, or until the patient's absolute lymphocyte count is consistently higher than 1,500.
- Tell the patient and the family that TMP-SMZ (Bactrim) may need to be discontinued briefly because it can prolong neutropenia should it occur.

**Expected Patient and Family Outcomes:**
- The patient and the family know about the risk factors for contracting PCP.
- The patient and the family comply with the prophylactic regimen.

## Oral Herpes Simplex

**Definition:** Reactivation of the herpes simplex virus (HSV) in the oral cavity.

**Clinical presentation:** Oral HSV presents as painful ulcers either intraoral or on the lips with vesicular or crusting lesions.

**Risk factors:** Risk factors include immune suppression, prior history of exposure, and predisposition to oral ulcers.

**Medical management:** Treatment includes good oral hygiene and administration of oral acyclovir. Prophylactic treatment may be necessary to prevent repeated reactivation of the herpes virus.

## Oral Thrush

**Definition:** *Oral thrush* is defined as overgrowth of oral yeast or fungus, commonly Candida albicans.

**Clinical presentation:** Oral thrush presents as scattered white plaques that cannot be removed by rinsing or brushing. Plaques can cause some tenderness or changes in taste. Thrush can also extend down into the esophagus, causing throat burning, irritation, or dysphagia.

**Risk factors:** Oral yeast, or thrush, grows in states of immune suppression or as a result of prolonged antibiotic therapy. If left untreated, yeast can extend through the bloodstream, sinuses, or intracranially.

**Medical management:** Simple oral thrush can be treated with antifungal medications such as nystatin or fluconazole. After treatment, old toothbrushes should be replaced. Extensive involvement of fungal infection requires more aggressive treatment.

**Nursing Assessment and Interventions:**
*Assessment.*
- Assess intraoral cavity daily.
- Encourage good oral hygiene.
- Administer medications as prescribed.

*Interventions.*
- Instruct families about the importance of good mouth care. Oral gingiva is very vascular, and oral bacteria or fungus can enter the bloodstream, exacerbating complications. Oral lesions tend to flare when blood counts are low.
- Instruct patients and families to report oral plaques, ulcers, or painful lesions.
- Instruct patients about the rationale for compliance with medications for oral infections.

**Expected Patient and Family Outcomes:**
- The patient and the family adhere to good mouth care.
- The patient and the family report oral lesions as soon as possible.
- The patient and the family adhere to medications as prescribed.

## Varicella Zoster (Chicken Pox) and Herpes Zoster (Shingles)

*Chicken pox* is a common childhood illness of the herpes virus group that is manifested by pruritis, fever, and clear, vesicular lesions. Although it is rare, a systemic illness such as pneumonia, hepatitis, or encephalitis can occur. The incubation period is 10–21 days, and the host is infectious approximately 24–48 hours prior to the onset of lesions. The contagious period ends after all lesions have crusted over and no further lesions develop. After an infection, the virus remains latent in the nerve tissues and can be reactivated during times of stress or if a person is immunocompromised. The subsequent rash is recognized as *herpes zoster*, a painful, vesicular clustering of lesions along a nerve pathway and is most often unilateral.

**Risk factors:** A person is at risk if he or she has had no previous immunity to varicella, is immunocompromised, or is exposed to someone with a varicella infection. Patients who have had varicella in the past can have viral reactivation as herpes zoster when in states of stress or immune compromise.

**Medical management:** Management measures include documenting a patient's immune status by testing for varicella titers. An infusion of intravenous immunoglobulin (IVIG) should be given as soon as possible after exposure (but no later than 96 hours afterward). An oral or intravenous course of acyclovir (Zovirax) is given for 7 days when a child develops chicken pox or herpes zoster while receiving treatment, or within 6 months after treatment has ended. Antihistamine therapy is given for pruritis. Medications for pain management frequently are needed for patients with shingles.

**Potential complications:** Complications can include systemic (i.e., pulmonary, hepatic, central nervous system) involvement, prolonged interruption of cancer treatment, or death.

**Nursing Assessment and Interventions:**
*Assessment.*
- Assess the patient's varicella titer.
- Document varicella titer in the patient's medical record.
- Monitor response to antiviral therapy.
- Assess rash for potential secondary bacterial infection.

*Interventions.*
- Teach the family about what constitutes an exposure and the importance of avoiding exposure (**Table 5-1**).
- Instruct the family about how these diseases are spread by direct contact with patients with varicella zoster, occasionally by airborne spread of respiratory secretions, and, rarely, from zoster lesions.
- Alert authorities at the patient's school to notify the students' parents if there is a chicken pox outbreak.
- Tell the family to notify the child's healthcare provider when an exposure occurs to ensure a timely administration of IVIG.
- Teach the family to recognize the signs and symptoms of a more serious progression of disease.
- Encourage the habit of frequently washing hands thoroughly.

**Expected Patient and Family Outcomes:**
- The patient and the family know about the potential seriousness of varicella infections.
- The patient and the family comply with the recommendations for treatment related to an exposure or outbreak.

## Immunizations

Live, attenuated vaccines and inactive or killed vaccines help provide immunity for specific diseases frequently associated with childhood (e.g., measles, mumps, and rubella). In an immunocompromised child, a live vaccine actually can cause the disease and result in a potentially fatal outcome. Inactivated vaccines can be ineffective because the host is unable to develop a cell-mediated response.

## Immunization Issues for Patients, Their Siblings, and Peers

Patients may receive killed (i.e., inactivated) vaccines and influenza vaccine while in therapy. All routine immunizations can resume 3–12 months after treatment is completed, depending upon individual situations. Patient-related precautions include not permitting a patient to assist with changing the diaper of an infant who has been vaccinated with oral polio vaccine. Conversely, if a patient who is not immune to chicken pox is exposed to someone with a vesicular rash who has received VARIVAX, it is not considered a varicella exposure. Administration of IVIG is not indicated in this situation because the risk of transmission is extremely low. It has been suggested that children with acute lymphoblastic leukemia in remission be considered for VARIVAX vaccination. Although the risk of natural varicella outweighs the danger presented by the attenuated vaccine virus, vaccination is currently not the standard practice.

It is recommended that all household members receive an influenza vaccine. They may also have all routine childhood immunizations, including chicken pox vaccine. A patient's siblings or other children living in the house should receive an inactivated polio virus vaccine.

### Nursing Assessment and Interventions

**Assessment:**
Review the patient's immunization status with the patient and the family.

**Intervention:**
Teach the patient and the family about the issues related to immunizations (see **Table 5-2**).

### Expected Patient and Family Outcomes
The patient and the family know the potentially serious side effects of immunizations in an immunocompromised host.

---

### Table 5-1. Exposure to Chicken Pox

Chicken pox, also called varicella, is a contagious disease, which means it can be caught by spending 1 hour or more in the same room with someone who is contagious. Chicken pox is contagious about 24–36 hours before the first spot appears. It continues to be contagious until all the sores have scabs on them. The chicken pox rash usually develops 10–21 days after exposure. In addition, a child who breaks out into a vesicular rash following VARIVAX immunization is considered to be mildly contagious. Contact should be avoided, when possible, but it is not necessary for the immunosuppressed child to receive treatment.

Symptoms of chicken pox may include a runny nose, watery eyes, tiredness, and a fever. Within a day or two a rash develops. There are three types of sores: small red spots, raised red areas, or fluid-filled blister-like sores that break open and scab over. The chicken pox rash usually starts on the stomach, chest, back, or scalp. It then spreads over the rest of the body. A person who has had chicken pox usually develops immunity to the disease, which means that most people get chicken pox only once.

A child who is receiving chemotherapy or who is immunocompromised has a harder time fighting infections. Therefore, the following information is important to know about their care.

The physician or nurse should be called right away if the child was with someone for 1 hour or longer who has the chicken pox rash or who broke out in a rash 24–36 hours later. It is very important to call the child's healthcare provider as soon as the child was exposed. (If the family finds out at night, they can wait until the morning.)

Some people who have a low resistance to infections require a special medicine after they are exposed to chicken pox. This special medicine, called intravenous immunoglobulin (IVIG), will lower the risk of a severe infection but may not prevent the person from getting the chicken pox. It is important that the person receive IVIG within 96 hours of exposure.

A blood test can be done about 6 weeks after a person has recovered from chicken pox to determine if he or she has immunity. As long as a person does not have immunity, he or she will require IVIG with each chicken pox exposure until chemotherapy has stopped or the immune system has recovered for 6–12 months.

> **Table 5-2. Issues Related to Immunizations**
>
> Children who have decreased immunity are not able to fight infection in the same way as a child with a normal immune system. For this reason, live-bacteria and live-virus vaccinations are contraindicated for patients with suppressed immune systems. Inactivated vaccines may be administered, but it should be understood that the child's immune response may be inadequate. Inactivated vaccines include diphtheria-tetanus-pertussis (Tri-Immunol), hepatitis B (Engerix-B), inactivated polio virus (IPV; Polivax), pneumococcal (Pneumovax), and influenza virus (Fluogen) vaccines.
>
> A definite recommendation for initiation of immunizations after treatment for cancer varies according to the diagnosis and intensity of treatment. Most institutions restart immunizations within 6–12 months after cessation of treatment (American Academy of Pediatrics, 2006).
>
> **Siblings and Household Contacts**
> Siblings can receive live immunizations without harm to their immunocompromised brother or sister as can other people in the house who have contact with the child. The exception is that siblings and household contacts should receive IPV because live polio vaccine strains are transmissible. Varicella vaccine (VARIVAX) is recommended for these people as well.
>
> **Friends, Classmates, and Daycare Contacts**
> It is unnecessary to avoid or prevent contact with friends or classmates after they have been vaccinated. If a person develops a vesicular rash after receiving the varicella vaccine, physical contact with the immunocompromised child should be avoided, if possible, until the rash resolves. However, it is not necessary to administer IVIG if exposure inadvertently occurs, as the risk of infection transmission is low. Immunocompromised children should avoid contact with the stool (i.e., do not assist with diaper changing) of anyone who has received the live polio virus (OPV) because live polio virus is excreted in the stool for several weeks. In rare cases, oral polio virus has been excreted in the stool for more than 2 months (American Academy of Pediatrics, 2006).
>
> Adapted from material in *Redbook 2006: Report of the committee of infectious diseases* (27th ed.), by American Academy of Pediatrics, 2006, Elk Grove Village, IL: Author.

# Central-Nervous-System Complications

*Linda Madsen*

Central-nervous-system (CNS) complications from disease and treatment pose a significant challenge to patients, families, and healthcare providers. These complications cause a wide range of issues, depending on the specific location in the CNS that has been injured. A child's age and developmental stage can increase the difficulty healthcare providers have in recognizing and managing these problems.

## Diabetes Insipidus

### Definition
*Central diabetes insipidus* (DI) is a disorder that causes a decreased production of the antidiuretic hormone (ADH) vasopressin, resulting in the interruption of tubular reabsorption of water by the kidneys. Without reabsorption, excessive water is excreted in the urine. Osmoreceptors in the brain regulate the synthesis and release of ADH in the hypothalamus. ADH travels through the pituitary stalk to the posterior lobe of the pituitary, where it is stored until it is released into circulation. In patients with DI, the hypothalamus is unable to produce sufficient ADH.

### Risk Factors
Risk factors include CNS tumors, surgery, or radiation therapy, which can affect the hypothalamic-pituitary axis (HPA). Postoperative swelling occurs 24–48 hours after surgery, temporarily decreasing the production of ADH. Langerhans cell histiocytosis; midline, supratentorial, or infratentorial brain tumors (i.e., pituitary tumors, hypothalamic tumors, pineal tumors, craniopharygiomas, germ-cell tumors, and third-ventricular tumors); CNS leukemia; and radiation therapy to the HPA all increase the risk of DI.

### Clinical Presentation
The symptoms of DI are polyuria, nocturia, polydipsia, a specific gravity of less than 1.005, hypernatremia, hypokalemia, and lethargy.

### Medical Management
A complete history is taken and a physical examination, including neurologic assessment, is performed. Evaluation and management of the underlying cause does not always reverse the condition. A fluid deprivation test is used to establish the diagnosis by measuring serum and urine osmolality and vasopressin levels in response to fluid restriction. If a patient's urine concentration or osmolality does not increase despite fluid restriction, the diagnosis is confirmed. Steroids may be given to reduce inflammation after surgery. Fluid balance is strictly monitored and maintained. Desmopressin (DDAVP), a synthetic vasopressin, is administered to act on the kidneys, causing them to reabsorb water.

### Potential Complications
The potential complications of DI are severe dehydration and hypovolemia leading to shock or hypernatremia, as well as hypokalemia that could progress to seizures.

### Nursing Assessment and Interventions
**Assessment:**
- Strictly monitor the patient's fluid intake and output.
- Weigh the patient twice a day.
- Closely monitor urine and serum sodium and osmolality and urine-specific gravity during evaluation and early management.
- Assess for neurologic changes.
- Assess the educational and support needs of the patient and the family.

**Interventions:**
- Fluids are replaced as needed.
- DDAVP is administered orally, intranasally, subcutaneously, or intravenously. After DDAVP is given, it is important not to fluid overload the patient.
- Educate the patient and the family regarding the basic pathology and etiology of DI.
- Teach the patient and the family about the technique and schedule of administering DDAVP and the signs and symptoms of breakthrough diuresis or overdose of DDAVP.
- Encourage the patient and the family to obtain a Medical-Alert bracelet.
- Inform the patient and the family that DDAVP dose adjustments may be needed during illness.

- Develop strategies for patients with abnormal thirst mechanisms to maintain normal hydration.
- Ensure that the patient has unlimited access to a bathroom and to oral fluids at day care or school.

### Expected Patient and Family Outcomes
- The patient and the family know about the disease process.
- The patient and the family can independently adjust the patient's DDAVP dose.
- The patient and the family adhere to follow-up recommendations.
- Appropriate fluid balance is maintained.

## Cranial Nerve Deficits

### Definition
*Cranial nerve deficits* are caused by impingement or invasion of the nerves arising from the brain stem that results in specific functional deficits (**Figure 5-1**).

### Risk Factors
The risk factors associated with cranial nerve deficits are primary or metastatic tumors of the CNS (e.g., brain-stem gliomas, pontine tumors, medulloblastomas, ependymomas, pineal tumors, pituitary tumors, optic gliomas, CNS lymphomas and leukemias, parameningeal or nasopharyngeal rhabdomyosarcomas, soft tissue sarcomas, neuroblastomas, nasopharyngeal carcinoma, neurofibromatosis, and retinoblastoma); resection of the tumor; radiation to the head; and chemotherapeutic agents, including vincristine (Oncovin), vinblastine (Velban), taxanes, cytarabine (Cytosine Arabinoside), cisplatin (Platinol), and ifosfamide (Ifex).

### Clinical Presentation
The symptoms vary, depending on which nerves are affected (**Table 5-3**). Parinaud syndrome, which is manifested by convergence nystagmus, no upward gaze, and increased pupillary reaction to accommodation to light, is often associated with pineal tumors. Horner syndrome, which is manifested by miosis, ptosis, exophthalmos, anhydrosis (decreased sweating), and constriction of the pupils, is often associated with hypothalamic tumors, tumors of the brain stem or the upper-cervical cord, and neuroblastoma. Certain chemotherapy agents, such as the vinca alkaloids, can affect the cranial nerves after the first dose or worsen with cumulative dosing.

### Medical Treatment
A complete medical history, physical examination, and neurologic examination should be performed. Surgical resection, radiation, or chemotherapy may be used to alleviate pressure on the nerves. Speech and occupational therapy are implemented to evaluate the effects of the cranial-nerve deficits on function and to rehabilitate the patient or help him or her to develop compensatory strategies. Chemotherapy-dosage adjustments may be needed if the deficit is significant and related to the chemotherapy.

### Potential Complications
Potential complications include muscle atrophy, corneal abrasions, facial palsy, and persistent deficits that inhibit function (e.g., dysphasia, altered taste resulting in poor nutrition, visual deficits, facial sensation, and mobility and hearing impairments).

### Nursing Assessment and Interventions
**Assessment:**
- Assess the extent of the deficit and its effects on the patient's functioning.
- Assess the patient for deficits before administering agents that pose a risk of cranial-nerve dysfunction.
- Assess the chronicity of the deficits.
- Assess the patient's and the family's coping abilities to support a child with deficits.
- Assess the learning needs of the child and the family and their need for safety measures.

**Interventions:**
- Assist with adaptation of activities of daily living.
- Protect eyes when blink-reflex defect occurs.
- Assist with occupational and speech therapy to reinforce and support rehabilitation strategies.

**Figure 5-1. Cranial Nerves: Ventral Surface of the Brain Showing Attachment of the Cranial Nerves**

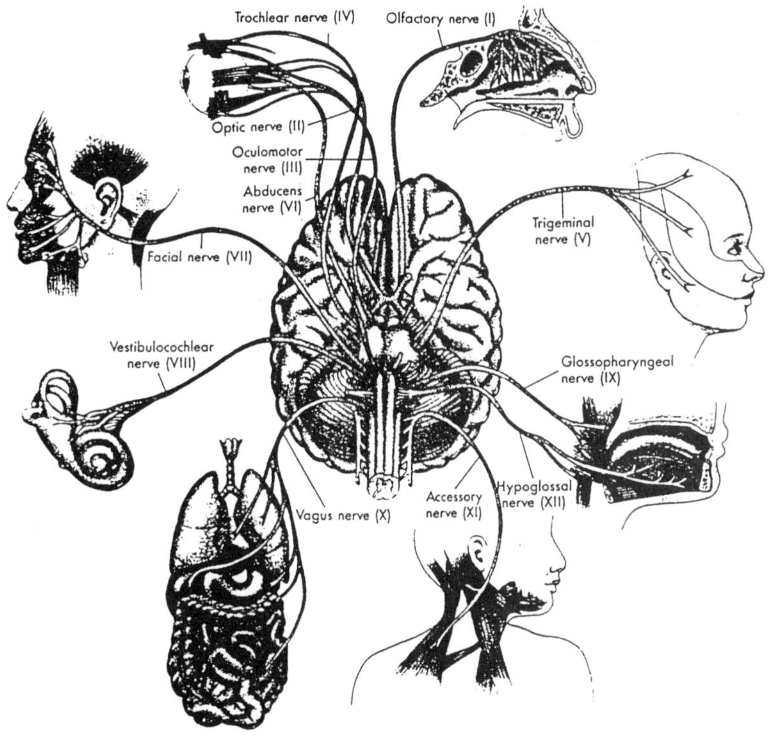

From *Anatomy and Physiology* (p. 345), by G. A. Thibodeau & K. T. Patton, 1992, St. Louis: Mosby. Copyright 1992 by Mosby. Reprinted with permission.

### Table 5-3. The Central Nervous System: Cranial Nerves and Their Functions

| Number | Nerve Name | Function | Deficits and Findings |
|---|---|---|---|
| I | Olfactory | Smell | Loss or change in smell |
| II | Optic | Vision | Loss of acuity, optic atrophy, altered visual fields |
| III | Oculomotor | Pupil constriction, eyelid movement, extraocular movements | Ptosis, dilated pupils, altered ocular muscle function (often causing double vision), poor near vision, nystagmus |
| IV | Trochlear | Downward and inward eye movement | Altered ocular muscle function and nystagmus |
| V | Trigeminal | Motor function of the jaw and sensation of the eye and face | Numbness, poor blink reflex, weakened chewing |
| VI | Abducens | Lateral eye movement | Altered ocular muscle function and nystagmus |
| VII | Facial | Movement of the forehead, eyes, mouth, taste of the anterior two thirds of the tongue | Facial paralysis, drooping mouth, sagging lower lid, flat nasolabial fold |
| VIII | Acoustic | Hearing and balance | Sensorineural hearing loss, tinnitus, vertigo, nausea and vomiting, ataxia |
| IX | Glossopharyngeal | Sensory functions of the pharynx and posterior tongue, includes taste | Altered taste and sensation of the throat |
| X | Vagus | Sensory and motor function of the pharynx and larynx, movement of palate | Hoarseness, altered gag reflex, altered swallowing function, dysphonia, vocal cord paralysis |
| XI | Spinal | Motor function of sternomastoid and trapezius muscles | Head tilt to one side, weakness of the shoulder muscles |
| XII | Hypoglossal | Motor function of the tongue | Tongue movement, dysarthria, dysphagia |

- Notify the child's physician if complications develop.
- Provide a safe environment for the patient during ambulation; help the patient distinguish hot from cold and detect other changes in sensation.
- Provide the patient with nutritional supplements or enteral feeding if needed.
- Provide home-safety instruction (i.e., assess and adapt the home environment as needed); educate the family about necessary adaptations and rehabilitation strategies; provide for ongoing occupational and speech therapy if needed; intervene when necessary to facilitate the patient's reentry to school; and help with educational planning.

### Expected Patient and Family Outcomes
- The patient and the family adhere to the recommendations for rehabilitative therapy.
- A safe environment is provided in the home and in modes of transportation.
- The patient has good hygiene, skin care, and nutrition.
- The patient attains optimal functioning despite deficits.

## Cognitive Deficits and Behavioral Changes

### Definition
*Cognitive deficits* are changes in or losses of intellectual and developmental functioning. *Behavioral changes* relate to the patient's personality and to social functioning.

### Risk Factors
Risk factors are medications that alter mood (e.g., steroids, procarbazine [Matulane], ifosfamide [Ifex]), and supportive-care medications including sedating antiemetics, pain medications, and antidepressants. Intrathecal chemotherapy and cranial radiation can affect intellectual functioning (see Section X, "Late Effects of Childhood Cancer"). Effects of radiation are highest for the youngest patients and can decline over time.

Other risk factors include tumors or resections of tumors, including craniopharyngioma, hypothalamic, and optic-pathway tumors (which can be associated with memory deficits, personality changes, or cognitive abnormalities), pontine tumors (which can be associated with personality changes), hemispheric gliomas (which can be associated with poor academic performance and/or personality changes), posterior fossa tumors (which can be associated with emotional lability and declining academic performance), frontal lobe tumors (which can be associated with behavioral problems), and brain stem gliomas (which can be associated with depression and irritability). Hydrocephalus is associated with cognitive challenges, especially if longstanding.

Encephalitis and meningitis are additional factors that create an increased risk for cognitive declines. Stress brought on by hospitalization, diagnosis, treatments, and pain are also risk factors.

### Clinical Presentation
The signs and symptoms can include a decline in school performance failure to achieve or a loss of developmental milestones; a change in personality and temperament (e.g., irritability, drastic mood swings, fatigue, lethargy, depression, emotional lability,

apathy); short-term memory loss; diencephalic syndrome (e.g., failure to thrive; emaciation in a euphoric infant with an increased appetite or caloric consumption and hyperkinesis); and increased intracranial pressure, which may be manifested by early-morning vomiting or headaches.

## Medical Management

Medical management consists of a complete medical history, physical examination, and diagnostic testing, as indicated, to evaluate the underlying cause. Surgical resection and placement of a ventriculostomy or ventriculo-peritoneal shunt may be needed to alleviate pressure. Radiation, chemotherapy, or both are given when indicated to reduce the mass. Steroids may be given to reduce inflammation after surgery. In addition, concomitant medications that can contribute to behavioral changes or cognitive decline must be carefully evaluated. Medications can be ordered to moderate ongoing mood disorders or to regulate problematic behavior. Neuropsychological evaluations should be done regularly to determine the extent of the patient's deficits and to help plan educational or behavioral interventions to maximize the patient's potential. The effects of radiation on the developing brain must be considered, and tumor management is adapted whenever possible to minimize the effect on the growing brain. Careful treatment of pain and referral for psychological support is often needed.

## Potential Complications

Possible complications are a worsening symptomatology; permanent impairment; social isolation, poor peer relationships, or both; a developmental crisis; family stress; and poor self-esteem.

## Nursing Assessment and Interventions

**Assessment:**
- Assess the patient's behavioral and cognitive functioning over time.
- Assess the impact of the child's behavior on family stress and functioning, as well as on his or her self-image and relationships.
- Assess the impact of cognitive functioning on the child's academic and developmental performance.
- Assess the side effects of medications that can alter behavior or impair learning ability or intellectual performance.

**Interventions:**
- Plan for the patient's reentry to school to ease his or her adaptation. The child may require an individual education plan if learning/rehabilitation or behavioral issues are significant.
- Assess early changes that indicate worsening symptoms or a recurrence of cognitive deficits or changes in behavior.
- Discuss strategies for managing behavior.
- Provide anticipatory guidance for the parents (i.e., review the potential side effects of medications, discuss how to identify symptoms that could indicate the patient's worsening status, and help identify resources to alleviate the family's stress).
- Encourage regular neuropsychological evaluations.
- Educate the child and the parents about school issues and reintegration.
- Encourage early intervention for cognitive and behavioral issues.
- Encourage the patient to interact with both unaffected peers and those who have experienced similar problems.

## Expected Patient and Family Outcomes
- The patient and the family know about potential cognitive deficits.
- The patient adopts a healthy lifestyle despite deficits.
- The patient and the family comply with recommended therapeutic interventions.

# Posterior Fossa Syndrome

## Definition

*Posterior fossa syndrome* consists of transient, or occasionally permanent, deficits after posterior fossa surgery. This syndrome often results in mutism or speech disturbance, dysphasia, decreased motor function, weakness, emotional lability, and cranial-nerve palsies, which usually present 24–48 hours after surgery and can last for approximately 2–6 months.

## Risk Factors

Risk factors are posterior fossa tumors (e.g., medulloblastoma or primitive neuroectodermal tumor, astrocytoma, brain-stem glioma, ependymoma), large tumor resection, surgical manipulation of the floor of the fourth ventricle, hydrocephalus, cerebellar insult, meningeal spread of tumor, cerebellar atrophy, and vascular disturbances.

## Clinical Presentation

The signs and symptoms may include, but are not limited to, facial weakness, nystagmus, emotional lability and irritability, mutism or difficulty verbalizing, inability to follow verbal commands, random movements, weakness of the arms and legs, dysphasia, hemiparesis, and absence of bladder or bowel control. The patient typically awakens after surgery functionally intact and begins to lose function within days.

## Medical Management

The patient is given a complete physical and neurologic examination, as well as a thorough examination to assess his or her swallowing ability and vocal-cord function. Hydrocephalus is treated if necessary. Referrals for occupational therapy, physical therapy, and speech therapy are made. Enteral or parenteral feeding may be necessary if the patient is dysphasic. Patients also may benefit from taking glucocorticoids.

## Potential Complications

Complications may include permanent functional impairment, aspiration, inability to maintain airway, muscle atrophy, nutritional deficiency, cognitive decline, and family dysfunction.

## Nursing Assessment and Interventions

**Assessment:**
- Assess early changes in the patient's neurologic status.
- Monitor the patient's fluid status.
- Assess the patient's gag reflex, vocal characteristics, and cognitive and swallowing abilities.
- Assess the effects of the deficits on the patient's personal safety.
- Assess the educational, psychological, and social support needs of the patient and the family.
- Assess the difference between irritability related to the syndrome and irritability related to pain. Irritability can be extreme and very stressful for the family.

**Interventions:**
- Prepare the families of high-risk patients before surgery for the possible onset of the syndrome.
- Provide support for the family; provide reassurance that symptoms typically improve over time, although in some situations they do not totally resolve.
- Implement safety precautions related to preventing aspiration, impaired motor function, and unsteady gait.
- Provide skin care.
- Implement enteral or parenteral feedings as appropriate.
- Support adaptive communication strategies.
- Assess and adapt the home environment as appropriate.
- Educate the family about needed adaptations and support rehabilitation strategies.
- Provide for ongoing occupational therapy and speech therapy if needed.
- Help plan for the patient's reentry to school, including adaptation to school and remediation if needed.

### Expected Patient and Family Outcomes
- The patient and the family understand the implications of deficits.
- The patient and the family comply with recommended therapeutic interventions.
- The patient and the family can identify and use available resources.

## Ototoxicity

*Wendy Landier*

### Definition
*Ototoxicity* is damage to the hearing organ that is associated with a therapeutic agent, resulting in hearing loss or vestibular (balance) changes. The type of hearing loss associated with ototoxic pharmacologic agents is sensorineural (resulting from damage to the cochlea/inner ear) and is usually irreversible (see **Figures 5-2** and **5-3**). Hearing loss associated with radiation, tumor, or surgical procedures may involve both conductive and sensorineural components. Ototoxicity has the potential to adversely affect a child's social, emotional, and intellectual development.

### Risk Factors
Potentially ototoxic agents commonly used in pediatric oncology include platinum-based chemotherapy (e.g., cisplatin and myeloablative doses of carboplatin), aminoglycoside antibiotics (e.g., gentamicin, tobramycin, amikacin), loop diuretics (e.g., furosemide), and radiation therapy to the ear, midbrain, or brain stem. Patients who are at increased risk for ototoxicity include those who are younger than 4 years of age when the ototoxic agent is administered and patients who receive high cumulative doses of platinum chemotherapy, high doses of radiation to the cochlea, surgery adjacent to the eighth cranial nerve, or therapy with multiple ototoxic agents. Other risk factors include the diagnosis of a central nervous system tumor, diminished renal function, rapid intravenous administration of the ototoxic agent, and preexisting hearing loss.

### Clinical Presentation
Symptoms of early hearing loss may include tinnitus or vertigo or both, difficulty in hearing when there is background noise, inattentiveness, or failure to turn toward sounds. However, many children have no symptoms of early hearing loss. Therefore, audiologic monitoring is required for all children receiving potentially ototoxic agents. Methods of audiologic evaluation include pure-tone audiometry (i.e., standard audiograms and behaviorally based assessments used with children who can cooperate with testing) or brain stem auditory-evoked response (i.e., electrophysiologic measurement of hearing used with infants or children who are unable to cooperate with standard testing). All patients who receive ototoxic agents should undergo periodic audiologic evaluations by an experienced pediatric audiologist.

### Medical Management
Patients with identified hearing loss should be referred to a pediatric otologist or audiologist for evaluation and fitting of appropriate hearing aids. Frequent follow-up assessments (i.e., every 6 months) for retesting and refitting of hearing aids are essential, especially for younger, growing children. Because hearing loss associated with ototoxicity usually is irreversible, preventive measures are undergoing evaluation, including shielding or modifying radiation fields to limit cochlear exposure and modifying therapeutic protocols to make possible earlier detection of ototoxicity and subsequent dose reduction or substitution of less ototoxic agents when feasible.

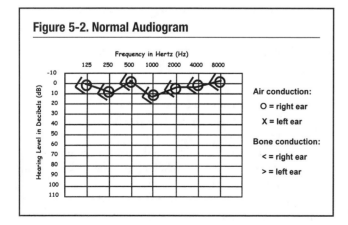

**Figure 5-2. Normal Audiogram**

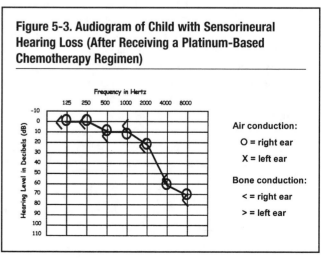

**Figure 5-3. Audiogram of Child with Sensorineural Hearing Loss (After Receiving a Platinum-Based Chemotherapy Regimen)**

### Nursing Assessment and Interventions

**Assessment:**
- Assess risk factors for ototoxicity in all patients who are receiving potentially ototoxic agents.
- Ensure that all such patients are appropriately monitored (i.e., periodic audiologic evaluations and frequent monitoring of aminoglycoside levels).

**Interventions:**
- Avoid rapid intravenous administration of ototoxic agents such as loop diuretics, aminoglycosides, or platinum chemotherapy.
- Ensure that preventive measures are implemented when medically indicated (e.g., prompt dose modification of aminoglycosides, if indicated, per blood levels; early dose modification of platinum chemotherapy per protocol guidelines if hearing loss is detected).
- Advise patients and parents about otoprotective strategies (i.e., using earplugs in noisy environments to prevent noise-induced hearing loss and avoiding ototoxic medications when alternatives are available).
- For children with hearing loss
  - ensure the patient receives a referral for a hearing-aid evaluation.
  - ensure the parents and the patient learn how to properly clean and care for the hearing aid and that they understand the importance of replacing batteries on a regular basis (most require replacement every 1–2 weeks).
  - familiarize the parents and the patient with options regarding communication methods (e.g., auditory/verbal, cued speech), and assistive devices (e.g., FM amplification system, telephone amplifiers, text telephones, adaptive appliances).
  - familiarize the parents and the patient with community and educational resources (e.g., in-home speech therapy, specialized classroom accommodations).

## Endocrine Abnormalities

*Rebecca A. Monroe*

Treatment for various hematologic and oncologic diseases commonly can induce hormone alterations. The primary endocrine effects from chemotherapy are related to the type of drug, the dose, the duration of treatment, and the age and sex of the patient. Endocrine effects from radiation therapy are related to the total dose of radiation, patient age, and location of treatment. Changes in endocrine function can occur months or years after treatment.

### Hormone Alterations

#### Definition

*Hormone alterations* are abnormally high or low levels of hormones secreted by the body. They occur because of neuroendocrine damage caused by the tumor or cancer treatment and can result in complications such as hypothyroidism, gonadal dysfunction, and growth-hormone deficiency (see Section X, "Late Effects of Childhood Cancer").

### Risk Factors

There are treatment-related and disease-related risk factors.

**Treatment-related factors:** These risk factors include those associated with radiation therapy (e.g., dose, patient's age, and radiation treatment site) and those associated with chemotherapy (e.g., alkylating agents, nitrosoureas). Alkylating agents can produce gonadal atrophy that can permanently alter reproductive function.

**Disease-related factor:** Tumor location is the disease-related factor.

### Clinical Presentation

The signs and symptoms of hormone alterations can include abnormal thyroid levels; fatigue; change in bowel habits; dry skin; delayed development of secondary sexual characteristics; precocious puberty; irregular menses; amenorrhea; hormone levels (e.g., follicle-stimulating hormone [FSH], luteinizing hormone [LH], testosterone, estradiol, growth hormone) that are abnormal for the patient's age; a decrease in linear growth; elevated levels of antidiuretic hormone; osteopenia or osteoporosis; and dyslipidemias (see Section X, "Late Effects of Childhood Cancer," for further discussion).

### Medical Management

The patient should be given a complete physical examination and a health history should be taken in addition to assessments of growth and secondary sexual maturation. Hormone replacement may be indicated after the patient has been evaluated by an endocrinologist.

### Potential Complications

Complications may include an increase or decrease in hormone levels, alterations in linear growth, abnormal bone metabolism, precocious puberty or alterations in sexual maturation, hypothyroidism, temporary amenorrhea or irregular menses, premature menopause, infertility, syndrome of inappropriate antidiuretic hormone secretion, and metabolic syndrome.

### Nursing Assessment and Interventions

**Assessment:**
- Obtain and compare serial measurements of the patient's height and weight throughout therapy and after therapy is concluded.
- Obtain serum hormonal evaluations (i.e., T3, free T4, TSH, LH, FSH) throughout therapy and after therapy is concluded, especially if the patient received radiation therapy to the hypothalamic-pituitary axis or thyroid gland.
- Monitor alterations in lipid levels secondary to hormonal changes.
- Obtain bone-mineral-density studies.
- Assess the patient's sexual development using the Tanner staging system.
- Assess a female patient's menstrual history at each visit.

**Interventions:**
- Provide ongoing education about the effects of the disease and its treatment.
- Encourage and support a multidisciplinary approach to endocrine problems related to the disease, the treatment, or both.

### Expected Patient and Family Outcomes
- The patient and the family comply with the multidisciplinary plan of care.
- The patient understands the need for long-term compliance and follow-up.

## Fertility Preservation

A patient's disease and treatment may have an impact on his or her fertility status. The infertility risk from cancer treatment is dependent on the type of treatment (e.g., chemotherapy, radiation, or both), treatment doses and duration, type of chemotherapy (e.g., alkylating agents, nitrosoureas), location of radiation (e.g., total body irradiation, testes in males, pelvic region and/or abdomen in females), and patient's age.

Fertility preservation remains a controversial issue. Questions that must be answered include: Is it appropriate to delay therapy to undergo fertility-preservation procedures? What happens to the patient's frozen reproductive tissue, gametes, or embryos in the event of the patient's death? The answers to these questions are unique to each individual and must be made in collaboration with the patient's medical team.

Patients and parents should be advised that insurance companies may not cover fertility-preservation procedures. The expenses associated with fertility preservation, in addition to storage fees, can be costly.

Gender-specific fertility-preservation options include the following:

### Males
Sperm cryopreservation is the traditional method of fertility preservation for postpubertal males. Currently, there are no established fertility-preservation options for prepubertal males. However, techniques involving testicular-tissue cryopreservation, and testicular germ-cell harvesting are being explored and may offer hope in the future.

### Females
Ovaries may be protected by oophoropexy or by shielding the ovaries to reduce radiation exposure. Embryo cryopreservation is also an established method of fertility preservation; however, it requires that the patient be postpubertal and have time to undergo hormonal stimulation and oocyte harvesting. In addition, the patient must have a partner or donor who can provide sperm to fertilize the eggs prior to cryopreservation. Such requirements pose many obstacles for young patients. Researchers are exploring techniques such as hormonal suppression of ovarian activity, oocyte cryopreservation, and ovarian-tissue cryopreservation; however, these techniques remain experimental.

### Nursing Assessment and Interventions
**Assessment:**
- Assess the patient's knowledge about his or her fertility status in relation to the disease, the treatment, or both.
- Assess the patient's sexual development using the Tanner staging system.

  **Interventions:**
- Arrange for private, uninterrupted discussions regarding fertility issues. Provide written educational material if available.
- Prior to the initiation of therapy, provide education about possible fertility-status changes and reproductive organ changes (e.g., impaired uterine development, orchiectomy) related to the disease and treatment, and educate the patient about possible fertility-preservation options.
- Refer to specialists (e.g., urologist, reproductive endocrinologist) as necessary.
- Encourage and support a multidisciplinary approach to fertility issues.

### Expected Patient and Family Outcomes
- The patient and the family understand potential risks to the patient's fertility status.
- The patient understands his or her fertility preservation options and is given the opportunity to pursue such options if medically appropriate. See Section X, "Late Effects of Childhood Cancer," for a further discussion.

# Cardiac and Pulmonary Complications

*Vicki Schaefers*

Cardiac and pulmonary side effects can be directly related to the underlying disease, but they are more commonly associated with specific therapies or an infectious process. A combination of these factors places a patient at greater risk for complications. Acute episodes of cardiopulmonary toxicities frequently evolve into chronic conditions (see Section X, "Late Effects of Childhood Cancer" for more details).

## Acute Cardiomyopathy
### Definition
*Cardiomyopathy* is a defect of the heart muscle that results from damage to cardiac myocytes; it causes loss of muscle fibers and shifts in intracellular calcium (see Section X, "Late Effects of Childhood Cancer").

### Risk Factors
Chemotherapy-related risk factors include cumulative doses of anthracyclines (the doses must be lowered if radiation treatment also is used), single agents (e.g., cyclophosphamide [Cytoxan]) as well as combination chemotherapy, and combination chemotherapy and radiation. Other risk factors are radiation therapy to the mediastinum, surgery for removal of a tumor in the chest wall or thorax, underlying cardiac disease, administration of intravenous (IV) products that cause fluid overload, anemia, age (particularly when a patient is younger than 4–5 years of age), and the use of glucocorticoids, which can cause hypertension.

### Clinical Presentation
The signs and symptoms of acute cardiac myopathy can include hypertension or hypotension, chest pain, decreased activity level, fatigue, tachycardia, shortness of breath, nonproductive cough, distention of the neck vein, pedal edema, cardiomegaly, gallop rhythm of the heart, and hepatomegaly.

## Medical Management
Medical management consists of performing a complete physical examination and taking a health history to review potential risk factors, establishing baseline cardiac status, obtaining information about prior therapies (including the cumulative dose of radiation and chemotherapy and patient's age when therapy was administered), assessing for routine monitoring of cardiac status, and assessing the child's activity level. Pharmacologic management consists of adjusting the rate, schedule, and dose of chemotherapy and prescribing any needed antiarrhythmic drugs. Blood-product transfusions also may be given if the patient is anemic, and oxygen therapy can be given if necessary. Cardioprotective agents (e.g., dexrazoxane [Zinecard]) have been shown to protect the heart from cardiac toxicity while not compromising the treatment effect. The dose of dexrazoxane is determined as a ratio with 10 mg of dexrazoxane given for each 1 mg of doxorubicin.

## Potential Complications
Complications can include disturbances in the cardiac rhythm, congestive heart failure, or death.

## Nursing Assessment and Interventions
**Assessment:**
- Identify the patient's risk factors for developing acute cardiomyopathy.
- Assess the patient for clinical manifestations of congestive heart failure (e.g., tachycardia, shortness of breath, gallop heart rhythm, hepatomegaly, pedal edema, distention of the veins in the neck).
- Monitor the patient's vital signs and assess the heart rate for normal rhythm and regularity.
- Assess electrocardiogram, echocardiogram, and 24-hour Holter monitor data, and evaluate the results of chest radiograph according to the treatment protocol or as ordered.

**Interventions:**
- Administer prescribed medications.
- Teach the family about medication-administration techniques.
- Teach the patient and the family about the signs and symptoms of congestive heart failure.

## Expected Patient and Family Outcomes
- The patient has minimal complications related to acute cardiomyopathy.
- The patient and the family can verbally identify the risk factors associated with acute cardiomyopathy.

# Pneumonitis

## Definition
*Pneumonitis* is an inflammation of the lung that is caused by infectious agents, irritants, or both.

## Risk Factors
The risk factors are neutropenia, bacterial agents (i.e., Pneumocystis carinii, Hemophilus influenza, Streptococcus pneumoniae, mycobacterium), viral agents (e.g., cytomegalovirus, herpes zoster, chicken pox, respiratory syncytial virus, Epstein-Barr virus), chemotherapy (e.g., busulfan [Myleran], melphalan [Alkeran], methotrexate [Mexate], bleomycin [Blenoxane]), radiation therapy to the lungs, and underlying respiratory disease.

## Clinical Presentation
Patients may present with dyspnea, persistent dry cough, malaise and/or fatigue, fever, moist rales, and a pleural friction rub. Tachypnea, cyanosis, and decreased oxygen saturation are late signs of impaired lung status.

## Medical Management
Prophylactic trimethoprim-sulfamethoxazole (Bactrim), pentamidine (Pentam-300), or dapsone (Avlosulfon) is used to prevent Pneumocystis carinii. Antibiotics are given for bacterial infections. Patients should receive an influenza vaccine annually. For symptomatic patients, blood cultures, a chest X ray, pulmonary function tests, and pulse oximetry monitoring are performed routinely. Bronchodilators may be prescribed. Oxygen and ventilator assistance are given if needed.

## Potential Complications
Complications include pulmonary fibrosis or death.

## Nursing Assessment and Interventions
**Assessment:**
- Monitor the patient's respiratory rate and effort.
- Assess the patient for signs of pulmonary toxicity.
- Assess the patient for dyspnea, nonproductive cough, rales, and tachypnea.

**Interventions:**
- Place emphasis on activities the patient can accomplish with minimal exertion.
- Discuss the importance of frequent rest periods, especially during periods of exertion, such as walking.
- Provide measures to decrease dyspnea, such as elevating the head of the patient's bed.

## Expected Patient and Family Outcomes
- The patient and the family understand the causes of pneumonitis.
- The patient experiences minimal discomfort.
- The patient and the family recognize and implement measures to reduce the patient's oxygen expenditure.
- The patient and the family identify symptoms or changes that necessitate an immediate medical evaluation.

# Pulmonary Fibrosis

## Definition
*Pulmonary fibrosis* is the formation of fibrous scar tissue in the lungs as a consequence of an inflammation, an injury, or both.

## Risk Factors
The risk factors are chemotherapy (e.g., busulfan [Myleran], methotrexate [Mexate], melphalan [Alkeran], bleomycin [Blenoxane]), radiation therapy to the lungs, radiation therapy in combination with chemotherapy, previous lung biopsy, underlying pulmonary disease, and smoking.

## Clinical Presentation
A patient may present with respiratory distress (e.g., tachypnea, dyspnea, cough, hypoxemia, increased respiratory effort) or chest pain, or interstitial infiltrates may be seen on a chest X ray.

## Medical Management

A patient should be given a complete routine physical examination, and a health history should be taken. These measures establish the patient's baseline pulmonary status, provide information about prior therapies—including cumulative doses of radiation and chemotherapy—and provide a review of potential risk factors.

The patient's pulmonary status, including pulmonary function, pulse oximetry, and chest X ray, is routinely monitored. The patient's activity level and respiratory status are assessed. For symptomatic patients, corticosteroids may be used; oxygen therapy should be given only if clinically indicated.

## Potential Complications

Complications include pulmonary hypertension or death.

## Nursing Assessment and Interventions

**Assessment:**
- Maintain complete and current treatment records, including information on prior therapies, doses, and test results.
- Monitor the patient for signs and symptoms of congestive heart disease and respiratory distress.
- Provide laboratory results and information on the patient's status to the physician and the patient's family.
- Monitor the patient's IV fluid rate to avoid fluid overload.
- Strictly maintain intake and output records.
- Weigh the patient daily.

**Interventions:**
- Teach the family how to modify the patient's activities according to his or her cardiopulmonary status.
- Instruct the family about the correct use of medications and prescribed therapies, and explain their side effects.
- Give written and verbal information to the patient and the family about potential future risk factors during times of increased cardiovascular stress caused by conditions such as pregnancy, illness, heavy weightlifting, or anesthetization.

## Expected Patient and Family Outcomes

- The patient and the family verbalize understanding of the potential complications of the disease and the treatment related to the cardiopulmonary system.
- The patient and the family understand the need for long-term follow-up.
- The patient and the family adhere to the recommended therapy.

# Gastrointestinal Complications

*Ruth Landers and Joan O'Hanlon-Curry*

Gastrointestinal (GI) complications associated with cancer treatment are common in children. The mucosal cells in childrens' GI tracts are rapidly dividing cells and are particularly sensitive to chemotherapeutic agents and radiation therapy. The cellular destruction of cancer treatment results in mucositis, an inflammatory response. Disruption of this mucosal barrier places an immunocompromised child at increased risk for pain, ulceration, bleeding, dehydration, malnutrition, and opportunistic infection.

## Mucositis and Esophagitis

### Definition

*Oral mucositis*, or *stomatitis*, is an inflammation or an ulceration of the mucous membranes of the oral cavity (i.e., the lips, tongue, palate, buccal mucosa, gingiva, and floor of the mouth). Esophagitis is mucositis of the esophagus.

### Risk Factors

Risk factors are trauma to the oral cavity, esophagus, or both because of surgical manipulation; cytotoxic therapy, such as anthracyclines and antimetabolites; radiation therapy to the head, neck, chest wall, and mediastinum (e.g., mantle radiation in lymphoma patients); radiation-induced xerostomia due to mucosal atrophy and fibrosis of the salivary glands; graft-versus-host disease; immunosuppression; local irritants including alcohol, tobacco, commercial mouthwashes, and spicy or hot foods; malnutrition; dehydration; dental caries; and gastroesophageal reflux.

### Clinical Presentation

**Mucositis:** A patient may have pale, ridged, erythematous, ulcerated, or bleeding mucous membranes and gingiva; dry, blistered, or cracked lips; whitish plaques with slightly raised, indurated borders caused by Candida albicans fungus; or ulceration of the oral mucosa caused by herpes simplex virus. Oral discomfort may cause difficulty in opening the mouth, speaking, or swallowing. The patient may experience difficulty in eating and drinking because of local discomfort and may develop alterations in taste. In addition, a patient may exhibit psychosocial withdrawal due to pain, an inability to communicate, and loss of oral gratification (especially in infants and toddlers).

**Esophagitis:** Patients can have burning retrosternal chest pain (i.e., heartburn) when stomach acid comes into contact with inflamed esophageal tissue or if *Candida* infection is present. Other symptoms include nausea, bloating, early satiety, or coughing.

### Assessment

Some method of consistent assessment of the oral cavity is necessary. Many centers use the *Common Terminology Criteria for Adverse Events*, established by the National Cancer Institute, to assess toxicity during clinical trials. Other groups have begun to establish content validity of other indices that may prove useful for assessing the oral cavity in children and young adults. One of these instruments is the Oral Assessment Scale, which was developed for use in adults but is now undergoing modification for use in pediatrics (Gibson et al., 2006).

### Medical Management

Treatment can include oral rinses (e.g., chlorhexidine [Peridex], normal saline solution, baking soda solution) after meals, at bedtime, and as needed to clean the oral mucosa, remove debris, and reduce the incidence of plaque and dental caries. Fluoride rinses and saliva substitutes are used for xerostomia or dry mouth. Antifungal treatments include nystatin (Mycostatin) suspension, clotrimoxazole (Mycelex) troches, and mouthwashes (e.g., amphotericin-B, nystatin), as well as fluconazole (Diflucan) or amphotericin B (Fungizone) to treat systemic candidiasis. Acyclovir (Zovirax) is used as a treatment for herpetic lesions and as a prophylaxis in patients who have had bone-marrow transplants. Other measures include intravenous fluid therapy in the acute phase when oral therapy is not adequate, parenteral nutrition if mucositis persists and weight loss becomes a problem, and consultation with a dentist and a dietitian.

**Pain control:** Local palliation can be provided with topical agents such as viscous lidocaine, diphenhydramine (Benadryl), and sucralfate (Carafate). Histamine antagonists and antacids relieve gastric and lower esophageal irritation. Centrally acting analgesics range from acetaminophen (Tylenol) to continuous narcotic infusion, with the choice depending on the severity of the mucositis or esophagitis.

## Potential Complications

Complications include viral, bacterial, or fungal infection; malnutrition; cachexia; dehydration; GI bleeding; and esophageal stricture.

## Nursing Assessment and Interventions

**Assessment:**
- Assess the patient's oral cavity by following the guidelines listed in **Table 5-4**.
- Assess for functional impairment in speech, swallowing, and drooling.
- Monitor the patient's fluid and dietary intake.
- Weigh the patient daily.

**Interventions:**
- Provide care in a nonthreatening manner to optimize compliance.
- Promote meticulous oral care. For younger children, recommend the use of sponges or toothettes (foam brushes) for swabbing affected areas. Recommend that the patient brush his or her teeth with a soft-bristle brush, floss when oral tissues are healthy and platelet count is acceptable, and use toothettes to cleanse, moisten, and apply medications to the oral cavity. (The latter recommendation applies especially to patients with thrombocytopenia). Swish-and-spit medications are reserved for use by older children.
- When the patient's speech is impaired, use communication methods that are appropriate for his or her age and developmental stage.
- Instruct the patient to avoid food or drink for 30 minutes after using oral rinses or antifungal medications to maximize their effects.
- Evaluate the patient's pain frequently and provide topical and systemic analgesia as indicated.
- Give pain medications before mealtime to decrease pain during eating.
- Encourage the patient to drink fluids unless they are contraindicated.
- Instruct the patient to avoid hot, dry, spicy foods.
- Encourage the patient through gentle reassurance and psychosocial support.
- Encourage routine dental exams and use of prophylaxis.

## Expected Patient and Family Outcomes

- The patient has good oral hygiene habits.
- The patient and the family identify oral medications that are appropriate for the patient's needs.
- The patient and the family recognize situations that require prompt professional intervention (e.g., inadequate oral intake, fever, pain).

## Diarrhea

### Definition

*Diarrhea* is an increase in the quantity, frequency, or fluid content of stool that differs from the usual pattern of bowel elimination. Diarrhea is caused by changes in intestinal absorption and motility.

### Risk Factors

Risk factors include manipulation of the bowel during surgery and resection of a significant portion of the small bowel, which can lead to decreased reabsorption and result in diarrhea and electrolyte loss. Chemotherapy agents that can cause bowel irritation include 5-fluorouracil (5-FU), cisplatin (Platinol), cytarabine

### Table 5-4. Assessment of the Oral Cavity

| Site | Grade 1 | Grade 2 | Grade 3 | Grade 4 |
| --- | --- | --- | --- | --- |
| Lips | Smooth, moist, and intact/pink | Slightly dry, wrinkled, and inflamed | Dry, rough, swollen, and inflamed | Very dry, inflamed, cracked, ulcerated, and bleeding |
| Tongue | Smooth, firm, pink, and intact | Dry, pink with some reddened areas | Raised red papillae, patchy ulcerations | Confluent ulcerations, inflamed, bleeding |
| Teeth | Clean without debris | Slightly dull with some debris present | Dull with more than half of teeth covered in debris | Very dull, covered in debris; bleeds easily |
| Gums | Intact, pink | Slightly inflamed with minimal swelling, may have slight bleeding with teeth brushing | Inflamed, swollen, and moderate bleeding with minimal trauma | Very inflamed and swollen, may have continuous oozing without trauma |
| Saliva | Sufficient quantity, thin | Slightly thickened with decreased quantity | Thick, ropy, mouth may appear dry | Very thick, ropy, or mucoid appearing; mouth very dry |

Grade 1 = No mucositis   Grade 3 = Moderate mucositis
Grade 2 = Mild mucositis   Grade 4 = Severe mucositis

Criteria based on NCI Common Terminology Criteria for Adverse Events

(cytosine arabinoside), mechlorethamine (nitrogen mustard), methotrexate (Mexate), anthracyclines such as doxorubicin (Adriamycin) or daunomycin (Cerubidine), and topoisomerase I inhibitors (e.g., irinotecan, topotecan). Radiation to the abdomen, pelvis, or the lower thoracic and lumbar spine increases the incidence of diarrhea. Other risk factors are biologic response modifiers such as interleukin-2 and interferon; intestinal infections secondary to mucositis and neutropenia (e.g., rotavirus, E. coli, shigella, salmonella, giardia); medications such as metoclopramide (Reglan), laxatives, antacids, electrolyte supplements, and antibiotics; dietary causes, including lactose intolerance, caffeine, alcohol, spicy and fatty foods, raw vegetables and fruits, tube feedings, and feeding supplements; and conditions such as endocrine tumors, graft-versus-host disease, and hyperthyroidism.

### Clinical Presentation

A patient may have frequent loose stools, perineal irritation, rectal excoriation or ulceration, abdominal cramping, hyperactive bowel sounds, fever, or mucus or blood in the stool. Sloughing of the gastrointestinal lining also may be detected in the stool. The patient may show signs of lethargy and dehydration, electrolyte imbalance, and poor nutrition (e.g., poor skin turgor, weight loss, hypotension, dry mucous membranes, and edema).

### Medical Management

Medical management consists of restoring and maintaining fluid and electrolyte balance, nutrition, normal bowel function, protecting skin integrity, and providing comfort. Parenteral therapy is given as indicated. Antidiarrheal medications (e.g., loperamide, octreotide) are given with caution because the patient may have a bowel obstruction or the diarrhea may be caused by an infection. Stool cultures should be taken if the presence of a microorganisim is suspected. Antispasmodic medications may be indicated to relieve abdominal pain, tenesmus, or both. Vancomycin (Vancocin) or metronidazole (Flagyl) is the antibiotic therapy for Clostridium difficile enteritis. The patient's platelet count may be maintained at more than 50,000 if blood is present in the stool. Sitz baths and barrier creams should be used to protect the perineum and anal/rectal area. The patient should have a diet specific to his or her individual needs.

### Potential Complications

Complications can include intestinal bleeding and infection, breakdown of rectal tissue, cellulitis or abscess, electrolyte imbalance, dehydration, malnutrition, and social withdrawal because of embarrassment and interruptions to daily functioning.

### Nursing Assessment and Interventions

**Assessment:**
- Monitor the volume, appearance, color, odor, and consistency of the patient's stool.
- Strictly monitor intake and output.
- Assess the patient frequently for signs and symptoms of dehydration and electrolyte imbalance.
- Weigh the patient daily or as frequently as his or her circumstances dictate.
- Assess the perianal region carefully for signs of skin breakdown.
- Perform a detailed abdominal assessment with attention to pain, bowel sounds, and girth.

**Interventions:**
- Administer GI and pain medications, as ordered, and monitor their effects.
- Encourage the patient to take fluids orally.
- Encourage the patient to eat a high-calorie, potassium-rich diet with adequate soluble fiber to provide bulk for enhanced fluid absorption in the gut.
- Gently and meticulously clean the patient's perianal area; do not rub the skin (it should be patted dry to prevent excoriation).
- Use alternative techniques to reduce the patient's stress and anxiety (e.g., relaxation, distraction, play therapy, and imagery).
- Control noxious odors to decrease nausea and vomiting.

### Expected Patient and Family Outcomes

- The patient and the family can identify methods of preventing and treating diarrhea.
- The patient and the family understand proper cleansing and personal hygiene methods of preventing and treating skin breakdown and perirectal cellulitis.
- The patient and the family recognize situations that require medical assistance (e.g., diarrhea unrelieved by usual interventions; dehydration).

## Constipation

### Definition

*Constipation* is the infrequent passing of hard, dry stool, often accompanied by straining, abdominal cramping, bleeding, and rectal discomfort.

### Risk Factors

Risk factors are obstruction or ileus; abdominal or pelvic surgery; postoperative adhesions; surgical trauma to the intestines, the rectum, or both; a treatment-related decrease in activity or immobility; spinal-cord decompression; neurotoxic effects of chemotherapy that decrease peristalsis (e.g., vinca alkaloids, vincristine [Oncovin], and vinblastine [Velban]); the side effects of drugs (e.g., narcotics, anticholinergics); poor dietary intake of fiber and fluids; metabolic conditions (e.g., hyperalcemia, hypokalemia, hypothyroidism); and an alteration in the defecation reflex due to discomfort, anxiety, lack of privacy, or change in environment.

### Clinical Presentation

A patient may have decreased or absent bowel sounds; generalized abdominal tenderness, distension, or both; decreased appetite; nausea; vomiting; pain and fear associated with difficulty in producing a stool; decrease in the normal frequency of stools; and hard, formed, and possibly blood-streaked stools.

### Medical Management

Surgery may be necessary to relieve an obstruction or to resect an invading tumor. Laxatives and stool softeners are given to relieve constipation and as a prophylaxis when constipation is anticipated. The patient should follow a high-fiber diet, increase fluid intake, and be encouraged to maintain or increase activity. Rectal manipulation, medication, and thermometers are contraindicated because of the increased risk of infection and bleeding.

## Potential Complications
Complications can include fecal impaction, paralytic ileus or intestinal obstruction, and perirectal abscess.

## Nursing Assessment and Interventions
**Assessment:**
- Monitor the frequency, volume, and consistency of the patient's stool output.
- Examine the patient's rectal area routinely for skin breakdown, fissures, hemorrhoids, swelling, or bleeding.
- Perform a complete abdominal assessment that includes level of pain, auscultation, palpation, and girth.

**Interventions:**
- Encourage the patient to drink fluids and eat a diet rich in fiber.
- Administer prescribed laxatives.
- Encourage the patient to ambulate and increase activity to alleviate gas pains and facilitate defecation.
- Report all adverse signs, including bleeding, increased abdominal pain, distension, and absent bowel sounds.
- Promote an environment of privacy and relaxation to enhance the patient's ability to maintain a normal bowel pattern.
- Encourage the patient to maintain a home-toileting routine (this is especially important to prevent regression in a child who has recently been toilet-trained).

## Expected Patient and Family Outcomes
- The patient and the family understand methods for preventing and treating constipation.
- The patient and the family can identify a regular bowel pattern.
- The patient and the family recognize the signs and symptoms of constipation that require medical attention.

# Perirectal Cellulitis

## Definition
*Perirectal cellulitis* involves inflammation and edema of the perineal and rectal area. Tears or fissures in the anorectal mucosa can cause perirectal cellulitis. Aerobic gram-negative bacilli and anaerobic bacteria are the most common infective organisms.

## Risk Factors
Risk factors include constipation or the passage of hard stool, causing trauma to the rectal mucosa; diarrhea involving caustic fluid that causes irritation and breakdown of perirectal tissue; perirectal mucositis associated with chemotherapy, radiation therapy, or both; chronic or profound neutropenia, thrombocytopenia, or both; rectal trauma (e.g., rectal stimulation, thermometers, suppositories); hemorrhoids; and anal fissures.

## Clinical Presentation
The patient may experience perineal and/or rectal discomfort. The patient also may develop fever and be afraid to defecate because of the resulting pain. A visual perirectal examination may reveal minimal irritation, fissures, gross swelling, and/or inflammation.

## Medical Management
Antibiotic treatment should be initiated at the first sign of discomfort or tenderness. Such treatment includes a specific antianaerobic agent (e.g., clindamycin [Cleocin], metronidazole [Flagyl]), and a broad-spectrum antibiotic. Other measures include administration of antipyretics, pain medications, stool softeners, sitz baths, or perineal irrigation 3–4 times a day. Dietary modifications may be required.

## Potential Complications
Complications include constipation and fecal impaction, tissue sloughing and necrosis, and infection that begins as a local abscess and leads to systemic sepsis. Mortality ranges from 8% to 36%; the primary cause of death is septic shock.

## Nursing Assessment and Interventions
**Assessment:**
- Inspect the patient's perirectal mucosa frequently for signs of irritation or skin breakdown.
- Monitor the patient for signs of infection or deteriorating integrity of tissue in the perirectal area.

**Interventions:**
- Administer prescribed medications to alleviate symptoms and control pain.
- Provide or encourage meticulous perineal hygiene, especially when the patient is neutropenic.
- Apply prescribed barrier creams and medicated creams.

## Expected Patient and Family Outcomes
- The patient, the family, or both can identify the risk factors for perirectal cellulitis.
- The patient practices good perineal hygiene.
- The patient, the family, or both can discuss measures for minimizing the risks associated with cellulitis.
- The patient, the family, or both can identify situations that require prompt professional intervention (e.g., pain, fever, erythema, tissue breakdown).

# Chemical or Reactive Hepatitis

## Definition
*Chemical* or *reactive hepatitis* is a nonviral inflammation of the liver caused by exposure to chemical or other environmental toxins, such as chemotherapy, biotherapy, and radiation.

## Risk Factors
Risk factors can include radiation to the liver or to the right side of the abdomen and chemotherapeutic agents (e.g., methotrexate [Mexate], chlorambucil [Leukeran], mercaptopurine [Purinethol], daunomycin [Cerubidine], doxorubicin [Adriamycin], and thioguanine [6-TG]). Intrahepatic chemotherapy, surgical resection of the liver followed by cancer treatment, underlying liver disease (e.g., infections, hepatitis, or hepatic candidiasis), and supportive-care medications, such as antimicrobials, anticonvulsants, and nonsteroidal anti-inflammatory agents, also can contribute to the development of hepatitis.

## Clinical Presentation
Patients may have pain in the right-upper quadrant; nausea; vomiting; dyspepsia; anorexia; fever; malaise; flu-like symptoms; jaundice (i.e., yellow sclera and conjunctiva, dark-orange urine, clay-colored stools); malabsorption (accompanied by diarrhea, weight loss, dehydration); bruising, bleeding, or both; pruritis;

and abnormalities in laboratory tests (e.g., elevated liver enzymes, prolonged prothrombin times).

### Medical Management
Agents that could cause the hepatotoxicity should be discontinued temporarily or permanently, and the use of additional hepatotoxic drugs should be avoided. Serum chemistries, liver transaminases, complete blood count, and coagulation profile should be monitored regularly. Abdominal ultrasound or liver biopsy may be required for further workup. Antiemetics and intravenous hydration should be given as needed for nausea and vomiting. Antipruritic agents and glucocorticoids can be given as well. Ursodiol can be used to treat hyperbilirubinemia. The patient also should be put on a low-fat, high-glucose diet with vitamin B and C additives, and physical activity should be limited.

### Potential Complications
Complications can include veno-occlusive disease, chronic active hepatitis, and cirrhosis.

### Nursing Assessment and Interventions
**Assessment:**
- Perform a routine physical assessment to detect jaundice and to determine the patient's neurologic status.
- Monitor the patient for signs of bleeding.
- Assess for pain and discomfort from itching.

**Interventions:**
- Encourage the patient to rest.
- Apply lotions and encourage the patient to take tepid baths to decrease pruritus.
- Instruct the patient to wear loose, light clothing.
- Encourage the patient to eat a low-fat, high-glucose diet.
- Administer analgesics, antipyretics, and antiemetics as ordered, and monitor their effects.

### Expected Patient and Family Outcomes
- The patient and the family know about potential complications.
- The patient and the family comply with the recommended care.

## Pancreatitis

### Definition
*Pancreatitis* is an acute or chronic inflammation of the pancreas.

### Risk Factors
Risk factors for pancreatitis are chemotherapy agents, specifically L-asparaginase (Elspar); radiation to the pancreas or to the left side of the abdomen; diabetes; tumor lysis syndrome; and use of an intrahepatic catheter.

### Clinical Presentation
The signs of pancreatitis can include epigastric or abdominal pain that radiates to the flank, back, or substernal area and is unrelieved by vomiting. They also can include abdominal rigidity, fever, tachycardia, hypotension, nausea and vomiting, elevated serum amylase and lipase, metabolic disturbances (e.g., hypoglycemia), signs and symptoms of shock, hypoactive bowel sounds, or ileus.

### Medical Management
Any treatment that could be the causative agent should be discontinued temporarily or permanently. Serum lipase and amylase and serum chemistries should be done. An abdominal ultrasound or computed tomography may be obtained. Pain relief is essential but may be problematic because some analgesics increase pain due to spasms of the sphincter of Odi. The patient should not take anything by mouth and may need a nasogastric tube. The patient should have a bland, low-fat diet when feeding is resumed. Fluid and electrolyte replacement and volume expanders should be given if the patient experiences shock. Physical activity should be limited.

### Potential Complications
Complications can include pancreatic abscess, pancreatic pseudocyst, and pancreatic necrosis.

### Nursing Assessment and Interventions
**Assessment:**
- Assess the patient's level of pain.
- Monitor the patient's vital signs.
- Assess the patient's level of consciousness and physical condition for signs of shock or electrolyte imbalance.

**Interventions:**
- Administer the appropriate analgesic and monitor its effect.
- Ensure that the patient receives appropriate oral and nasal care while a nasogastric tube is in place.
- Comfort and reassure the patient.

### Expected Patient and Family Outcomes
- The patient, the family, or both recognize the early symptoms of pancreatitis and seek early medical intervention.
- The patient complies with dietary and pharmacologic recommendations.

## Nausea and Vomiting

### Description
*Nausea* occurs when the vomiting center in the brain is stimulated, causing wavelike feelings of GI distress. *Vomiting* is the forceful expulsion of stomach contents. Nausea and vomiting related to chemotherapy and radiation therapy are mediated by the vomiting center in the brain (**Figure 5-4**). It occurs through several different mechanisms: (a) activation of the chemoreceptor trigger zone (CTZ) in the fourth ventricle of the brain, (b) peripheral stimulation by neurotransmitter receptors in the gut wall, (c) cortical pathway activation by learned response (i.e., anticipatory nausea and vomiting), and (d) vestibular pathway disruption related to motion and balance.

Nausea and vomiting are among the most common and feared side effects of cancer-related chemotherapy. Poorly controlled nausea and vomiting can result in dehydration, electrolyte imbalances, extended anorexia, esophageal tears, and significant distress. The consequences can include prolonged hospitalization, increased length of time between chemotherapy cycles, and patient-initiated discontinuation of treatment. Clinical research demonstrates that the cycle of nausea and vomiting is difficult to reverse once it has been established. The best form of management is prevention.

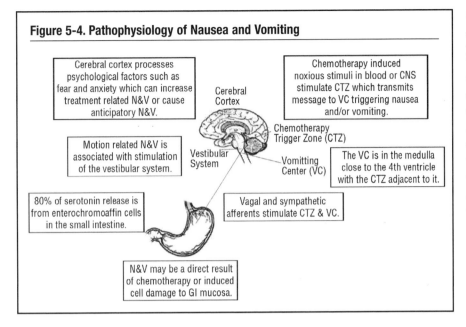

Figure 5-4. Pathophysiology of Nausea and Vomiting

## Risk Factors

All agents used in chemotherapy have the potential to cause nausea and vomiting. The emetogenic potential and patterns of vomiting varies among the different agents (**Table 5-5**). To determine the emetogenic potential, an understanding is required of the agent, the dosage, the duration of infusion, and the combination of drugs used. Radiation therapy also can cause nausea and vomiting when applied to the total body and to the head and abdomen. Cerebral edema contributes to the nausea associated with cranial radiation. Serotonin release from the intestine is likely to contribute to nausea associated with abdominal radiation.

Other factors that contribute to nausea are increased intracranial pressure secondary to brain tumors, metabolic disturbances, side effects of narcotics, younger age, and female gender.

## Patterns of Nausea and Vomiting

The acute pattern begins within several hours of chemotherapy and produces the most severe symptoms during the first 12–24 hours. It is usually self-limited and resolves within 24 hours.

The delayed pattern begins after chemotherapy has been administered and can last up to 2 weeks. It occurs when antiemetic therapy is insufficient, is given on a poorly planned schedule, or both.

The anticipatory pattern is a conditioned response and can occur any time after one course of chemotherapy. Risk factors include inadequate control of a previous chemotherapy episode that results in nausea and vomiting, age (usually young adults or adolescents), and preexisting anxiety, depression, or both. Triggers can include the sight of the hospital, clinic, or healthcare workers, or hospital-associated odors. The pattern usually is resistant to standard therapy. An oral dose of lorazepam (Ativan) given the night before and the morning of chemotherapy may decrease the pattern's incidence.

## Medical Management

Various neurotransmitters (e.g., serotonin, dopamine, histamine, norepinephrine, vasopressin) activate the CTZ and vomiting center. The goal of antiemetic therapy is to identify the emetic pathways and block the neurotransmitter release. The goals of successful antiemetic therapy are to minimize or prevent nausea and vomiting and enhance the patient's quality of life (See **Tables 5-6** and **5-7** and Section IV, "Childhood Cancer Treatment," for a description of the pharmacologic classification of these agents.) The principles related to using antiemetics are as follows:

- Drugs should be selected on the basis of their sites of action.
- Appropriate doses should be based on the patient's weight.
- Drugs should be scheduled according to their duration of action.
- Drugs should be scheduled according to the pattern of emesis.
- The frequency of emesis and the effectiveness of agents should be evaluated frequently.

### Table 5-5. Emetogenic Potential of Chemotherapeutic Agents

**Acute Symptoms**

*Highly emetogenic*
Actinomycin-D
Cisplatin (≥40 mg/m$^2$)
Cyclophosphamide (≥1 g/m$^2$)
Cytarabine (≥1 g/m$^2$)
Dacarbazine
Ifosfamide
Mechlorethamine

*Moderately emetogenic*
Anthracyclines (daunorubicin, doxorubicin, idarubicin)
Carboplatin
Cisplatin (<40 mg/m$^2$)
Cyclophosphamide (<1 g/m$^2$)
Cytarabine (IV <1 g/m$^2$, or IT)
Mercaptopurine (IV)
Methotrexate (IV >1 g/m$^2$)
Nitrosoureas (Carmustine, Lomustine)

*Mildly emetogenic*
Bleomycin
Epipodophyllotoxins (etoposide, teniposide)
Paclitaxel
Procarbazine
Topotecan
Vonblastine

*Nonemetogenic*
Asparaginase
Mercaptopurine (PO)
Methotrexate (low-dose IV, IM, PO, IT)
Steroids
Thioguanine
Vincristine

**Delayed Symptoms**

*Severe*
Cisplatin
*Moderate*
Cyclophosphamide

> **Table 5-6. Pharmacological Classification of Antiemetics**
>
> **Serotonin receptor antagonists (e.g., ondansetron [Zofran], granisetron [Kytril])**
> - Are highly selective antagonists of serotonin receptors but have no effect on dopamine receptors
> - Have a main site of action thought to be on vagal afferents in the small intestine
> - Have two main side effects: headache and a transient elevation of liver enzymes
>
> **Dopamine antagonists (e.g., phenothiazines: chlorpromazine [Thorazine] and prochlorperazine [Compazine])**
> - Alter the effects of dopamine (Intropin) in the CNS and block dopamine receptors in the chemoreceptor trigger zone
> - Have these main side effects: extrapyramidal effects, athetosis (i.e., involuntary movement of limbs and facial grimacing, oculogyric crisis, rhythmic protrusion of the tongue, bulbar-type speech, dystonic reaction), sedation, hypotension, arrhythmias, constipation, and dry mouth
>
> **Glucocorticoids (e.g., dexamethasone [Decadron], prednisolone [Pediapred, Hydeltra-T.B.A.])**
> - Are thought to interfere with the permeability of the blood-brain barrier to allow other antiemetic agents to act on the chemoreceptor trigger zone
> - Have these main side effects: depression, euphoria, hypertension, acne, and a cushingoid appearance
>
> **NK-1 antagonist (e.g., aprepitant [Emend])**
> - Is a selective high-affinity antagonist of human substance P/neurokinin (NK1) receptors
> - Has little or no affinity for serotonin, dopamine, and corticosteroid receptors
> - Has three main side effects: fatigue, diarrhea, and hiccups.

Nonpharmacologic interventions include relaxation exercises, distraction and guided imagery, self-hypnosis, and music therapy.

### Nursing Assessment and Interventions

**Assessment:**
- Monitor fluid balance.
- Document characteristics of emesis, including volume, color, and presence of blood.
- Report adverse signs and symptoms to the patient's physician and document findings in the patient's medical record.
- Assess the effectiveness of antiemetics on the basis of the patient's response.

**Interventions:**
- Formulate an individualized plan of care with the patient and family that is based on previous responses and personal coping skills.
- Explain the possible side effects of chemotherapy.
- Instruct the patient regarding the administration of antiemetics.
- Modify the treatment plan as needed.

### Expected Patient and Family Outcomes
- The patient has minimal nausea and vomiting caused by chemotherapy.
- The patient and the family understand the use of antiemetics and know how to administer them at home.
- The patient and the family know when to call for professional help during an episode of nausea and vomiting.

**Reference**

Gibson, F., Cargill, J., Allison, J., Begent, J., Cole, S., Stone, S., et al. (2006). Establishing content validity of the oral assessment guide in children and young people. *European Journal of Cancer, 42*, 1817–1825.

## Renal and Bladder Complications

*Ruth Anne Herring*

Abnormalities and impairments of renal function that occur are most often related to the pathophysiology of the disease process, the nephrotoxic agents that are used for treatment, abdominal or pelvic irradiation, or a combination of these factors. Renal- and bladder-related side effects can be transient, cumulative, permanent, or progressive.

### Kidney Impairment

#### Definition
*Kidney impairment* is the decreased ability of a kidney to perform the normal functions of electrolyte balance, eliminate waste products, and maintain the acid and base balance.

#### Risk Factors
Risk factors for renal impairment include primary tumors involving the kidney; treatment resulting in rapid tumor lysis; increased cellular metabolism; chemotherapy; other nephrotoxic medications (e.g., antibiotics); volume depletion, dehydration, or both; radiation therapy that includes kidneys within the treatment field; and sepsis.

#### Clinical Presentation
The laboratory findings for patients with kidney impairment can include elevated blood urea nitrogen (BUN), creatinine, and/or uric acid and alterations in levels of serum electrolytes, calcium, magnesium, and/or phosphates. Urine testing may reveal proteinuria, hematuria, and/or decreased urine creatinine clearance. Physical symptoms include increased weight, elevated blood pressure, tachycardia, tachypnea, oliguria, ascites or abdominal distention, and fatigue. Fluid intake and output may be unbalanced.

#### Medical Management
Renal function (e.g., urinalysis and serum BUN; creatinine and electrolyte results) should be assessed and evaluated before each course of chemotherapy (especially courses that include agents associated with increased renal toxicity). The potential for renal toxicity is increased when the baseline renal function is already reduced. A physical assessment should be made, and vital signs should be checked before treatment is started. The patient should have adequate hydration before receiving chemotherapy. Alkalinization, hyperhydration, or both should be instituted when certain agents (e.g., methotrexate [Mexate], cisplatin [Platinol]) are administered. Diuretic therapy should be given when it is indicated. Doses of other nephrotoxic agents (e.g., vancomycin

### Table 5-7. Antiemetic Agents for Children

**Mild-to-Moderate Emetogenic Chemotherapy**

| | Dose | Routes | Frequency | Side Effects |
|---|---|---|---|---|
| Prochlorperazine (Compazine) | 0.5 mg/kg | PO, IV | q 4–6 hr | EPS, agitation |
| Chlorpromazine (Thorazine) | 0.5 mg/kg | PO, IV | q 4–6 hr | EPS, agitation |
| Promethazine (Phenergan) | 0.5 mg/kg | PO, IV | q 4 hr | EPS, agitation |

**Mild-to-Severe Emetogenic Chemotherapy**

| | | | | |
|---|---|---|---|---|
| Metoclopramide (Reglan) | 1–2 mg/kg | IV | q 2–4 hr | EPS[a], sedation |
| Ondansetron (Zofran) | 0.15 mg/kg if given as three doses, or 0.45 mg/kg as one dose | PO, IV | qd, tid | Headache |
| Granisetron (Kytril) | 10 mg | PO, IV | qd | Headache |
| Aprepitant | 125 mg day 1, 80 mg day 2, 3 | PO | Daily | Somnolence, fatigue |
| Dexamethasone and aprepitant | 12 mg day 1, 8 mg day 2, 3 | IV | Daily | Facial flushing, hyperglycemia, electrolyte imbalance |
| Palonestron (Aloxi) | 0.25 mg | IV | Once 30 min before chemotherapy | Abdominal pain, dizziness, headache, fatigue |

**Supplemental Agents**

| | | | | |
|---|---|---|---|---|
| Diphenhydramine (Benadryl) | 1 mg/kg | PO, IV | q 4–6 hr | Sedation |
| Dexamethasone (Decadron) | 6 mg/m$^2$ as one dose, or divided tid | PO, IV | qd, tid | Facial flushing, hyperglycemia, electrolyte imbalance |
| Lorazepam (Ativan) | 0.025 mg/kg | PO, IV | q 6 hr | Sedation |
| Hydroxyzine (Vistaril/Atarax) | 1 mg/kg | PO, IV | q 4–6 hr | Sedation, headache |

*Note.* EPS = extra pyramidal symptoms; IV = intravenous; PO = by mouth, orally; q = every; qd = once a day; tid = three times a day.

[Vancocin], aminoglycosides, amphotericin) should be decreased or minimized whenever possible. Dialysis is instituted when patients have renal failure.

## Potential Complications

Complications may include dehydration or fluid overload; acute tubular necrosis; fluid and electrolyte imbalances; electrolyte wasting (e.g., hypokalemia, hypomagnesemia, hyponatremia, and/or hypophosphatemia); tumor lysis syndrome (e.g., hyperkalemia, hyperuricemia, hyperphosphatemia, and/or hypocalcemia); renal failure; and renal Fanconi syndrome. Renal Fanconi syndrome can persist for years after the patient completes therapy that includes ifosfamide or high-dose cyclophosphamide.

## Nursing Assessment and Interventions

**Assessment:**
- Assess the patient's vital signs and hydration status.
- Maintain accurate intake and output (maintain urine output of 1–2 ml/kg/hr or more during infusion of nephrotoxic chemotherapy and during the posthydration period).
- Weigh the patient daily, or twice a day if indicated, when he or she is receiving ifosfamide (Ifex) or high doses of cyclophosphamide (Cytoxan) or methotrexate (Mexate).
- Assess the patient's urine-specific gravity and pH, and assess for the presence of blood frequently while the patient is receiving nephrotoxic chemotherapy and during the posthydration period.
- Monitor the patient for symptoms of dehydration or fluid overload.
- Monitor for changes in the patient's serum chemistries.

**Interventions:**
- Maintain adequate patient hydration.
- Administer antiemetics to minimize emesis-related fluid and electrolyte losses.
- Educate the patient and the family about the importance of maintaining adequate hydration after discharge.
- Arrange for at-home intravenous hydration for the patient when it is needed.
- Instruct both the patient and the family to monitor the patient's urine output at home and to report changes in urine color, odor, and amount.
- Instruct the patient and the family about the importance of taking oral electrolyte supplements if prescribed.

## Expected Patient and Family Outcomes

- Both the patient and the family recognize the signs and symptoms of renal impairment and seek early intervention.
- Both the patient and the family understand the importance of maintaining adequate hydration through oral intake.

## Hemorrhagic Cystitis

### Definition
*Hemorrhagic cystitis* is a condition in which symptoms range from mild dysuria and urinary frequency to severe hemorrhage associated with significant damage to the epithelial lining of the bladder.

### Risk Factors
Chemotherapy (e.g., ifosfamide [Ifex], cyclophosphamide [Cytoxan]) and radiation therapy to the pelvis are risk factors. Adenovirus, cytomegalovirus, and polyomavirus can also cause hemorrhagic cystitis in severely immunosuppressed patients.

### Clinical Presentation
Symptoms include hematuria and dysuria.

### Medical Management
Prevention of hemorrhagic cystitis is a major goal and requires adequate patient hydration before, during, and after administration of ifosfamide (Ifex) and cyclophosphamide (Cytoxan). Mesna (Mesenex) should be administered in conjunction with cyclophosphamide or ifosfamide to protect the bladder by binding to acrolein (i.e., the metabolic byproduct of ifosfamide and cyclophosphamide that causes hemorrhagic cystitis). In addition, furosemide (Lasix) can be given to maintain urine output. Treatment of hemorrhagic cystitis depends on the degree of bleeding and can include increased hydration, blood product support, and/or continuous bladder irrigation.

### Potential Complications
Complications include bladder fibrosis, chronic hemorrhagic cystitis, urinary reflux, and hydro-nephrosis.

### Nursing Assessment and Interventions
**Assessment:**
- Maintain the patient's urine-specific gravity at less than 1.010.
- Perform urinalysis at least daily when the patient is receiving either cyclophosphamide or ifosfamide.
- Test urine for blood with every void.
- Assess the patient's intake and output and weights accurately.

**Interventions:**
- Maintain adequate patient hydration.
- If cyclophosphamide has been ordered to be given orally, schedule doses so that it is administered early in the day.
- Have the patient void every 1–2 hours while receiving chemotherapy regimens that include cyclophosphamide or ifosfamide and for 12–24 hours after completion of each dose of these agents.
- Instruct the patient and the family about the importance of adequate hydration and frequent voiding before and after receiving cyclophosphamide or ifosfamide.
- Assess the patient's ability to maintain adequate hydration at home.
- Instruct the patient to void every 1–2 hours during waking hours and just before bedtime for 12–24 hours after receiving cyclophosphamide or ifosfamide.
- Educate the patient and family about the signs and symptoms of hemorrhagic cystitis (e.g., hematuria or dysuria).
- Instruct the family to report any changes in their child's urine output, as well as occurrence of dysuria or hematuria.

### Expected Patient and Family Outcomes
- The patient and the family recognize the signs and symptoms of hemorrhagic cystitis and seek early medical intervention.
- The patient and the family understand the importance of maintaining adequate hydration.
- The patient and the family comply with recommended therapies.

## Skin Changes

*Robbie Norville*

Skin is a natural barrier to infection, and a break in this barrier increases the risk for infection. An immunocompromised child with cancer has a risk of developing serious infection from normal flora on the skin when a portal of entry is provided. Optimal hygiene and skin protection help to minimize the effect of cancer treatment on the skin.

### Altered Skin Integrity

#### Definition
*Altered skin integrity* is a disruption of the ability of the skin to serve as a protective barrier.

#### Risk Factors
As rapidly growing cells, skin is particularly susceptible to the effects of chemotherapy and radiation therapy. Risk factors include underlying or subcutaneous tumor; radiation therapy; chemotherapeutic agents; antibiotics; corticosteroids; procedures that disrupt skin integrity (e.g., injections, ostomies, excisions, central venous access devices, gastrostomy tubes); prosthetic devices; malnutrition; and immobility.

#### Clinical Presentation
The clinical presentation of alteration in skin integrity and cutaneous toxicity varies depending on the underlying cause. The effects of radiation on skin can include mild erythema, hyperpigmentation, moist and dry desquamation, tenderness, and pruritus at the site of the radiation field. Skin reactions called radiation recall can occur at previous radiation sites following subsequent chemotherapy administration. Presentation includes warmth, erythema, and dermatitis, which can progress to severe desquamation and ulceration. Agents associated with radiation recall include bleomycin (Blenoxane), dactinomycin (Actinomycin D), daunorubicin (Daunormycin), etoposide (VePesid), melphalan (Alkeran), and methotrexate (Mexate). Alopecia, which can occur as a result of chemotherapy, radiation, or both, usually begins 2–3 weeks after treatment. Alopecia can be patchy and is usually temporary, although permanent alopecia almost always occurs with radiation of more than 55 Gy. Photosensitivity can occur as a result of treatment with trimethoprim-sulfamethoxazole (Bactrim), methotrexate, 5-fluorouracil (Fluorouracil), and vinblastine (Velban). Depigmentation and hyperpigmentation are associated with methotrexate, bleomycin, 5-fluorouracil, busulfan (Myleran), cyclophosphamide (Cytoxan), and anthracyclines. Nail changes associated with chemotherapy can include banding, discoloration, and separation of the nail plate from the nail bed (onycholysis). Onycholysis can be painful and lead to infection.

Nail changes are associated with anthracyclines and taxanes. See **Table 5-8** for a list of skin reactions caused by chemotherapy agents. Delayed healing or an increased incidence of infection is associated with chemotherapy, radiation, or both; poor nutritional status; and glucocorticoid therapy. Friability of the skin may be a consequence of an underlying tumor and places the skin at risk of breakdown.

### Nursing Assessment and Interventions

**Assessment:**
- Perform a baseline assessment of the patient's skin, and assess daily to determine whether there are potential problem areas. Particular attention should be given to any disruption in skin integrity, radiated areas, skin folds and creases, perineal area, and areas overlying tumor masses.
- Assess the patient's understanding of alopecia, encourage a discussion of altered body image, and, if the patient desires it, refer him or her for a wig.
- Monitor the healing of the patient's wounds, including those caused by central venous access devices and gastrointestinal tubes, incision sites or wounds, and surgical sites, throughout the course of therapy.
- Examine the patient's skin at previously irradiated sites for signs or symptoms of radiation recall; provide appropriate treatment.

**Interventions:**
- Explain photosensitivity to the patient and the need to avoid excessive sunlight.
- Instruct the patient on the use of sunscreen. Recommend products with a sun-protection factor of 30 or greater.
- Teach the child and the family how to assess skin integrity and teach them appropriate skin-care techniques.
- Emphasize the importance of a good daily hygiene regimen and care of irradiated skin (**Table 5-9**).
- Report all changes in skin integrity to the patient's physician.

- Reposition the patient every 2 hours if his or her mobility is limited.
- Ensure that the patient receives adequate nutrition. Consider a nutritional consultation if he or she has persistent weight loss (i.e., a loss of 5% or more of body weight) or poor nutritional status.
- Consult a specialist in enterostomal therapy for patients who have particularly complex wound-management needs.

### Expected Patient and Family Outcomes
- The patient uses sunscreen when outdoors.
- The patient's skin remains intact and infection free.
- The patient and the family comply with necessary wound and ostomy care for the patient.

## Musculoskeletal Complications

*Sameeya N. Ahmed-Winston*

Musculoskeletal complications associated with treatment for cancer and hematologic disorders are common in children and adolescents. The comprehensive care of children with cancer requires an interdisciplinary approach across the continuum of

### Table 5-8. Skin Reactions Caused by Chemotherapy Agents

| Skin Reaction | Chemotherapy Agents |
|---|---|
| Radiation recall | Bleomycin<br>Dactinomycin<br>Daunomycin<br>Etoposide<br>Melphalan<br>Methotrexate |
| Photosensitivity | Bactrim<br>5-Fluorouracil<br>Methotrexate<br>Vinblastine |
| Hyperpigmentation | Anthracyclines<br>Bleomycin<br>Busulfan<br>Cyclophosphamide<br>5-Fluorouracil<br>Methotrexate |
| Nail changes | Anthracyclines<br>Taxanes |

### Table 5-9. Nursing Care of Irradiated Skin

**Prevention of Acute Radiation Dermatitis**

Assess patient for risk factors

Assess skin integrity

Avoid activities that increase risk of skin breaks
- Avoid friction, scrubbing, shaving, and use of abrasive skin-care products
- Minimize tape and gauze dressings

Avoid restrictive or tight-fitting clothing

Protect skin from temperature extremes and sun exposure

Ensure optimal skin care
- Cleanse skin and perineal area with unscented, mild, moisturizing soap and lukewarm water
- Cleanse scalp with mild shampoo and lukewarm water
- Avoid deodorants, perfumes, powders, or oil-based creams or lotions

**Treatment of Acute Radiation Dermatitis**

Dry desquamation
- Use hydrophilic moisturizing lotions frequently to keep skin moisturized
- Remove all skin care products before each radiation treatment
- Administer antipruritics

Moist desquamation
- Assess skin for signs and symptoms of infection
- Apply topical, normal saline soaks to affected area
- Follow soaks with moisturizing lotions or gels
- Avoid use of tape or adhesive dressings to affected area
- Apply hydrocolloid dressing to preserve moist environment and promote comfort
- Administer analgesics and antipruritics

care. Children with cancer, specifically those with musculoskeletal malignancies, experience side effects that can be directly related to their underlying disease but are more commonly associated with specific therapies including surgery, chemotherapy, radiation, and immunotherapy. Complications of aggressive combination therapy include limitation of movement, asymmetry, and alteration in body image and function related to limb-salvage and amputation procedures. Goals of management include minimizing the impairment and maximizing activity. In an increasing number of children, advances in surgical techniques involving limb reconstruction make it possible to perform limb-sparing procedures instead of amputation.

## Limitation of Movement and Asymmetry

Decreased range of motion (ROM) can occur in joints because of hematological disorders, malignancy, asymmetry of the extremity or trunk, and treatment-associated complications.

### Risk Factors
- Site of the disease
- Site and dose of radiation therapy
- Surgical excision of the tumor and surrounding tissue and bone
- Use of glucocorticosteroids
- Flexion deformity caused by asymmetrical growth of epiphyses

### Clinical Presentation
- Decreased ROM
- Direct or indirect (i.e., referred) pain
- Alteration in gait and asymmetry of limbs
- Scoliosis or kyphosis
- Changes in functional performance (e.g., weakness or atrophy of muscles)
- Changes in skin integrity
- Swelling caused by accumulation of fluid and blood

### Medical Treatment
- Detailed history and physical examination
- Functional evaluation
- Radiological evaluation (e.g., magnetic resonance imaging, computed tomography, X rays)
- Symptom management (e.g., with ice or heat, analgesics, antinflammatories, bed rest, non-weight bearing)
- Occupational therapy and physical therapy consultation
- Use of prosthetic devices (e.g., brace, splint, lift, crutches) or joint replacement

### Potential Complications
- Fracture
- Infection
- Avascular necrosis
- Altered gait and limb asymmetry
- Alterations in body image
- Decreased muscle tone
- Muscle weakness or atrophy
- Thrombosis

### Nursing Assessment and Interventions
**Assessment:**
- Perform ongoing functional assessments of the patient, including physical and psychosocial aspects.
- Perform accurate height and extremity measurements.

**Interventions:**
- Encourage the patient to comply with recommended rehabilitation.
- Provide appropriate skin care.
- Manage the patient's symptoms.
- Provide psychosocial support for the patient.
- Educate the patient and the family about home care.
- Coordinate the location and schedule for rehabilitation.
- Encourage necessary adaptations for the patient at school and at home.
- Provide information related to community services and support groups.

### Expected Patient and Family Outcomes
- The patient and the family understand the need for long-term follow-up.
- The patient and the family comply with needed therapies.

## Amputation and Limb-Salvaging Procedures

### Definition
*Amputation* is the surgical removal of tumor-bearing bone with a 6–7-cm margin proximal to the upper limit of the tumor. *Limb-salvage procedures* include rotational plasties, autologous grafts, vascularized grafts, allografts, endoprostheses, metallic prostheses, arthrodises, and/or allograft prosthetic composites.

Body-image disturbances can result from surgical procedures required to treat certain malignancies and certain hematological disorders. Attitudes about body image are dynamic, can change with interactions with different people and situations, and can be influenced by age and developmental level. As body image is an important part of one's self-concept, body-image disturbance can have a profound impact on how individuals view themselves overall.

### Risk Factors
- Fractures can prevent or delay limb-salvage procedures.
- Location and/or size of the tumor can prohibit a limb-salvaging procedure.
- Infections
- Life span of prosthetic devices used in limb reconstruction.
- Degree of tumor response to chemotherapy

### Medical Treatment
A multidisciplinary approach should include coordination of care with the surgeon, rehabilitation team, and oncology team. Symptom management and restoration of function should also be included in the medical-treatment plan.

### Potential Complications
- Fractures
- Joint dislocations
- Skin necrosis
- Wound infections
- Thrombosis
- Rejection of a graft
- Delayed complications such as arthritis, recurrence of local tumor, nonunion of osseous junctions, and late infections.

# Section V Side Effects of Treatment

## Nursing Assessment and Interventions

**Assessment:**
- Assess the patient's perception of change in structure or function of body part.
- Evaluate the patient's need for physical therapy, occupational therapy, or both.
- Assess the patient's perceived impact of change on activities of daily living (ADLs), social behavior, personal relationships, and occupational activities.
- Assess the impact of body-image disturbance in relation to the patient's developmental stage.

**Interventions:**
- Help the patient to incorporate actual changes into ADLs, social life, interpersonal relationships, and occupational activities.
- Acknowledge normalcy of the patient's emotional response to actual or perceived change in body structure or function.
- Encourage verbalization of positive or negative feelings about actual or perceived change.
- Provide comfort measures (see the discussion of surgery in Section IV, "Supportive Care").
- Support the patient in his or her use of assistive devices (e.g., crutches, prosthesis).

## Expected Patient and Family Outcomes
- The patient adjusts to the amputation and prosthetic device if one is used.
- The patient makes use of appropriate community resources.
- The patient and the family understand the need for long-term follow-up.
- The patient achieves maximum mobility.
- The patient demonstrates enhanced body image and self-esteem as evidenced by the ability to look at, touch, talk about, and care for an actual or perceived altered body part or function.

# Nutritional Complications

*Cheryl Rodgers*

Healthy children require adequate nutrition for normal growth and development and for maintaining good health. Children with hematologic and oncologic diseases have additional nutritional needs because of the demands of their disease and treatment regimen. These additional nutritional requirements are often difficult to achieve because of the multiple physical and psychological effects of their disease and/or treatment.

Children have minimal caloric reserves that, compared with adults, make them more susceptible to malnutrition. Malnourished children are prone to serious deficits in growth and development, poor disease outcomes, increased morbidity, decreased immune function, and decreased quality of life.

## Alteration in Nutrition

### Definition
An *alteration in nutrition* is any change in the process of consuming, digesting, or utilizing nutrients within the body.

### Risk Factors
Chemotherapy and radiation can cause significant damage to the mucosal cells throughout the gastrointestinal (GI) tract, resulting in multiple side effects such as nausea, vomiting, diarrhea, mucositis, and esophagitis, that can lead to poor oral intake and poor absorption of nutrients. In addition, some chemotherapy medications and radiation may damage the salivary glands, causing decreased saliva production, which can interfere with taste, ability to chew, and/or ability to swallow. Infections can irritate the GI mucosa and result in a decrease of oral intake or absorption of nutrients. Medications such as antibiotics and narcotics are commonly administered to children with various hematologic and oncologic diseases and may cause further irritation to the GI tract, which can increase GI symptoms and/or interfere with absorption of nutrients. Corticosteroids are another medication commonly used for the treatment of various diseases that can result in a patient gaining a significant amount of weight; however, steroids increase protein catabolism that can contribute to malnutrition. Uncontrolled symptoms, such as an acute pain crisis in a patient with sickle-cell disease, can make a patient reluctant to eat.

In addition, various psychological influences and social factors can significantly affect the desire and ability to eat. Psychological influences including fatigue, depression, and anxiety can cause a patient to experience a lack of energy or lack of desire to eat. A child may also use food as a means of control in his or her life because food may be the only form of choice that a child has during treatment for an oncologic or hematologic disease. Social factors include a change in environment and/or a change in the patient's caregiver that can affect how the foods are prepared and where and with whom the foods are eaten.

### Clinical Presentation
Patients with alterations in nutrition can have various clinical presentations. Cachexia is a complex metabolic process that results in rapid and profound loss of body weight, fat, and muscle. Presenting signs and symptoms of cachexia include significant anorexia, weight loss or emaciation, and metabolic abnormalities. Other nutritional disparities may not be as obvious. Vitamin and trace-element deficiencies have been noted in patients with poor oral intake or malabsorption and can cause changes in the appearance of the skin, eyes, lips, tongue, nails, or hair. In addition, alterations of metabolism in fat, protein, and carbohydrates have been noted in underweight or malnourished cancer patients that have caused them to have high serum-lipid levels, significant loss of fat and muscle mass, catabolic states, glucose intolerance, or insulin resistance.

### Nutrition Management
Management includes providing nutritional education to patients and families, performing thorough nutritional assessments, and tailoring nutritional interventions based on individual needs (see Section VI, "Supportive Care").

### Nursing Assessment and Interventions
**Assessment:**
- Assess the patient's baseline nutritional status.
- Determine the patient's nutritional risks.
- Obtain a nutritional history.
- Assess for use of complementary and alternative therapies.

- Perform a thorough physical examination.
- Obtain the child's anthropometric measurements and plot these data at regular intervals.
- Obtain laboratory measurements (e.g., protein markers, electrolytes, triglyceride, and glucose).
  **Interventions:**
- Educate the patient and the family regarding the nutrition-related effects of therapy.
- Offer the patient frequent small meals and snacks, including foods of various taste, color, and texture.
- Encourage meticulous oral hygiene for the patient.
- Provide symptom management as indicated.
- Educate family members about nutritional interventions to ensure compliance with therapy.
- Consult a dietitian regarding the patient's nutritional needs.
- Refer the patient for psychosocial support if necessary.

### Expected Patient and Family Outcomes
- The patient maintains a positive nutritional status.
- The patient and the family understand the effects of poor nutrition on the patient's tolerance of therapy and the fact that poor nutrition increases the side effects or toxic effects of treatment.
- The patient and the family comply with recommended nutritional guidelines.

## Growth and Developmental Complications

*Deborah J. Lee*

The period of infancy through adolescence is an important time for growth and development wherein profound physical growth, cognitive and motor-skill development, and self-identity acquisition occur. Children with hematologic or oncologic diseases can experience delays in growth and development as a result of their disease and/or treatment. These side effects can be minimal, moderate, or severe and can occur during treatment or years after all therapies are completed. Deviations in growth and development milestones need to be promptly identified and addressed.

### Risk Factors
Risk factors include treatment at a young age (i.e., younger than 6 years of age); treatment after the onset of puberty; intensive combination chemotherapy; radiation higher than 24 Gy to the spine, long bones, hypothalamic-pituitary region, head, or neck; chemotherapy combined with radiation; suboptimal nutrition; surgery; anemia; iron overload; and use of glucocorticoids. Long-term hospitalizations, decreased mobility, or the extent of illness may also affect cognitive development by preventing children from participating in school or learning activities.

### Clinical Presentation
A patient may initially present with minimal signs of cognitive changes, such as temporary confusion or short-term memory loss. A decline in school performance (often in math skills) and/or a decrease in generalized intelligence (a loss of 10–20 IQ points) may then be seen. Girls are at a higher risk than boys for general cognitive declines. There may be a decline in visual spatial skills and a slower information-processing rate. A patient may have a developmental delay, delayed gross-motor and/or fine-motor development, or delays in personal, social-skill, or language development. A brief summary of normal growth and developmental milestones is listed in **Table 5-10**.

Physical symptoms can include deficiencies in growth or thyroid hormone, malnutrition secondary to chronic illness, early onset of puberty, impaired spinal growth, poor vertebrae development or loss of vertebral height, atrophy of growth-arrest lines, kyphosis, osteoporosis, short stature, or dental and maxillofacial abnormalities (e.g., facial asymmetry or hypoplasia). Growth may be dramatically affected by radiation delivered directly to the bones, epiphyses, and surrounding soft tissues. These areas are most susceptible to damage during periods of rapid growth, such as puberty. There is also diminished growth in soft-tissue mass and muscle in the radiation fields, which may result in asymmetry of adipose tissue and obesity. Scoliosis has been seen in 67%–80% of patients treated with spinal radiation of 20 Gy–62 Gy. The scoliosis markedly progresses during pubertal growth spurts regardless of age at the time of treatment. Radiation to soft tissues (e.g., breast tissue) may produce asymmetry with consequent alterations in body image. Body image may also be affected in patients who have leg-length discrepancies as a result of amputation or limb-salvage procedures.

Neuroendocrine dysfunction can be manifested by luteinizing hormone (LH), follicle-stimulating hormone (FSH) deficiency, or both, demonstrated by failure to enter or progress through puberty, decreased libido, and primary amenorrhea. A thyrotropin deficiency results in poor linear growth, excessive weight gain, lethargy, and delayed puberty. An adrenocorticotropic hormone deficiency can be accompanied by decreased stamina or lethargy. Hyperprolactinemia can result in pubertal delay or arrest, as well as amenorrhea with or without galactorrhea. Patients who receive cranial radiation greater than 25 Gy may develop precocious puberty. If left untreated, those who develop secondary sex characteristics (before age 10 in males and before age 8 in females) may have halted growth as a result of the premature fusion of the epiphyses.

### Medical Management
Management includes measuring the patient's standing height every 3–6 months and plotting it on a standard growth curve. A sitting height measurement of patients who have received radiation to the spine, abdomen, or pelvis should be taken. Measurements of the ratio of the patient's weight to height and velocity of growth (i.e., cm/year) also should be made. Patients should be examined for scoliosis. Bone age and Tanner stage evaluation can be used to determine the child's physical age of development. Baseline and ongoing assessments of LH, FSH, testosterone, and estradiol levels should be performed. Patients should be evaluated by an orthopedist if receiving treatment before or during a period of rapid growth. Measurements of growing limbs should be monitored closely.

Because of the long-term effects of radiation to the thyroid gland or hypothalamus, thyroid functions should be assessed in patients who have received mantle, head and neck, spinal, or total

## Table 5-10. Growth and Development

| Age | Physical Development | Cognitive Development | Fine and Gross Motor Development | Sexual Development |
|---|---|---|---|---|
| **Infant (birth–1 year)** | Birth weight doubles by 1st year. Height increases by 50% of birth length by 1st year. | Progression from reflexive behavior to imitate activity<br>Follows moving objects; visual acuity 20/60<br>Localizes sound | Increased use of hands (i.e., pincer grasp)<br>Sits unsupported and walks independently or with minimal assistance | Tanner Stage I |
| **Toddler (1–3 years)** | Weight gain 1.8–2.7 kg per year. Height increases 7.5 cm per year. | Differentiation of self from others/objects<br>Acquires use of language<br>Develops depth perception; visual acuity 20/40 | Uses a pencil or crayon<br>Increased locomotion skills (i.e., walks alone, walks up and down stairs) | Tanner Stage I<br>Develops gender identity |
| **Preschooler (3–5 years)** | Weight gain 2–3 kg per year. Height increases 6.5–9 cm per year. | Increased use of language, sometimes without understanding<br>Begins comprehending time<br>Egocentric in thought and play | Increased fine muscle coordination (i.e., drawings advance from scribbles to pictures)<br>Refinement in eye-hand and muscle coordination (i.e., riding tricycle, skipping) | Tanner Stage I<br>Identifies with same-sex parent through sex-role imitation |
| **School age (6–12 years)** | Weight gain 2–3 kg per year. Height increases 5 cm per year. | Increased narrative skills and use of more complex grammar correctly<br>Learns to work with others; enjoys playing team sports | Handedness is established<br>Increased ability to write, draw, and develop skills for arts-and-crafts hobbies<br>Increased muscular coordination and control | Tanner Stage I–III<br>Develops sexual awareness |
| **Adolescent (12–20 years)** | Weight gain 7–25 kg in girls and 7–30 kg in boys during adolescence. Height increases 5–20 cm in girls and 10–30 cm in boys during adolescence. | Develops advanced reasoning skills and abstract thinking | Rapid body growth can cause clumsiness and poor coordination | Tanner Stage I–V<br>Develops sexual identity, relationships, and intimacy |

body irradiation. The growth-hormone status of patients who received radiation therapy to the hypothalamic-pituitary axis should be assessed when there is documented growth delay (see Section X, "Late Effects of Childhood Cancer," for further details). In addition, a neuropsychological evaluation should be done and an early educational intervention provided when appropriate.

### Nursing Assessment and Interventions

**Assessment:**
- Assess the younger (birth–age 6) patient's developmental level with a standardized screening tool such as the Denver Developmental Screening Test.
- Assess cognitive and academic abilities routinely and compare with baseline measurements.
- Measure the patient's height and weight and plot the values on standard growth curves.
- Assess the child's Tanner stage of development.
- Assess the patient's menstrual history.
- Inquire about school attendance and school performance.
- Identify children with a high risk for central-nervous-system sequelae (based on their young age at time of treatment or treatment regimens including cranial radiation, intrathecal chemotherapy, and high dose methotrexate).
- Assess the impact of the illness on the patient's growth and development.

**Interventions:**
- Initiate age-appropriate activities that foster motor and cognitive development.
- Initiate activities that provide visual, auditory, verbal, and tactile stimulation.
- Encourage physical activity and refer to physical therapists as indicated.
- Collaborate with the patient's family and friends in stimulating the child's development.
- Communicate with the healthcare team regarding developmental needs.
- Assess and monitor calorie counts. Referrals to a dietitian should be obtained as needed.
- Make appropriate referrals to neuropsychology and endocrinology, as indicated, to obtain baseline and ongoing evaluations.
- Provide education, support, and reassurance to the patient and the family.
- Encourage and facilitate reintegration into the school system.

### Expected Patient and Family Outcomes
- The patient continues to develop appropriately for his or her age.
- The patient is evaluated for developmental deficits or growth impairments.
- The patient and the family maintain ongoing contact with the healthcare team.
- The patient and the family develop effective coping mechanisms.
- The patient and the family demonstrate knowledge of, and participation in, appropriate interventions.

# Pain

*Eufemia Jacob*

## Definition
*Pain* is an unpleasant sensory and emotional experience associated with acute or potential tissue damage (see the discussion of procedure pain in Section VI, "Supportive Care," and of terminal pain in Section IX, "Care for the Terminally Ill Child and the Family"). Pain is a complex phenomenon that requires clinicians to have sufficient knowledge; comprehensive assessment skills, including effective communication; and a broad understanding of treatment options. Pain in children with hematologic and oncologic disorders can be complex, particularly when the disease is severe, as in sickle-cell disease, or advanced, as in cancer.

## Clinical Presentation
Pain can be acute, chronic, or both. The signs and symptoms of acute pain can occur suddenly. The pain can be self-limiting and can result in restlessness, anxiety, hypertension, tachycardia, and tachypnea. The causes of acute pain in children with cancer are recent surgery, invasive medical procedures, and side effects of treatment, which can include infection, mucositis, myalgias, or peripheral neuropathies.

The signs and symptoms of chronic pain include persistent pain that usually lasts for more than 6 months. The pain can be constant or intermittent, accompanied by minimal alterations in the patient's vital signs, and result in depression. The causes of chronic pain in children with cancer can include disease progression, phantom-limb sensations, infection, and postherpetic syndrome.

## Risk Factors
Disease-related risk factors are infiltration or compression of soft tissue, bone, or nerves by tumor, and stimulation of pain receptors by effusions or edema.

Treatment-related risk factors include invasive diagnostic or treatment procedures, as well as inflammation, mucositis, and infection.

## Types of Pain
To appreciate the complexity and challenges of pain, it is helpful to understand the different types of pain because the etiologies and treatment are very different. There are two major types of pain: nociceptive and neuropathic.

Nociceptive pain occurs when normal tissues are damaged. This type of pain is usually responsive to nonopioids and opioids (**Table 5-11**). Examples of nociceptive pain include the following:
- Somatic pain—arises from bones, joints, muscles, skin, or connective tissues; it is usually aching or throbbing in quality and is well localized. This type of pain generally responds to combinations of acetaminophen and codeine.
- Visceral pain—arises from the visceral organs, such as the gastrointestinal tract, liver, and pancreas. Often this type of pain is poorly localized and may feel like a vague, deep ache, sometimes cramping or colicky in nature. This type of pain is generally very responsive to opioids.

Neuropathic pain results from nerve damage, either in the peripheral nerves or the central nerves. Treatment of this type of pain is usually more difficult, as it is only partially responsive to acetaminophen, nonsteroidal antiinflammatory (NSAID) medications, or opioids and may respond better to other adjuvant medications (Table 5-11). Examples of neuropathic pain include the following:
- Centrally generated pain includes deafferentation pain, which occurs with injury to either the peripheral or central nervous system. An example is phantom pain, which reflects injury to the peripheral nervous system after amputation of a limb.
- Sympathetically maintained pain is associated with dysregulation of the autonomic nervous system. This type of pain occurs more commonly after fractures and soft-tissue injuries of the arms and legs, which may occur as a result of disease process or chemotherapy in patients with cancer or as a result of ischemia from vaso-occlusive painful episodes in patients with sickle-cell disease. Sympathetically maintained pain presents as extreme hypersensitivity in the skin around the injury and also peripherally in the limb. This type of pain is termed allodynia.

Neuropathic pain may originate from the peripheral nervous system or from the central nervous system. When a nerve becomes injured by degeneration, pressure, inflammation, or infection, it becomes electrically unstable and fires off signals in a completely inappropriate, random, and disordered fashion. These signals are then interpreted by the brain as pain and can be associated with symptoms of nerve malfunction such as hypersensitivity to touch, vibration, or hot and cold, as well as tingling, numbness, and weakness. Often there is referred pain to an area where that nerve would normally supplies. Nerve pain is often described as lancinating, shooting, burning, and hypersensitive.

## Physiologic Processes Underlying the Experience of Pain
Four physiologic processes underlie the experience of pain: (1) transduction occurs at the site of injury, (2) transmission occurs at the spinal tracts within the spinal cord, (3) perception occurs in the brain, and (4) modulation occurs in the brain stem and spinal cord.

### Transduction
When tissue is damaged by injury, infection, trauma, or surgery, some cells are damaged. These cells release chemical substances, such as prostaglandins, bradykinins, serotonins, substance P, and

### Table 5-11. Medications for Pain

| Pain Type | Medication Classification | Medication Type |
|---|---|---|
| Mild | Nonopioids | Acetaminophen |
|  |  | Ibuprofen |
|  |  | Ketoprofen |
|  |  | Naproxen |
|  |  | Ketorolac |
| Mild to moderate | Nonopioid combined with opioids | Hydrocodone + Acetaminophen |
|  |  | Hydrocodone + Ibuprofen |
|  |  | Oxycodone + Acetaminophen |
|  |  | Codeine + Acetaminophen |
| Moderate to severe | Opioids | Codeine |
|  |  | Hydrocodone/Oxycodone |
|  |  | Oxymorphone |
|  |  | Morphine |
|  |  | Hydromorphone |
|  |  | Fentanyl |
| Severe | Patient-controlled analgesia (PCA) | Morphine |
|  |  | Hydromorphone |
|  |  | Fentanyl |
| Poor or inadequate pain control | Adjuvant medications | Antidepressants: amitriptyline or nortriptyline |
|  |  | Anticonvulsants: gabapentin or carbamazepine |
|  |  | Anxiolytics: lorazepam or diazepam |
|  |  | Corticosteroids: dexamethasone |
|  |  | Others: clonidine, mexiletine, ketamine, lidocaine, or capsaicin cream |

Adapted from material in *Pediatric Dosage Handbook*, by C. Taketomo, J. Hodding, & D. Kraus, 2004, Hudson, OH: Lexi-Comp; *Guideline for the Management of Acute and Chronic Pain in Sickle Cell Disease*, by L. J. Benjamin, C. D. Dampier, A. K. Jacox, V. Odesina, D. Phoenix, B. Shapiro, et al., 1999, Glenview, IL: American Pain Society.

histamine, that activate or sensitize the nerve endings and cause pain. Treatment options can include NSAIDs such as ibuprofen and naproxen, or corticosteroids such as dexamethasone that interfere with the production of prostaglandins.

### Transmission

Pain signals are transmitted through the nerves that travel from the periphery to the central spinal cord, then into the brain stem and thalamus, and then to the cortex. C fibers are unmyelinated, small-diameter, slow-conducting fibers that transmit poorly localized, dull pain and are particularly sensitive to opioids. Delta fibers are sparsely myelinated, large-diameter, fast-conducing fibers that transmit well-localized, sharp pain. These fibers are less sensitive to opioids, but anticonvulsants or anesthetics can relieve some types of pain by blocking the transmission of the pain signals.

### Perception

The exact location in the brain where pain is perceived is not clear. The reticular system in the brain is responsible for the autonomic response to pain and warns us to attend to the pain. The somatosensory cortex localizes and characterizes the pain. The limbic system is responsible for the emotional and behavioral response to pain. Cognitive behavioral interventions, such as distraction, relaxation, and imagery can reduce the sensory components of pain and can direct the person's attention away from the pain sensation. A common misconception occurs when patients with sickle-cell disease rate their pain as high but are seen laughing, talking on the phone, or playing video games. The interpretation is that the patient is faking pain or inflating the pain rating; however, these activities may be distraction techniques.

### Modulation

Modulation refers to changing or inhibiting pain impulses. There is a pain pathway that involves nerve cells originating in the brain stem that descends to the dorsal-horn nerve cells in the spinal cord. These fibers release substances such as endogenous opioids, serotonin, norepinephrine, gamma aminobutyric acid (GABA), and neurotensin. All these substances occur naturally in the body, inhibit the transmission of pain, and produce analgesia. Modulation is thought to explain the wide variations in perception of pain from one person to another. Tricyclic antidepressants such as amitriptyline and desipramine interfere with the reuptake of serotonin and norepinephrine and prevent the feeling of pain. GABA is an inhibitory neurotransmitter and interferes with the transmission of pain. Baclofen is a substrate of GABA receptors and can produce analgesia for many pain conditions, particularly those that are accompanied by muscle spasms.

These four mechanisms (i.e., transduction, transmission, perception, and modulation) are the physiologic processes underlying nociceptive pain. The mechanisms are not as clear with neuropathic pain, wherein injury to nerves results in repetitive spontaneous transmission of pain.

A physiologic phenomenon can occur with repetitive painful stimuli that occur with the recurrent, painful episodes in sickle-cell disease, or with repetitive painful procedures such as lumbar punctures or bone-marrow aspirations that patients with cancer undergo. N-methyl-D-aspartate antagonists (NMDA receptors) may be responsible for the progressive increase in firing at the dorsal horn and result in repeated, prolonged, painful stimuli. The spinal cord becomes hypersensitive and excitable, leading to amplified and exaggerated responses. Many clinicians do not recognize that these events may be occurring in the spinal cord during the transmission of pain signals and could affect subsequent pain experiences.

## Negative Consequences of Unrelieved Pain

Pain related to surgery, tissue trauma, tumor growth, infection, injury, inflammation, or ischemia can trigger a number of physiologic stress responses in the human body.

These stress responses are protective in nature because they activate the sympathetic nervous system and alert the body to an impending or existing harm. The responses prevent further damage by minimizing blood loss, maintaining perfusion to vital organs, promoting healing, and fighting infection. However, pain and stress responses, especially when prolonged, also can produce a number of harmful effects and can have negative consequences. The harmful effects of unrelieved pain are many and involve multiple systems (**Table 5-12**). Effects of unrelieved pain in patients' quality of life vary and include sleeplessness, anxiety, fear, hopelessness, decreased physical activity, and interference with school and activities of daily living; they can also lead to thoughts of suicide. Poorly controlled acute pain also can predispose patients to debilitating chronic-pain syndromes. Some chronic pain states can be prevented with early and aggressive pain management.

## Nursing Assessment and Interventions

### Assessment

Pain should be assessed on the basis of the patient's developmental stage (**Table 5-13**). The initial assessment is often conducted by using the 0-to-10 numerical ratings scale for older children, the Wong-Wong-Baker faces pain-rating scale for younger children (see **Figure 5-5**), or the face, legs, activity, crying, consolability (FLACC) scale for nonverbal or preverbal children. A more comprehensive assessment may include the following components.

**Current, worst, and least pain:** In addition to asking how much pain a patient is currently experiencing, ask the patient to numerically rate (using a numerical-rating scale) what was the greatest amount of pain and what was the least amount of pain he or she has had in the past 24 hours. A rating of 6 for current pain

### Table 5-12. Effects of Unrelieved Pain

| System | Response to Unrelieved Pain | Clinical Effects | Response to Analgesics |
|---|---|---|---|
| Endocrine | Releases excessive amounts of ACTH, cortisol, ADH, growth hormone, catecholamines, and glucagons | Increased heart rate, increased respiratory rate, fever, poor glucose usage, destruction of carbohydrate, protein, and fat | Slows the metabolic response to stress |
| Cardiovascular | Activates the sympathetic nervous system | Increased heart rate, blood pressure, cardiac workload, and oxygen demand | Reduces cardiac workload, increases myocardial oxygen supply, and reduces thromboembolic complications |
| Respiratory | Limits thoracic and abdominal muscle movement leading to respiratory dysfunction | Decreased tidal volumes, vital capacity, and alveolar ventilation; can progress to atelectasis and pneumonia | Patients are able to stand, walk, cough, and breathe deeply better |
| Renal | Releases hormones that regulate urinary output, fluid, and electrolytes | Increased sodium, hypokalemia, fluid overload, increased cardiac workload and hypertension | Improves blood flow to the kidneys and maintains renal function |
| Gastrointestinal (GI) | Increased sympathetic nervous system activity; decreased gastric emptying and intestinal motility | Impaired GI function and paralysis | Improves GI blood flow |
| Musculoskeletal | Impaired mobility | Muscle spasm, impaired muscle function, fatigue, and immobility | Improves range of motion, ease of mobility, and independence |
| Cognition & Emotion | Sleeplessness | Altered mental and emotional status, altered temperament, increased vulnerability to stress | Promotes sleep and improves cognitive function |
| Immune | Suppressed immune function | Susceptibility to infection | Improves immune system |

is good, if the worst he or she has had in the past 24 hours was 8 and the lowest was 2. However, a rating of 6 is not good if his or her pain had been 6 in the past 24 hours, in the past 7 days, or during the past month. It is important to examine changes and trends, not only in current pain, but also in worst and least pain. Examining trends in pain over time allows for finding periods when pain peaks and troughs and determining whether these peaks and troughs are associated with medications, activities, or other events that can aggravate or minimize pain.

**Pain location:** Body-outline diagrams for assessing the location of pain are useful not only for indicating the extensiveness of the pain but also for determining the specific location of the pain. When pain is not seen, it may be more difficult to believe and treat. A body-outline diagram may help clinicians to understand the extensiveness of the pain. The body-outline diagram also may be useful in patients who are not able to explain their pain using words or numbers. Some patients are not able to quantify their pain and become frustrated when asked to rate their pain on a numerical rating scale; however, they may be able to mark the areas on the body-outline diagram without difficulty. In addition, clinicians may not able to assess a non-English-speaking patient's pain, and the patient may not complain of pain and therefore may be at high risk for receiving inadequate treatment.

**Medications:** Asking patients what medications they have used to relieve pain may yield information on adherence and outcomes. Patients may not be adherent to their medication regimen because of intolerable side effects (e.g., nausea, itching, drowsiness) or other reasons. Teaching patients about the negative consequences of pain may improve compliance; however, if intolerable side effects are experienced, changing medication or adding adjunctive medications should be considered. Clinicians may label patients as "drug seeking" when they make a request for a specific pain medication (or amount of medication; e.g., "The only thing that helps is 20 mg of morphine."). However, patients, especially after dealing with chronic pain, should be regarded as experts in their own pain management; they know what it takes to relieve their pain. If drug-seeking behavior is suspected, clinicians should administer the pain medication first, then make a referral to an addiction-medicine specialist so that the patient can obtain an appropriate diagnosis and treatment plan.

**Relief provided by medications:** In addition to asking about the pain intensity on a numerical rating scale, another useful assessment may be a pain-relief measure. Asking the patient, "How much did the medicines help with your pain on a scale from 0 = did not help at all to 10 = helped a lot" may offer a different way for some patients to think about their pain and enable them to self-evaluate the effectiveness of medications.

**Interference of pain with function:** Questioning patients about how much pain interferes with normal activities such as walking, sleeping, eating, and playing allows for a more thorough assessment. This is important because the goal of pain management may not necessarily be to decrease pain intensity but rather to increase patients' ability to sleep at night or participate in their activities of daily living. Sometimes there is not one medication or "magic pill" that completely eliminates pain. However, strategies such as cognitive behavioral interventions can increase patients' pain tolerance and improve their functional ability to engage in activities they enjoy.

**Pain quality:** A challenge in assessment is distinguishing between neuropathic types of pain, wherein nerve tissues are involved, and nociceptive types of pain, wherein inflammation or ischemia is involved (**Table 5-14**). In patients 8 years and older, a word-descriptor list can be used to describe different qualities of pain.

### Interventions

- Plan for managing pain by considering a patient's individual characteristics and cultural beliefs, considering the patient's pain threshold based on his or her current use of pain medications, assessing the patient's current or past use of illicit drugs or alcohol, addressing the patient's fears related to using drugs, and assessing the anxiety levels of the patient and the family.
- Educate the patient and the parents about pain management and the differences between acute and chronic pain.
- Discuss painful procedures honestly with the patient and the family and prepare them for the procedures (see Section VI, "Supportive Care").
- Document the patient's pain and evaluate interventions.

### Pain Management

Initial management often includes the administration of nonopioids and NSAIDs for mild pain; a combined formulation of acetaminophen and opioids such as acetaminophen with codeine or oxycodone for moderate pain; and intravenous opioids such as morphine, hydromorphone, or fentanyl for severe pain. However, patients with hematologic and oncologic disorders

**Table 5-13. Pain Assessment by Developmental Level**

| Developmental Level | Expression of Pain |
|---|---|
| Infant | An infant may cry intensely, be inconsolable, draw his or her knees to the chest, exhibit hypersensitivity or irritability, or be unable to eat or sleep. |
| Toddler | A toddler may be verbally aggressive, exhibit regressive behavior or withdraw, or guard the painful area. |
| Preschooler | A preschooler may verbalize the intensity of the pain, view the pain as punishment, and understand that there can be a secondary gain associated with the pain. |
| School-age child | A school-age child verbalizes pain, can use an objective measurement of pain, and resists movement. The child also can be influenced by cultural beliefs and can experience nightmares associated with pain. |
| Adolescent | An adolescent can verbalize pain but may not request pain medications or may deny the pain in the presence of peers. An adolescent also can experience changes in sleep patterns and in appetite or display regressive behavior in the presence of family members. |

### Figure 5-5. Wong-Baker Faces Pain Rating Scale

| 0 | 1 | 2 | 3 | 4 | 5 |
|---|---|---|---|---|---|
| Face 0 is very happy, because he doesn't hurt at all. | Face 1 hurts just a little bit. | Face 2 hurts a little more. | Face 3 hurts even more. | Face 4 hurts a whole lot. | Face 5 hurts as much as you can imagine, although you don't have to be crying to feel this bad. |

From *Wong's Essentials of Pediatric Nursing* (6th ed., p. 1301), by D. L. Wong, M. Hockenberry-Eaton, D. Wilson, M. L. Winkelstein, & P. Schwartz, 2001, St. Louis: Mosby, Inc. Reprinted with permission.

### Table 5-14. Type, Location, and Quality of Pain

| Type of Pain | Location | Pain Quality |
|---|---|---|
| Musculoskeletal | Long bones, shoulder, pelvis, hips, neck, or chest wall | Sharp, throbbing, achy, or pressure-like; worsened by movement or weight bearing |
| Visceral | Usually occurs in the abdomen but may radiate to groin, shoulder, or back | Cramping, colicky, dull, aching; pain lessens by bending over or curling up |
| Postsurgical | Depends on location of surgery | Tight and constricting, or constant and aching; worse with movement |
| Neuropathic | May radiate along the nerve root | Varies according to the specific nerve regions involved |
| Intercostal Nerves/Ribs | May radiate along the nerve root | Burning, shooting, aching, pressure-like; may be worsened by deep breathing or moving |
| Brachial Plexus | Located in shoulder and arms, and radiates down arm | Burning, shooting, numbness, tingling; hyperalgesia (extreme sensitivity to touch); allodynia (distress from stimuli) |
| Lumbar Plexus | Radiates down thigh, groin, or back of thigh | Burning, shooting, numbness, tingling, or prickling; leg edema (late sign) |
| Sacral Plexus | Midline of lower back | Burning, shooting, dull, aching; may have bowel and bladder dysfunction |
| Spinal Cord | Cervical, thoracic, or lumbosacral areas | Dull, aching, sharp with movement, tight, band-like; worsens when lying down, coughing, sneezing, or weight bearing; can rapidly progress from pain to sensory loss and motor-function loss |

may have pain that is more complex and requires multimodal approaches to management. If a patient-controlled-analgesia (PCA) device is used for patients, clinicians need to perform daily evaluation of medication use to ensure that the patient receives adequate doses and adequate relief. In addition, clinicians should educate the patient and family members regarding use of the device to ensure their understanding. As the patient's pain changes, changes in PCA settings, along with reinforcement of education regarding its use, may be needed.

Preemptive analgesia (i.e., giving the patient pain medications before he or she experiences pain) has been thought to be effective in some cases. This practice is implemented commonly prior to surgeries and limb amputation in cancer patients. It is generally difficult to use with sickle-cell pain because that type of pain is unexpected and unpredictable; however, it can be used to prevent pain from escalating to its peak.

In some instances, pain can be undertreated because of parents' and providers' misconceptions; they may have exaggerated fears of addiction or respiratory depression. Addiction and respiratory depression are rare in patients who have a physiologic basis for their pain. If respiratory depression does occur, it is reversible with the administration of naloxone. Patients with addiction problems are more complex to treat and may require larger amounts of analgesics than would be required for nonaddicted patients. It is more common for patients whose pain is undertreated to exhibit behaviors (e.g., hypervigilance, clock watching) that are similar to those of patients with addiction. This phenomenon is called *pseudoaddiction*. These patients often may have received home medications in higher equianalgesic doses (**Table 5-15**) than the prescribed intravenous morphine during hospitalization, and thus may complain that the medications do not work. Clinicians need to pay careful attention to titration of

### Table 5-15. Equianalgesic Conversions and Weaning Opioids

**Equianalgesic Conversions**

| Medication | Dosing |
|---|---|
| Morphine to hydromorphone | Start new opioid at 50% of equianalgesic dose. Titrate to desired effect. |
| Morphine to methadone | Start at 25% of equianalgesic dose. Titrate to desired effect. |
| Morphine to codeine | 1 mg IV morphine = 20 mg PO codeine |
| IV morphine to oral morphine | 1 mg IV morphine = 3 mg PO morphine |
| Morphine to hydrocodone | 1 mg IV morphine = 3 mg PO hydrocodone |
| Morphine to oxycodone | 1 mg IV morphine = 3 mg PO oxycodone |

**Weaning Opioids**

| Medication | Dosing |
|---|---|
| Tapering opioids, if patient received longer than 1 week | IV dose is decreased by 50% for 2 days; then taper by 25% every 2 days. Opioids may be stopped when dose is equianalgesic to 0.3 mg/kg/day of PO morphine in patients <10 kg or 15 mg/day of PO morphine in patients >50 kg. |
| Discontinuing opioids | IV dose is decreased by 50% and PO acetaminophen with codeine or PO morphine is initiated. |

*Note.* IV = intravenous; PO = oral.

medications at the time of admission, starting from previous equianalgesic home doses and weaning schedules, and ensure appropriate conversions to minimize the risk of behaviors that mimic addiction. If addiction is suspected, appropriate referral should be made to an addiction-medicine specialist rather than minimizing the administration of analgesics. It is safe to use analgesic drugs for controlling pain, and given the negative consequences associated with pain, it may be unsafe to allow patients to experience prolonged pain by not controlling or treating it.

Pain in children with hematologic and oncologic disorders such as sickle-cell disease and cancer is complex. Multiple dimensions need to be assessed and multitreatment modalities need to be incorporated. Medications alone may not penetrate into all the pain-signaling pathways. Cognitive behavioral interventions, psychosocial interventions, and physiotherapies may help to decrease pain intensity and help with relaxation, coping, and improving function. Other dimensions may be used for setting goals and evaluating the effectiveness of treatment regimens.

### Expected Patient and Family Outcomes

- The patient and the family are active participants in the pain-management process.
- The patient and the family understand the goals of pain management.
- The patient's medications are administered early in the pain cycle and on a regular schedule.
- The patient experiences pain control with minimal sedation or other side effects.
- The patient and the family recognize the need for changes in the pain-management regimen when indicated by a change in the patient's pain level.
- The patient and the family understand how to appropriately manage the side effects of analgesics.
- The patient and the family are satisfied with pain-control measures.

## Oncologic Emergencies

*Rita Secola and Debbie Reid*

*Oncologic emergencies* are life-threatening events that can occur during a child's course of treatment for cancer. Some emergencies manifest at the time of diagnosis, as a direct result of cancer treatment, or when cancer recurs.

### Hyperleukocytosis

#### Definition
Hyperleukocytosis is a condition in which the peripheral white blood cell count is greater than 100,000/mm$^3$, causing increased blood viscosity and blast-cell aggregates and thrombi in the microcirculation.

#### Risk Factors
The risk factors are acute lymphoblastic leukemia, seen in 10% of patients; acute nonlymphoblastic leukemia, seen in 20% of patients; and chronic myelogenous leukemia in the acute phase, seen in 100% of patients.

#### Clinical Presentation
The signs can include shortness of breath, tachypnea, cyanosis, blurred vision, papilledema, agitation, ataxia, confusion, delirium, and stupor.

#### Medical Management
Patients typically receive intravenous (IV) hyperhydration (approximately 3,000 mL/m2/day), sodium bicarbonate, and allopurinol (Zyloprim) or rasburicase (Elitek). In addition, metabolic abnormalities are aggressively corrected. Other measures often include blood-product support, leukopheresis, exchange transfusions, and chemotherapy.

## Potential Complications

Patients can experience central-nervous-system (CNS) hemorrhage, pulmonary leukostasis, metabolic alterations, and renal failure.

## Nursing Assessment and Interventions

**Assessment:**
- Assess and monitor the patient's urine output, observe for hematuria and/or a pH <7.0 or >7.5.
- Observe the patient's respiratory status for dyspnea, tachypnea, and pulmonary congestion.
- Assess the patient for signs or symptoms of bleeding.
- Evaluate the patient's neurologic status and level of consciousness.
- Monitor the patient's weight closely.
- Perform a guaiac test on the patient's stools.
- Provide timely intensive care unit (ICU) consultations as indicated.

    **Interventions:**
- Report critical changes in the patient's symptoms to his or her physician.
- Explain the purpose of the monitoring to the patient and the patient's family.

## Expected Patient and Family Outcomes

- The patient and the family understand the implications of hyperleukocytosis and the potentially life-threatening situation that it presents.
- The patient and the family participate in making decisions about treatment and care.
- The patient and the family list the signs and symptoms that should be reported to the healthcare team.

## Acute Tumor Lysis Syndrome

### Definition

*Acute tumor lysis syndrome* (TLS) is a significant complication associated with initial chemotherapy for various subtypes of lymphomas and leukemias and other tumors with high growth fraction. *TLS* is defined as severe metabolic abnormalities that include hyperuricemia, hyperphosphatemia, hypocalcemia, and hyperkalemia. These metabolic abnormalities are a direct result of the death and degradation of tumor cells and the release of their contents into circulation. One abnormality or a combination of abnormalities may occur and lead to acute renal failure and potentially life-threatening cardiac dysfunction (**Figure 5-6**). Laboratory findings include: uric acid >8 mgm/dL; potassium >6 mEq/L); phosphorous >10 mgm/dL; calcium <8 mgm/dL; and elevated blood urea nitrogen (BUN) and creatinine levels.

### Risk Factors

Patients with a disease that exhibits a high proliferation rate and a high tumor-growth fraction and who are highly sensitive to cytotoxic therapy (especially those with acute lymphoblastic leukemia [ALL], acute myelogenous leukemia, and non-Hodgkin's lymphoma [NHL]) are at risk for TLS. Specifically, patients with T-cell ALL, Burkitt and other B-cell NHL, a significantly elevated white blood count (WBC), an elevated uric acid level >8 mgm/dL, and lactate dehydrogenase (LDH) >2 times the normal institutional upper limits are at higher risk for developing TLS. The extreme rapidity of tumor breakdown that occurs in these types of diseases can quickly overwhelm the body's homeostasis. Additional risk factors for developing TLS are found in patients with a large tumor burden with lymphadenopathy, mediastinal mass, hepatosplenomegaly, large tumor, and renal insufficiency. TLS also has been noted in neuroblastoma, small-cell lung carcinoma, multiple myeloma, and other solid tumors.

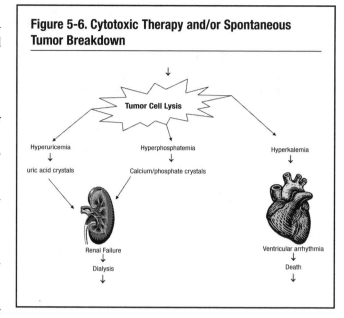

**Figure 5-6. Cytotoxic Therapy and/or Spontaneous Tumor Breakdown**

### Clinical Presentation

TLS has a rapid onset and may manifest at prediagnosis, at 6–48 hours after initial treatment, and up to 7 days thereafter. It is imperative to identify patients at risk and to complete a detailed history. Symptoms may include abnormal laboratory findings (e.g., elevated WBC, phosphorus, uric acid, potassium, BUN, creatinine, and LDH and decreased calcium); flank pain; hematuria; decreased urine output; lethargy; nausea and/or vomiting; edema; muscle cramps and twitching; numbness and tingling; carpopedal spasms; seizures; diarrhea; respiratory distress; abdominal fullness or ascites; and irregular heartbeat.

### Medical Management

Early identification of high-risk patients with preexisting hyperuricemia, as well as those taking prophylactic measures to prevent TLS, is critical for reducing the morbidity associated with the disease and for obtaining optimal patient outcomes. The single most important intervention is hydration.

- Administer intravenous hydration with D5 1/4 NS (without potassium) at 3 L/m$^2$/day to attain a urine output of greater than 100 cc/m$^2$/hr and a urine-specific gravity of less than 1.010.
- Force diuresis (e.g., with LASIX or mannitol) if clinically indicated.
- Manage hyperkalemia (i.e., remove sources of potassium, diuretics, Kayexalate, glucose/insulin IV infusion, IV calcium gluconate, sodium bicarbonate IV push, and hemofiltration/dialysis).

- Manage hyperuricemia (e.g., with alkalinization IV NaCCO3 40 mEq/L, allopurinol orally 100 mg/m$^2$/dose 3 times a day [maximum dose 800 mg/day], or rasburicase [Elitek] 0.15 or 0.2 mg/kg/dose IV every day for 1–5 days).
- Manage hyperphosphatemia (use oral phosphate binder, implement dietary phosphate restriction, remove phosphate-containing medications, provide IV glucose/insulin infusion).
- Manage hypocalcemia (treat hyperphosphatemia, keep serum bicarbonate <30, infuse calcium gluconate IV).
- Provide timely renal or ICU consultations as indicated.
- Consider leukopheresis or exchange transfusion if warranted to reduce tumor burden.
- Establish metabolic stability prior to the start of cytotoxic therapy.

## Nursing Assessment and Interventions
- Give strict attention to fluid balance.
- Maintain strict input and output; maintain urine output at greater than 3–5 cc/kg/hr.
- Monitor urine-specific gravity (keep >1.010) and urine pH (keep at 7.0–7.5) every 4 hours.
- Assess vital signs at least every 4 hours.
- Obtain "tumor lysis" laboratory specimens at least every 6–12 hours as ordered, and evaluate values promptly.
- Perform ongoing respiratory assessments.
- Perform ongoing assessments for edema.
- Monitor weight three times a day.
- Provide ongoing neurologic assessments (i.e., for loss of consciousness, weakness, muscle twitching, numbness, and tingling, seizures).
- Provide ongoing gastrointestinal (GI) assessment (for nausea, vomiting, diarrhea).
- Provide ongoing assessment for Chvostek-Weiss (unilateral facial spasm) and Trouseau (carpopedal spasms) signs.
- Maintain seizure precautions.
- Monitor for abnormal cardiac rate or rhythm (e.g., peaked T waves, widened QRS, ventricular arrhythmias).
- Administer IV hydration, as ordered, without potassium.
- Administer alkalinization/allopurinol and/or rasburicase (Elitek) as ordered.

If these metabolic abnormalities cannot be controlled, more severe complications can occur, including the need for hemofiltration, dialysis, or both, or heart block or cardiac arrest.

## Expected Patient and Family Outcomes
- The patient and the family can verbalize their understanding of the seriousness of TLS.
- The patient has minimal symptoms of TLS, or the TLS is under control.
- The patient does not experience any life-threatening events related to TLS.

# Septic Shock

## Definition
Septic shock is a systemic response to pathogenic microorganisms and endotoxins in the blood that are usually gram-negative and arise from endogenous flora. Septic shock can lead to decreased tissue perfusion, cellular hypoxia, and death. Septic shock also is defined as sepsis with hypotension (i.e., systolic blood pressure <90 mm Hg or a reduction from baseline of 40 mm Hg) despite adequate fluid resuscitation, along with perfusion abnormalities that may include but are not limited to lactic acidosis, scant urination, or an acute alteration in mental status.

## Risk Factors
Risk factors include prolonged neutropenia (i.e., lasting more than 7 days), an absolute neutrophil count lower than 100 mm$^3$, breaks in skin and mucus-membrane integrity, use of invasive devices, malnutrition, and asplenia.

## Clinical Presentation
Not all children with sepsis develop shock. Many times the febrile patient with neutropenia does not have the clinical symptoms of sepsis or shock until after antibiotics are initiated.

Sepsis should be considered a possibility whenever a patient presents with a known or suspected infection and with two or more of the following symptoms: fever or hypothermia, unexplained tachycardia and tachypnea, signs of peripheral vasodilation, leukocytosis, or leukopenia, and reduced mental alertness. Severe sepsis is the diagnosis if any organ failure is confirmed.

If left untreated, or if the child is not responsive to treatment, then shock progresses. When shock is classified by etiology, the terms *hypovolemic, caridogenic,* and *distributive* are used. Hypovolemic shock is the most common manifestation of shock and is usually due to inadequate intravascular volume relative to vascular space (i.e., dehydration, hemorrhage, inflammatory condition [e.g., sepsis]). Distributive shock results from the inappropriate distribution of blood volume (e.g., in sepsis or anaphylaxis). Cardiogenic shock is caused by myocardial dysfunction. Shock also is classified by its effects on blood pressure as compensated shock (e.g., early shock, tachycardia, and poor perfusion with normal blood pressure) or decompensated shock (e.g., late shock, weak central pulses, altered level of consciousness, oliguria, and hypotension). Septic shock is diagnosed when there is severe sepsis and hypotension despite fluid resuscitation, or when blood pressure is maintained with vasoactive drug support.

## Medical Management
Early recognition and prompt treatment of sepsis or septic shock are essential to the patient's survival.

Volume resuscitation is the most important intervention for patients with septic shock. Maintaining cardiovascular volume with isotonic or crystalloid boluses of 20 cc/kg over 5–20 minutes and to 60 cc/kg or greater during the first hour often is required to help stabilize the child. However, when volume resuscitation is inadequate to restore blood pressure, vasoactive drugs are recommended. The only proven treatment for septic shock is the early administration of antimicrobials, preferably with broad-spectrum antibiotics (see Section VI, "Supportive Care"), until the causative pathogen is identified.

## Potential Complications
CNS complications include a decreased level of consciousness, anxiety, restlessness, confusion, disorientation, lethargy, and, in some cases, coma. Respiratory effects can include tachypnea, rales, wheezing, dyspnea, cyanosis, and pulmonary congestion. Cardiac difficulties comprise tachycardia, thready pulse, narrowing pulse pressure, decreased peripheral circulation, and cool, clammy skin. Renal complications are manifested by oliguria and anuria and can result in renal failure. Hematologic complications consist of bleeding or disseminated intravascular coagulation (DIC) or both. Complications result from the progression of shock and can lead to multiorgan failure and death if not treated promptly.

## Nursing Assessment and Interventions
**Assessment:**
- Monitor the patient's physical status and vital signs continuously to assess for subtle changes in condition, and be aware that changes in a child's vital signs lag behind deteriorations in physical status.
- Strictly monitor the patient's fluid intake and output.

**Interventions:**
- Obtain blood cultures immediately and administer IV antibiotics promptly when a patient is febrile and neutropenic.
- Provide support for the patient and the family. (See also Section VI, "Supportive Care.")

## Expected Patient and Family Outcomes
- The patient and the family understand the signs and symptoms of early infection and seek prompt medical attention.
- The patient has minimal complications related to septic shock.

# Disseminated Intravascular Coagulation

## Definition
*DIC* is the consumption of coagulation factors that are greater than the body's ability to replace them, thus inhibiting coagulation. Alterations in blood-clotting mechanisms are manifested by decreased platelets, increased prothrombin, and decreased fibrinogen, which result in diffuse intravascular coagulation and tissue ischemia.

## Risk Factors
Risk factors are malignancy, infection, and trauma. Promyelocytic leukemia is the most common malignancy associated with DIC at initial diagnosis. The overall most common cause of DIC in children with cancer is gram-negative sepsis.

## Clinical Presentation
A patient can have petechiae, ecchymosis, and purpuric rash. There also can be diffuse uncontrolled bleeding, a platelet count <20,000/mm$^3$, prolonged prothrombin time and partial thromboplastin time, increased D-dimer assay, decreased antithrombin III levels, below-normal fibrinogen, and increased fibrin-degradation products.

## Medical Management
Treatment consists of symptom management and replacement of blood products (e.g., fresh-frozen plasma, cryoprecipitate, transfusions of platelet and packed red blood cells). Heparin, once a mainstay of DIC management, now is rarely used.

## Potential Complications
Complications include bleeding from puncture sites, GI bleeding, hematuria, oliguria, dyspnea, tachypnea, tachycardia, diminished peripheral circulation, restlessness, confusion, and lethargy.

## Nursing Assessment and Interventions
**Assessment:**
- Monitor the patient for signs and symptoms of DIC.
- Assess the following for presence and amount of bleeding: urine, stool, emesis, and needle-puncture sites.
- Assess changes in laboratory values.
- Assess tissue perfusion, including color, temperature, and peripheral pulses.

**Interventions:**
- Apply direct pressure to active bleeding sites.
- Administer pain medications as needed.
- Elevate the sites of active bleeding when the patient can tolerate this measure.
- Administer blood products as ordered.
- Provide support for the patient and the family.
- Teach the patient and the family measures to use to prevent bleeding.

## Expected Patient and Family Outcomes
- The patient and the family can identify risk factors for the development of DIC.
- The patient has minimal complications related to DIC.

# Typhlitis

## Definition
*Typhlitis* is a bacterial invasion of the cecum that leads to necrotizing colitis. Tissue involvement ranges from inflammation to full-thickness infarction or perforation or both. *Clostridium septicum* and *Pseudomonas aeruginosa* are the most common organisms associated with typhlitis.

## Risk Factors
Risk factors are severe neutropenia, high-risk acute leukemia, induction therapy for acute myelogenous leukemias, infection, and mucositis.

## Clinical Presentation
Symptoms can include profound neutropenia; fever; severe abdominal pain in the right-lower quadrant; distended abdomen; high-pitched, diminished, or absent bowel sounds; nausea; vomiting; and diarrhea.

## Medical Management
Management consists of broad-spectrum antibiotic coverage, supportive management, and radiological evaluation. Surgical intervention may be indicated in the following situations: persistent GI bleeding despite resolution or correction of clotting abnormalities; evidence of free intraperitoneal perforation; clinical deterioration requiring support with vasopressors and hyperhydration, which suggests uncontrolled sepsis from infarction; and symptoms of an intraabdominal process that requires surgical intervention in a patient without neutropenia.

### Potential Complications

Complications can include sepsis, necrosis of the cecum, temporary or permanent ostomy, and death.

### Nursing Assessment and Interventions

**Assessment:**
- Perform a physical assessment of the patient to evaluate bowel sounds and the degree of abdominal pain.
- Assess the patient's vital signs for indications of septic shock.
- Measure the patient's abdominal girth.
- Assess the patient for nausea, vomiting, and diarrhea.

**Interventions:**
- Provide pain management.
- Provide skin, oral, and perianal care for the patient.
- Provide support for the patient and the family.

### Expected Patient and Family Outcomes
- The patient and the family can identify the risk factors for typhlitis.
- The patient and the family seek early medical intervention for symptoms of severe abdominal pain, with or without fever.

## Spinal-Cord Compression

### Definition

*Spinal-cord compression* is a neurologic emergency that occurs in approximately 4%–5% of patients with malignancies, either at the time of initial diagnosis or at recurrence. In most cases it is usually not life threatening but can cause moderate-to-severe neurologic morbidity. Prompt assessment and intervention must be provided as needed to preserve neurologic function. Compression can occur as a result of tumor invasion of the vertebrae, resulting in collapse of the spinal cord or increased pressure in the spinal canal. Some primary tumors also can invade the spinal cord.

### Risk Factors

Risk factors are primary CNS tumor of the spinal cord, neuroblastoma, lymphoma, and metastatic sarcoma.

### Clinical Presentation

Patients may exhibit local, referred, or diffuse pain in the neck or back. Back pain occurs in 80% of children with compression. Other signs are motor deficits, including weakness, ataxia, hypotonic or hyporeflexic muscular reactions; paralysis; muscle atrophy; and sensory deficits, such as bowel or bladder dysfunction, paresthesia, loss of pain sensation, and loss of temperature sensation. Specific symptoms depend on the location and extent of tumor involvement.

### Medical Management

The patient should be given a diagnostic evaluation that includes a detailed neurologic examination and a magnetic resonance imaging or computed tomography scan of the spine or both. The underlying disease may be treated with high doses of glucocorticoids, which are administered to reduce the edema and pain; emergent radiation therapy to the primary or metastatic lesion, which results in a rapid decrease in the size of radiosensitive tumors; chemotherapy; and surgical decompression involving a laminectomy.

### Potential Complications

Complications are temporary or permanent sensory or motor changes or both, paralysis, muscle atrophy, a decrease in or loss of bowel or bladder function, and sexual impotence.

### Nursing Assessment and Interventions

**Assessment:**
- Perform a comprehensive assessment of the patient.
- Observe the patient for early signs and symptoms, such as neck or back pain, motor weakness, and loss of sensation.
- Perform frequent neurologic checks.
- Observe the patient for motor or sensory deficits.

**Interventions:**
- Help the patient with positioning and range of motion.
- Discuss with the patient safety issues related to altered mobility.
- Provide a regimen for skin care.
- Initiate consultation with a physical therapist and occupational therapist after the patient's condition has been stabilized.
- Educate the patient and the family about how to maintain the patient's independence within the limitations caused by the compression.
- Provide supportive care for the patient and the family.

### Expected Patient and Family Outcomes
- The patient and the family can identify the symptoms associated with spinal-cord compression and know the importance of seeking early medical intervention.
- The patient remains as independent as possible.
- The patient and the family participate in a rehabilitation program as indicated.
- The patient and the family use available community resources.

## Syndrome of Inappropriate Antidiuretic-Hormone Secretion

### Definition

The antidiuretic hormone acts on the distal renal tubules and collecting ducts to increase permeability, thus increasing water absorption. Excess production of antidiuretic hormone (ADH) from tumors that stimulate the posterior pituitary gland results in excessive water retention. The syndrome of inappropriate antidiuretic-hormone secretion (SIADH) is caused by a continuous release of ADH without a relationship to plasma osmolality. SIADH is associated with a decrease in urine output and an increase in weight without edema, leading to hyponatremia and water intoxication.

### Risk Factors

Risk factors may be related to disease or treatment. The most common malignancies associated with SIADH are central nervous system tumors, Hodgkin's disease, and non-Hodgkin's lymphoma. Infectious causes are primarily pulmonary fungal or bacterial infections. Medications such as steroids, narcotics, thiazide diuretics, anesthetic agents, cisplatin, cyclophosphamide, and vincristine have been linked with SIADH. In addition, overhydration with hypotonic solutions may be a causative factor.

## Clinical Presentation

The signs of early SIADH (i.e., serum Na+ less than 130 mEq/L) are thirst, anorexia, headache, muscle cramps, weakness, and lethargy.

The signs of midcourse SIADH (i.e., serum Na+ less than 125 mEq/L) are nausea, vomiting, hyporeflexia, and confusion.

The signs of late SIADH (i.e., serum Na+ less than 120 mEq/L) are seizures, coma, and death.

## Medical Management

The underlying disease must be treated. Management of symptoms includes following the patient's serum chemistries as well as urine Na+ and urine osmolality and restricting fluids for patients with serum Na+ greater than 125 mEq/l. Corrections occur slowly over 7–10 days. Hypertonic saline solution may be administered for severe SIADH (i.e., serum Na+ less than 120 mEq/L).

## Potential Complications

Complications can include weakness, fatigue, altered mental status, nausea and vomiting, diarrhea, abdominal cramping, thirst, oliguria, weight gain, myalgias, muscle cramping, progressive lethargy, coma, and seizures.

## Nursing Assessment and Interventions

**Assessment:**
- Determine whether the patient is at risk for SIADH.
- Perform a comprehensive physical assessment of the patient.
- Monitor strictly the patient's fluid intake and output.
- Monitor laboratory values.
- Weigh the patient daily.

**Interventions:**
- Ensure that the orders for fluid restriction are followed.
- Educate the patient and the family about the importance of fluid restriction.

## Expected Patient and Family Outcomes

- The patient and the family can identify the risk factors associated with SIADH.
- The patient and the family report the signs and symptoms of SIADH in a timely manner.
- The patient has minimal complications related to SIADH.

# Anaphylaxis

## Definition

*Anaphylaxis* is an immediate hypersensitivity reaction to a foreign protein that can occur within seconds or minutes after exposure. An anaphylactic reaction is potentially life threatening because it may result in respiratory or cardiac-system dysfunction or both. Generally, the more rapid the onset of a reaction, the more severe it will be.

## Risk Factors

Risk factors are IV administration of medications or chemotherapeutic agents, antibiotics (i.e., trimethoprim-sulfamethoxazole [Bactrim], penicillin [Pen-Vee-K], and amphotericin B [Fungizone]); blood-product infusions; intravenous immune globulin; chemotherapy agents (i.e., L-asparaginase [Elspar], etoposide [VP-16], teniposide [VM-26]); and radiologic contrast media.

## Clinical Presentation

Symptoms of anaphylaxis can range from small urticarial lesions (i.e., hives) to a systemic response.

Anaphylaxis manifests in the cutaneous system in the form of pruritis, erythema, urticaria, and angioedema; in the CNS by anxiety and agitation; in the respiratory system by hoarseness, coughing, sneezing, dyspnea, laryngeal edema, stridor, and cyanosis; in the cardiovascular system by tachycardia, hypotension, and decreased peripheral perfusion; and in the GI system by nausea, vomiting, and diarrhea.

## Medical Management

Test doses of high-risk medications should be administered to prevent anaphylaxis, and patients should be pretreated with diphenhydramine (Benadryl), hydrocortisone (Solu-Cortef), or both. Supportive management of anaphylactic reaction includes administration of epinephrine and oxygen as well as intubation when required. Patients should be observed for a minimum of 4 hours after a mild anaphylactic reaction. A more severe reaction may require hospitalization. Patients receiving PEG-asparaginase are at risk for delayed or prolonged reactions.

## Potential Complications

Patients can experience mild-to-moderate discomfort or respiratory arrest, or they can develop cardiorespiratory arrest that results in death.

## Nursing Assessment and Interventions

**Assessment:**
- Assess the patient's risk for anaphylaxis.
- Document in the patient's chart allergies and previous history of reactions.
- Ensure that an emergency cart and an oxygen delivery system are readily available.

**Interventions:**
- Educate the patient and the family about the potential risk of allergic reactions.
- Stop IV infusion as soon as symptoms appear.
- Maintain IV access.
- Evaluate the patency of the patient's airway and assess vital signs.
- Notify a physician immediately.
- Administer emergency drugs as ordered or per institutional protocol.
- Remain calm.
- Instruct the patient of appropriate actions to take if a suspected allergic reaction occurs at home.
- Inform patients about the risk of delayed reactions when given PEG-asparaginase.

## Expected Patient and Family Outcomes

- The patient and the family know the patient's allergy history.
- The patient and the family recognize the symptoms of anaphylaxis (i.e., itching, hives, difficulty breathing, anxiety, restlessness).
- The patient maintains a patent airway and has minimal complications from anaphylaxis.

# Bibliography

## Bone-Marrow Suppression
Walsh, T., Roilides, E., Groll, A., Gonzalez, C., & Pizzo, P. (2006). Infectious complications in pediatric cancer patients. In P. A. Pizzo & D. G. Poplack (Eds.), *Principles and practice of pediatric oncology* (5th ed., pp. 1269–1329). Philadelphia: Lippincott Williams & Wilkins.

## Central-Nervous-System Complications
Baillieux, H., De Smet, H. J., Lesage, G., Paquier, P., De Deyn, P. P., & Marien, P. (2006). Neurobehavioral alterations in an adolescent following posterior fossa tumor resection. *Cerebellum, 5*, 289–295.

Wilson, P. E., Oleszek, J. L., & Clayton, G. H. (2007). Pediatric spinal cord tumors and masses. *Journal of Spinal Cord Medicine, 30*, S15–S20.

Wolfe-Christensen, C., Mullins, L. L., Scott, J. G., & McNall-Knapp. R. (2007). Persistent psychosocial problems in children who develop posterior fossa syndrome after medulloblastoma resection. *Pediatric Blood and Cancer, 49*, 723–726.

## Ototoxicity
Huang, E., Teh, B. S., Strother, D. R., Davis, Q. G., Chiu, J. K., Lu, H. H., et al. (2002). Intensity-modulated radiation therapy for pediatric medulloblastoma: Early report on the reduction of ototoxicity. *International Journal of Radiation, Oncology, Biology, Physics, 52*, 599–605.

Knight, K. R., Kraemer, D. F., & Neuwelt, E. A. (2005). Ototoxicity in children receiving platinum chemotherapy: Underestimating a commonly occurring toxicity that may influence academic and social development. *Journal of Clinical Oncology, 23*(34), 8588–8596.

Kushner, B. H., Budnick, A., Kramer, K., Modak, S., & Cheung, N. K. (2006). Ototoxicity from high-dose use of platinum compounds in patients with neuroblastoma. *Cancer, 107*(2), 417–422.

Landier, W. (2004). Monitoring and management of ototoxicity. In A. J. Altman (Ed.), *Supportive care of children with cancer: Current therapy and guidelines from the Children's Oncology Group* (3rd ed., pp. 130–138). Baltimore: The Johns Hopkins University Press.

Landier, W., & Merchant, T. (2005). Adverse effects of cancer treatment on hearing. In C. L. Schwartz, W. L. Hobbie, L. S. Constine, & K. S. Ruccione (Eds.), *Survivors of childhood and adolescent cancer: A multidisciplinary approach* (2nd ed., pp. 109–123). Heidelberg, Germany: Springer-Verlag.

Punnett, A., Bliss, B., Dupuis, L., Abdolell, M., Doyle, J., & Sung, L. (2004). Ototoxicity following pediatric hematopoietic stem cell transplantation: A prospective cohort study. *Pediatric Blood and Cancer, 42*(7), 598–603.

## Endocrine Abnormalities
Brougham, M. F. H., Kelnar, C. J. H., & Wallace, W. H. B. (2002). The late endocrine effects of childhood cancer treatment. *Pediatric Rehabilitation, 5*(4), 191–201.

Brydøy, M., Fosså, S. D., Dahl, O., & Bjøro, T. (2007). Gonadal dysfunction and fertility problems in cancer survivors. *Acta Oncologica, 46*(4), 480–489.

Keene, N., Hobbie, W., & Ruccione, K. (2000). Hormone producing glands. In N. Keene, W. Hobbie, & K. Ruccione (Eds.), *Childhood cancer survivors: A practical guide to your future* (pp. 259–286). Sebastopol, CA: O'Reilly.

Kenney, L. B., Laufer, M. R., Grant, F. D., Grier, H., & Diller, L. (2001). High risk of infertility and long term gonadal damage in males treated with high dose cyclophosphamide for sarcoma during childhood. *Cancer, 91*, 613–621.

Oberfield, S. E., & Sklar, C. A. (2002). Endocrine sequelae in survivors of childhood cancer. *Adolescent Medicine, 13*(1), 161–169.

Perkins, J. L., Kunin-Batson, A. S., Youngren, N. M., Ness, K. K., Ulrich, K. J., Hansen, M. J., et al. (2007). Long-term follow-up of children who underwent hematopoietic cell transplant (HCT) for AML or ALL at less than 3 years of age. *Pediatric Blood Cancer, 49*(7), 958–963.

Thomson, A. B., Critchley, H. O. D., Kelnar, C. J. H., & Wallace, W. H. B. (2002). Late reproductive sequelae following treatment of childhood cancer and options for fertility preservation. *Best Practice and Research Clinical Endocrinology and Metabolism, 16*(2), 311–334.

Tournaye, H., Goossens, E., Verheyen, G., Fredericks, V., De Block, G., Devroey, P., et al. (2004). Preserving the reproductive potential of men and boys with cancer: Current concepts and future prospects. *Human Reproduction Update, 10*(6), 525–532.

Vadaparampil, S. T., Clayton, H., Quinn, G. P., King, L. M., Nieder, M., & Wilson, C. (2007). Pediatric oncology nurses' attitudes related to discussing fertility preservation with pediatric cancer patients and their families. *Journal of Pediatric Oncology Nursing, 24*(5), 255–263.

## Cardiac and Pulmonary Complications
Adamson, P. C., Balis, F. M., Berg, S., & Blaney, S. M. (2005). General principles of chemotherapy. In P. A. Pizzo & D. G. Poplack (Eds.), *Principles and practice of pediatric oncology* (5th ed., pp. 290–365). Philadelphia: Lippincott Williams & Wilkins.

Loerzel, V. W., & Dow, K. H. (2003). Cardiac toxicity related to cancer treatment. *Clinical Journal of Oncology Nursing, 7*, 557–562.

## Gastrointestinal Complications
Eilers, J., & Million, R. (2007). Prevention and management of oral mucositis in patients with cancer. *Seminars in Oncology Nursing, 23*, 201–212.

Riola, F., & Fatigoni, S. (2006). New antiemetic drugs. *Annals of Oncology, 17*, 96–100.

Schwarzberg, L. S. (2007). Chemotherapy-induced nausea and vomiting: Which antiemetic for which therapy? *Oncology, 21*, 946–953.

Smith, A. R., Repka, T. L., & Weigel, B. J. (2005). Aprepitant for the control of chemotherapy induced nausea and vomiting in adolescents. *Pediatric Blood and Cancer, 45*, 857–860.

## Renal and Bladder Complications
Kelly, K. M. (2003). Clinical emergencies in children with cancer. In M. A. Weiner & M. S. Cairo (Eds.), *Pediatric hematology/oncology secrets* (pp. 187–190). Philadelphia: Hanley & Belfus.

## Skin Changes
McNees, P. (2006). Skin and wound assessment and care in oncology. *Seminars in Oncology, 22*(3), 130–143.

McQuestion, M. (2006) Evidence-based skin care management in radiation therapy. *Seminars in Oncology, 22*(3), 163–173.

Viale, P. H. (2006). Chemotherapy and cutaneous toxicities: Implications for oncology nurses. *Seminars in Oncology Nursing, 22*(3), 144–151.

## Musculoskeletal Complications

Lewis, V. O. (2007). What's new in musculoskeletal oncology? *The Journal of Bone and Joint Surgery, 89,* 1399–1407.

Link, M., Gebhart, M., & Meyers, P. (2006). Osteosarcoma. In P. A. Pizzo & D. G. Poplack (Eds.), *Principles and practice of pediatric oncology* (5th ed., pp. 1074–1115). Philadelphia: Lippincott Williams & Wilkins.

Rodriguez-Merchan, E. C. (2003). Management of musculoskeletal complications of hemophilia. *Seminars in Thrombosis and Hemostasis, 29,* 87–95.

Suell, M. N., & Mueller, B. U. (2007). *Bone and joint complications in sickle cell disease.* Retrieved May 26, 2008, from www.uptodate.com.

## Nutritional Complications

Bechard, L., Adiv, O., Jaksic, T., & Duggan, C. (2006). Nutritional supportive care. In P. A. Pizzo & D. G. Poplack (Eds.), *Principles and practice of pediatric oncology* (5th ed., pp. 1330–1347). Philadelphia: Lippincott Williams & Wilkins.

Han-Markey, T. (2000). Nutritional considerations in pediatric oncology. *Seminars in Oncology Nursing, 16*(2), 146–151.

Jacob, E., Miaskowski, C., Savedra, M., Beyer, J., Treadwell, M., & Styles, L. (2006). Changes in sleep, food intake, and activity levels during acute painful episodes in children with sickle cell disease. *Journal of Pediatric Nursing, 21*(1), 23–34.

Nitenberg, G., & Raynard, B. (2000). Nutritional support of the cancer patient: Issues and dilemmas. *Critical Reviews in Oncology/Hematology, 34,* 137–168.

Rust, D., Simpson, J., & Lister, J. (2000). Nutritional issues in patients with severe neutropenia. *Seminars in Oncology Nursing, 16*(2), 152–162.

## Pain

Jacob, E. (2004). Neuropathic pain in children with cancer. *Journal of Pediatric Oncology Nursing, 21*(6), 350–357.

Jacob, E. (2007). Pain in children. In M. J. Hockenberry, D. Wilson, & M. L. Winkelstein (Eds.), *Wong's nursing care of infants and children* (8th ed., pp. 205–256). St. Louis: Mosby.

McMahon, S., & Koltzenburg, M. (2005). *Wall and Melzack's textbook of pain.* Philadelphia: Elsevier Health Sciences.

Melzack, R., & Wall, P. (2003). *Handbook of pain management: A clinical companion to the textbook of pain.* Philadelphia: Elsevier Health Sciences.

Renn, C. L., & Dorsey, S. G. (2005). The physiology and processing of pain: A review. *AACN Clinical Issues, 16*(3), 277–290.

Rosenow, J. M., & Henderson, J. M. (2003). Anatomy and physiology of chronic pain. *Neurosurgery Clinics of North America, 14*(3), 445–462.

Zempsky, W. T., Schechter, N. L., Altman, A. J., & Weisman, S. J. (2004). The management of pain. In A. J. Altman (Ed.), *Supportive care of children with cancer* (3rd ed., pp. 200–220). Baltimore: The Johns Hopkins University Press.

## Oncologic Emergencies

Cairo, M., & Bishop, M. (2004). Review of tumor lysis syndrome (TLS): New treatment strategies and proposed classification. *British Journal of Haematology, 127,* 3–11.

Reingold, S. R., & Lange, B. J. (2005). Oncologic emergencies. In P. A. Pizzo & D. G. Poplack (Eds.), *Principles and practice of pediatric oncology* (5th ed., pp. 1202–1230). Philadelphia: Lippincott Williams & Wilkins.

Secola, R., Cairo, M., Militano, O., & Bergeron, S. (2006). *COG nursing clinical practice tumor lysis syndrome guidelines.* Retrieved May 26, 2008, from www.childrensoncologygroup.org.

# Section VI  Supportive Care

Cheryl Rodgers

## Section Outline

Psychological Preparation and Support for Painful Procedures

Sedation for Painful Procedures

Central Venous Access Devices

Nutritional Support

Treatment of Infections

Blood Product Support

Bibliography

# Psychological Preparation and Support for Painful Procedures

*Catherine Fiona Macpherson*

## Principles of Treatment
Psychological preparation and support for painful procedures can decrease children's distress, which helps them cope more effectively. Developing strategies for managing a painful procedure creates a foundation for effective coping with future painful procedures.

## Role of Treatment
Painful procedures occur frequently during the treatment of cancer and can also occur during the treatment of hematologic diseases, requiring caregivers to help children cope effectively.

## Types of Preparation
(See **Table 6-1** for detailed guidelines.)
- Provide developmentally appropriate information regarding the procedure.
- Teach developmentally appropriate coping strategies to be used during the procedure.
- Use medical play as developmentally appropriate, and involve a child-life specialist or another psychosocial support professional.
- Provide information to family members if they want to participate in preparing the child for the procedure.

## Nursing Assessment and Interventions

### Assessment
**Prior to the preparation session:**
- Assess the child's chronological age and cognitive level.
- Ask the child and the family about the child's past procedure experiences, responses, use of coping strategies, and effectiveness of those strategies.
- Consider the potential influences of the child's personality and culture, as well as the family's feelings about the procedure.
- Determine the role the family wants to assume, such as being present during the procedure, coaching, or entering the room after the procedure. Support any role the family can assume.

**During the preparation session:**
- Assess the child's baseline understanding of the procedure, including any misconceptions, by asking the child how the procedure will be done, what he or she will feel, who will be present, where the procedure will take place, and how long it will last.
- Continue to assess the child's understanding during the preparation session. Ask questions in different ways to determine whether the child really understands and is not just repeating what he or she has been told, or ask the child to tell you what he or she would tell another child to prepare him or her for the procedure.

**After the procedure:**
- Assess the child's perception of the procedure.
- Assess with the child the effectiveness of his or her coping strategies.
- Reassess the child's understanding of the procedure over time, even for a procedure frequently experienced, because the child's understanding, as well as his or her needs for preparation and support, may change.

### Interventions
- Choose an environment free of distractions.
- Choose the most appropriate time for preparation (the younger the child, the closer to the time of the procedure the preparation should be done).
- Prepare the child for all procedures, even those the staff considers routine and nonthreatening. Even when time does not allow for formal preparation, children still benefit from some type of preparation, either immediately before or during a procedure.
- Be aware that some children seek information while others avoid it; attempt to provide information but do not force it.
- Match preparation and support with the child's coping style.
- Present information in a developmentally appropriate manner.
- Tell the child why the procedure needs to be done to alleviate any misconceptions.
- Give the child information about the sequence of events and sensations to expect during the procedure to foster realistic expectations.
- Tell the child what he or she will be asked to do during the procedure.
- Explain how long the procedure will last, using a time frame with which the child is familiar, such as the length of a favorite TV show.
- Ensure that all information, including that regarding potential pain, is honest and accurate.
- Encourage the child to express his or her feelings and concerns about the procedure.
- Provide opportunities for hands-on learning by encouraging medical play.
- Be extremely cautious about language; avoid using words with double meanings, such as "shot" and "push."
- Choose words that convey a less frightening message, such as "gently slide the needle in" rather than "stick the needle in," or "warm" or "sting" rather than "burn."
- Use medical terms, but define them so the child can understand them.
- Teach coping strategies:
  - Explain the rationale for using coping strategies.
  - Provide suggested coping strategies for procedures; such as distraction, imagery, relaxation, and positive self-statements.
  - Encourage the use of a combination of cognitive and behavioral coping strategies for greater effect.
- Encourage the child to practice the strategies that have been chosen.
- Promote coping during the procedure:
  - Provide positive reinforcement during the procedure to enhance compliance and to help the child use coping strategies. Avoid saying "good girl" or "good boy," so that children do not equate compliance with being a good person; define the behavior that is being reinforced (e.g., "I really like the way you are holding so still.").

## Table 6-1. Developmental Considerations for Psychological Preparation and Support

| Stage | Developmental Characteristics | Concerns Related to Healthcare Experiences | Suggestions |
|---|---|---|---|
| Infant | Is in the sensorimotor stage<br>Is establishing a "self" versus others<br>Forms attachments to favorite toys<br>Attends to a variety of visual, auditory, and tactile stimuli | Separation anxiety (8–24 months)<br>Stranger anxiety | Include parents as often as possible.<br>Prepare parents for tests and procedures.<br>Encourage parents to support the child during the procedure.<br>Maintain the crib as a safe place where no procedures are performed. |
| Toddler | Engages in preoperational thinking<br>Is egocentric<br>Can understand only concepts that he or she has experienced<br>Mixes reality and fantasy<br>Has a limited concept of time<br>Has very little understanding of anatomy<br>Has limited verbal skills<br>Has limited self-expression skills<br>Believes in imminent justice | Pain as "punishment"<br>Fear of needles<br>Separation<br>Disruptive changes in familiar routines | Be truthful about pain.<br>Be honest.<br>Prepare the child for a procedure with tangible equipment and allow the child to manipulate safe equipment.<br>Use dolls for preparation, not the child's transitional object (favorite toy).<br>Provide simple explanations and information.<br>Reassure the child that he or she is not being punished.<br>Emphasize that there will be an end to the procedure.<br>Clarify any misconceptions created by the child's fantasies.<br>Provide only realistic choices.<br>Maintain the bed as a place that is safe from invasive procedures. |
| Preschool-Age Child | Is in the preoperational stage<br>Has better developed verbal skills than toddlers<br>Uses play for self-expression<br>Is egocentric<br>Is acquiring a sense of initiative<br>Engages in magical thinking<br>Uses and repeats words that he or she does not understand | Fear of needles<br>Magical thinking<br>Fear of a new environment<br>Fear of the unknown<br>Fear of loss of control and body mutilation (a fear of older preschoolers) | Encourage questions.<br>Address the child's fantasies.<br>Reassure the child that the procedure is not being done to blame or punish.<br>Use visual aids for teaching.<br>Allow the child to manipulate safe equipment.<br>Be honest.<br>Allow the child to "play out" events.<br>Maintain the bed as a place that is safe from invasive procedures. |
| Primary-School-Age Child | Is at the stage of concrete operations<br>Can think and reason logically but not abstractly<br>Has a good concept of time<br>Seeks autonomy and independence<br>Understands cause and effect | Loss of control<br>Bodily injury or mutilation<br>Fear of death<br>Fear of incompetency | Be honest.<br>Offer help so the child can work through feelings and establish coping strategies early.<br>Address the child's concerns about mutilation.<br>Allow for realistic choices.<br>Focus the child's preparation on sensory information and behavioral expectations.<br>Use pictures, body outlines, dolls, or models for preparation. |
| Adolescent | Is at the stage of formal operations<br>Thinks abstractly<br>Engages in some magical thinking<br>Is establishing his or her own identity<br>Considers socialization with peers important<br>Understands the body and bodily functions | Loss of control<br>Privacy<br>Loss of skills<br>Body image<br>Perception of peers<br>Loss of independence | Allow for choices.<br>Develop trust.<br>Stress the importance of compliance.<br>Promote peer contacts.<br>Include the adolescent in decision making.<br>Begin the preparation with reason, then use concrete details.<br>Maximize the adolescent's independence.<br>Respect the adolescent's privacy. |

- Give the child realistic choices (e.g., "Which arm should I use for the blood pressure cuff?") to provide him or her with some control.
- Give the child a role during the procedure, such as holding the gauze or adhesive bandage.
- Consider providing a small reward following the procedure.
- Encourage family presence during the procedure and give a family member a role, such as coaching the child in use of the chosen coping strategies.
• Avoid using the child's bed for invasive procedures whenever possible to maintain the bed as a place of safety and security for the child.
• Consider using pharmacologic interventions in combination with psychological preparation and support for painful procedures.

## Expected Patient and Family Outcomes
• The child has a developmentally appropriate understanding of the procedure.
• The child has coping strategies to employ during the procedure.
• The child copes effectively during the procedure.

# Sedation for Painful Procedures

*Catherine Fiona Macpherson*

## Principles of Treatment
Sedation levels range from minimal to moderate (i.e., conscious sedation), to deep, and to general anesthesia. The level of sedation required for a procedure depends on the nature of the procedure. Noninvasive, nonpainful procedures, which require only the child's cooperation and immobilization, may be accomplished with minimal sedation. However, invasive and significantly painful procedures that require the child's cooperation and immobilization necessitate at least moderate sedation. See **Table 6-2** for definitions of levels of sedation.

## Role of Treatment
Procedural pain is often identified as the most distressing aspect of the cancer experience for the child and the family. It is reasonable to assume that procedural pain is also a significant source of distress for children with hematologic diseases who undergo painful procedures. The use of moderate sedation may reduce the pain and distress that children associate with invasive and significantly painful procedures, such as bone-marrow aspirations, and may also prevent children from developing negative expectations about their repeated exposure to these procedures during treatment.

## Drugs
Safe and effective sedation depends on (a) selecting the most appropriate drug for the nature of the procedure, (b) using the lowest effective drug dose, and (c) using the fewest number of drugs necessary. A combination of an analgesic and a sedative (with potential anxiolytic and amnestic effects) is recommended for painful procedures. Knowledge of each drug's onset, peak, and duration of action is necessary. Each drug should be titrated to effect. Intravenous administration of drugs, rather than oral, intranasal, or intramuscular administration, may provide more predictable and rapid onset, shorter duration of action, and more precise titration to effect.

### Table 6-2. Definition of Sedation Levels

| Level of Sedation | Definition |
|---|---|
| Minimal | "A drug-induced state during which patients respond normally to verbal commands; although cognitive function and coordination may be impaired, ventilatory and cardiovascular functions are unaffected."* |
| Moderate | "A drug-induced depression of consciousness during which patients respond purposefully to verbal commands, either alone or accompanied by light tactile stimulation... No intervention is required to maintain a patent airway and spontaneous ventilation is adequate. Cardiovascular function is usually maintained."* |
| Deep | "A drug-induced depression of consciousness during which patients cannot be easily aroused but respond purposefully after repeated verbal or painful stimulation... Patients may require assistance in maintaining a patent airway, and spontaneous ventilation may be inadequate. Cardiovascular function is usually maintained... deep sedation may be accompanied by partial or complete loss of protective airway reflexes."* |

*(Cote, Wilson, & Work Group on Sedation, 2006, p.2589)

## Potential Complications
Sedation occurs on a continuum and children often pass from the intended level to a deeper level. Therefore, it is essential that healthcare professionals involved in the sedation of children are able to rescue the child from a level of sedation deeper than that intended for the procedure. The ability to rescue requires both the ability to recognize the level of sedation and the ability to provide cardiopulmonary support. Continuous monitoring and observation by a healthcare professional not involved in performing the procedure provides for rapid and accurate identification of complications and initiation of rescue interventions. The risks of sedation may be minimized by consideration of underlying medical conditions that may interact with the sedation process. The most common serious complications of sedation are airway compromise and respiratory depression (resulting in airway obstruction), hypoventilation, hypoxemia, and apnea. Hypotension and cardiopulmonary arrest may result from failure to recognize and treat respiratory complications. Although rare, seizures and allergic reactions are also possible. Children younger than 6 years of age and those with developmental delays may require more sedation to achieve cooperation and immobilization. Unfortunately, these children are particularly vulnerable to the effects of sedation medications on respiratory drive, airway patency, and protective reflexes. Most sedation complications can be effectively managed by repositioning the child to open the airway, stimulating the child to breathe, administering supplemental oxygen, using suction, providing bag-mask ventilation, and administering reversal agents for the drugs.

## Nursing Assessment and Interventions

The American Academy of Pediatrics (AAP) has established guidelines for monitoring pediatric patients during and after sedation for procedures. These guidelines apply to all providers in all settings. Individual institutions may develop specific sedation protocols for institutional use based on these guidelines. The AAP guidelines (Cote, Wilson, & Work Group on Sedation, 2006) include detailed descriptions of (a) how to identify safe candidates for minimal, moderate, and deep sedation; (b) the role of a responsible adult caregiver in accompanying the child to and from outpatient sedation; (c) the facilities, personnel, age- and size-appropriate equipment, and drugs necessary for monitoring and rescuing the sedated patient; (d) recommendations for fasting from food and liquids prior to sedation; and (e) guidelines for documentation before, during, and after sedation.

General monitoring guidelines include continuous monitoring of oxygen saturation and heart rate and intermittent monitoring of respiratory rate, blood pressure, and head position for airway patency during the procedure and until the child has fully recovered from sedation.

General recovery parameters include satisfactory and stable airway patency, oxygen saturation, and cardiovascular function; intact protective reflexes; and return of the child to his or her baseline level of consciousness. A child who receives reversal agents (e.g., naloxone, flumezenil) requires longer monitoring after sedation, as the duration of the reversal agent may be shorter than that of the drugs used for sedation, which can result in resedation.

## Expected Patient and Family Outcomes

- The child experiences minimal pain and distress related to the procedure.
- The child receives effective sedation with no complications.

### Reference

Cote, C. J., Wilson, S., and Work Group on Sedation. (2006). Guidelines for monitoring and management of pediatric patients during and after sedation for diagnostic and therapeutic procedures: An update. *Pediatrics, 118,* 2587–2602.

# Central Venous Access Devices

*Joetta D. Wallace*

## Principles of Treatment

Intravenous (IV) access is needed when caring for children with cancer and serious blood diseases. The need to frequently obtain blood samples and administer chemotherapy, iron chelating products, supportive medications, fluids, and blood products necessitates readily available access.

## Role of Treatment

Central venous access devices (CVADs) minimize the need for venipunctures, thereby reducing patient discomfort. These devices minimize the emotional trauma associated with venipuncture and the placement of peripheral IV lines. Veins that are used frequently for administering chemotherapy are prone to scarring; thus, CVADs provide a safe administration route for vesicant chemotherapy. Placement of a CVAD before beginning treatment, regardless of white blood cell count, has been found to be safe. Most centers attempt to place the CVAD as soon after the diagnosis as possible, rather than waiting until peripheral sites can no longer be accessed. A recent study by Tremolada et al. (2005) has shown that the number of days from the CVAD placement significantly affects how a child copes and also predicts the child's quality of life, which also predicts parental trust in the medical care.

## Types of CVADs

The two main types of CVADs are external catheters and implanted subcutaneous ports. Each type has advantages and disadvantages; and matching the right CVAD to each patient requires a multidisciplinary approach that includes the physician, nurse, surgeon, child-life specialist, and family. Careful consideration must be given to the child's age, the treatment planned, limitations on bathing and activity, ability of the family to participate in care of the device, geographical location, skill of healthcare providers near the family's home, and insurance reimbursement for supplies.

### Tunneled External Devices—Broviac, Hickman, Groshong, and Permcath

These external central venous catheters (See **Figure 6-1** for Hickman) are surgically placed with cutdown or percutaneous technique, threaded internally into a major blood vessel, and advanced until the tip reaches the junction of the superior vena cava (SVC) and right atrium. The catheter is tunneled from the entrance site through subcutaneous tissue or fascia and brought out through the skin (i.e., the exit site) on the chest. A Dacron cuff is located on the outside of the catheter and positioned halfway between the insertion site and exit site. The cuff encourages fibrous tissue adherence, helps to secure the catheter to the site, and decreases the risk of bacteria entering central circulation. The catheter can be viewed on an X ray or fluoroscope because it is radiopaque.

### Groshong

The Groshong (**Figure 6-2**) central venous catheter does not require routine heparinization. Its advantage is that it has a small self-sealing end that can be flushed with normal saline (NS). The manufacturer recommends flushing with heparin twice per month. Some centers have reported valve failure in its small-lumen catheters.

### Permcath

This CVAD is similar to a Vascath or Quinton catheter or a Powercath and is routinely used for dialysis. Because of its rigid wall construction, it can withstand pressure from an apheresis machine, making it appropriate for patients undergoing stem-cell collection in preparation for a peripheral blood stem-cell transplant. It is placed by a surgical technique similar to that used when placing Hickman and Broviac catheters. A disadvantage is the difficulty in securing the device due to its lack of flexibility under a dressing. Because of the stiff nature of the tubing, there is a relatively increased risk of breakage that cannot be repaired.

## Nontunneled External Devices—Peripherally Inserted Central Catheter

A peripherally inserted central catheter (PICC) is a threadlike, flexible device that is placed peripherally through a basilic or median cubital vein and advanced to the SVC. It is usually not tunneled under the skin but is placed directly into the vein like a venipuncture. Its advantage is that it can be placed outside of the operating room by nurses trained in its placement. It can provide an economical and safe method of IV access for short and intermediate use. Also, there are reports of successful long-term (i.e., longer than 60 days) use of these devices.

There are both advantages and disadvantages of using catheters.

**Advantages:**
- They are available as single-lumen or multiple-lumen catheters. Multiple-lumen catheters are recommended for patients on aggressive regimens who may require simultaneous supportive therapies, such as parenteral nutrition, blood products, and antibiotics.
- Access is accomplished without a needle stick. Needleless supplies are now routinely available.
- Immediate use is available after placement.
- Repairs for most line breaks are possible with special kits and trained personnel.
- Removal can be done in an outpatient setting with local anesthetic.

**Disadvantages:**
- Daily flushing with NS or heparin is required. Routine dressing changes and cap changes must be performed by the family. These skills must be taught and reinforced.
- Dressing changes involve a moderate amount of tape, the removal of which can be as traumatic as a needle stick for some children.
- Placement by a surgeon is required.
- Some centers restrict activities such as swimming and contact sports.
- There may be an impact on the child's body image because the device is visible.
- Accidental dislodgement is a frequent concern, especially in infants and toddlers.
- There is an increased risk of infections and complications with multiple-lumen devices.
- Some third-party payers do not cover the disposable medical supplies that are needed, such as the dressing, tape, etc. This expense must be borne by the family and can be prohibitive.

## Implanted Venous Access Device or Port

These are surgically implanted central catheters whose placement is similar to that of an external central venous line. The implanted venous access device (IVAD) connects to a port that has a self-sealing silicone septum encased in titanium and attached to tubing (**Figure 6-3**). The tubing is threaded into the SVC to the junction of the SVC/renal artery, in the same way as the external devices, but instead of exiting the skin, the port portion is secured in a subcutaneous pocket on the patient's upper chest or abdomen. The IVAD is accessed with a special noncoring Huber needle, which is attached to tubing. This needle can be secured and left in place for up to a week before a needle change is needed. As with external devices, there are advantages and disadvantages with IVADs.

**Figure 6-1. Hickman® Dual-Lumen Catheter**

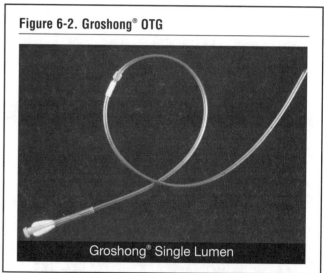

*Courtesy of Bard Access Systems*

**Figure 6-2. Groshong® OTG**

*Courtesy of Bard Access Systems*

**Figure 6-3. Catheter with a Titanium Port**

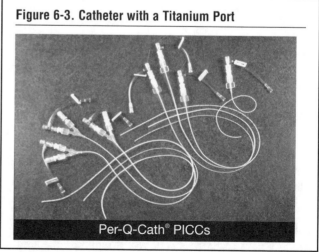

*Courtesy of Bard Access Systems*

**Advantages:**
- IVADs are especially useful when therapy is needed only intermittently, as in monthly red blood cell transfusions for patients with sickle-cell disease who are on chronic transfusion protocols, patients with hemophilia who are on prophylaxis programs, or patients with cancer who are receiving chemotherapy only every 2–4 weeks.
- No home supplies are required and no home maintenance is needed other than routine observation for signs of infection, because IVADs are implanted completely under the skin.
- They may be accessed for up to a week as needed.
- Routine flushing with heparin is required only once a month or after the device is accessed for blood draws or infusions.
- They are much less visible on children, possibly resulting in less impact on body image.
- Fewer infections and complications are reported with IVADs.

**Disadvantages:**
- Accessing a port requires a needle stick. This discomfort can be minimized with the use of an anesthetic cream or spray, but for some children, anxiety about the needle can be considerable. Child-life specialists are especially helpful in preventing and alleviating this concern.
- Special skill is required to access an IVAD. Nurses, and families if indicated, must learn the sterile technique. If the child lives in a rural location, the special needles required and personnel trained in IVAD access may not be readily available.
- Removal requires surgery and general anesthesia.
- Scarring and keloid formation from repeated port accesses may be more prominent.

## Potential Complications Associated with CVADs

### Infection
Infection associated with the device is the most common problem with CVADs. The incidence is between 2% and 60%, depending on the study, device, and patient characteristics. The signs and symptoms of an infection must be readily recognized and treated aggressively with appropriate antibiotics. Infection can occur inside the device, at the exit site, or in the tunnel or pocket surrounding the CVAD. Many infections can be cleared and catheters salvaged, but persistent or recurrent infections necessitate removal of the line and replacement only after eradication of the infection has been documented. Every effort to preserve the CVAD should be undertaken, especially in children for whom venous access will be required for most of their lives, such as patients with hemophilia, thalassemia, or sickle-cell anemia.

### Occlusion
Occlusion is the second most common complication associated with CVADs. The ease with which the CVAD can be flushed depends on whether the occlusion is partial or complete. Occlusions can be caused by a thrombus in the line or at the end of the catheter; by the fibrin sheath around the catheter tip, which allows fluids to flow through the CVAD but inhibits blood withdrawal; or by precipitate caused by the administration of medications with incompatible fluids. Elimination of the occlusion to restore function to the device may be accomplished with fibrinolytic (e.g., t-PA, alteplase) and non-thrombolytic (e.g., ethanol, sodium bicarbonate) agents.

### Malposition
A malposition can be caused by the CVAD being pulled on, migration of the catheter, or improper placement of the catheter. Indications that the catheter is not correctly placed include inability to withdraw blood or flush the line, patient's complaint of pain when the device is flushed, and swelling or discoloration along the tubing or port. Use of the CVAD must be suspended until the correct location can be ensured. Sometimes it is necessary to replace the CVAD.

### Break in the CVAD
An external break can result in blood loss, an air embolism, or sepsis. An internal break can cause infiltration or extravasation of a medication, or the patient may experience edema at the site or chest pain when the CVAD is flushed. External breaks can sometimes be repaired, whereas internal breaks require replacement of the line.

## Nursing Assessment and Interventions

### Assessment
- Participate in determining which CVAD is best for the patient by considering the family's ability to manage a catheter, the patient's body image, and the treatment plan.
- Assess what the patient and the family know about the device and the care they will be expected to deliver.
- Assess the exit site for signs of infection (e.g., erythema, tenderness, swelling, drainage, foul odor).
- Evaluate the CVAD for patency (i.e., it flushes without resistance or discomfort and has positive blood return).
- Observe the patient for facial swelling, distension of the neck vein, tachycardia, and shortness of breath, all of which could indicate SVC thrombosis.
- Ensure that the device is properly secured. To prevent dislodgment, an external catheter should be coiled under the dressing, and the IV tubing connected to the CVAD should be taped and pinned to the patient's clothing.
- Evaluate the integrity of the venous access device (i.e., monitor for kinking or twisting or leaking of fluid or blood).
- Ensure that the port needle is correctly placed to prevent infiltration or extravasation when vesicant chemotherapy is infused.
- Assess the CVAD dressing. Is it intact? When was it last changed?
- Evaluate the injection caps at the end of the line. Are they intact? Is there any leaking? Is there residual blood in the cap? When were the caps last changed?

### Interventions
Care of the CVAD is one of the most controversial management issues in pediatric oncology. No national standards exist, but there are a multitude of institutional practices. Manufacturers of CVAD products can also provide guidelines for care. The following interventions are examples of guidelines for CVAD care:
- Flush the lines with heparin regularly, according to institutional guidelines.

- Broviac and Hickman catheters—Catheter flushes range from 10 to 100 units/ml of heparin, using 3–5 ml per flush, one to three times a day. It is important to exert positive pressure with the flush as it completes to help decrease the potential for clot formation at the tip of the catheter.
- Groshong catheter—This type of catheter does not require daily heparin flushes and can be flushed routinely with saline. However, the manufacturer recommends heparin flushes at least twice a month.
- Permcath—Institutions use 100 or 1,000 units of heparin as a flush. When using 1,000 units, the clinician should withdraw the heparin from the line before flushing or administering medications so that the patient does not develop a systemic effect from the heparin. The line should be flushed by using a positive-pressure technique.
- Ports—To flush the device, use 10–100 units of heparin. If a port is to be deaccessed, 5 ml of 100 units/ml of heparin often is used. Ports can be deaccessed for a month.

- Site care should be provided according to institutional policy or as determined from a patient assessment.

  One method of site care is to clean the site with 2% aqueous chlorhexidine (Chloroprep) and let it dry. A chlorhexidine-impregnated patch (Biopatch) can be placed at the exit site and covered with an occlusive dressing (e.g., Tegaderm, Bioclusive, Opsite). The tubing is coiled off the exit site and taped separately to provide slack from the site if the tubing is accidentally pulled. Dressings are changed when wet or soiled and regularly up to once a week. Injection caps at the end of the lumens are changed using an aseptic technique according to the institution's policy (caps usually are replaced weekly). Injection caps that leak or that retain blood after a blood draw can become infected and should be changed promptly.
- External breaks—Using a kit provided by the manufacturer, a repair in a central venous line can be made with sterile technique and according to institutional policy. Until the repair is made, clamp the line that is distal to the break and cover the end with sterile gauze to prevent an air embolism, excessive blood loss, or further contamination.
- Assess for internal breaks and occlusions—Signs of an internal displacement or a break can include a patient's complaint of chest or head discomfort, swelling around the exit site, or an inability to flush the CVAD or to aspirate blood. It is important to make a prompt evaluation using a chest X ray or cathetergram (dye study) or both. Signs of extravasation are erythema near the exit site or a patient's complaints of a burning sensation or pain in the chest or abdomen when a vesicant or irritant chemotherapy is infused through the CVAD. In this case, the chemotherapy infusion should be stopped immediately and as much of the vesicant as possible should be aspirated from the CVAD. If an antidote for the extravasated chemotherapy is recommended, it should be administered into the surrounding tissue (see Section IV, "Childhood Cancer Treatment"). A plastic surgeon may need to be contacted to debride the wound.
- CVAD occlusions—For blood-clot and fibrin-sheath occlusions, a fibrinolytic agent, such as 1 mg/1 ml of Alteplase, may be instilled into the line and allowed to dwell for 1 hour. If the patency of the catheter is not resolved, a chest X ray or cathetergram should be done to document the clot. Based on the cathetergram results, a second dose of a fibrinolytic agent may be instilled.
  - Occlusions occasionally result from precipitate (i.e., from medications or parenteral nutrition) in a CVAD. For a mineral precipitate, 0.2–1 ml of 0.1% hydrochloric acid (equal to the internal volume of the device) should be instilled and allowed to stand for 20 minutes to 1 hour. Many drugs are incompatible with heparin. For a medication precipitate, 1 mEq/ml of sodium bicarbonate should be instilled. For a lipid precipitate, 70%–95% ethyl alcohol or sodium hydroxide should be instilled. Many institutions use protocols with algorithms to manage occluded lines or lines that flush but do not have a blood return (**Figure 6-4**).
- Teach the patient and family about the care of a CVAD, the risks (i.e., infection, occlusion, displacement), and troubleshooting. This instruction must be started before the line is placed and completed before discharge. Reinforcement of instruction throughout hospitalization and with each readmission is indicated. The patient, the family, or both must demonstrate the ability to provide competent catheter care. Ongoing education and evaluation are important whenever the patient returns to the hospital or clinic. Involvement of a child-life specialist in preparing the child for surgery as well as for the CVAD itself is beneficial.
- Inform the patient that the external device must be covered with an occlusive dressing while he or she showers and that the dressing must be changed after showering. Many institutions recommend that patients with external devices do not go swimming because of the risk of infection.
- Communicate with the appropriate home-health agency (if necessary) about providing the patient with home supplies for line care and possible follow-up at his or her home.

## Expected Patient and Family Outcomes

- The patient and the family can competently perform line care (i.e., flushing, cap changes, dressing changes).
- The patient and the family understand the increased risk of infection with a CVAD, a port, or a PICC line, and they understand why competent care of the line is essential. They recognize signs and symptoms of infection in the line, at the exit site, or along the tunnel.
- The family should demonstrate or explain the steps to take if the line breaks or becomes dislodged.
- The risks associated with having a CVAD are minimized as a result of proper care and prevention strategies.

**Reference**

Tremolada, M., Axia, V., Pillon, M., Scrimin, S., Capello, F., & Zanesco, L. (2005). Parental narratives of quality of life in children with leukemia as associated with the placement of a central venous catheter. *Journal of Pain and Symptom Management, 30*(6), 544–552.

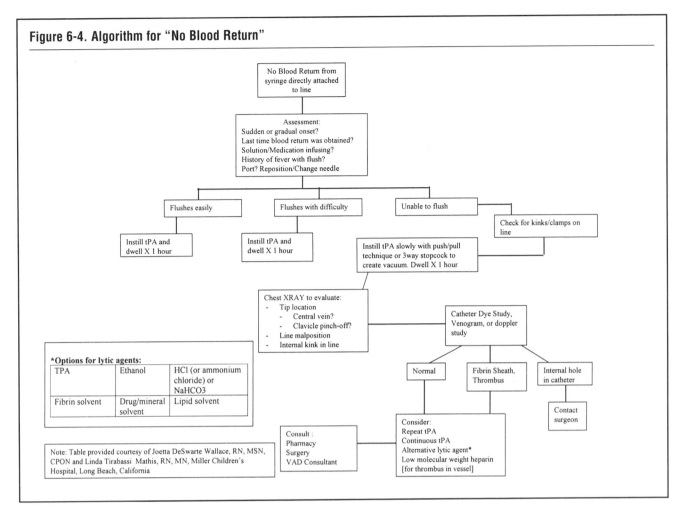

Figure 6-4. Algorithm for "No Blood Return"

## Nutritional Support

*Cheryl Rodgers and Sara Gonzalez*

### Principles of Treatment

The goals of nutritional support for oncology and hematology patients include preserving nutritional status or reversing nutritional deficiencies, preserving lean body mass, minimizing nutrition-related side effects, and maximizing the patient's quality of life. Nurses play an important role in anticipating potential risk factors, assessing and identifying symptoms, and initiating appropriate interventions promptly.

### Nutritional Needs

Several methods are available for estimating energy requirements in children, including the recommended dietary allowance, estimated energy requirement, and dietary reference intakes. However, these estimates were developed as recommendations for healthy populations, so they may not accurately predict the needs of sick children. A child's protein and caloric needs typically increase during illness because of physiological stress and increased catabolism from additional energy and protein requirements needed for tissue healing. The resting energy expenditure (REE), developed by the World Health Organization (WHO), can be useful for calculating the daily caloric needs of children. REE can be defined as the amount of energy required to maintain normal homeostatic function during periods of rest. The estimates of REE for different age groups, along with appropriate activity and stress factors (**Table 6-3**), are useful for accurately determining energy requirements for acutely ill patients. Energy and protein requirements may be increased by 15% to 50% to compensate for patients' previous weight losses, malnutrition, or metabolic changes.

### Nutritional Assessment

Nutritional status should be assessed at the time of diagnosis and regularly throughout therapy to identify patients at nutritional risk, determine the causes of poor oral intake or malnutrition, assess the efficacy of nutritional support, and identify patients who may benefit from dietary counseling from a registered dietitian. The current literature reflects controversy regarding the most accurate methods of conducting a nutritional assessment. However, assessments can be useful if they are obtained consistently over time, rather than only comparing single measurements with age-specific norms.

### History

Obtaining a patient's history is one of the most important methods for acquiring information during a nutritional assessment. Nutritional history should include recent changes in diet; past and current appetite levels; food allergies or intolerances; typical food-preparation methods; use of vitamins, herbs, or other dietary supplements; recent weight changes; bowel history; and

> **Table 6-3. Estimating Daily Calorie Needs in Children 1 Year of Age or Older**
>
> For children 1 year of age or older, compute the estimated resting energy expenditure (REE) based on the World Health Organization (WHO) equations below.
> *W = body weight in kilograms.*
>
> | Age Range (Years) | Male | Female |
> |---|---|---|
> | 1–3 | 60.9 W − 54 | 61 W − 51 |
> | 3–10 | 22.7 W + 495 | 22.5 W + 499 |
> | 10–18 | 17.5 W + 651 | 12.2 W + 746 |
> | 18–30 | 15.3 W + 679 | 14.7 W + 496 |
>
> REE = _____
>
> Next, multiply REE by an activity/stress factor.
>
> (REE) × (1.3) for a well-nourished child at bed rest with mild to moderate stress (mild surgery)
>
> (REE) × (1.5) for a very active child with mild to moderate stress, an inactive child with severe stress (trauma, sepsis, cancer, extensive surgery), or a child with minimal activity requiring catch-up growth
>
> (REE) × (1.7) for an active child requiring catch-up growth or an active child with severe stress
>
> From *Energy and Protein Requirements* (FAO/WHO/ UNV Expert Consultation Technical Report Series 724); (p. 71), by the World Health Organization (WHO), 1985, Geneva, Switzerland: Author. Copyright 1985 by WHO. Adapted with permission.

past and current gastrointestinal (GI) symptoms. A food record can be helpful for assessing current nutritional intake; however, a 24-hour diet recall usually does not accurately represent a patient's intake because under- and overreporting of food consumption are common. Instead, a prospective food diary, in which patients or family members record all oral intake for 3 to 7 days, is a more reliable method for obtaining valid information. To ensure proper interpretation, a registered dietitian should perform the analysis of the food diary.

### Physical Examination
Findings from a physical examination can help to identify nutrition-related problems. Examination of a patient's mouth and throat can lead to the discovery of mucositis and/or esophagitis, either of which can have a significant impact on a patient's willingness and ability to eat. Observation is a useful tool for identifying changes in body composition. Although obesity and wasting may be easy to identify, other, more subtle characteristics of the patient's nutritional status, such as edema, dehydration, and poor fat or muscle mass, can be noted during examination. Micronutrient deficiencies can cause subtle changes in the appearance of a patient's skin, eyes, lips, tongue, nails, and hair.

### Anthropometric Measurements
Weight and length/height measurements taken over time are important components of nutritional monitoring and provide a great deal of information for the least amount of inconvenience and cost. Weight changes can be an indicator of an acute change in energy stores, although weight can fluctuate significantly depending on the patient's hydration status. Length should be measured for infants and toddlers who are unable to stand, whereas height can be measured for children age 2 years and older who are able to stand. Length/height is a good indicator of chronic nutritional status but will not change as rapidly as weight, so it is not as helpful for assessing acute nutritional changes. Weight-for-height/length ratios reflect body weight in proportion to length/height, and ratios can be plotted on growth curves published by the National Center for Health Statistics for comparison with the general population. Weight-for-length growth curves should be used when length is obtained, and body mass index growth curves should be used when height is obtained. Monitoring trends in weight-for-height ratios can help distinguish stunted growth (i.e., chronic malnutrition) from wasting (i.e., acute malnutrition). Head circumference is a useful measurement until head growth slows at about 3 years of age. Midarm circumference (MAC) and skin-fold triceps readings (SFT) are quick, noninvasive measurements that enable muscle mass and body fat monitoring for children of all ages. Anthropometric measurements can vary tremendously based on the technique, the accuracy of the equipment, and the level of cooperation from the patient, all of which can affect the accuracy of the results. It is important to redo questionable measurements and remove any outlier readings when comparing results over time.

### Laboratory Measurements
Monitoring laboratory values is another method commonly used for assessing a patient's nutritional status. Serum protein markers such as albumin, prealbumin (also called transthyretin), transferrin, and retinol-binding protein can be used to evaluate the patient's nutritional status. Protein markers with shorter half-lives, retinol-binding protein, and prealbumin are better indicators of recent diet changes and current protein status. However, many factors, including common hematologic and oncologic complications, such as kidney or liver dysfunction, presence of infection or inflammation, hydration status, and the use of corticosteroids, can affect laboratory values. Such factors should be taken into account when using protein markers for assessment of nutritional status. In addition, it is important to evaluate triglyceride and cholesterol levels as part of a complete nutritional assessment. Assessment of other chemistry levels—including blood and urine sodium, potassium, chloride, bicarbonate, glucose, calcium, phosphorus, and magnesium; kidney function tests, such as creatinine and blood urea nitrogen; and liver function tests, such as alkaline phosphatase, alanine aminotransferase, aspartate aminotransferase, g-glulamyltransferase, and bilirubin—are also important to measure in order to obtain a thorough nutritional assessment.

### Nutritional Interventions
The goal of nutritional intervention is to prevent or reverse malnutrition. Many types of nutritional interventions, from minor dietary alterations to more aggressive techniques such as nutritional support, can be implemented. Providers should attempt to use the least invasive method possible to meet the nutritional requirements of the patient. Patients and their families should be included in the discussion when determining a method of nutritional support, because their cooperation is essential to ensure compliance with the therapy.

## Symptomatic Relief

Patients often experience undesirable symptoms related to their hematologic or oncologic disease and treatment. Patients often refuse or are unable to eat when experiencing unpleasant symptoms such as pain, nausea, vomiting, or constipation. It is necessary to treat these symptoms to help increase the patient's desire and ability to eat. **Table 6-4** lists nursing interventions that may help control common GI symptoms.

## Dietary Adaptation

Making modifications to a patient's diet can help increase his or her oral intake. Patients should avoid foods with unpleasant smells or tastes. Small, frequent meals are often better tolerated than large, heavy meals. A high-calorie, high-protein diet can help patients meet nutritional needs with smaller quantities of food. High-calorie condiments, such as butter or cheese, can be added to food to increase the patient's caloric intake and may increase the food's flavor. Patients with cancer often desire sweet and salty foods because of taste changes caused by chemotherapy, and intake of these foods should be encouraged as tolerated.

## Oral Supplementation

Often dietary changes alone are inadequate to meet patients' nutritional needs. In such instances, high-calorie, high-protein oral supplements may help to provide additional calories and protein without significantly increasing the volume that needs to be consumed. Oral supplements vary according to protein, lactose, fat, mineral, gluten, and fiber content and come in a variety of forms, including liquid, powder, or bar (See **Table 6-5**).

## Appetite-Stimulant Medications

Although the exact mechanism of action involved in appetite stimulation is not completely understood, several medications, such as cyproheptadine, megestrol acetate, and dronabinol, may be prescribed in an attempt to increase a patient's appetite. Cyproheptadine is a 5-HT2 receptor antagonist that affects the appetite center of the hypothalamus to stimulate appetite. Megestrol acetate is a synthetic progesterone whose precise mechanism with respect to appetite is unknown; however, it causes many patients to experience significant improvement in appetite. Dronabinol binds to cannabinoid receptors, which inhibit the release of neurotransmitters that cause nausea and vomiting and

### Table 6-4. Nursing Interventions for Common Gastrointestinal Symptoms

| Symptom | Intervention |
|---|---|
| **Anorexia/Early satiety** | Offer small, frequent meals and have snacks readily available<br>Drink minimally during meals<br>Offer high-calorie oral supplements<br>Provide a comfortable, relaxing environment while eating<br>Appetite stimulant medication may be indicated |
| **Nausea/Vomiting** | Provide small, frequent meals<br>Offer bland and cold foods (hot foods may make nausea worse)<br>Avoid foods that are fatty, fried, greasy, very sweet, spicy, or have strong odors<br>Do not force the patient to eat<br>Rest after meals<br>Encourage use of relaxation or distraction |
| **Dysgeusia (taste changes)** | Tart foods (e.g., oranges or lemonade) may taste better<br>Marinate meat in fruit juice, salad dressing, or sweet-and-sour sauce<br>Offer chicken, turkey, eggs, dairy, or fish for protein if beef tastes strange<br>Use herbs or seasonings to add flavor<br>Offer fluids with meals |
| **Mucositis** | Offer soft foods<br>Avoid foods and drinks that can irritate the mouth (e.g., citrus fruits; tomato products; spicy, salty, hot, rough, or dry foods)<br>Mix food with butter, gravy, or sauce to soften and make swallowing easier<br>Use a straw to drink liquids<br>Perform mouth care frequently |
| **Xerostomia (dry mouth)** | Drink fluids frequently<br>Sweet and tart foods can help saliva production<br>Suck on hard candy or popsicles or chew gum<br>Add sauce, gravy, or salad dressing to food |
| **Diarrhea** | Offer small, frequent meals<br>Avoid milk and milk products if lactose worsens the diarrhea<br>Avoid excessive juice consumption and greasy, fatty, fried, high-fiber foods if they worsen diarrhea<br>Drink large amounts of fluid to replenish fluid losses<br>Provide rectal skin care as indicated<br>Provide antidiarrhea medication if indicated |
| **Constipation** | Offer a high-fiber diet and drink large amounts of fluid; offer prune juice<br>Encourage physical activity (even just walking can help)<br>Laxative or stool softener may be needed |

### Table 6-5. Enteral Products for Infants and Children

#### Infant Formulas (birth–1 year)
*Human breast milk is ideal for infants and should be used whenever possible. If breast milk is unavailable or contraindicated, most infants tolerate standard formula. Infant formulas are generally 20 kcal/oz, but they can be concentrated up to 30 kcal/oz.*

| Standard | Premature | Soy* | Semi-Elemental* | Elemental* | Specialty |
|---|---|---|---|---|---|
| (Contain lactose & milk protein) | (Specially designed for premies) | (Contain soy instead of milk protein) | (For milk protein allergy or malabsorption) | (For severe allergies or malabsorption) | (For infants with specific needs or disease states) |
| Enfamil | Enfacare | Good Start | Alimentum | Elecare | Similac PM 60/40 |
| Good Start | NeoSure | Supreme Soy | Nutramigen | Neocate | Enfamil AR |
| Similac | | Isomil | Pregestimil | | Similac Lactose-Free* |
| | | Prosobee | | | |

#### Pediatric Formulas (1–10 years)

| Standard* | With Fiber* | Semi-Elemental* | Elemental* | Specialty* |
|---|---|---|---|---|
| Kindercal | Kindercal with fiber | Peptamen Jr | Elecare | Compleat Pediatric |
| Nutren Jr | Nutren Jr with fiber | Pepdite Jr | Neocate Jr | |
| PediaSure | PediaSure with fiber | Vital Jr | E028 Splash | |
| Resource Just for Kids | Resource Just for Kids with fiber | | Vivonex Pediatric | |

#### Adult Formulas (children 10 years and older)

| Standard | High Fiber* / High Calorie/High Protein* | Semi-Elemental* | Elemental* | Specialty* |
|---|---|---|---|---|
| Boost* | Boost with fiber | Peptamen | Reabilan | Compleat |
| Carnation Instant Breakfast | Boost Plus | Peptamen 1.5 | Tolerex | Nepro |
| Ensure* | Boost High Protein | Peptinex DT | Vivonex Plus | NutriHep |
| Nutren 1.0* | Ensure Plus | Vital HN | Vivonex TEN | Portagen |
| Osmolite* | Ensure with fiber | | | Pulmocare |
| Resource Fruit Beverage* | Jevity | | | Renalcal |
| | Nutren with fiber | | | Suplena |
| | Nutren 1.5 | | | |
| | Nutren 2.0 | | | |
| | Scandishake | | | |

#### Modular Additives
*Most modular additives can be added to formula (except for fats). Modulars can be helpful if the nutrient density needs to be increased without increasing volume significantly. Use caution with infants.*

| Carbohydrate* | Protein* | Fat* | Fiber* | Thickeners* | Human Milk Fortifiers |
|---|---|---|---|---|---|
| Polycose powder | Beneprotein | MCT Oil | Benefiber | Rice cereal | Enfamil HMF |
| Corn syrup | Casec | Microlipid | | Simply Thick | Similac HMF |
| Dextrose | Promod | Vegetable oil | | Thick-it | Similac Natural Care Advance |
| Cornstarch (not for infants <6 months) | | | | Thicken-up | |

#### Oral Rehydration Solutions* *(Often used to treat mild or moderate dehydration)*
Enfalyte, Liquilytes, Pedialyte, Rehydralyte

*Note.* Formulas can be consumed orally or through a tube feed. Semi-elemental or elemental formulas are used when standard formulas cannot be tolerated.
*Lactose-free formula for children who may become lactose intolerant.

---

can also improve the appetite. These medications can cause adverse side effects and, therefore, should be used cautiously.

### Artificial Nutrition
If a patient is unable to meet his or her nutritional needs orally, artificial nutrition, in the form of either enteral or parenteral nutritional support, is warranted. Unless oral feeding is contraindicated, patients and families should be advised that children receiving supplemental nutrition should be encouraged to eat.

### Enteral Nutrition
If oral feeding is inadequate for meeting nutritional needs, enteral nutrition should be considered. Unless contraindicated, enteral nutrition is generally the preferred method of nutritional support because it preserves GI integrity and prevents bacterial translocation of the gut; however, enteral nutrition requires that the patient's GI tract be intact to absorb nutrients. Nasogastric (NG) tubes can be placed for short-term use, while nasoduodenal and

nasojejunal tubes are generally used for longer periods or if NG feeds are not well tolerated. The type and size of the tube is based on the size of the child and viscosity of the formula. If enteral nutritional support is expected to continue for more than 4 weeks, a gastrostomy or jejunostomy tube is preferable. Complications related to gastrostomy or jejunostomy tubes can include cellulitis and other infections, despite good hygiene practices. Skin irritation and excoriation at the placement site can be reduced with appropriate use of topical or oral antibiotics.

Formula choice is based upon the patient's GI function and the nutrient composition of the formula. Unflavored products are usually better tolerated than flavored products because they have a lower osmolality. Two types of feeding schedules can be used: bolus (also called intermittent) feedings and continuous infusion. Bolus feeds are given intermittently throughout the day, are more similar to a normal feeding pattern, and are usually more convenient for the patient. Continuous feeds are administered as a steady infusion and can be cycled to allow the patient to eat during off-times. Many patients tolerate continuous feedings better than bolus feedings, particularly if they are nauseated. If a patient has had minimal oral intake for less than 3 days, full-strength formula at 1–2 cc/kg/hr may be started. Feedings may be increased by 1–2 cc/kg/hr per day, as tolerated, until the goal is achieved. If the patient has had minimal oral intake for more than 3 days, or if GI problems exist, half-strength formula at 1–2 cc/kg/hr can be started. The concentration should be advanced to full strength after 12–24 hours; the rate then should be increased by 1–2 cc/kg/hr per day to goal. If the patient's fluid needs are not met with oral intake and tube feeding, extra free water should be provided as flushes or added to the feedings. The tube should be flushed frequently with water before and after administration of all medications and daily to maintain patency. It may be necessary to administer some medications several hours before or after tube feeds to prevent drug-nutrient interactions.

### Total Parenteral Nutrition/Hyperalimentation

Parenteral nutrition is indicated when oral or enteral feedings, or a combination of both, are unable to meet a patient's nutritional needs. Total parenteral nutrition (TPN) can be used to meet 100% of the patient's nutritional needs without exacerbating GI symptoms and distress; however, parenteral nutrition requires close monitoring and frequent laboratory evaluations. TPN requires a central venous catheter, which is essential if parenteral nutrition is to be used for an extended period. Peripheral parenteral nutrition can be administered temporarily (i.e., less than 3 weeks) through a peripheral venous line to provide a nutrient solution containing 10% dextrose and 2% amino acids, but, to prevent vein damage, osmolality should not exceed 1,000 mOsm.

Parenteral nutrition can cause early satiety and decreased oral intake in patients. Cyclical feeds may be used to allow for greater oral intake during daytime hours. Other complications of TPN can include infections, hepatotoxicity, and metabolic abnormalities. Hypoglycemia can occur if TPN is suddenly discontinued; therefore, the rate should be decreased gradually when stopping the infusion. If hyperglycemia occurs, the dextrose concentration can be decreased or insulin can be administered.

## Nutritionally At-Risk Patients

Patients are identified as being at nutritional risk if they meet any of the following criteria:
- weight loss of 5% of pre-illness body weight
- weight-for-length or body mass index <10th percentile for age
- voluntary food intake of <70% of estimated requirements for 5 or more days
- anticipated gut dysfunction for more than 5 days.

Nutritionally at-risk patients typically require immediate nutritional support to correct their current or impending malnutrition. When treating a malnourished patient, it is important to consider the potential for refeeding syndrome. Refeeding syndrome creates acute, and often significant, electrolyte changes when enteral or parenteral nutritional support is initiated in malnourished patients. When the nutritional support is initiated, there is a sudden shift from fat to carbohydrate metabolism. This results in an increase in insulin secretion, which stimulates cellular uptake of phosphate, leading to profound hypophosphatemia that is often accompanied by hypokalemia and hypomagnesemia. This phenomenon usually occurs within 4 days of initiation of feeds and can result in multiple complications, including muscle weakness, immune dysfunction, cardiac failure, respiratory distress, and death. To prevent refeeding syndrome, artificial feedings should be initiated at a reduced caloric rate (i.e., 25%–50% of estimated requirements) and advanced slowly. In addition, serum electrolytes should be measured before starting feeds and repeated at least daily for 4 days after feeding is started. If refeeding syndrome occurs, nutrition support should be stopped immediately, and electrolyte imbalances should be corrected. After serum electrolytes have normalized, feeds can be restarted at a low rate.

## Expected Patient and Family Outcomes
- The patient undergoes thorough nutritional assessments throughout treatment.
- The patient receives appropriate nutritional supplementation throughout treatment.
- The patient and the family are knowledgeable about the nutritional options available during treatment.
- The patient has minimal complications associated with nutritional supplementation.

# Treatment of Infections

*Pat Wills Alcoser*

## Principles of Treatment

Chemotherapy and radiation for cancer therapy and hematopoietic stem-cell transplantation (HSCT) disrupt normal hematopoiesis, causing pancytopenia and placing patients at significant risk for infections (See **Table 6-6** for a list of common infections, associated organisms, and treatment options). Corticosteroids, used in some treatment regimens, cause additional general immune suppression. Infections can be life threatening if not treated appropriately and aggressively. Antibiotic, antifungal, and antiviral medications are essential components of care (See **Table 6-7**).

### Table 6-6. Selected Infections, Commonly Associated Organisms, and Treatment Options

| Infection | Commonly Associated Organisms | Treatment Options |
|---|---|---|
| **Central Line Bacteremia** | **Gram Positive** <br> *Staphylococcus aureus, Staphylococcus epidermidis, Enterococcus* | Vancomycin, nafcillin |
| | **Gram Negative** <br> *Enterobacter, E. coli, Pseudomonas, Klebsiella* | Timentin, amikacin, cefotaxime, cefuroxime, tobramycin |
| | **Fungal** <br> *Candida* | Amphotericin |
| **Rhinorrhea** | **Viral** <br> Respiratory syncytial virus (RSV) | Ribavirin, Synagis |
| | Influenza, parainfluenza | Tamiflu, amantadine |
| **Pneumonia** | **Bacterial** <br> *Streptococcus pneumoniae, Mycobacterium, Mycoplasma, Legionella* | Cefotaxime, clindamycin, trimethoprim/sulfamethoxazole (TMP-SMX), erythromycin |
| | **Fungal** <br> *Cryptococcus, Histoplasma, Coccidioides, Candida, Aspergillus* | Amphotericin, fluconazole, voriconazole |
| | **Viral** <br> RSV <br> *Cytomegalovirus* (CMV), adenovirus | Ribavirin, Synagis, ganciclovir, Foscavir |
| **Mucositis, Esophagitis** | **Viral** <br> Herpes simplex virus (HSV) | Acyclovir |
| | **Fungal** <br> *Candida* | Nystatin, fluconazole, amphotericin |
| **Necrotizing Gingivitis** | **Bacterial Gram-Negative Anaerobes** <br> *Bacteroides, Clostridium, Peptostreptococcus* | Clindamycin, metronidazole, imipenem |
| **Sinusitis** | **Gram Positive** <br> *Streptococcus pneumoniae, Haemophilus influenzae, Moraxella catarrhalis* | Amoxicillin/clavulanate, TMP-SMX |
| | **Gram Negative** <br> *Pseudomonas aeruginosa* | Aztreonam, ceftazidime, meropenem, piperacillin, Timentin, tobramycin |
| | **Fungal** <br> *Aspergillus, zygomycetes, Fusarium* | Amphotericin, voriconazole |

*(continued)*

## Risk Factors Associated with Infection

Multiple risk factors associated with disease and treatment can increase the risk of infection in patients. Certain malignancies are associated with additional immune deficits. Hodgkin's disease, T-cell malignancies, and Burkitt's lymphoma pose greater risks for viral and fungal infections because of abnormalities in their cellular immune systems.

Neutropenia and lymphopenia place patients at risk for complications related to infections. Severe neutropenia is an absolute neutrophil count (ANC) <500, whereas moderate neutropenia is defined as an ANC <1,000. High-dose chemotherapy regimens can cause neutropenia for 21 to 28 days from the first day of administration. HSCT recipients are immune compromised for at least 1 year or longer posttransplant if they remain on immune-suppression medications. Latent organisms, such as herpes zoster, pneumocystis pneumonia, herpes simplex, and cytomegalovirus, can reactivate in states of immune suppression.

Alterations in normal mucosal and skin barriers can allow

## Table 6-6. Selected Infections, Commonly Associated Organisms, and Treatment Options (continued)

| Infection | Commonly Associated Organisms | Treatment Options |
|---|---|---|
| Cutaneous/Skin | **Bacterial** **Gram Positive** *Staphylococcus aureus, Staphylococcus epidermidis,* methicillin-resistant *Staphylococcus aureus* (MRSA) | Clindamycin, TMP-SMX |
| | **Bacterial** **Gram Negative** *Pseudomonas aeruginosa, Stenotrophomonas maltophilia* | Aztreonam, ceftazidime, meropenem, piperacillin, Timentin, tobramycin |
| | **Viral** Varicella zoster | Acyclovir |
| | **Fungal** *Candida* | Amphotericin, voriconazole |
| Typhlitis, Pseudomembranous Colitis | **Gram Negative** *Pseudomonas aeruginosa, Clostridium difficile* | Ceftazidime, metronidazole, cefepime, imipenem, meropenem |
| Perirectal Cellulitis/ Abscess | **Bacterial** **Gram-Negative Aerobic Bacilli** *Pseudomonas aeruginosa, Klebsiella pneumoniae, E. coli* | Ceftazidime, cefepime, amikacin, cefotaxime, meropenem |
| | **Gram-Negative Anaerobes** *Bacteroides, Clostridium, Peptostreptococcus* | Metronidazole, clindamycin, imipenem |
| Urinary Tract | **Gram-Negative Aerobic Bacilli** *E. coli, Klebsiella, Proteus, Pseudomonas aeruginosa* | Augmentin, cefuroxime, cefoxitin, ceftriaxone, nitrofurantoin, ciprofloxacin, gentamicin, levofloxacin |
| Hemorrhagic Cystitis | **Viral** Adenovirus, BK virus, CMV | Ribavirin, cidofovir, ganciclovir, Foscavir |
| Ventriculoperitoneal Shunts/Meningitis | **Bacterial** **Gram Positive** *Staphylococcus epidermidis, Staphylococcus aureus, Enterococcus,* alpha-hemolytic streptococci | Vancomycin |
| | **Bacterial** **Gram Negative** *E. coli, Klebsiella pneumoniae, Pseudomonas aeruginosa* | Ceftazidime, cefepime, amikacin, cefotaxime, meropenem |
| | **Fungal (brain abscess)** *Candida albicans, Aspergillus* | Amphotericin |
| | **Protozoan** Toxoplasmosis | Pyrimethamine, sulfadiazine, folic acid |

bacteria to enter the bloodstream. Implanted devices, such as central venous catheters, shunts, and prosthetic devices, are also portals of entry for microorganisms.

Poor nutrition adds additional risk for infection. Bacterial translocation across the gastrointestinal tract is often a cause of bacteremia.

Patients who have had a splenectomy are at risk for infection from encapsulated organisms.

## Clinical Presentation

General signs and symptoms of infection include the following:
- Fever, defined as a temperature of ≥ 101 °F

### Table 6-7. Antibiotic Classes and Side Effects

#### Aminoglycosides
Aminoglycosides are bactericidal antibiotics active against many aerobic gram-negative and some aerobic gram-positive bacteria. Anaerobes are resistant because transport of aminoglycosides into cells is oxygen dependent. Aminoglycosides in combination with penicillins or vancomycin act synergistically to kill gram-positive bacteria. Aminoglycosides are inactive against fungi and viruses.

| Drugs | Side Effects |
|---|---|
| Gentamicin<br>Tobramycin<br>Amikacin | Ototoxicity is directly proportional to amount of drug given.<br>Renal toxic. Monitor levels. Dosing adjustment required for renal impairment.<br>Side effects include drop in blood counts, neurological changes such as headaches, gait changes, paresthesias, and tremors. |

#### Extended Spectrum Penicillins
Extended spectrum penicillins are bactericidal and are active against enteric gram-negative bacilli, most gram-positive and gram-negative aerobic cocci, some gram-positive aerobic and anaerobic bacilli, and gram-negative aerobic and anaerobic bacilli. More resistant to inactivation by beta-lactamase-producing gram-negative bacteria. Inactive against mycobacteria, *Mycoplasma*, *Rickettsia*, fungi, and viruses.

| Drugs | Side Effects |
|---|---|
| Penicillin G<br>Nafcillin<br>Ampicillin<br>Ticarcillin<br>Piperacillin | Side effects include altered taste, dizziness, irritability, seizures, nausea, vomiting, diarrhea, changes in liver and kidney function, hypokalemia, and superinfection. |

#### Cephalosporins
Cephalosporins are bactericidal. They are classified as first, second, third, and fourth generation based on spectrum of activity.
First generation cephalosporins are active only against gram-positive bacteria.
Second generation cephalosporins are active against gram-positive and gram-negative bacteria.
Third generation cephalosporins are less active against gram-positive bacteria and have extended spectrum against gram-negative organisms.

| Drugs | Side Effects |
|---|---|
| **First Generation**<br>Cefazolin (Ancef) | Side effects include nausea, vomiting, diarrhea, changes in liver and kidney function tests, dizziness, headache, and pancytopenia. |
| **Second Generation**<br>Cefoxitin | Side effects include hypersensitivity reactions and superinfection. Dosing adjustment required for renal impairment. |
| **Third Generation**<br>Cefotaxime<br>Ceftazidime | Side effects include phlebitis, leukopenia, thrombocytopenia, and superinfection. |

#### Macrolide Antibiotics
Active against gram-positive organisms, *Staphylococcus aureus* (except MRSA), *Streptococcus*, and *Mycobacterium*.

| Drugs | Side Effects |
|---|---|
| Erythromycin<br>Clarithromycin<br>Azithromycin | Associated with prolonged QTc, elevated liver transaminases and hepatic impairment, abdominal cramping, diarrhea, myelosuppression, superinfection, and Stevens-Johnson syndrome. |

#### Other Antibiotics
Useful against aerobic gram-positive bacteria, *Staphylococci*, and *Streptococci*.

| Drugs | Side Effects |
|---|---|
| Vancomycin<br>Clindamycin | Monitor for antibiotic-associated colitis, which can be fatal.<br>Hypotension associated with both. Vancomycin also associated with erythematous reaction known as Red Man's syndrome. May need slower infusion time with premedications. Vancomycin is also renal toxic and neurotoxic. Clindamycin associated with Stevens-Johnson syndrome. |

#### Carbepenems
Carbepenems are beta-lactam antibiotics with an extended spectrum of coverage to include gram-positive organisms (including *Enterococcus faecalis* and *Listeria*), gram-negative organisms (including *Haemophilus influenzae* and *Neisseria gonorrhea*, Enterobacter, and *Pseudomonas aeruginosa*), and anaerobes (including *Bacteroides fragilis*).

| Drugs | Side Effects |
|---|---|
| Imipenem<br>Meropenem | Adverse events include anaphylaxis, central nervous system effects (seizures, confusion), and superinfection. Dosing adjustment in renal impairment. |

*(continued)*

### Table 6-7. Antibiotic Classes and Side Effects *(continued)*

#### Antifungal Agents

| | |
|---|---|
| Amphotericin B<br>Liposomal complex amphotericin<br>Fluconazole<br>Itraconazole<br>Voriconazole<br>Caspofungin | Alert to dosing differences between amphotericin B and the liposomal complex amphotericin.<br>Anaphylaxis precautions with amphotericin.<br>Monitor electrolytes and renal function daily with amphotericin.<br>Monitor liver function studies with azoles. Voriconazole associated with alterations in vision. |

#### Antiviral Agents

Used for prophylaxis or treatment of viral reactivation.

| | |
|---|---|
| Acyclovir: Herpes simplex virus<br>Ganciclovir: Cytomegalovirus<br>Foscarnet: Cytomegalovirus, herpes simplex virus | Renal toxic, monitor for electrolyte imbalances. Associated with blood dyscrasias, monitor blood counts. Acyclovir and foscarnet associated with headaches. Ganciclovir associated with fever. |

#### Antipneumocystis Agents

Pneumocystis pneumonia is a protozoan organism latent in the immune-competent person that reactivates and can cause fatal pneumonia in the immune-suppressed patient.

| | |
|---|---|
| Trimethoprim-Sulfamethoxazole<br>Pentamidine<br>Dapsone<br>Atovaquone | Trimethoprim-Sulfamethoxazole is associated with blood dyscrasias and liver toxicity. Also associated with Stevens-Johnson syndrome.<br>Inhaled pentamidine is associated with bronchospasm; patients should receive a pre- and posttreatment bronchodilator.<br>Severe hypotension associated with rapid IV infusion of pentamidine.<br>Dapsone is associated with methomoglobinemia and blood dyscrasias. Hemolysis seen in patients with glucose-6-phosphate dehydrogenase deficiency.<br>Atovaquone associated with headache, insomnia, anxiety, nausea, vomiting, and diarrhea. |

*Note.* IV = intravenous; MRSA = methicillin-resistant *Staphylococcus aureus*; QTc = heartrate-corrected QT interval.

- Chills in addition to fever indicate a higher probability of multiorganism or gram-negative sepsis.
- Pain, inflammation, erythema, warmth, or purulent drainage (may be subtle or absent due to neutropenia)
- Other symptoms with or without fever are indicators for the site of origin of the infection.
- Bacteremia—history of fever and/or chills after flushing central lines may indicate blood and central-line infection.
- Pneumonia—productive or nonproductive cough, chest pain, rales or rhonchi, malaise, anorexia
- Otitis media—earache, hearing loss, irritability, drainage
- Mucositis—ulcerations, vesicles, pustules, sore throat, hoarseness, drooling, pain
- Esophagitis—retrosternal burning, chest pain, odynophagia, anorexia, dehydration
- Sinusitis—nasal or postnasal drainage, cough, headache, tooth pain, sore throat; tenderness in frontal, maxillary, or ethmoid area
- Cutaneous (i.e., skin) infections—vesicles (unilateral nerve distribution indicative of zoster), tingling, pruritus, pustules, inflammation, warmth, pain, bleeding, rash, skin plaques, erythema, desquamation
- Typhlitis—right-lower-quadrant pain, fever, diarrhea or constipation, guarding, prostration
- Pseudomembranous colitis—abdominal pain, diarrhea (bloody or mucoid), nausea, vomiting
- Urinary tract infection (UTI)—abdominal or suprapubic pain, urinary frequency and/or urgency, dysuria, hematuria, malodorous urine. Flank pain or back pain may indicate kidney infection.
- Perirectal cellulites or abscess—pain with or without erythema, induration, fissure, pain on defecation, rectal itching
- Ventricular peritoneal (VP) shunt infection—headache, vomiting, meningeal signs (e.g., irritability, neck stiffness, or neck pain), other neurological changes.

## Diagnostic Workup

The diagnostic workup varies according to the patient's presenting signs and symptoms but commonly includes one or more of the following:

- Complete blood count—determines degree of neutropenia and other cytopenias
- Creatinine, BUN, electrolytes—determine hydration and renal function
- Liver transaminases—determines hepatoxocity or hepatitis
- Amylase and lipase—evaluate for pancreatitis if abdominal pain is present
- Urinalysis and culture—determine UTIs

- Chest X ray or computed tomography (CT) scans—evaluate for pneumonia or other potential source of infection
- Stool cultures—evaluates causes of diarrhea
- Nasal wash—evaluates for viral infections if rhinorrhea, nasal congestion, or cough is present.

## Medical Treatment

Treatment for infections includes administration of broad-spectrum antibiotic therapy until the causative pathogens are identified or cultures return a negative result.

## Nursing Assessment and Interventions

### Assessment
- Obtain baseline then frequently monitor vital signs, including temperature, blood pressure, heart rate, respiratory rate, pulse oximetry, and capillary refill. A drop in blood pressure, increase in heart rate, increase in respiratory rate, prolonged capillary refill (i.e., >3 seconds), decreased pulse oximetry, and confusion indicate septic shock.
- Obtain a detailed history. Components of the history should include
  - Onset and duration of fever; administration of acetaminophen or other fever-reducing medications
  - Associated symptoms
  - Chills, especially if associated with flushing central line
  - Pain—location (ears, head, neck, chest, abdomen, rectum)
  - Nausea, vomiting, diarrhea
  - Dysuria or hematuria
  - Location of rash, lesions, or other changes in skin integrity
  - Changes in level of consciousness
  - Cough, rhinorrhea, or shortness of breath
  - Medications—Review medication list, time last taken. Assess compliance with pneumocystis carinii pneumonia (PCP) prophylaxis and pneumococcal prophylaxis or both.
  - Date of last chemotherapy or length of time post-HSCT to anticipate extent of neutropenia or immune suppression
  - Prior history of organ dysfunction (renal or hepatic compromise).
- Head-to-toe physical assessment from oral mucosa to perirectal area with attention to primary complaints

### Interventions
- Obtain blood work as indicated.
- Obtain blood cultures from each central-line lumen and Port-A-Cath.
- Obtain urinalysis and urine culture.
- Culture any sites of drainage.
- Administer antibiotics promptly (see **Table 6-8** for principles of antibiotic therapy).
- Administer intravenous fluids for bolus or maintenance as ordered.
- Administer antifungal or antiviral therapy as indicated.
- Obtain chest X rays or CT scans as ordered.
- Prepare patient for diagnostic procedures (i.e., lumbar puncture or VP shunt tap) if indicated.
- Perform ongoing assessments to identify changes in status or new associated symptoms.

---

**Table 6-8. Principles of Antibiotic Therapy**

- Know baseline allergies.
- Monitor for allergic reaction to antimicrobials.
- Know baseline renal and hepatic status.
- Pay attention to dose adjustments for renal or hepatic impairment.
- Double check dosing with formulary.
- Monitor for drug interactions.
- Monitor culture and sensitivity results.
- Monitor drug levels as indicated.
- Know that prolonged fever with no response to antibiotic therapy may indicate fungal infection.

---

- Communicate test results to physician as soon as they are available.
- Inform patient in developmentally appropriate manner the reason that tests or procedures are being performed.
- Inform and educate parents about patient's status and treatment plan. Provide reassurance and alleviate any parental guilt.
- Reevaluate understanding of immune compromise related to treatment.
- Reeducate about signs and symptoms of infection and monitoring of temperature.
- Reeducate about rationale for PCP or pneumococcal prophylaxis.
- Assess and reeducate parent's understanding of central-line care.

### Expected Patient and Family Outcomes
- The patient recovers from infectious episode with minimal complications.
- The patient and the family adhere to prophylactic medication regimens.
- The patient and the family learn appropriate central-line care.
- The family recognizes signs of infection and knows when to seek medical attention.

# Blood Product Support

*Teresa M. Conte*

## Definition

Blood components are products derived from human whole blood, which, when broken down, form red blood cells (RBCs), platelets, white blood cells (WBCs), and plasma. Plasma can be further processed to obtain cryoprecipitate. Oncologic and hematologic diseases often produce various hematologic deficiencies that result from an increased loss, increased destruction, or decreased production of a blood component. Many children with cancer and hematologic diseases require infusions of one or more blood components during the course of their treatment.

## Indications for Blood Product Infusions

Indications for infusions of blood products are to restore blood volume, improve oxygen-carrying capacity, minimize bleeding, correct coagulopathies, and/or replace plasma proteins. Often, different diseases have different transfusion parameters that dictate when transfusion of blood components is necessary.

## Pathophysiology of Blood Component Deficits

In children with cancer, tumor cells can replace normal cells within the bone-marrow space. Bone-marrow production becomes suppressed because of chemotherapy, radiation therapy, or both. Kidney damage, a side effect of several chemotherapeutic agents such as cisplatin (Platinol), cyclophosphamide (Cytoxan), and ifosfamide (Ifex), also may result in reduced production of erythropoietin, which assists in the formation of red cells.

Children who have hematologic diseases may need transfusion support depending on the type of disease they have. Some diseases, such as Fanconi's anemia, Diamond-Blackfan anemia, Shwachman-Diamond syndrome, Kostman's syndrome, and Pearson's syndrome often can result in bone-marrow failure, requiring transfusion of various blood products. Other hematological disorders such as sickle-cell anemia, aplastic anemia, and thalassemia may require transfusion of blood products at various times during the course of the illness.

## Sources of Blood Components

The two sources of blood components are donor and autologous. Donor blood components are collected from volunteer donors for transfusion to another person and may be donated for a specific recipient (i.e., a designated donor). Autologous blood is collected from the patient and stored for later reinfusion.

## Types of Blood Components

### Whole Blood

Whole blood contains RBCs, WBCs, platelets, and plasma. Whole blood is rarely administered but may be used to restore RBCs and volume when massive blood loss has occurred. Occasionally, it may be used for exchange transfusions.

**Volume guide:** Volume is 20 ml/kg initially to replace massive blood loss.

**Crossmatching:** Donor and recipient blood must be ABO identical and Rh compatible.

### Packed RBCs

Packed RBCs (PRBCs) are cells used to improve tissue oxygenation and correct anemia without causing a significant increase in blood volume. In children receiving chemotherapy to treat cancer, transfusion of PRBCs usually occurs when the hemoglobin is <8 gm/dL. Children receiving radiation therapy optimally have a hemoglobin of 10 gm/dL to maximize the oxygen-carrying capacity of the body prior to radiation. Children with thalassemia receive transfusions of PRBCs when their hemoglobin is <7 gm/dL. Children with sickle-cell disease are transfused with PRBCs only when necessary, because transfusions in these patients can lead to infection, iron overload, or alloimmunization.

PRBCs are prepared by removing the plasma portion of whole blood. The PRBCs are divided into units, each of which contain anywhere from 200 cc to 600 cc. If the entire unit is not needed, the blood bank can split the unit into smaller portions called alloquots. The shelf life of PRBCs is 21–42 days. After they have been transfused, their life span is approximately 30 days.

**Volume guide:** The volume guide for pediatric patients shows that 10 ml/kg will increase Hgb 3 g/dl; 15 ml/kg is the maximum amount given in a single transfusion.

**Crossmatching:** Crossmatching is done within 72 hours prior to transfusion. The donor's and patient's blood must be ABO identical and Rh compatible.

**Transfusion time:** Transfusion of each unit or alloquot of PRBCs takes between 1 and 2 hours. A transfusion must be completed within 4 hours of the blood's removal from a blood bank. Some children with severe anemia or fluid overload may require slower transfusion times to reduce the potential for cardiac overload. Other patients, such as those who are actively hemorrhaging, may require faster transfusions.

**Special preparation:** Patients who have had severe transfusion reactions to PRBCs receive PRBCs that have been washed. This process occurs in the blood bank and reduces the amount of WBCs, protein, and cellular waste in the unit. Washing the PRBCs changes their expiration time. PRBCs expire 24 hours after they are washed and placed into a bag and 4 hours after they are washed and placed into a syringe. Washed PRBCs are placed in a bag that looks noticeably different from "regular" PRBCs.

**Filter:** A 40-μ microaggregate (leukopore) filter must be used for all PRBC transfusions.

### Platelets

One unit of platelets is obtained from 500 ml of fresh whole blood. An apheresis unit is equal to 6–8 random donor units.

Platelets are suspended in a small amount of plasma and stored at room temperature on an agitator for up to 5 days. The types of platelet preparations are as follows:
- Random-donor platelets, which combine alloquots of platelets from different donors and expose the recipient to multiple foreign antigens
- Single-donor platelets, which minimize a recipient's exposure to foreign antigens
- Human lymphocyte antigen (HLA)-matched platelets, which are obtained by apheresing an HLA-identical donor to further minimize a recipient's exposure to foreign antigens.

One unit of platelets should increase a patient's peripheral blood level by 10,000 cells/mm$^3$. Platelets are administered when a patient is actively bleeding or when his or her platelet count is less than 10,000 cells/mm$^3$. Platelet infusions may be given prophylactically in children with vascular brain tumors if the count is less than 50,000 cells/mm$^3$. Platelets are also given prophylactically when the count is less than 50,000 cells/mm$^3$ in children with cancer who undergo surgery or invasive procedures. Children with platelet disorders such as idiopathic thrombocytopenia purpura usually receive platelets when the count is 35,000 or less.

Platelet counts can be drawn 60 minutes after an infusion. Failure to achieve adequate increases in circulating platelet counts often is due to infection, fever, disseminated intravascular coagulation (DIC), splenomegaly, or formation of antibodies to antigens in the donated blood. Exposure to multiple tissue antigens leads to formation of antibodies to the antigens, which results in a patient's inability to experience a platelet rise after platelet transfusion.

**Volume guide:** Pediatric volume is 10 ml/kg or 1 random unit per year of age. Adult volume is 6–10 units.

**Crossmatching:** Crossmatching is not required, but ABO-identical and Rh-compatible platelets are preferable.

**Transfusion time:** The transfusion time should be as fast as the patient can tolerate but should be within 4 hours after the platelets are released from a blood bank.

During transfusion, it is recommended that the bag and volume-control chamber (burretrol) be gently agitated every 30 minutes to prevent platelets from clumping or sticking to the bag and tubing.

**Special preparation:** For patients who have had severe transfusion reactions to platelets, the blood bank administers saline-suspended platelets. Saline suspension of the platelets reduces the number of WBCs in the unit and removes cellular waste. This process removes the plasma from the platelets, so it reduces the amount of fluid, not the amount of platelets, that are in a unit.

## Granulocytes

Granulocytes may be used to treat patients who are severely neutropenic and have ANCs of <500 x $10^9$ with documented infections, especially those caused by gram-negative organisms or fungal infections that do not respond to medicine. Granulocytes are not recommended for patients whose bone-marrow functions are not likely to recover.

Granulocytes are collected from a single donor and stored at room temperature. They contain large numbers of leukocytes, many platelets, and some RBCs.

Febrile and allergic reactions are common, as the recipient's antibodies react to the antigens on the donor leukocytes. Diphenhydramine (Benadryl), acetaminophen (Tylenol), or hydrocortisone (Solu-Cortef) may be ordered before a transfusion to prevent these reactions. Infusions can lead to pulmonary sequestrations, especially if the recipient is receiving antifungal medications such as amphotericin, ambisome, or abelcet. It is recommended that granulocyte infusions be separated from antifungal-medication infusions for a period of hours; however, individual institutions may have their own guidelines for this. Because of their low survival time after infusion, high degree of toxicity, and limited clinical evidence of benefit, granulocytes are rarely used.

**Volume guide:** The volume usually is 1 unit per day until the patient's condition improves, and signs of neutrophil recovery are apparent.

**Crossmatching:** Crossmatching is required because there are many RBCs contained within the volume of granulocytes to be transfused. The donor and the recipient must be ABO identical and Rh compatible.

**Transfusion time:** Granulocytes are transfused over 2–4 hours (5 ml/kg/hr). A standard-sized filter (i.e., 170 μ) should be used for administering granulocytes. **A 40-μ microaggregate filter should not be used because it will filter out the granulocytes.** Granulocytes are not kept in the general blood bank inventory. The blood bank must make special arrangements for obtaining granulocytes from donors. The donation must be prearranged, so it is important that the treatment team and the blood bank maintain ongoing communication to ensure that the granulocytes will be available when needed.

## Fresh-Frozen Plasma

Plasma is the clear-fluid portion of blood that remains when RBCs are removed from whole blood. Fresh-frozen plasma (FFP) is separated and frozen less than 6 hours after collection. FFP contains plasma proteins and stable coagulation factors (i.e., fibrinogen and factor IX) and unstable coagulation factors (i.e., factor V and factor VIII). FFP contains approximately 1 unit/ml of each coagulation factor. It is used to replace coagulation factors in bleeding patients with multiple coagulation-factor deficiencies resulting from liver disease, DIC, or dilutional coagulopathy (e.g., because of massive blood replacement). The U.S. Food and Drug Administration recently approved frozen plasma (FP) as a new option for patients. The new product is plasma that is frozen within 24 hours of collection. The main difference between FFP and FP is that FP has a lower amount of factor VIII.

**Volume guide:** The volume is 10–30 ml/kg.

**Crossmatching:** Crossmatching is not required. However, the patient and the donor must be ABO identical. Rh compatibility is not required because the product does not contain RBCs.

**Transfusion time:** FFP is transfused over 2–4 hours. It must be infused within 6 hours of the time it is thawed.

## Albumin (5% or 25% solution) and Plasma Protein Fraction (5% solution)

Albumin contains 96% albumin and 4% globulins, and plasma protein fraction (PPF) contains 83% albumin and 17% globulins. Both are treated with heat to destroy viruses. Albumin and PPF are used to treat patients who are both hypovolemic and hypoproteinemic. Both treatments must be used with caution in patients susceptible to fluid overload.

**Volume guide:** The volume is 0.5–1 g/kg = 10 ml/kg of 5% solution; 1 g/kg = 4 ml/kg of 25% solution.

**Crossmatching:** Crossmatching is not required.

**Transfusion time:** The transfusion rate for a 5% solution is 1–2 ml/minute (60–120 ml/hr) or more rapid if the patient is in shock. The transfusion rate for a 25% solution is 0.2–0.4 ml/minute (12–24 ml/hr).

## Cryoprecipitate

Cryoprecipitate is prepared by thawing FFP. The cryoprecipitate is used to replace fibrinogen and clotting factor deficiencies. It contains clotting factors VIII and XIII, fibrinogen, and von Willebrand factor.

**Volume guide:** The dosage varies depending on a patient's disease and condition. Doses are usually repeated every 8–12 hours until bleeding stops or the desired factor VIII level is attained.

**Crossmatching:** Crossmatching is not required. ABO compatibility is suggested, not required.

**Transfusion time:** The transfusion time is 1–2 hours, but the cryoprecipitate must be transfused within 6 hours of the time the frozen plasma is thawed.

## Clotting Concentrates

Factor VIII and factor IX clotting concentrates are used to treat specific clotting deficiencies. They provide a known dosage in a small volume. One unit provides the amount of factor activity that is normally present in 1 ml of normal plasma.

**Volume guide:** 1 unit/kg of factor VIII should increase a patient's plasma level by 2%; 1 unit/kg of factor IX should increase a patient's plasma level by 1%.

**Crossmatching:** Crossmatching is not required.

**Transfusion time:** The transfusion time is 5–15 minutes. The factor is withdrawn from a vial using a filter needle.

## Special Component Preparations

### Irradiated Blood Products

T lymphocytes that are present in the blood of a donor can cause graft-versus-host disease (GVHD) in an immunocompromised recipient. Immunocompromised recipients include patients with malignancies, chemotherapy recipients, bone-marrow-transplant candidates, and neonates. The lymphocytes in the donor's blood attack the recipient's tissue, which is unable to reject incompatible foreign cells, resulting in GVHD. Irradiation of a donor's blood makes the WBC lymphocytes nonviable. All donor blood components are irradiated by a blood bank just before transfusion.

### Leukocyte-Reduced Blood Products

Leukocyte-reduced RBCs and platelets are indicated for all patients receiving chemotherapy and for individuals who have repeated febrile reactions associated with RBC transfusions, platelet transfusions, or both. Patients who receive frequent transfusions may become alloimmunized to leukocyte antigens and sometimes to platelet antigens. This sensitization can manifest itself as a febrile transfusion reaction or refractoriness to a transfusion of platelets or both. Leukocyte reduction also decreases the risk of transmitting cytomegalovirus (CMV) to the recipient.

Leukocytes can be removed from the blood products by centrifugation, filtration, or washing the RBCs in saline solution. Washed RBCs are preferable for patients with severe allergic reactions to transfusions.

### Cytomegalovirus-Negative Components

CMV is an easily transmitted virus that can cause serious infections and possibly even death in immunosuppressed individuals or premature infants. The virus can persist in a carrier state in the blood of a previously infected person even though antibodies are present. It is generally accepted that leukocyte reduction during the collection process is an effective method of reducing CMV transmission to a CMV-negative recipient. Bone-marrow-transplant candidates who are CMV negative and neonates who weigh less than 1,250 grams at birth usually receive CMV-negative blood components.

### Other Considerations

Patients may require blood products that have had certain antigens removed. These are listed on the unit of blood itself. Just as children with cancer require irradiated blood products, children with sickle-cell disease require sickle-negative blood. Other special antigen removal, such as Kell, may be necessary and is based on the individual receiving the transfusion.

## Potential Complications

### Febrile Response

Symptoms include fever, chills, muscle pain, chest pain, flushing, and headache.

### Allergic Reaction

Symptoms include itching, hives, dyspnea, wheezing, respiratory arrest, and cardiac arrest.

### Circulatory Overload

Symptoms include hypertension, hypotension, bradycardia, tachycardia, cyanosis of the extremities, and clammy skin.

### Sepsis

Symptoms include fever, chills, bleeding, DIC, nausea and vomiting, diarrhea, and abdominal cramping.

## Nursing Assessment and Interventions

### Assessment

**Before the Transfusion:**

- Assess the child's pretransfusion status, including weight, clinical condition, laboratory values, indications for component therapy, previous transfusion history, and indications for premedication.
- Confirm that consent for the transfusion of blood products has been obtained and is current.
- Assess the child's and the family's understanding of the transfusion process.
- Assess the child's intravenous access and patency of his or her veins.
- Verify the physician's orders, including the type of component, special requirements (e.g., irradiated blood products, leukocyte-reduced blood products), the number of millimeters or units to be given, the date and time they are to be administered, and the duration of the infusion.
- Verify that the patient has an active type and screen in the blood bank. A type and screen last for 72 hours and may be repeated as necessary.
- Administer any premedications as ordered.
- Perform a baseline assessment and check the patient's vital signs before beginning the infusion.
- Verify the following with a second healthcare provider in the presence of the patient, according to institutional policy:
  – The type of product, blood group, and Rh type
  – The patient's identification band containing his or her name and medical record number
  – The transfusion service record or labels on the bag match pertinent identification, compatibility, crossmatching (if required), ABO group, unit number, expiration date of the product, lot numbers (if provided), and any other information on or attached to the product.

**During the Transfusion:**

- Monitor the patient according to institutional policy; at a minimum, this includes observing the patient for the first 15 minutes and reassessing the patient's vital signs every hour during the transfusion.
- Monitor the patient for any possible transfusion reaction throughout the duration of the transfusion.

- Notify the next nurse assuming care of the patient that the patient received a transfusion, so that the patient will continue to be monitored for any delayed reactions.

## Interventions
- Take the following actions when there is a suspected transfusion reaction:
  - Stop the transfusion.
  - Draw 3–5 ml and discard the blood specimen, flush the IV line with saline, and maintain venous patency.
  - Notify the physician and the blood bank.
  - Assess the patient's condition and vital signs.
  - Check the blood bag for a compatibility label and the patient identification label for clerical errors.
  - Return the untransfused portion, with tubing set, to the blood bank.
  - Obtain blood and urine samples from the patient.
  - Document the reaction in the patient's medical record. Include the date and time the transfusion began, venipuncture sites, venous access device, the unit number of the blood component, type of product and filter used, times of any filter and/or tubing changes, the volume infused, vital signs, observations of the patient's tolerance, education provided to the patient and the family, and any medications that were omitted or given to the patient.

## Expected Patient and Family Outcomes
- The child and the family understand the purpose of the infusion of the blood product.
- The child and the family understand the signs and symptoms of a transfusion reaction.
- The blood component is infused safely.

# Bibliography

### Psychological Preparation and Support for Painful Procedures
Chen, E., Joseph, N. H., & Zeltzer, L. K. (2000). Behavioral and cognitive interventions in the treatment of pain in children. *Pediatric Clinics of North America, 47,* 513–525.

Christensen, J., & Fatchett, D. (2002). Promoting parental use of distraction and relaxation in pediatric oncology patients during invasive procedures. *Journal of Pediatric Oncology Nursing, 19,* 124–132.

Collins, J. J., & Weisman, S. J. (2003). Management of pain in childhood cancer. In N. L. Schechter, C. B. Berde, & M. Yaster (Eds.), *Pain in infants, children, and adolescents* (2nd ed., pp. 517–538). Philadelphia: Lippincott Williams & Wilkins.

Finley, G. A., & Schechter, N. L. (2003). Sedation. In N. L. Schechter, C. B. Berde, & M. Yaster (Eds.), *Pain in infants, children, and adolescents* (2nd ed., pp. 563–577). Philadelphia: Lippincott Williams & Wilkins.

### Sedation for Painful Procedures
Collins, J. J., & Weisman, S. J. (2003). Management of pain in childhood cancer. In N. L. Schechter, C. B. Berde, & M. Yaster (Eds.), *Pain in infants, children, and adolescents* (2nd ed., pp. 517–538). Philadelphia: Lippincott Williams & Wilkins.

Cravero, J. P., & Blike, G. T. (2004). Review of pediatric sedation. *Anesthesia and Analgesia, 99,* 1355–1364.

Doyle, L., & Colletti, J. E. (2006). Pediatric procedural sedation and analgesia. *Pediatric Clinics of North America, 53,* 279–292.

Finley, G. A., & Schechter, N. L. (2003). Sedation. In N. L. Schechter, C. B. Berde, & M. Yaster (Eds.), *Pain in infants, children, and adolescents* (2nd ed., pp. 563–577). Philadelphia: Lippincott Williams & Wilkins.

### Central Venous Access Devices
Anton, M., & Massicotte, M. (2001). Venous thromboembolism in pediatrics. *Seminars in Vascular Medicine, 1,* 111–122.

Carr, E., Jayobose, S., Stringel, G., Slim, M., Ozkaynak, M., Tugal, O., et al. (2006). The safety of central line placement prior to treatment of pediatric acute lymphoblastic leukemia. *Pediatric Blood and Cancer, 47*(7), 886–888.

Goes, C., & Ronan, J. (2004). Central venous access. In A. J. Altman (Ed.), *Supportive care of children with cancer* (3rd ed., pp. 269–278). Baltimore: Johns Hopkins University Press.

Maki, D. G., Stolz, S. M., Wheeler, S., & Mermel, L. A. (1997). Prevention of central venous catheter-related bloodstream infection by use of an antiseptic-impregnated catheter: A randomized, controlled trial. *Annals of Internal Medicine, 127,* 257–266.

Matsuzaki, A., Suminoe, A., Koga, Y., Hatano, M., Hattori, S., & Hara, T. (2006). Long-term use of peripherally inserted central venous catheters for cancer chemotherapy in children. *Supportive Care in Cancer, 14*(2), 153–160.

Pearson, M., & Abrutyn, E. (1997). Reducing the risk for catheter-related infections: A new strategy. *Annals of Internal Medicine, 127,* 304–306.

Zaoutis, T. E., Greeves, H. M., Lautenbach, E., Bilker, W. B., & Coffin, S. E. (2004). Risk factors for disseminated candidiasis in children with candidiasis. *Pediatric Infectious Disease Journal, 23,* 635–641.

### Nutritional Support
Barale, K., & Charuhas, P. (2005). Oncology and hematopoietic cell transplantation. In P. Samour & K. Kings (Eds.), *Handbook of pediatric nutrition* (3rd ed., pp. 459–481). Sudbury, MA: Jones and Bartlett Publishers, Inc.

Bechard, L., Adiv, O., Jaksic, T., & Duggan, C. (2006). Nutritional supportive care. In P. Pizzo & D. Poplack (Eds.), *Principles and practice of pediatric oncology* (pp. 1330–1347). Philadelphia: Lippincott Williams & Wilkins.

Fuhrman, M., Charney, P., & Mueller, C. (2004). Hepatic proteins and nutrition assessment. *Journal of the American Dietetic Association, 104*(8), 1258–1264.

Kraft, M., Btaiche, I., & Sacks, G. (2005). Review of the refeeding syndrome. *Nutrition in Clinical Practice, 20*(6), 625–633.

Nitenberg, G., & Raynard, B. (2000). Nutritional support of the cancer patient: Issues and dilemmas. *Critical Reviews in Oncology/Hematology, 34,* 137–168.

Wang, Z., Heshka, S., Zhang, K., Boozer, C., & Heymsfield, S. (2001). Resting energy expenditure: Systemic organization and critique of prediction methods. *Obesity Research, 9,* 331–336.

## Treatment of Infections

American Academy of Pediatrics. (2006). *2006 Red Book: Report of the Committee on Infectious Diseases* (27th ed.). Elk Grove Village, IL: American Academy of Pediatrics.

Gilbert, D. N., Moellering, R. C., Eliopoulos, F. M., & Sande, M. E. (2005). *The Sanford Guide to antimicrobial therapy*. Hyde Park, VT: Antimicrobial Therapy, Inc.

Kline, N. (2007). Prevention and treatment of infections. In C. R. Baggott, K. P. Kelly, D. Fochtman, & G. V. Foley (Eds.), *Nursing care of children and adolescents with cancer* (3rd ed., pp. 266–278). Glenview, IL: Association of Pediatric Hematology/Oncology Nurses.

Walsh, T., Roilides, E., Groll, A., Gonzalez, C., & Pizzo, P. (2006). Infectious complications in pediatric cancer patients. In P. Pizzo & D. Poplack (Eds.), *Principles and practice of pediatric oncology* (5th ed., pp. 1269–1329). Philadelphia: Lippincott Williams & Wilkins.

## Blood Product Support

Conte, T., & Wallace, J. (2007). Supportive care. In K. Wilson & R. Bryant (Eds.), *Foundations of pediatric hematology nursing: A comprehensive orientation and review course*. Glenview, IL: Association of Pediatric Hematology/Oncology Nurses.

Fitzpatrick, L. (2002). Blood products. *Nursing, 32*(5), 36–42.

Herberg, A. (2003). Blood product administration. In V. R. Bowden & C. Smith Greenberg (Eds.), *Pediatric nursing procedures* (122–132). Philadelphia: Lippincott Williams & Wilkins.

Miller, R. L. S. (2002). Blood component therapy. *Urologic Nursing, 22*(5), 331–342.

Norville, R., & Bryant, R. (2007). Blood component deficiencies. In C. R. Baggott, K. P. Kelly, D. Fochtman, & G. V. Foley (Eds.), *Nursing care of children and adolescents with cancer* (3rd ed., pp. 347–364). Glenview, IL: Association of Pediatric Hematology/Oncology Nurses.

# Section VII  Psychosocial Issues

Mary C. Hooke

## Section Outline

Development of Infants (Birth–1 Year)

Development of Toddlers (1–3 Years)

Development of Preschoolers (4–6 Years)

Development of School-Age Children (7–12 Years)

Development of Adolescents (13–18 Years)

Development of Young Adults (18–25 Years)

Family Systems

Family Resources

Cultural Care

Spirituality

School Reentry and Attendance

Professional Nurse-Patient Relationships

Bibliography

# Development of Infants (Birth–1 Year)

*Mary C. Hooke*

## Normal Development

### Psychosocial Stage of Trust Versus Mistrust
Infants work to develop a sense of trust while overcoming a sense of mistrust. Infants trust that their needs for food, comfort, stimulation, and caring will be met. Mistrust develops in response to a lack of trusting experiences.

### Cognitive Stage
This is the sensorimotor stage during which simple learning takes place through sensory experiences and exploration. Infants progress from reflex behaviors to simple repetitive acts and imitative activities. Infants work toward developing a sense of object permanence.

### Emotional and Social Characteristics
Infants' temperaments or behavioral styles influence their human interactions.

### Body Image and Sense of Self
Infants' sensorimotor experiences provide the first perceptions of their own body, and the mouth is an infant's primary area of pleasure. Infants develop an awareness of their hands and feet, with which they suck or play. They acquire a sense of object permanence through sensorimotor development. At this point infants recognize themselves as distinct from their parents.

### Fears
Infants' fears of strangers and of separation from their parents are important to the development of healthy parent-child attachments. Infants also may have fears related to loud noises, bright lights, sudden movements, animals, and heights.

### Significant Relationships
An infant's attachment to a mothering figure is of primary importance. By 6 months, an infant shows a distinct preference for his or her mother and shows attachment to the father by 7 months.

### Risks to Infants with Cancer or a Blood Disorder
Hospitalization often causes these infants to be separated from their parents for significant periods. Disease (e.g., cancer, sickle-cell disease, hemophilia) and/or its treatment can cause side effects such as fatigue, pain, central-nervous-system (CNS) changes, immobility, and mucositis (cancer), which can interfere with sensorimotor experiences and the infant's development. Hospitalization and treatment also bring about changes in the routines and patterns that provide security to an infant. Furthermore, treatment involves experiences that infants fear, such as those involving separation, strangers, loud noises, bright lights, and sudden movements.

## Nursing Assessment and Interventions

### Assessment
- Assess the relationship between the infant and the parent (i.e., bonding behaviors, responsiveness, interplay between the parent and the child).
- Assess the infant's level of development by using assessment tools such as the Ages and Stages Questionnaires (Squires, Potter, & Bricker, 1999).
- Assess the infant's sensorimotor experiences:
  - Have oral-motor experiences and pleasure been affected by the disease or treatment?
  - Is the infant able to roll and move his or her hands and feet to the mouth?
  - Has the infant experienced complications or received therapies that can affect neurological function (e.g., CNS bleed, stroke, intrathecal [IT] medications, therapies that cross the blood-brain barrier, radiation therapy)?

### Interventions
- Encourage the development of trust.
- Encourage the parents to visit and room with the infant.
- Allow the parents to hold the infant as much as possible.
- Encourage comforting touch.
- Perform examinations as quickly as possible.
- Provide sensorimotor experiences for the infant.
- Provide pleasurable visual, auditory, tactile, taste, and movement mechanisms for the infant's stimulation.
- Encourage the development of the infant's oral-motor pleasure through actions such as sucking and oral intake.
- Consult with an occupational therapist or a speech therapist if the infant's oral functioning is impaired.
- Consult with a physical therapist and an occupational therapist if the infant has developmental delays or is at risk because of disease complications or therapy.
- Encourage age-appropriate developmental skills.

## Expected Patient and Family Outcomes
- The outcomes of nursing interventions have been evaluated, and the plan of care has been adjusted accordingly.
- A comprehensive developmental assessment is completed every 2 months and as needed for infants who have developmental delays or impairments.
- The patient achieves his or her potential developmentally despite challenges.

## Reference
Squires, J., Potter, L., & Bricker, D. (1999). *The ASQ user's guide for the Ages and Stages Questionnaires®: A parent-completed, child-monitoring system.* Baltimore: Paul H. Brookes.

# Development of Toddlers (1–3 Years)

Mary C. Hooke

## Normal Development

### Psychosocial Stage of Autonomy Versus Shame and Doubt
Toddlers develop a sense of independence and self-mastery. They discover that their behavior is their own and has predictable effects on others. They learn that gratification must sometimes be delayed, and limits on their behavior will be set. Continued dependence at this stage can cause them to have a sense of doubt about their ability to control their own actions.

### Cognitive Stage
Toddlers continue to develop in the sensorimotor phase of cognitive development (12–24 months), during which they increase their understanding of object permanence and a sense of cause and effect through trial and error. Toddlers develop their language skills (i.e., they develop mental symbolism); they show curiosity and engage in experimentation, exploration, and mimicry. They are egocentric in their thinking. During the later, preoperational phase, toddlers become preconceptual thinkers. They increase their ability to use speech, but they continue to be egocentric in thought, play, and behavior. Toddlers do not think logically but, rather, can be magical in their thinking based on their perception of an event.

### Emotional and Social Characteristics
Toddlers may express their frustration through temper tantrums as they strive for autonomy. They respond with negativism to requests and questions. They are vulnerable to stress because of their limited ability to cope.

### Body Image and Sense of Self
Toilet training is the major task for toddlers. During this stage in their development, they learn the names of body parts and their purposes, and they learn to recognize differences between the sexes. They are unable to understand the concepts of body integrity and internal organs. They find intrusive experiences and procedures very threatening. Toddlers are able to separate from their parents for brief periods but are fearful of strangers when their parents are not present. They learn that they are individuals separate from others, but they perceive that the world revolves around them.

### Fears
Toddlers fear separation from their parents. They fear strangers, especially when their parents are not present. They also may fear sleep, animals, and loud noises.

### Significant Relationships
Parents are the primary people of importance in a toddler's life. Interactions with other people, however, start to become more important for toddlers. They demonstrate parallel play with other children.

### Risks to Toddlers with Cancer or a Blood Disorder
Hospitalization may cause separation from parents and the introduction of strangers, both of which are major sources of fear and stress for toddlers. Disease (e.g., cancer, sickle-cell disease, hemophilia) can cause side effects, such as fatigue, pain, isolation, CNS changes, and immobility, which can interfere with a toddler's normal needs for exploration, experimentation, and development of autonomy. A toddler's normal negativism and temper tantrums can be exacerbated by a sense of loss of control, pain, and the side effects of medications such as steroids.

Toddlers are unable to understand what cancer is and how treatment works. They have limited verbal skills with which to explain their perceptions and sensations to others. Disease treatment and hospitalization also cause changes in discipline and routines that normally provide toddlers with a sense of security. A toddler can fail to achieve success in toilet training because of regression, illness, bladder abnormalities, and high levels of intravenous hydration. A chronic illness and its treatment can encompass this entire developmental stage.

## Nursing Assessment and Interventions

### Assessment
- Use developmental tools such as the Ages and Stages Questionnaires (Squires, Potter, & Bricker, 1999) to assess the toddler's developmental level.
- Interview the family about the toddler's normal behavior, routines, sleep patterns, fears, security objects, toilet training, ability to communicate and use language, responses to limits and discipline, and effective comfort measures.
- Assess the toddler's responsiveness to interactions with his or her parents.
- Assess for the impact of disease and treatment on the toddler's current developmental level (e.g., regression in achievement of milestones, language, or toilet training).
- Assess whether the toddler has experienced complications or received therapies that can affect neurological function (e.g., a CNS bleed, stroke, intrathecal medications, therapies that cross the blood-brain barrier, radiation therapy).

### Interventions
- Use assessment data from an interview with the toddler's parents for individualizing the patient's care plan to maintain consistency; address topics such as the toddler's normal behavior, routines, fears, toilet training, limits, and discipline.
- Encourage independence by providing opportunities for the toddler to participate in care and by offering appropriate choices.
- Encourage mobility and independence by allowing the toddler to engage in physical activity or to move around using a wagon or stroller.
- Encourage the toddler's need to explore, play, and experiment with the environment while at the same time providing safe boundaries.
- Arrange for rehabilitation services for toddlers who have developmental delays or are at risk because of disease complications or therapy.
- Provide the toddler with consistency in caregivers to promote the development of trusting relationships.
- Provide opportunities for play to help the toddler work through fears; consult child-life resources about the use of therapeutic play.

- Support the parents in their toilet-training efforts with the toddler by providing frequent opportunities for toileting and the use of training pants instead of diapers.
- Provide simple explanations describing sensations and desired behavior, because a toddler does not understand causal relationships.
- Teach parents about the toddler's response to illness and ways to promote the toddler's development during the illness; use resources for education such as child-life specialists and child psychologists.
- Discuss the toddler's need for socialization with the parents, and develop creative ways to meet these needs when the toddler is at home.

### Expected Patient and Family Outcomes
- The outcomes of nursing interventions are evaluated, and the plan of care has been adjusted accordingly.
- A comprehensive assessment of development is completed every 2–6 months and as needed for toddlers who have developmental delays or impairments.
- The patient achieves his or her potential developmentally despite challenges.

### Reference
Squires, J., Potter, L., & Bricker, D. (1999). *The ASQ user's guide for the Ages and Stages Questionnaires®: A parent-completed, child-monitoring system*. Baltimore: Paul H. Brookes.

## Development of Preschoolers (4–6 Years)

*Mary C. Hooke*

### Normal Development

#### Psychosocial Stage of Initiative Versus Guilt
Preschoolers develop mastery over their physical skills and are energetic learners. They feel satisfaction in their play and work. If they overstep the limits of appropriate behavior, they feel guilty.

#### Cognitive Stage
Preschoolers move from preconceptual thought processes that are egocentric and symbolic to intuitive thought that enables them to think and verbalize their mental processes. They are beginning to consider other viewpoints during this stage. Preschoolers use magical thinking when relating one event to another and believe that thoughts are all-powerful. Preschoolers have only a limited understanding of time and relate it to a specific event (e.g., lunchtime). They also attribute lifelike qualities to inanimate objects and believe that everyone thinks as they do.

#### Emotional and Social Characteristics
Preschoolers have increased mastery over their fear of strangers and separation; however, they find prolonged separation to be stressful and need their parents' support. They are more social and willing to please than toddlers. They have internalized the standards of their culture. They find support in security objects and can work through fears and anxieties through play.

#### Body Image and Sense of Self
During this stage, children are beginning to understand the concepts of desirable and undesirable appearances. They are at risk for developing their own prejudices or experiencing the prejudices of others. They develop their sexual identity through identification with the parent of their sex and imitate roles (e.g., what mothers and fathers do) through play. Preschoolers continue to have a poor sense of their internal anatomy and its functions and find intrusive procedures to be frightening.

#### Fears
Preschoolers may be afraid of the dark, of being left alone, and of having their body mutilated. They are fearful of pain as well as the objects and people associated with pain. They also are afraid of witnessing others in pain.

#### Significant Relationships
Preschoolers' parents and family continue to be of primary importance to them. They may attend an early-childhood program and kindergarten, which provide opportunities for social development with their peers and significant adults other than their parents.

#### Risks to Preschoolers with Cancer or a Blood Disorder
The experience of having cancer and undergoing treatment separates a preschooler from social relationships that are important for the development of social skills. Cancer therapy can cause side effects, such as fatigue, pain, isolation, and immobility, which can interfere with a preschooler's energetic play and work and deprive him or her of developmental experiences and a sense of accomplishment. Central nervous system toxicities also can interfere with a preschooler's cognitive development.

Hospitalization can cause prolonged, stressful periods of separation from parents. Furthermore, preschoolers with cancer may have decreased opportunities to be with both parents, especially if one parent takes on the role of primary caregiver. This circumstance can affect the development of the child's sexual identity. Preschoolers also may develop a poor sense of body integrity if they have experienced physical impairments. In addition, their tendency to engage in magical thinking places them at risk for increased fears. If they witness someone else's pain or injury, they may develop fears about experiencing that pain or wound because of their ability to imagine an event without having experienced it.

### Nursing Assessment and Interventions

#### Assessment
- Use parental history and developmental milestones to assess the preschooler's current developmental level.
- Assess the impact of disease and treatment on the preschooler's current developmental level.
- Assess whether the preschooler received neurotoxic therapies (e.g., intrathecal medications, therapies that cross the blood-brain barrier, radiation therapy).
- Interview family members about the preschooler's normal behavior, routines, sleep patterns, fears, coping skills, security objects, toileting and hygiene skills, concerns about himself or herself, limits and discipline, and comfort measures.

- Assess the responsiveness of the interaction between the parents and the preschooler.
- Listen to the preschooler's conversations and observe his or her play; assess the child's understanding of his or her disease and its treatment.
- Observe for fearful or anxious behavior, and try to determine the source of the child's fear.

### Interventions
- Individualize the patient's care plan to include information from the interview with the parents; address information about the preschooler's normal routines, self-care skills, fears, coping, comfort measures, bathroom routines, and security objects, as well as limits and discipline.
- Encourage the child's mastery of self-care skills, and promote independence in activities of daily living.
- Provide opportunities for stimulating play and success while providing safe boundaries.
- Arrange for neuropsychology consultation and rehabilitation services for the preschooler who has developmental delays or is receiving neurotoxic therapies.
- Consult child-life resources when using therapeutic play to learn about illness and promote the child's adaptive skills.
- Provide simple, brief explanations about treatments and experiences while keeping in mind the limits of a preschooler's understanding of time.
- Maintain the child's bed and room as safe areas; protect the child from witnessing pain in other children.
- Discuss with the parents their child's need for socialization and devise creative ways to meet them.
- Use a school reentry program for a child who is returning to a preschool group or kindergarten (see the subsection "School Reentry and Attendance"); provide guidance and assistance as the child makes the transition, and help the child with appearance and adjustment issues.
- Teach the parents about preschoolers' responses to illness and ways to promote their child's development during illness; use resources such as child-life specialists and child psychologists for education.

### Expected Patient and Family Outcomes
- The outcomes of nursing interventions are evaluated, and the plan of care is adjusted accordingly.
- A comprehensive developmental assessment is completed every 6 months and as needed for preschoolers who have developmental delays or impairments.

## Development of School-Age Children (7–12 Years)

*Linda Madsen*

### Normal Development

#### Psychosocial Stage of Industry Versus Inferiority
The challenge for children at this stage is to become proficient at accomplishing tasks as they become increasingly independent from their parents. At this time the peer group is a source of feedback for socially acceptable behavior, and conformity to the group is valued. If a child is unable to perform tasks in the social, physical, and academic realms, he or she can develop feelings of inadequacy that lead to a sense of inferiority. A sense of industry is developed if competence at these skills is adequate. The overall goal for children at this stage is to answer the question, "What can I do?"

#### Cognitive Stage
This is the stage of concrete thinking or concrete operations. Children at this stage are able to conceptualize and think through concepts without having had a corresponding experience upon which to rely. They are able to classify, sort, and order things; perform inductive reasoning; and understand the concepts of reversibility and object conservation. Children at this stage also see things in absolute terms and consider rules to be inflexible. Their primary focus is on mastery of school subjects and productive development of skills.

#### Emotional and Social Characteristics
Children at this stage are beginning to place importance on peer relationships and approval. Their peers give them feedback about acceptable behavior. They value conformity; an individual's physical differences may be threatening to the group. They wish to please and try to be cooperative. Confidence often exceeds a child's true capabilities at this age. They need privacy and strenuous physical activity. Their self-esteem is linked to their competence at performing tasks.

#### Fears
Children at this stage have fears about losing control, being faced with the physical aspects of illness, failing to accomplish tasks, and being isolated from their peers.

#### Significant Relationships
Children at this stage of development have significant relationships with their parents and other family members, school staff, and peers.

#### Risks to Children with Cancer or a Blood Disorder
**Lost productivity:** This risk is associated with absence from school, weakness, fatigue, decreased endurance, or disability that interferes with normative functions and the lowered expectations placed on them by the significant adults in their lives. Central-nervous-system toxicities also can interfere with the school-age child's cognitive development.

**Poor peer relationships due to isolation from the group:** Sick children may fail to interact with the group because of frequent absences from school and inability to participate in social activities. Poor self-esteem because of physical changes can lead children to isolate themselves and perceive themselves as being different from the group. The peer group also might reject these children, because they perceive them as being different.

**A sense of loss of control:** Children may feel that they have lost control over their emotions because of having to undergo painful procedures and stressful situations. Children who have experienced a loss of physical function or endurance or who have experienced weakness may feel a loss of body integrity. They also may sense that they are incapable of functioning independently if they have experienced a loss of function or weakness or if their parents overprotect them.

**A sense of inferiority resulting from unrealistic expectations:** Parents and teachers may have unrealistically high or low expectations that are inconsistent with the child's true abilities.

**Information deficit:** Children may feel responsible for the diagnosis. As they grow older, children may need new information to successfully deal with the new challenges related to their illness.

## Nursing Assessment and Interventions

### Assessment

- Assess current growth and development.
- Determine level of success in interpersonal relationships, and evaluate these key relationships through questioning and observation:
  - the extent of contact with peers in school and during outside activities
  - the level of involvement in school and extracurricular activities
  - the quality of peer relationships
  - the level of inclusion in the peer group.
- Assess the parents' and teachers' ability to normalize and adapt their expectations.
- Assess the effect of changes on self-image by using verbal and nonverbal cues:
  - the extent of physical limitations
  - the perception of these limitations
  - the effects of the limitations on activities of daily living.
- Assess for signs that the child is using healthy strategies for coping, and assess his or her level of adjustment by observing and questioning the child and the family about
  - the child's ability to incorporate the changes imposed by the disease and its treatment into the activities of daily living
  - the child's level of involvement with his or her own care
  - the child's personal affect
  - the child's ability to establish normalcy in relationships and activities.
- Determine whether school-related issues exist, such as attendance and the child's ability to maintain his or her previous academic performance.
- Assess whether the school-age child has received neurotoxic therapies (e.g., intrathecal medications, therapies that cross the blood-brain barrier, radiation therapy).
- Assess level of knowledge and information needs about the disease and its treatment through discussions with the child and the family; consider the child's previous experiences and any past illnesses.

### Interventions

- Foster the child's sense of mastery and development of self-esteem:
  - Give the child tasks and actively involve the child in his or her own care.
  - Encourage play so that the child can master skills and overcome fears related to the diagnosis and treatment.
  - Encourage the child to share knowledge about the condition so that he or she can appear more confident in the eyes of peers.
  - Encourage the child to participate in hobbies, sports, social events, and schoolwork that highlight his or her strengths.
  - Encourage activities that draw upon fine and gross motor skills to develop physical skills.
- Foster normalcy whenever possible:
  - Encourage the child to maintain routines and usual activities.
  - Be flexible, within reason, with the timing of treatments and tests.
  - Encourage the parents to maintain discipline and consistency in their approach to parenting.
  - Encourage parents to maintain their expectations about academic achievements in school and at home.
  - Encourage the child to maintain relationships with peers and family members.
  - Encourage the child to maintain his or her usual level of responsibility within the family.
- Foster positive peer relationships:
  - Encourage the child to maintain contact with peers through visits, involvement with social activities, phone calls, videotapes, videophone, and letters.
  - Encourage socialization with peers, including those with cancer (e.g., in camps or a playroom, shared social activities).
  - Teach the child how to cope with teasing and name calling.
- Foster the development of healthy coping:
  - Encourage play that will help the child maintain control during invasive procedures.
  - Prepare the child for procedures by explaining the sensations that he or she will feel, the reasons for them, and how they will occur; offer visual aids and strategies that the child can use to maintain self-control.
  - Help the child save face when the child loses his or her composure.
  - Praise the child for any signs of helpful behavior or positive coping.
  - Explain the cause of the disease and alleviate any feelings of responsibility and guilt the child might have.
  - Encourage open and honest communication, and serve as a role model for this behavior.
- Facilitate the child's educational endeavors:
  - Use games to teach concepts.
  - Explain new information while building upon past experiences.
  - Educate teachers and school officials about the importance of normalizing their expectations and providing tutors when they are needed.
  - Facilitate prompt reentry into school.
  - Encourage daily attendance at school.
  - Educate classmates about the child's condition and needs, dispel any myths they might have, and elicit their support.
  - Arrange for neuropsychology consultation and interventions if the child has developmental delays or is receiving neurotoxic therapies.
- Foster the child's independent functioning:
  - Avoid unnecessary restrictions.

- Encourage involvement in tasks related to the treatment and reporting of side effects.
- Encourage the parents to give the child freedom and responsibility to learn about his or her illness and its management.
- Allow the child to have control over some aspects of care.
- Offer the child choices about tasks that must be accomplished, such as receiving medication, whenever possible.
- Encourage self-care activities, such as dressing and brushing teeth.
- Encourage the child to do as much for himself or herself as possible.
- Have a physical therapist and an occupational therapist work on the child's muscle strength, mobility, and ability to perform activities of daily living as appropriate.
- Ensure that the child maintains a balance between rest and play.
- Help maintain the child's privacy.

## Expected Patient and Family Outcomes

- The outcomes of the nursing interventions are evaluated, and the plan of care is adjusted.
- The assessment is comprehensive, and reassessments are made on an ongoing basis.

# Development of Adolescents (13–18 Years)

*Linda Madsen*

## Normal Development

### Psychosocial Stage of Identity Versus Identity Confusion

The challenge for adolescents is to establish their own identity by examining and integrating their values and beliefs with those of society. Physical changes are rapid during this time; society's reactions to these changes acutely influence adolescents' self-concepts. The peer group is instrumental in helping an adolescent shape and try out future roles. The goals during this stage are to be able to start to make choices about an occupation and to form meaningful relationships outside the family. The framework is to develop values and ideologies that further the individual's future. An adolescent's overall goal is to answer the question, "Who am I?"

### Cognitive Stage

Adolescents are capable of abstract thought. They are also at the stage of formal operations, or the ability to reason and make predictions about things beyond their actual experience or knowledge. They can engage in introspection and are able to enhance the development of their values and beliefs. During this new intellectual stage in their development, they question theories and generate hypotheses.

### Emotional and Social Characteristics

Teenagers' developing independence is their key characteristic. They vacillate between dependent and independent functioning. They believe that people around them are aware of all their flaws—social, emotional, intellectual, and physical—leading them to feel embarrassed about minor issues. They are egocentric and idealistic and are careful critics of the world and people around them, seeing the world primarily from their own perspective.

The dominant focus for adolescents is to be accepted by and included in their peer group, which provides feedback about normative behavior. Their position in the peer-group structure has a great influence on their sense of self-esteem. They value conformity. An individual's physical differences may be threatening to the group.

Adolescents need privacy. Body-image issues are acutely important; teens are extremely self-conscious about changes in their bodies and feel that others are acutely aware of these changes. Body image and the way the teenager feels about body functioning and effectiveness is linked to his or her sense of worth. Developing positive self-esteem requires others' recognition and approval of one's accomplishments. Teenagers have a tendency to feel personally inadequate; at the same time, they find it difficult to admit to needing information or assistance.

Teenagers tend to focus on immediate or short-range goals and are interested in immediate gratification. They are emotionally labile because of hormonal changes. Engaging in risk-taking behavior is common among adolescents, who tend to believe that bad things "won't happen to me" (i.e., the concept of the "personal fable"). This attitude also can contribute to poor adherence to treatment.

### Fears

Teenagers fear rejection by their peers, loss of self-control, loss of identity, loss of their ability to attain future goals, and loss of previously acquired independence.

### Significant Relationships

The most significant relationships teenagers have are with their peers, adult role models, and their families.

### Risks to Teenagers with Cancer or a Blood Disorder

**Loss of control and independent functioning:** Teenagers with cancer or blood disorders have an imposed dependence upon their caregivers, which can be exacerbated if their parents tend to overprotect them.

**Devastating impact of alterations in body image or the ability to identify with peers:** Teenagers' inability to identify with their peers and be accepted as part of the group can be detrimental to their self-esteem. Among the physical changes that can occur in teens with cancer are hair loss, moon face, acne, weight gain or loss, surgical incisions, and amputation, as well as a dependence on central lines and feeding tubes. Patients with hemoglobinopathies can experience pubertal and growth delays. All of these diseases can also result in functional limitations, such as hemiparesis, joint pain or disease, or fatigue and weakness. Cognitive challenges can set the teen even farther apart from the peer group.

**Poor peer relationships due to isolation from the group:** Because of frequent absences from school and social events, teens might have too little interaction with their peers. In addition, poor self-esteem because of alterations in body image may lead a teen to avoid his or her peer group.

**Rebellion and lack of adherence to treatment or supportive care:** In their desire to be like their peers, teens may rebel and refuse to comply with their treatment or supportive care. Other factors associated with treatment nonadherence include a teenager's normal short-range focus and risk-taking behavior.

**Loss of or change in the teen's goals for the future:** Because of the rigors of therapy, permanent disability or change in body functioning, or complications of disease or treatment, teens' goals for their future may have altered. Goals also may change because they have shifted their priorities after facing a life-threatening or life-altering disease.

**Information deficits:** Information deficits can occur because of teens' characteristic inability to admit to their knowledge gaps. A large volume of information is needed for patients to successfully manage their treatment.

## Nursing Assessment and Interventions

### Assessment
- Assess current growth and developmental level.
- Determine the patient's level of success in interpersonal relationships, and evaluate key relationships through questioning and observation.
- Assess the teen's ability to speak for himself or herself and participate significantly in decision making, and assess the parents' ability to respect the teen's decisions.
- Identify key support people within the family, community, healthcare, and school settings.
- Interpret verbal and nonverbal cues about the effect of body-image changes on the patient's self-concept. Take into account the extent of the changes to the body, the patient's perspective on these changes, and the amount of interest the patient has in his or her appearance.
- Assess the patient and the family for healthy coping strategies and their level of adjustment by observing and questioning the following areas:
  - the ability to incorporate into daily life the changes imposed by the disease and treatment
  - the level of the family's involvement in the teen's care and the teen's level of independence
  - the quality of the teen's relationships and level of involvement in his or her peer group
  - the ability to establish normalcy in relationships and activities
  - the level of participation in high-risk activities
  - the teen's personal affect and level of interest and involvement in life
  - the teen's interest in, knowledge about, and involvement in managing his or her disease.
- Assess through discussion with the patient, family, and school staff the teen's ability to maintain academic performance and attendance and whether he or she has taken an interest in planning for the future.
- Assess the impact of the disease and treatment on the teen's future goals and aspirations.
- Assess the teen's level of sexual involvement and functioning to determine educational needs regarding sexuality, which should include
  - the use and importance of birth-control measures, especially when teratogenic medications and imaging are used
  - the role of heredity in reproductive decision making for patients with hemoglobinopathy and hemophilia
  - the use and importance of precautions against sexually transmitted diseases (STDs), including human immunodeficiency virus (HIV)
  - the potential effects of cancer treatment and priapism on fertility and sexual functioning in patients with sickle-cell disease.
- Assess the teen's ability to adhere to the treatment plan through ongoing dialogue about treatment and lifestyle considerations. Is he or she able to fit it into a new "normal" routine?
- Assess the patient's level of knowledge and desire for information about the disease and its treatment by having a discussion with the patient about his or her previous experience.

### Interventions
- Support the adolescent's autonomy:
  - Encourage the teen to take an active role in managing the disease.
  - Encourage caregivers to allow the teen freedom and responsibility to learn and manage as many aspects of the illness as possible but to remain involved and maintain an oversight/support role.
  - Encourage collaborative decision making with the healthcare team.
  - Allow the teen control over as many aspects of his or her care as possible.
  - Respect the teen as an individual separate from parents by addressing questions directly to him or her and providing opportunities for him or her to discuss concerns without parents being present.
- Encourage self-care and maintenance of independence:
  - Educate teen about early recognition and careful, proactive management of side effects/complications, such as pain, fatigue, and nausea, to minimize their effects on the teen's well-being.
  - Encourage the teen to do as much as possible for himself or herself.
  - Encourage the patient to accept help when he or she needs it. Emphasize that such acceptance is a sign of strength and maturity and that there are times when a problem is too difficult to solve alone.
  - Facilitate physical and occupational therapy referrals, if needed, to maintain or improve muscle strength, mobility, and the ability to perform activities of daily living.
  - Encourage the teen to break out of the "sick role" and be as involved in life as is feasible.
  - Respect the teen's wishes concerning the amount of assistance he or she needs.

- Encourage normalcy whenever possible:
  - Facilitate maintenance of routines and usual activities.
  - Be flexible with the timing of treatments and testing whenever possible.
  - Encourage parents and teachers to maintain reasonably normal performance expectations.
  - Encourage parents to maintain discipline and be consistent in their approach to parenting.
  - Encourage the teen to maintain relationships with the important people in his or her life.
- Encourage socialization and social support:
  - Foster positive peer relationships (e.g., match patients on a one-on-one basis with peers who have similar diseases or experiences).
  - Provide information about online chat rooms for teens with specific diseases.
  - Provide opportunities for socialization with other patients such as retreats, camps, common inpatient and outpatient meeting places, and social events.
  - Encourage contact with peers at home and school through phone calls, visits, letters, the Internet, and attendance at social activities when usual attendance is not possible.
  - Look past the disease and get to know the teen as an individual.
- Foster the development of healthy self-esteem by promoting a positive body image:
  - Maintain the teen's privacy.
  - Encourage activities that enhance personal hygiene and appearance.
  - Encourage the teen to get up and dressed every day, even when hospitalized.
  - Encourage the patient to prepare for hair loss by selecting attractive head coverings (e.g., wigs, hats, scarves).
  - Facilitate control of acne.
  - Encourage dress and cosmetics that minimize attention to scars, pigment changes, and weight changes.
  - Emphasize, when appropriate, the temporary nature of the changes to the body.
  - Encourage activities that focus and build on strengths.
- Support adolescent hope and coping:
  - Provide nursing care using a calm, competent approach. Facilitate the open expression of feelings, anxieties, beliefs, goals, and needs. Listen and respond honestly and be nonjudgmental. Alleviate symptoms promptly, and anticipate needs.
  - Use humor and maintain a lighthearted approach. Let the patient tease you, if appropriate.
  - Be flexible and do not hover over the teen.
  - Explore interests and aspects of their world that do not involve the illness.
  - Maintain a positive, optimistic attitude.
  - Provide hopeful stories of others in similar situations.
  - Convey genuine concern for the individual's well-being.
  - Provide opportunities for spiritual support. Honor the patient's beliefs and values.
  - Teach the teen to put his or her disease in perspective by accepting what is uncontrollable and focusing on what he or she can control. Offer a broader perspective.
  - Help develop a realistic focus and plan for the future using a goal-oriented approach. Help the teen see his or her strengths and ways in which he or she can contribute to a healthy future. Give honest, positive feedback.
  - Provide psychological preparation for invasive and disfiguring procedures. Teach relaxation and imagery techniques to help the teen cope with side effects, pain, and anxiety.
  - Model and encourage open and honest communication.
  - Normalize fears and concerns. Emphasize that a diminished sense of physical well-being is normal during treatment and complications.
  - Allow the teen time alone for self-reflection, introspection, and thought.
  - Help the teen discover the strength for coping that he or she already possesses.
  - Approach teaching and the provision of support by explaining the common concerns and feelings of people in similar situations.
  - Suggest hand-holding and other strategies that minimize anxiety and help the teen maintain control during painful procedures.
- Focus on wellness in the areas of adequate nutrition; rest and activity patterns; responsible sexual behavior; and avoidance of smoking, drinking alcohol, and using illicit drugs:
  - Explain how the individual can take control in all these areas to be as well as possible.
  - Explain that pacing one's activities and resting frequently can lessen the effects of fatigue.
  - Teach the importance of birth control and taking precautions against STDs. Educate the teen about fertility and sexual functioning as they relate to therapy and the potential short-term, late effects of therapy and complications of disease. Teach him or her about the hereditary aspects of hemoglobinopathies and hemophilia.
- Facilitate a focus on education and career issues. Show the teen how to adapt these goals when necessary.
- Encourage attendance at school, or facilitate tutoring when attendance is not feasible:
  - Assist with school accommodations as needed for disabilities or treatment.
  - Provide programming for school reentry if the teen wishes it.
- Educate the individual about the disease and treatment, including areas he or she can affect:
  - Provide multiple opportunities over the course of care for the teen to learn with staff.
  - Reinforce the importance of taking medications at home and adhering to the treatment plan. Partner with the adolescent to strategize ways to fit this into his or her daily routine.
  - Suggest books, articles, videos, and computer resources for independent learning.

- Look for signs that additional information may be needed. Clarify misinformation, dispel myths, and provide in-depth information for those who seek it.
- Encourage the teen to discuss with the healthcare team any information he or she finds independently. Some sources may be inaccurate or incomplete or may be misunderstood by the teen.
- Provide resources for learning about and writing advance directives (e.g., a living will).

### Expected Patient and Family Outcomes
- The outcomes of the interventions are evaluated, and the plan of care is adjusted.
- Comprehensive ongoing assessments are made.
- The patient achieves his or her potential developmentally despite challenges.

## Development of Young Adults (18–25 Years)

*Linda Madsen and Mary C. Hooke*

### Normal Development

#### Psychosocial Stage of Intimacy Versus Isolation
The goals of young adulthood focus on committing oneself to concrete affiliations and partnerships. This stage builds on the identity established during adolescence. The egocentrism of adolescence is replaced by reciprocity in relationships. A young adult learns to develop an intimate, interpersonal relationship in which it is possible to merge his or her identity with someone else without fear of losing the sense of self. The adolescent who does not have a secure identity will have difficulty developing intimacy in young adulthood. Relationships will remain shallow, and the young adult will experience a sense of isolation and loneliness.

#### Cognitive Development
Piaget describes formal operational thought as the ability to reason about what is possible as well as what is real. Formal operational thought includes the ability to reason about hypotheses related to objects and problems, both present and future, and to reflect on the uniqueness of one's own thoughts and perspectives. Adolescents should develop to this level, but typically they reason in egocentric and narrow ways. They may reason that the best solutions to global problems (e.g., overpopulation, pollution) are the logical ones and be unable to appreciate mitigating factors, such as world politics and culture differences. As the adolescent becomes a young adult, the quality of thought may not change, but the quantity of what is reasoned will increase.

#### Emotional and Social Characteristics
Young adults are focused on developing adult identities. They are beginning to realize their potentials and to set and work on goals. They are transitioning from the relatively egocentric focus of adolescence to a more outward focus as they realize their interdependence with society. They begin to explore their place in society and how their individuality relates to relationships with other people. Significant others—partners, spouses, friends, and family—may include their own children, coworkers, or members of the community. The ability to form intimate and caring relationships with others is key. Relationships are more mature and based on independent individuals finding connectedness, which is the foundation for deeper commitments. Initial exploration toward career goals lays the groundwork for a career.

The individual begins to strive toward financial, psychological, and physical independence and autonomous living. He or she is becoming accountable for his or her choices and the consequences of those choices. The young adult must deal with life's challenges and problems largely independently. The individual receives help only when necessary, when self-determination and resources are overwhelmed by the complexity of the challenges he or she faces.

The young adult begins to internalize morals and ideals. The goal is to be socially, physically, and intellectually competent to accomplish tasks. The well-adjusted young adult is able to maintain individuality and independence while remaining connected to the family. He or she has a sense of self-confidence and competence, character, connection to the larger world, and caring or compassion toward others. To successfully complete development, the healthy, productive young adult must
- find a valued place in a constructive group
- learn how to form close, durable human relationships
- feel worthwhile as an individual
- achieve a reliable basis for making informed choices
- know how and when to use support systems
- express constructive curiosity and exploratory behavior
- find ways to be useful to others
- believe in a promising future with real opportunities.

### Fears
The young adult facing a diagnosis or relapse of cancer may fear isolation and loneliness as well as a loss of independence (both physical and psychological), self-determination, usefulness, and future goals and aspirations. The patient may fear becoming less physically attractive or a burden to a spouse or romantic partner. The patient may worry about his or her future fertility or about children he or she already has. Educational or career plans may need to be put on hold. The necessity of maintaining employer-provided health insurance can limit career options. However, treatment can make it difficult for the patient to continue working. Treatment expenses or the loss of his or her job or supportive relationships can force the young adult to depend on his or her parents financially. Mortality comes into the young adult's reality at a time when planning for the future normally is the primary focus.

### Risks to the Young Adult with Cancer or a Blood Disorder
**Altered body image:** Altered physical appearance or body image can have a devastating impact on the young adult's ability to pursue or maintain intimate relationships. In the young adult with cancer, physical attractiveness can be affected by acne, hair loss, moon face, weight changes, surgical incisions, and loss of limb function. Patients with hemoglobinopathies may have experienced pubertal and growth delays that can affect them as young adults. Cancer and blood disorders can result in functional limitations, including fatigue, weakness, pain, and neurological changes. These

physical changes can potentially inhibit the individual's perceived or real ability to pursue romantic relationships.

**Isolation from school/work/community:** Such isolation may mean the loss of opportunities to develop relationships with others and pursue and explore career goals.

**Loss of ability to maintain or develop intimacy with significant others:** Real or perceived changes may lead to isolation. The patient may be deprived of opportunities to explore social relationships or lack the energy to do so.

**Change of goals or timeline for achieving goals:** The complications of living with cancer can cause a change in the timeline for goal achievement or a complete inability to attain previously planned goals. Goals also might change because facing a life-threatening or life-altering disease may cause a young adult to realign his or her priorities.

**Loss of independent functioning:** Perceived or necessary financial, social, or physical dependence may be overemphasized because some families tend toward overprotection.

## Nursing Assessment and Interventions

### Assessment
- Assess the patient's current growth and developmental level.
- Determine the patient's level of success in interpersonal relationships, and evaluate key relationships through questions and observation.
- Assess the extent of the patient's peer contacts and involvement in work, school, community, and outside activities.
- Assess the patient's ability to make independent decisions and the ability of the patient's parents and significant others to respect those decisions.
- Identify key support persons within the family, community, healthcare, school, and work settings.
- Interpret verbal and nonverbal cues about the effect of body-image changes on the patient's self-concept. Take into account the extent of the changes to the body, the patient's perspective on these changes, and the amount of interest the young adult has in his or her appearance.
- Assess the patient, family, and, if applicable, the significant other for healthy coping strategies and their level of adjustment by observing and questioning the following areas:
  - the ability to incorporate into daily life changes imposed by the disease and treatment
  - the level of the family's involvement in the patient's care
  - the patient's level of independence
  - the ability to establish normalcy in relationships and activities
  - the level of participation in high-risk activities
  - the young adult's personal affect and level of interest and involvement in managing his or her disease.
- Assess the young adult's ability to maintain work and/or academic performance and attendance and level of interest in planning for the future.
- Assess the impact of the disease and its treatment (including side effects and late effects) on the young adult's future goals and aspirations.
- Assess caregiving resources for patients who are responsible for their own children.
- Assess the young adult's level of sexual involvement and functioning to determine educational needs regarding sexuality, which should include
  - the use and importance of birth-control measures, especially when teratogenic medications and imaging are used
  - the use and importance of taking precautions against STDs, including HIV
  - the potential effects of cancer treatment and priapism on fertility and sexual functioning in patients with sickle-cell disease
  - the role of heredity in reproductive decision making for patients with hemoglobinopathy and hemophilia.
- Assess the young adult's ability to adhere to the treatment plan through ongoing dialogue about treatment information and lifestyle considerations.
- Assess the patient's level of knowledge and desire for information about the disease and its treatment by having a discussion with the patient about his or her previous experiences.
- Assess the patient's knowledge of advance directives.
- Assess the patient's readiness to transition to adult healthcare systems and his or her ability to act as his or her own advocate in the healthcare system.

### Interventions
- Support the young adult's autonomy:
  - Encourage the young adult to take an active role in managing the disease.
  - Transition patients who need ongoing disease management to adult healthcare providers.
  - Encourage self-advocacy and collaborative decision making with the healthcare team.
  - Allow the young adult control over as many aspects of care as possible.
  - Respect the patient's privacy, keeping discussions with him or her confidential, and share information with support persons only if the patient has given permission to do so.
- Encourage self-care and maintenance of independence:
  - Educate about early recognition and careful, proactive management of potential complications of the disease and side effects of treatment to minimize their effect on the individual's well-being.
  - Encourage the young adult to do as much for himself or herself as possible.
  - Help the patient accept help when he or she needs it. Emphasize that such acceptance is a sign of strength and maturity and that there are times when a problem is too difficult to solve alone.
  - Facilitate physical and occupational therapy referral, if needed, to maintain or improve muscle strength, mobility, and the ability to perform activities of daily living.
  - Encourage the young adult to break out of his or her role as "the sick one" and to be as involved in life as possible.
  - Respect the individual's wishes concerning the amount of assistance he or she needs.

- Encourage normalcy whenever possible:
  - Facilitate the maintenance of the patient's routines and usual activities.
  - Be flexible, whenever possible, with the timing of treatments and testing.
  - Encourage family, teachers, and colleagues to maintain reasonably normal school and work expectations.
  - Encourage the patient to maintain important relationships.
  - Encourage the patient to fulfill his or her responsibilities.
  - Encourage the young adult to care for his or her children and to obtain child care when needed.
- Encourage socialization and social support:
  - Foster positive peer relationships.
  - Provide information about online chat rooms for patients with the same disease type as the young adult.
  - Provide opportunities for socialization with other patients, such as retreats, young-adult conferences, common inpatient and outpatient meeting places, and social events.
  - Encourage contact with peers at home, work, and/or school through phone calls, visits, letters, the Internet, and attendance at social activities.
  - Facilitate the patient's ability to have time alone with his or her significant other.
- Foster the development of healthy self-esteem through a positive body image:
  - Maintain privacy.
  - Encourage activities that enhance hygiene and personal appearance.
  - Encourage the patient to get up and dressed every day, even when hospitalized.
  - Encourage activities that focus on and build strengths.
  - For the young adult with cancer
  - Encourage the patient to prepare for hair loss by selecting attractive head coverings (e.g., wigs, hats, scarves).
  - Facilitate control of acne.
  - Encourage dress and cosmetics that minimize attention to scars and changes in pigment and weight.
  - Emphasize the temporary nature of the changes to the body.
  - Support the young adult's hope and coping skills.
  - Provide nursing care using a calm, competent approach. Facilitate the open expression of feelings, anxieties, beliefs, goals, and needs. Listen and respond honestly, and be nonjudgmental. Alleviate symptoms promptly and anticipate needs.
  - Use humor and have a lighthearted approach. Let the patient tease you, if appropriate.
  - Maintain a positive, optimistic attitude.
  - Provide hopeful stories of others in similar situations.
  - Convey genuine concern for the individual's well-being.
  - Provide opportunities for spiritual support. Honor the patient's beliefs and values.
  - Teach the young adult to put the disease in perspective by accepting what is uncontrollable and focusing on what he or she can control. Offer a broader perspective.
  - Help the individual develop a realistic focus and plan for the future using a goal-oriented approach. Help the individual see his or her own strengths and how he or she can contribute to a healthy future. Give honest, positive feedback.
  - Provide psychological preparation for invasive and disfiguring procedures. Teach relaxation and imagery techniques to cope with side effects, pain, and anxiety.
  - Model and encourage open and honest communication.
  - Normalize fears and concerns. Stress that a diminished sense of physical well-being is normal during treatment.
  - Enable the patient to take time alone for self-reflection, introspection, and thought.
  - Help the young adult identify and build the strengths for coping that he or she already possesses.
  - Approach teaching and the provision of support by explaining the common concerns and feelings of people in similar situations.
  - Facilitate the use of relaxation and imagery techniques for coping with side effects, pain, and anxiety.
  - Suggest hand-holding and other strategies that minimize anxiety and help the patient maintain control during painful procedures.
- Focus on wellness, such as adequate nutrition; rest and activity patterns; responsible sexual behavior; and avoidance of smoking, alcohol, and illicit drug use:
  - Explain how the individual can take control in all of these areas to remain as healthy as possible.
  - Teach that staying active and exercising decreases fatigue.
  - Teach the importance of birth control and precautions against STDs. Educate the young adult about fertility and sexual functioning as they relate to therapy and the potential short-term and late effects of therapy and complications of disease. Teach about the hereditary aspects of hemoglobinopathies and hemophilia.
  - Facilitate a focus on education and career issues. Show how to adapt goals, when necessary.
- Encourage the patient to attend school, or facilitate tutoring when attendance is not feasible.
  - Assist the patient in obtaining the necessary documentation for work or school if medical treatment or assistance with disabilities is needed.
  - Educate the young adult about the disease and treatment, including areas he or she can affect.
  - Provide multiple opportunities over the course of treatment for the patient to learn with staff.
  - Reinforce the importance of taking oral medications at home and adhering to the treatment plan. Partner with the patient to strategize ways to fit this into the routine of life.
  - Suggest books, articles, videos, and computer resources for independent learning.
  - Look for signs that additional information may be needed. Clarify misinformation, dispel myths, and provide in-depth information for those who seek it.
  - Encourage the young adult to discuss with the healthcare team any information he or she finds independently. Some sources may be inaccurate or incomplete or may be misunderstood by the patient.

– Provide resources for learning about and writing advance directives.

## Expected Patient and Family Outcomes

- The outcomes of the interventions are evaluated, and the plan of care is adjusted.
- Comprehensive, ongoing assessments are made.
- The patient achieves his or her potential developmentally despite challenges.

# Family Systems

*Lona Roll*

## Definition

The diagnosis of cancer or chronic illness in a child or adolescent is a critical life event for the entire family. A complete assessment of the family requires a multidisciplinary approach that involves all members of the healthcare team and their evaluations of different aspects of the family's dynamics.

The Institute for Family-Centered Care (2007) recognizes that patient- and family-centered care is an innovative approach to the planning, delivery, and evaluation of health care that is grounded in mutually beneficial partnerships among patients, families, and providers. Family-centered care applies to patients of all ages and is based on the core concepts of dignity and respect, information sharing, participation, and collaboration.

The definition of family is complex and ultimately resides with the family itself. Identifying key members of the family, how they interact, and who ultimately will be responsible for the care of the child or adolescent permits the nurse to plan interventions tailored to that family's particular needs and level of comprehension. Family approaches to the presence of cancer or chronic illness in a child or adolescent vary depending on the stage of development of the illness and the degree of support that is available.

Understanding the coping strategies that family members have used in previous situations can help a nurse support the family through many challenges. Coping is a response to a stressful event that can be viewed as a process leading to a desirable outcome. Coping strategies change over time. There is no objective definition of "good coping" or "bad coping"; these strategies should be appraised in light of their outcomes.

People use coping strategies based upon their appraisal of a stressful situation. For example, some parents seek information when faced with an unknown challenge as a way of taking control of the situation. Others may find that some form of denial or avoidance helps them through a difficult situation. Problems may arise when one parent uses a coping strategy that is at odds with that of the other parent.

The research program of Knafl and Deatrick (2006) has focused on how families manage their child's serious illness as well as their family life. They have identified general issues common to all families. These include how family members define and manage their situation, the consequences they perceive for family and life, and the outcomes for individual and family functioning. The Family Management Style Framework is a tool that can be used for assessing families. In its current form, the framework uses interviews and observation skills to assess and interpret how the family is managing (Deatrick, Thibodeaux, Mooney, Schmus, Pollack, & Davey, 2006). Ogle (2006) has organized a table (see **Table 7-1**) that identifies five family-management styles with themes and subthemes that can help pediatric hematology/oncology nurses develop nursing interventions that are individualized to the strengths and management difficulties of the families for whom they care.

The family system is a dynamic, changing system. The nursing process in relation to family assessment should be used for each stage of the illness, including diagnosis, treatment, end of treatment, relapse, and terminal care. Assessment of the child and the family throughout the illness process is essential for maximizing their ability to cope and adjust.

## Nursing Assessment and Interventions

The assessments and interventions for the child with cancer are used with families whose child has a chronic hematologic illness, such as sickle-cell disease or hemophilia. The goal of this lifelong care is to maximize the child's cognitive, physical, and psychosocial potential.

### Assessment

Assessment of a family of a child diagnosed with cancer or a chronic hematologic illness is an ongoing process in which all members of the multidisciplinary team (i.e., medical, nursing, psychology, social work, child-life staff) participate.

**At the time of diagnosis:** The initial assessment at the time of diagnosis unfortunately must occur at a time when the family is undergoing a major crisis.

- Assess the following characteristics of the family:
  - family composition (i.e., who the members of the family are)
  - occupation and educational levels of family members
  - cultural and religious traditions
  - communication and interaction patterns (i.e., how members relate to each other and express their emotions)
  - decision-making and problem-solving dynamics (i.e., who makes and enforces family rules and follows through on family members' problems).
- Assess the family-management style in relation to how the parents define the child's illness, their management approach, and the consequences they perceive for the future.
- Assess family members for shock, disbelief, and fear:
  - Do family members ask for second or third opinions?
  - Do they seek medical information?
  - Do they use protective mechanisms to soften the reality of the cancer diagnosis?
- Assess for expressions of guilt and anger:
  - Family members may direct their anger at the treatment team or, many times, at those who initially informed them of the diagnosis.
  - Parents may express feelings of guilt and ask why their child has cancer, what they could have done to have caused it, and why they did not detect it earlier.
  - In the case of genetically transferred hematologic disorders, parents may feel guilty about passing the disorder on to their child.

- Assess for factors that may make it difficult for families to cope, such as having a single-parent or stepfamily structure, preexisting physical or mental health problems, economic problems, language differences, or isolation from cultural supports.

**During treatment:** The assessment of the family's adaptation to living with illness should continue during the child's treatment. The assessment should include
- the family's management style in relation to the child's living at home again after inpatient care, caring for the child, and sharing the burden of care
- the family's return to a normal routine
- the family's compliance with maintaining the child's medical regimens
- the ability of the patient's siblings to adapt to and cope with their new lifestyle.

**After cancer treatment ends:** This assessment should include the family's reaction to the end of the child's treatment routine and the family's fears about relapse in the absence of active treatment. Continue the ongoing assessment and follow-up with the patient to monitor for potential long-term effects of the cancer therapy.

**During a cancer relapse:** This period is viewed as the most difficult time for many families, because they are aware of the struggles ahead and the decreased likelihood of a patient's long-term survival. This assessment should include
- the family's need for further preparation regarding their child's possible need for more intensive chemotherapy
- the family's support system (i.e., who has proven to be a strong support for the family and can continue to help it during this very trying time).

**During end-of-life care:**
- Assess the family's coping abilities and whether they need and desire further, possibly unconventional treatment or have accepted that all further care will be terminal care.
- Determine the family's desires concerning where the child should die (i.e., at home or in a hospital) when such a choice is possible (see Section IX, "Care for the Terminally Ill Child and the Family").
- Assess the needs of the patient's siblings and extended family. For further details, see the discussion of terminal care in Section VIII, "Patient and Family Education."

## Interventions

Psychosocial interventions for the family of a child diagnosed with cancer or a chronic hematologic condition require planning and support from the entire treatment team, including professionals from the areas of medicine, nursing, psychology, social work, and child life, who must work together to develop coordinated approaches for each family.

**At the time of diagnosis:**
- Help the family meet its basic needs, including those involving sleeping arrangements, food, clothes, and care of the patient's siblings.
- Help the family interpret medical information; ideally, the primary nurse is present at the initial discussion with the family to clarify the information that is presented.
- Explain and review hospital routines and the care being given to the child.

### Table 7-1. Family Management Styles—Themes and Sub-Themes Currently Being Empirically Refined

| Conceptual Component | Theme | Family Management Styles | | | | |
|---|---|---|---|---|---|---|
| | | Thriving | Accommodating | Enduring | Struggling | Floundering |
| Defining | Child identity | Normal | Usually normal | Normal, tragic | Variable | Tragic, problem |
| | Illness view | Life goes on | Usually life goes on | Variable | Serious, hateful | |
| | Management mind-set | Confident | Mothers confident | Confident, burdensome | Mothers burdened, fathers confident | Burdensome, inadequate |
| | Parenting mutuality | Yes | Usually yes | Usually yes | Usually no | Usually no |
| Management | Parenting philosophy | Accommodative | Usually accommodative | Accommodative, protective | Usually accommodative | Usually missing, inconsistent |
| | Management approach | Proactive | Usually proactive | Usually proactive | Usually proactive | Usually reactive |
| Perceived Consequence | Difficulty managing family/illness | No | No | Variable | Usually mothers, uncommon in fathers | Usually yes |
| | Future expectations | Positive outlook: favorable illness course, diminishing impact | Usually positive outlook: favorable illness course, diminishing impact | Variable outlook regarding illness course and impact | Mothers usually negative outlook: unfavorable illness course, escalating impact; fathers usually positive outlook | Negative outlook: unfavorable illness course, escalating impact |

From "Clinical Application of Family Management Styles to Families of Children with Cancer," by S. K. Ogle, 2006, *Journal of Pediatric Oncology Nursing, 23*(1), 28–31. Copyright 2006 by SAGE Publications. Reprinted with permission.

- Encourage the parents to maintain their parenting role by comforting the child, explaining the diagnosis to him or her, and setting limits on the child's behavior as needed.
- Encourage the parents to include siblings in the family's experience; help them explain diagnoses and procedures in terms they can understand; encourage sibling visitation.
- Prepare the family for the child's transition to the home:
  - Begin early in the child's hospitalization to provide information related to the patient's eventual discharge.
  - Reassure the parents that they still are the best caregivers for their child.
  - Reassure the parents that someone from the treatment team is always available for them when they are at home.

**During treatment:**
- Continue to help the family understand the treatment protocol.
- Help the family identify the side effects of the treatment and appropriate interventions.
- Reassure the family that it is doing well in interpreting events that occur in relation to the sick child (i.e., do some hand-holding with the family).
- Help the parents reestablish their protective, nurturing role:
  - Provide opportunities for the family to work on reestablishing family life patterns, and address each family member's needs.
  - Stress the importance of the child's return to school for education, normalcy, and peer interactions.
  - Stress the importance of including siblings in discussions about the child's illness, and include them in the child's care.

**At the end of cancer treatment:**
- Prepare the parents for the transition from treatment to survival and the task of "getting on with life."
- Encourage the parents to view their child as normal. Remind them that their outlook and attitudes influence their child's self-perception.
- Review the follow-up plan and reassure the parents that the child will continue to be followed closely by the treatment team for signs of relapse or late effects of therapy.

**During a cancer relapse:**
- Provide empathy and support to family members as they adjust to the initial shock of the child's relapse.
- Provide information to the family about new treatment plans.
- Arrange assistance for family members if they must travel to another treatment center with the child for specialized care.
- Explain the meaning of relapse and new treatment options to the extended family and to other support systems.

**During end-of-life care:** See Section IX, "Care for the Terminally Ill Child and the Family," for a discussion of interventions.

## Expected Patient and Family Outcomes

- A multidisciplinary team approach is used to assess family coping and use of resources at each stage of care.
- Families are able to move through all stages of the diagnosis and treatment of the child or adolescent with cancer or a chronic hematologic illness, and their psychological-care needs are met by a multidisciplinary team.

### References

Deatrick, J. A., Thibodeaux, A. G., Mooney, K., Schmus, C., Pollack, R., & Davey, B. H. (2006). Family management style framework: A new tool with potential to assess families who have children with brain tumors. *Journal of Pediatric Oncology Nursing, 23*(1), 19–27.

Institute for Family-Centered Care. (2007). What is patient-family-centered health care? Retrieved May 25, 2008, from www.familycenteredcare.org.

Knafl, J. A., & Deatrick, J. A. (2006). Family management style and the challenge of moving from conceptualization to measurement. *Journal of Pediatric Oncology Nursing, 23*(1), 12–18.

Ogle, S. K. (2006). Clinical application of family management styles to families of children with cancer. *Journal of Pediatric Oncology Nursing, 23*(1), 28–31.

# Family Resources

*Suzanne L. Nuss*

Many childhood malignancies that were once considered fatal are now curable. Blood disorders, such as sickle-cell disease and hemophilia, that were once life limiting are now chronic diseases that require ongoing care into adulthood. Because of this, pediatric hematology/oncology patients today require nursing interventions that were not needed in the past. Prevention of acute and late effects of the disease and its treatment, maintenance of wellness in the child during and after therapy, and support of the efforts of patients' families as they cope with a chronic, life-threatening illness are major functions of nursing.

Nursing strategies for promoting the family's role as primary caregivers for the child include recognizing and accepting diverse styles of family coping, helping families recognize their strengths and methods of coping, reassuring parents that their roles are important and essential, promoting family-centered care, and communicating with local healthcare teams to offer continuity of care (Scott-Findlay & Chalmers, 2001; Walker, Wells, Heiney, & Hymovich, 2007).

It is important to stress that the patient's entire family is affected by the diagnosis of a chronic illness. Preexisting factors, such as cultural influences, employment situations, family dynamics, home environment, finances, socioeconomic situations, or support systems, affect how a family functions or copes. If any of these factors are unstable when a cancer diagnosis is made, the entire family system can break down. Nurses have a responsibility to perform a thorough assessment to determine the types of resources that a family may require to cope with the cancer experience of one of its members.

## Nursing Assessment and Interventions

### Assessment

**The home environment:** All children with cancer or blood disorders have special needs; however, those from rural areas must deal with adverse circumstances not encountered by children from urban areas, where the university-based tertiary medical centers that provide the majority of pediatric hematology/oncology care are located. Adverse circumstances include lack of tertiary health care and the need to travel long distances for treatment, necessitating the family to take on more responsibility for the child's care (Scott-Findlay & Chalmers, 2001). In response to the special needs of these children, the National Association of Children's Hospitals and Related Institutions (NACHRI) has developed recommendations for caring for children with cancer in the home setting (NACHRI Patient Care Oncology FOCUS Group, 2000). These recommendations are also applicable to children with blood disorders.

- Assess the accessibility of the child's home in relation to the child's special needs:
  - Is the home easy to enter and exit?
  - Does the home have stairs? Is the child capable of climbing stairs? Is the caregiver capable of carrying the child if the child is unable to climb stairs?
- Assess the level of cleanliness of the child's home:
  - How clean is the environment? Are there pest infestations or rodents?
  - Is there an area where Hickman-catheter care can be performed or intravenous medications can be given?
  - Does the home have running water?
- Determine the proximity of the child's home to the treatment center, and assess the family's plan for the child in an emergency situation, such as a high fever or neutropenia.
- Assess the family's transportation needs:
  - Does the family have access to a car? Is the car reliable?
  - Does the family have access to public transportation if it is needed?
  - If the patient needs to be taken to the hospital by ambulance, is the treatment center the closest hospital, or do advance arrangements need to be made with an ambulance company?
- Does the family have a telephone? If not, is there a phone nearby that can be used in an emergency?

**Finances and medical coverage:** According to Scott-Findlay and Chalmers (2001), rural families who lived long distances from the medical center experienced "great financial hardship" (p. 215) because of excessive travel to and from the tertiary care center (including fuel and car maintenance), lodging, and meals. In addition, patients who live in rural areas often are from farm families. Consequently, time away from the farm for treatments adds to the financial burdens of these families. Often there is little or no financial assistance to help families defray these additional expenses.

- Determine whether the family has medical insurance; if not, determine whether the family should be referred to a financial counselor or social worker.
- Make an assessment of possible incidental expenses the family could incur (e.g., buying meals, paying for housing near the medical center). Does the family have the funds to cover these incidental expenses?
- If the family has medical insurance, determine whether the policy covers home care; if so, determine what is covered, including the number of hours of nursing care:
  - How much must the family pay on its own before the insurance will pay all of the child's medical expenses? Does the family have the funds to cover these out-of-pocket expenses?
  - Does the family's insurance program include a prescription plan?
  - Does the insurance company require precertification for all hospital admissions? If so, who will ensure that precertification is done?

**Family dynamics:** In American society, individualism, competition, nuclear families, and an orientation toward the future are highly valued. Despite these values of the dominant culture, many diverse groups continue to maintain their ethnic self-identity, values, norms, behaviors, and language. People from diverse ethnic groups may place a higher value on the needs and traditions of the group, such as conformity, extended family, and mutual empathy. A thorough assessment of the family dynamics must be made so that the family can be supported appropriately.

- Assess the family's primary cultural influences:
  - Are there any types of restrictions?
  - Does the family's culture prevent family members from asking questions?
- Determine the parents' employment status:
  - Do the parents work?
  - Must they work for financial reasons?
  - Will the parent(s) continue to work?
  - Do they have flexible work hours?
  - Will the parents be able to leave work for emergencies?
- Assess the composition of the family constellation:
  - Who lives in the household?
  - What is the developmental stage of the family?
- Determine whether there are other children in the family and whether other family members are also receiving medical care.
- Determine the level of the parents' involvement in their children's care:
  - Are two parents living with the family, or is the child from a single-parent household?
  - If this is a single-parent family, does the parent have to work for financial reasons and medical benefits?
  - When the patient is hospitalized, who will provide care for the patient's siblings, if there are any?
- Assess various members' roles within the family structure:
  - What roles did the family members play before the cancer diagnosis?
  - Will family members' roles change as a consequence of the child's illness?
  - How will those role changes need to be renegotiated when treatment is completed?
- Determine whether the family has any spiritual concerns:
  - Does the family rely on religion, spirituality, or both?
  - Does the family have the support of the religious community to which it belongs?
- Assess the stability of the family. Does the family have any preexisting, ongoing concerns (e.g., marital difficulties, financial concerns)?

**Resources:** The coping strategies and available support systems for each patient and family vary. The way in which patients or families accept assistance also varies. The major strategies that parents use to cope with their children's illnesses include reading books about different aspects of childhood cancer, talking with a counselor during times of stress, talking with another parent whose child has cancer, and attending group meetings. Many parents also obtain information from the Internet. Caution must be advised, however, as not all of the information that is found on the Internet is accurate or reliable. Although many community-based resources are available to help patients and families with treatment, rehabilitation, and financing, patients and their families frequently are unaware of these services. A thorough assessment of the family's resources should be made.

- Determine the family's availability (i.e., are members available to learn about the child's illness and treatment).
- Assess the family's emotional capabilities (i.e., are members emotionally capable of absorbing the information).
- Establish whether there are existing support systems for the family (e.g., friends, other family members, clergy, teachers).
- Determine how much the family understands about the child's illness and treatment.
- Determine whether the family has communication barriers. Do the members of the healthcare team and the family speak the same language? If not, is an interpreter readily available?
- Ascertain whether family members have any learning disabilities that might prevent them from learning about the child's disease and its treatment.
- Determine whether the family perceives a need for support; if so, is it willing to accept support?
- Find out whether any other family members have illnesses or physical limitations. Does the primary caregiver have any medical conditions or physical limitations that might prevent him or her from caring for the patient?
- Assess the family's coping skills:
  – Has the family ever experienced a stressor of this magnitude?
  – Do family members have similar or different coping skills?

### Interventions
**The home environment:**
- Refer the family to a social worker as needed (e.g., to arrange for new housing or to arrange for use of a telephone).
- Be prepared to anticipate situations beforehand (e.g., make arrangements with a local ambulance service to take the child to the treatment center and not to the closest hospital, as some are required to do).
- Offer suggestions (e.g., if the house is not clean, suggest keeping one area clean for use when changing the dressing for a patient with a Hickman catheter).

**Finances and medical coverage:**
- Refer the family to a social worker as needed (e.g., if the family is medically indigent or needs assistance with housing and meals to be with a child hospitalized far from home).
- Provide information about organizations that offer financial assistance (e.g., Leukemia Society of America, pharmaceutical companies that may offer free medication for children in hardship situations).
- Determine who will be responsible for precertification (i.e., a family member or a nurse).

**Family dynamics:**
- Learn about the family's specific culture, including restrictions that might have an impact on health care.
- Include siblings as much as possible in teaching sessions, family meetings, and support groups.
- Be as flexible as possible, especially in accommodating the parents' work schedules.
- Offer anticipatory guidance with respect to role changes that may occur within the family.
- Include the family's religious community in providing support to the family.
- Refer the family to a social worker as needed.

**Resources:**
- Include the family's existing support systems to the extent possible.
- Use interpreters, as necessary, when a language barrier exists.
- Offer information about support groups.
- Introduce parents new to the experience of having a child with cancer to parents who have undergone a similar experience.
- Individualize plans of care to take advantage of family members' effective coping skills and to minimize any detrimental strategies.
- Offer teaching sessions as often as necessary and in different formats (e.g., group sessions, one-on-one sessions, teaching packets).
- Offer information on outside community resources.

## Expected Patient and Family Outcomes
**The home environment:**
- The home is accessible and clean.
- The family has access to a telephone, either in the home or nearby.
- A plan is in place for ambulance transportation in case of an emergency, if the child's home is not near a treatment center.
- The family has access to a car or to public transportation if the treatment center is nearby.

**Finances and medical coverage:**
- Social-services staff are involved if the family does not have medical insurance or is not eligible for Medicaid benefits.
- The family experiences minimal out-of-pocket expenses.
- The family does not become overburdened financially.

**Family dynamics:**
- The plan of care is tailored to the family's culture.
- The parents and siblings verbalize their support.
- The parents have minimal absences from work.
- All family members adjust to their role changes with minimal anxiety.
- The family's religious community is included in the plan of care.
- Social-services staff is included in the plan of care, as necessary.

**Resources:**
- The family makes use of its available resources.
- The family demonstrates an understanding of the illness and its treatment.
- The family exhibits effective coping skills and strategies.

### References
National Association of Children's Hospitals and Related Institutions (NACHRI) Patient Care Oncology FOCUS Group. (2000). Home care requirements for children and adolescents with cancer. *Journal of Pediatric Oncology Nursing, 17,* 45–49.

Scott-Findlay, S., & Chalmers, K. (2001). Rural families' perspectives on having a child with cancer. *Journal of Pediatric Oncology Nursing, 18,* 205–216.

Walker, C. L., Wells, L. M., Heiney, S. P., & Hymovich, D. P. (2007). Family-centered psychosocial care. In C. R. Baggott, K. P. Kelly, D. Fochtman, & G. V. Foley (Eds.), *Nursing care of children and adolescents with cancer* (3rd ed., pp. 365–390). Glenview, IL: Association of Pediatric Hematology/Oncology Nurses.

# Cultural Care

*Jane Hennessy*

## Definition

The rapidly increasing diversity of client populations is challenging healthcare professionals to develop a better understanding of the role that culture plays in clients' beliefs, responses, and behaviors regarding health and illness. Many misunderstandings between clients and professional healthcare providers can be attributed to the fact that each uses different culturally based concepts and reasoning processes to determine and manage health and illness states. By understanding and appreciating the impact of culture on health behavior, healthcare professionals are able to explore ways of identifying and incorporating patients' and families' belief systems about health into the plan of care in a culturally sensitive yet clinically effective manner.

The literature demonstrates the tremendous controversy that exists regarding the exact definitions of *culture, ethnicity, minority status,* and *ancestry. Culture* can be defined as "the sum total of socially inherited characteristics of a human group that comprises everything which one generation can tell, convey, or hand down to the next" (Fejos, 1959, p. 44). Endelman and Mandel (1986) define culture as learned patterns of living, including health beliefs and behaviors, that have been handed down from generation to generation. Culture also has been described as patterned ways in which humans have learned to think about and act in their world.

*Ethnicity* focuses on the cultural characteristics of a particular group and the norms, values, attitudes, and behaviors that are typical of an ethnic group and that stem from a common culture of origin transmitted across generations. Ethnicity is closely tied to culture, ethnic identity, and minority status. A person's ethnic identity is that aspect of self that includes a sense of membership in an ethnic group and the attitudes and feelings associated with that membership.

*Minority status* refers to the status of the ethnic group within the larger society. It implies less power, disproportionately low representation of group members in positions of authority and leadership, unequal social and economic position, and more experiences with prejudice and discrimination than the majority population.

*Ancestry* is defined as an individual's specific nationality, group, or country from which the person or his or her parents or ancestors resided before immigrating to the United States. It is important to recognize that although many culturally diverse groups share the characteristics of a dominant culture, they may continue to maintain their own ethnic identification, values, language, and behaviors. For example, Hispanics commonly are considered to be one ethnic group but, in fact, they represent many different countries, dialects, religions, and cultural identities.

Culture encompasses not only the concept of ethnic background, but also the many subcultures to which an individual is exposed (e.g., rural, urban, immigrant, native, laborer, professional). Likewise, cultural background cannot be viewed as being mutually exclusive of personal, familial, and social experiences when considering the framework of an individual patient's perception of health and illness.

## Demographics of Ethnic Populations

Since 1970, diversity in the racial and ethnic makeup of the U.S. population has been increasing. The 2000 census shows that the Caucasian race group remains the largest but accounts for a smaller proportion of the total population than it once did (i.e., 80.3% of the population in 1990; 75.1% in 2000). The African American population remained relatively stable; it constituted 12.1% of the population in 1990 and 12.3% in 2000. The proportion of Asians and Pacific Islanders has increased from 2.9% of the total population in 1990 to 3.8% in 2000. Alaska Native and American Indians accounted for 0.8% of the population in 1990 and 0.9% in 2000, and those claiming some other race accounted for 3.9% of the population in 1990 and 5.5% in 2000. People who declared that their ancestry includes two or more races accounted for 2.4% of the population in 2000. In 1980, the U.S. census asked people for the first time if they had Hispanic ancestry and included individuals of any racial background. Since 1980, this population has almost doubled in size—in 2000, it comprised 12.5% of the U.S. population, or 35.3 million people (Hobbs & Stoops, 2002).

## Cancer Survival and Diversity

*Healthy People 2010: Understanding and Improving Health* describes a statistical disparity in cancer deaths (U.S. Department of Health and Human Services [HHS], 2000). African Americans are more than twice as likely to die of cancer as are Pacific Islanders, Asians, Hispanics, or American Indians; they are approximately 34% more likely to die of cancer than Caucasian Americans (HHS).

It has been suggested that preventive measures such as changes in dietary habits and quitting smoking can decrease cancers by 50%. Cancer survival rates also may be increased by improving access to healthcare resources. This access can be increased by making certain that information given is appropriate linguistically and culturally and that all groups have access to both prevention and treatment options (HHS, 2000).

In December 2000, the HHS Office of Minority Health issued standards for delivering appropriate health care to people who belong to racial, cultural, linguistic, or ethnic minorities. These standards are guidelines meant to help healthcare agencies establish programs that meet the needs of the minority populations they serve. The guidelines address the need for competent interpreter services and for health agencies to monitor the changing cultural composition of the communities they serve (Shaw-Taylor, 2002). Despite the issue of these standards, the *Midcourse Review of the Healthy People 2010* found that the goals of prevention and eliminating health disparities in the control of cancer were not being met, and data have shown an increase in disparity (HHS, 2007). According to the HHS (2000), higher income, health insurance, and ongoing health care are predictive of the ability to obtain quality health care. Eleven million children in the United States are not covered by health insurance. According to the National Health Interview Survey conducted during the first three months of 2007, 41.9 million people were not insured at the time they were interviewed. Of children younger than 18 years, 8.5% were uninsured during the time of the survey, indicating a decrease in uninsured children since 1997 (Cohen & Martinez, 2007).

## Clinical Trials and Minority Groups

Minority and economically disadvantaged populations are underrepresented in national clinical trials (Hightower, 2006). Information and an understanding of the ethnic and cultural environment of these populations, as well as the barriers they face with regard to participation in clinical trials, are required if recruitment and minority-inclusion levels are to be improved.

Barriers to participation include health providers neglecting to invite the patient to the trial, physical access, and affordability (e.g., lost work time, transportation costs), as well as patient and family perceptions of health and specific attitudes toward research trials. Other barriers are fear and mistrust, insufficient recruitment efforts, consent information that has not been translated into the language used by the patient, and insufficient availability of valid and culturally appropriate questionnaires and sampling tools.

The National Institutes of Health–funded clinical trials mandate the inclusion of ample numbers of minorities. Factors that could facilitate participation include adequate information and education about the risks, benefits, costs, and required time commitment; peer-group norms that are supportive of the goals of the trials; endorsement of the goals of the clinical trials by church, cultural, or social groups and by employers; improved access to the healthcare system and specific locations where trials are being conducted; a perceived benefit to the individuals from their participation; and minimal actual cost to individuals or families with respect to time lost from work or associated transportation and child-care needs.

## Culture and the Family

The family is the basic unit of every society and the basic unit for the transmission of culture. In some cultures, the family is central; in others, it is peripheral to a greater governing body. Depending on its cultural norms, a family can act as the primary decision-making body for all of its members, or it can defer to the individual the right to decide. In American society, decision making does not rest with a single authority—sometimes it is in the hands of the individual, sometimes the family makes the decision, and at other times neither the individual nor the family has the final say. In many other societies in which the rules clearly state that the family makes the decision for the individual, there may be a designated decision maker, or consensus may be reached through family discussions. In these societies, it is rare for an outside authority to interfere in family matters.

American society is a composite of many often conflicting cultures with different values and beliefs. When different values clash in a way that may be important to society as a whole (e.g., parents who are Jehovah's Witnesses who object to a healthcare professional's decision to provide their child with a blood transfusion), the state may become the decision maker and determine which value is correct. Thus, the right to make decisions regarding their children can be taken away from parents.

Healthcare professionals who work primarily with children and adolescents must assess the strengths, culture, and structure of each family and must be aware of the role these play in healthcare decision making. A compromise must be achieved when potentially conflicting cultural beliefs exist, especially when dealing with issues of informed consent, treatment planning, and end-of-life decisions.

## Culturally Sensitive Care in Hematology/Oncology

Communication is the basis of any relationship between a healthcare professional and a patient and his or her family. Language can be a critical barrier to effective communication, but issues related to education level, income, and socioeconomic status also figure prominently.

Professionals in healthcare settings must do the following:
- Educate themselves regarding the cultural characteristics of their targeted populations.
- Identify the points of access and key leaders in the targeted ethnic communities.
- Develop institution-based programs targeted at overcoming economic and logistical barriers in these specific ethnic groups.
- Provide professional translation services that incorporate training in medical translation.

## Assessment of Culture and Perceptions of Health and Illness

Culture influences illness and health behaviors. Illness behaviors can be influenced by a culture's definition of the appropriate steps to take in seeking health care. Culture also can affect beliefs about the cause of illness, symptom presentation and interpretation, and expectations and decision making regarding treatment.

At the time of assessment, a nurse must keep in mind the beliefs and assumptions that healthcare providers bring to the workplace. Assessment can be made easier by remembering that in all cultures parents communicate with their children and respond to a child's distress. How parents communicate or answer a cry varies from culture to culture (Trawick-Smith, 2006).

## Nursing Assessment and Interventions

A cultural assessment and related interventions at the time of an initial diagnosis, during treatment planning and intervention, at relapse, and/or at the terminal phases of illness enhance overall compliance with the treatment plan and contribute to comprehensive, high-quality care.

### Assessment
**At the initial diagnosis:**
- Assess the patient's and the family's preferred pattern of communication (i.e., verbal or nonverbal) as well as their language preferences.
- Learn about the parenting and child-rearing practices of the family, and assess the impact these may have on the patient's future compliance with and adherence to the treatment plan.

- Identify potential culturally driven barriers to communication, compliance, acceptance of the diagnosis, and adherence to the treatment plan.
- Explore the family's ethnic beliefs regarding cancer and its causes and treatments.
- Assess the focus of control (e.g., is it in the hands of the individual, the medical professional, a healer, a divine power).
- Identify potential financial, transportation, or other logistical barriers that may impede care.

**During treatment planning and intervention:** Identify the primary caretaker(s) as well as the primary decision maker(s) within the family structure.

**At the time of relapse or during the terminal phases of illness:**
- Assess the child's interpretation of the pain experience in the context of cultural norms and beliefs.
- Reevaluate and document the family's beliefs and wishes regarding the rights of the child to information and inclusion in the decision-making process.
- Become familiar with ethnic-specific mourning and grieving practices, as well as with dying and burial traditions and beliefs.
- Consider the following when assessing a child's pain, evaluating its intensity, or developing treatment strategies:
  – cultural beliefs regarding demonstrating pain (i.e., emotionally or stoically)
  – cultural acceptance of medications via oral, intravenous, or invasive routes
  – the use of alternative methodologies to manage the child's pain.

### Interventions
**At the initial diagnosis:**
- Provide culturally appropriate and language-appropriate information, patient education, treatment-related information, and informed-consent materials.
- Respect the parenting and child-rearing practices of the family as much as possible.
- Discuss in detail the family's diet and nutritional practices, paying particular attention to herbal or other medicinal practices, views regarding nutrition for infants and toddlers, and beliefs regarding the relationship between diet and the causes of illnesses.

**During treatment planning and intervention:**
- Enlist the influential members of the family unit or ethnic community (e.g., religious leaders, community gatekeepers, healers) to assist the family with decision making. Arrange to have these key people at the informed-consent and treatment-planning conferences whenever it is appropriate and desired by the family.
- Discuss the family's cultural beliefs regarding the rights of children, including their right to assent and consent and to be included in making day-to-day decisions.
- Discuss with the child and the family the comfort measures and remedies they used to manage the illness prior to the diagnosis, and incorporate these practices into the treatment plan whenever possible.
- Avoid using family members as interpreters during sensitive conversations (e.g., those regarding treatment options, informed consent, end-of-life decisions). Relatives or close friends may have an unknown level of competency; violate the family's confidentiality and privacy; tend to take a protective role; or omit, change, or add valuable information.
- Encourage patients and their families to share their cultural beliefs regarding intrusive or invasive procedures.
- Recognize that patients from some ethnic groups do not trust their healthcare institutions or services for a variety of reasons (e.g., they see them as too invasive, they are unable to recognize the metaphysical or natural causes for diseases, they have fears related to the status of their U.S. residency).

**At the time of relapse or at the end of life:**
- Recognize that some patients and families may have a religiously based belief that suffering is a necessary or inevitable part of life, and they may not wish curative or palliative therapy to be administered.
- Discuss with the child and the family their beliefs regarding the use of alternative therapies; help the family distinguish between a palliative and curative intent.
- Help patients die in a manner that is consistent with their values and the way they have lived.

## Expected Patient and Family Outcomes
The patient and the family receive culturally sensitive cancer care that incorporates their cultural beliefs and values into the management plan, minimizes barriers to prompt and effective intervention, and facilitates access to state-of-the-art and research-based treatment.

### References
Cohen, R. A., & Martinez, M. E. (2007). *Health insurance coverage: Early release of estimates from the National Interview Survey.* Retrieved October 26, 2007, from www.cdc.gov/nchs/nhis.htm.

Endelman, C., & Mandel, C. (1986). *Health promotion throughout the lifespan.* St. Louis: Mosby.

Fejos, P. (1959). Man, magic, and medicine. In I. Goldstein (Ed.), *Medicine and anthropology* (pp. 46–53). New York: International University Press.

Hightower, D. (2006). Minority participation in clinical trials. *Benchmarks, 6*(4). Retrieved May 25, 2008, from www.cancer.gov/newscenter/benchmarks-vol6-issue4/page1.

Hobbs, F., & Stoops, N. (2002). *Demographic trends in the 20th century* (Census 2000 Special Reports, Series CENSR-4). Washington, DC: U.S. Government Printing Office.

Shaw-Taylor, Y. (2002). Culturally and linguistically appropriate health care for racial or ethnic minorities: Analysis of the U.S. Office of Minority Health's recommended standards [Electronic version]. *Health Policy, 62,* 211–221.

Trawick-Smith, J. (2006). *Early childhood development: A multicultural perspective* (4th ed.). Upper Saddle River, NJ: Pearson Education.

U.S. Department of Health and Human Services. (2000). *Healthy people 2010: Understanding and improving health* (2nd ed.). Washington, DC: U.S. Government Printing Office.

U.S. Department of Health and Human Services. (2007). *Midcourse review healthy people 2010.* Retrieved October 26, 2007, from www.healthypeople.gov/data/midcourse/html/default.htm.

# Spirituality

*Kristin Stegenga*

## Definition

Providing a single definition of spirituality is challenging because the experience of spirituality is deeply personal and subjective. Among the definitions offered is one by the National Cancer Institute (2006) which defines *spirituality* as "having to do with deep, often religious, feeling and beliefs, including a person's sense of peace, purpose, connection to others and beliefs about the meaning of life." It is the dimension of the self that seeks to connect with God or the divine. Assigning meaning to the experiences of life is also part of spirituality. It is present in and experienced by both adults and children. Spirituality crosses the boundaries of culture and religion and can be experienced within or without a specific culture or organized religion.

*Religion*, by contrast, is a set of beliefs, language, and rituals that are used to express spirituality in a structured format. These elements are often shared by a religious community. Members share a set of beliefs, often come together to worship, and share a spiritual life.

Children are particularly open to spirituality. They often draw upon spiritual beliefs and experiences when they experience distress. They may use their spirituality to deal with what is happening to them and may make meaning and derive comfort and resilience from this.

The diagnosis of an acute or chronic life-threatening illness is a time of crisis for both the patient and the family. Sometimes a diagnosis such as this strengthens an individual's or family's spirituality, and other times it can rock the very core of the individual's or family's beliefs.

Nurses are encouraged to assess spiritual thoughts and beliefs as part of the holistic care that they strive for in pediatric hematology/oncology practice. This assessment can help the nurse understand the needs of the patient and family within the context of the whole person. Many tools are available for assessing spirituality. One tool is FICA (**f**aith or beliefs, **i**mportance and influence, **c**ommunity, and **a**ddress), proposed by Puchalski and Romer (2000). Another tool is the HOPE questions, which assess for sources of hope, meaning, comfort, strength, personal spirituality, and organized religion, as well as several other related constructs (Anandarajah & Hight, 2001). Barnes, Plotnikoff, Fox, and Pendleton (2000) developed the Seven Questions for Learning About Connections Families and Children Make Among Spirituality, Religion, Sickness and Healing. Nurses are encouraged to further explore these and other tools to establish greater comfort with assessing for the spirituality as well as the spiritual needs of their patients.

## Nursing Assessment and Interventions

### Assessment
- Observe the patient's room for spiritual or religious articles, symbols, etc.
- Observe the patient's and family's use of prayer or other religious or spiritual rituals within the healthcare setting.
- Assess for spiritual needs at diagnosis and throughout care provision.
- Observe for behaviors that might indicate spiritual distress (e.g., hopelessness, fear, anger, loneliness, depression).

### Interventions
- Communicate respect for individual expressions of spirituality.
- Offer chaplain or other spiritual-support services.
- Refer patients or families who exhibit or express spiritual distress to hospital-support services or their own community faith leader.
- Facilitate open communication among the patient, family, medical team, and faith community as appropriate.

## Expected Patient and Family Outcomes
- The patient's symptoms of spiritual distress improve.
- The patient and the family are able to identify and claim sources of hope and strength.
- The patient and the family maintain or develop spiritual or religious practices.
- The patient and the family move from spiritual distress to spiritual equilibrium.
- A trusting relationship develops among the nurse, the patient, and the family.

## References

Anandarajah, G., & Hight, E. (2001). Spirituality and medical practice: Using the HOPE questions as a practical tool for spiritual assessment. *American Family Practice, 172,* 390–391.

Barnes, L. L., Plotnikoff, G. A., Fox, K., & Pendleton, S. (2000). Spirituality, religion, and pediatrics: Intersecting worlds of healing. *Pediatrics, 106,* 899–908.

National Cancer Institute (2006). *Spirituality in cancer care.* Retrieved October 8, 2007, from www.cancer.gov/cancertopics/pdq/supportivecare/spirituality/Patient.

Puchalski, C., & Romer, A. L. (2000). Taking a spiritual history allows clinicians to understand patients more fully. *Journal of Palliative Medicine, 3,* 129–138.

# School Reentry and Attendance

*Lauri A. Linder*

School reentry and attendance are important components of care for children and adolescents with cancer and hematologic disorders. Improved survival rates have led to placing more emphasis on promoting school reentry and attendance. Regular school attendance is an important factor in children's and adolescents' preparation for a productive future. School supports the achievement of normal tasks of growth and development not only through academic achievement but also through interactions with peers and personal development. Pediatric hematology/oncology nurses have an opportunity and a responsibility to support children and families with an outlook toward the child's future by promoting school attendance and participation.

For children and adolescents with cancer, the severity of the illness at the time of diagnosis, as well as the intensity of the treatment protocol, may limit the extent to which school attendance is possible. Many children and adolescents are unable to maintain full-time school attendance after their diagnosis and initiation of treatment. Others, such as those with brain tumors, may experience permanent disability related to their illnesses that further restricts resumption of preillness school attendance. Lack of regular school attendance places the child or adolescent at risk for falling behind in his or her classroom studies, underachievement, and lower self-esteem. Limited school attendance also results in further isolating the child from his or her peers.

Children and adolescents with hematologic disorders also face unique challenges in maintaining regular school attendance. Among children and adolescents with hemophilia, increased school absences are associated with a greater number of bleeding episodes and disease-related physical limitations. Increased absenteeism is also associated with poorer math, reading, and total achievement scores (Shapiro et al., 2001). Children and adolescents with sickle-cell disease not only are at risk for increased absenteeism related to disease-related symptoms but also are vulnerable to central-nervous-system complications arising from recurrent microinfarction and hypoxia.

Children and adolescents with cancer or hematologic disorders have as much need for and draw as much benefit from school as their healthy peers. Continuing school attendance conveys a strong message that life goes on, that there is hope, and that there are expectations for the future. School provides young people with the opportunities and resources to develop the intellectual and interpersonal skills they need to cope successfully with their illness and to function in the world. Healthcare professionals must be prepared to anticipate the social, emotional, and cognitive needs of these individuals, who most likely will grow into adulthood and become productive citizens.

For a child or adolescent with cancer, the intensity and frequency of treatments may limit full-time school attendance and participation in school-related activities. Modifications in the child's or adolescent's educational program may be indicated to foster the individual's success and ability to keep up with his or her peers. In the United States, Section 504 of the Rehabilitation Act of 1973 provides for appropriate modifications within the educational program to accommodate the special needs of children or adolescents with chronic diseases or disabilities. The scope of services offered to these children and adolescents, however, varies among states (United States Department of Health and Human Services, 2008).

Facilitating successful school reentry and/or continued attendance is a collaborative, multidisciplinary effort. Nurses first must identify other interdisciplinary team members who are or who should be involved in this endeavor. These may include education specialists, child-life specialists, social workers, psychologists, rehabilitation therapists, and neuropsychologists, as well as physicians and nurses. The child's or adolescent's teachers and other relevant school staff should be involved in preparing for the child's return. The child or adolescent along with his or her parents also should be included in any planning efforts.

Many treatment centers have developed school-reentry programs to ease the child's, or adolescent's transition back to school or to promote ongoing school attendance. Even if such programs do not exist in a patient's particular setting, nurses can still be involved in facilitating the return to school and promoting ongoing success in the classroom setting.

## Nursing Assessment and Interventions

### Assessment

When assessing a child's or adolescent's readiness for and needs related to school, nurses must consider various factors.

- Assess previous school history:
  - Has the child or adolescent attended school regularly?
  - Has the child or adolescent been absent recently due to illness or illness-related symptoms?
  - How do the child or adolescent and family view the importance and benefits of school?
  - Is the child or adolescent being home schooled?
- Anticipate the treatment schedule:
  - How long will the treatment last?
  - How frequent are treatments anticipated to be?
  - Does the treatment plan require frequent or extended hospitalizations or both?
  - How often might regular school attendance reasonably be expected?
- Assess the child or adolescent for any special learning needs related to the illness or its treatment:
  - Is there a likelihood that the child's or adolescent's illness could result in immediate or future learning difficulties?
  - Is there a likelihood that treatment, such as radiation or surgery, could cause immediate or future learning problems?
  - Would the child or adolescent benefit from baseline neuropsychological testing in anticipation of potential changes in cognitive abilities (and therefore learning abilities)?

### Interventions

Successful planning for school reentry or promoting regular school attendance depends on both medical and developmental issues. For children younger than 11 years, a large part of school involves learning to make friends and developing physical skills. Preteens and adolescents have made friends and are at the stage of seeking their friends' ongoing approval and support. Planning for the return to school must include preparing the child or adolescent and his or her classmates and friends. These efforts can be accomplished collaboratively by the nurse, a member of the psychosocial team, or both.

Implementation of an educational plan for the child's or adolescent's school is the next step in this collaborative process. Benefits of such programs include increased accuracy of knowledge regarding the medical condition and its associated treatment, decreased absenteeism, and the increased satisfaction of the child or adolescent and his or her parents. Classroom visits provide opportunities to present accurate information and to clarify misconceptions classmates may have about the impact of the illness and its treatment on their affected classmate and on themselves.

Components of successful programs have included (a) obtaining parental permission to contact the school, (b) contacting the school to communicate an interest in offering an educational program, (c) providing a session for faculty and school staff, (d) providing a session for the child's peers, and (e) providing follow-up with the child or adolescent and his or her family (Koontz, Short, Kalinyak, & Noll, 2004). When planning such sessions, the nurse should determine whether the child or adolescent wishes to participate in sessions for his or her peers. Some children and adolescents may wish to be an active part of the peer-education program and others may not. Having the child or adolescent present reinforces for children and adults alike the message of hope and the expectation of a future for the child or adolescent. An approach that combines some education about the illness with students' participation in brainstorming, problem solving, and role playing can promote the development of empathy among peers and help dispel the negative stigma and fear that often accompany an unfamiliar diagnosis.

Concrete materials can be sent before the visit for students and school staff to review, or they can be used at the time of the visit and left to review later to reinforce the content of the visit. Photos of the child or adolescent, the treatment center, and the child or adolescent with healthcare providers provide a meaningful connection between the information presented and the classmates. The Internet is another source of information and provides a means of communication between the ill child, classmates and teachers, parents, and school personnel. Other resources are available through national and local health departments and associations (see **Table 7-2**).

An instruction sheet for the teacher and other school staff can be helpful for supporting a child's or adolescent's success in attending school. Such a form can outline the treatment plan and identify special considerations, including physical limitations, and instructions for coping with commonly occurring symptoms such as fever, nausea, and fatigue, as well as exposure to chicken pox or other infectious diseases. Instructions also should include an action plan for emergencies involving central-venous-access devices. Such a plan also supports appropriate follow-up during the school year by establishing a process of ongoing communication between the school and the treatment facility. The plan also should identify a primary contact person at both the treatment center and the school. Parents should be included in this arrangement. The benefits of such a plan include increasing opportunities for early intervention if problems should arise. It also presents timely opportunities for further assessments of the child and referrals to developmental, educational, or mental-health services.

**Communicating with the classroom teacher:**
- Clarify the child's or adolescent's diagnosis and treatment as well as anticipated frequency of absences.
- Identify the need for a tutor if or when the child or adolescent is homebound or hospitalized. Check state laws and school-district policy regarding the time frame of absences and provision of tutor services. These laws and policies vary from state to state and from district to district.
- Determine whether a visit to the class by representatives from the treatment facility is feasible.
- Identify the child's or adolescent's daily or weekly school schedule so that medical appointments can be planned with the least amount of interruption in school attendance.

**Coordinating the classroom visit:**
- Identify representatives from the healthcare institution who can visit the classroom, and schedule a visit.
- Communicate any potential medical or psychosocial issues with the appropriate school staff (e.g., school nurse, counselor) to identify and solve potential problems associated with school reentry and/or continued attendance.
- Notify the family about the scheduled date and time of the visit.

**Preparing the child or adolescent and the family:**
- Solicit the child's or adolescent's input into the content of the school visit and the extent to which he or she wishes to participate.

### Table 7-2. Educational Resources for Families

| Resources | Title | Contact |
|---|---|---|
| Organizations | Learning Disabilities Association of America | www.ldanatl.org |
| | Surviving and Moving Forward: The SAMFund for Young Adult Survivors of Cancer | www.thesamfund.org |
| Publications | Cancervive Parent's and Teacher's Guide for Kids with Cancer | www.cancervive.org |
| | Educating the Child with Cancer: A Guide for Parents and Teachers | www.candlelighters.org |
| | The Jester Lost His Jingle | Jester Books |
| | Learning & Living with Cancer: Advocating for Your Child's Educational Needs | The Leukemia and Lymphoma Society, www.lls.org |
| | Our Child Has Cancer: What Do We Do About School? | 602/300-0831 |
| | What Is Cancer Anyway: Explaining Cancer to Children of all Ages | Published by Dragonfly |
| Puppet Program | The Kids on the Block Puppets | The Kids on the Block, Inc., 800/368-KIDS (5437), www.kotb.com |
| Videos | "Back to School: Teens Prepare for School Re-Entry" | www.starbright.org |
| | "Emily's Story: Back to School After Cancer" | www.cancervive.org |
| | "Making the Grade: Back to School After Cancer" | www.cancervive.org |
| | "Why, Charlie Brown, Why?" | No longer being produced. Many major treatment centers may have copies. |

- Help the child or adolescent identify current and potential concerns related to being at school.
- Consider role playing the actual entrance into the classroom on the first day back to help promote a sense of readiness and confidence.
- Identify the siblings' concerns and the possible need for a visit to their classrooms.
- Acknowledge the parents' fears and concerns about their child's attendance at school.

## Expected Patient, Family, and School Outcomes

- The nurse coordinates a plan with the child or adolescent, the parents, and school staff for assessing the effectiveness of the intervention.
- The child or adolescent and his or her family provide anecdotal reports during routine medical visits, reporting not only their response to initial school reentry but also their perceptions of the ongoing adjustment of the child or adolescent and his or her peers.
- School staff inquire whether the child has been ridiculed or teased by peers and how involved and welcome the child or adolescent feels at school.
- Appropriate school staff are able to answer questions that may arise from peers about the chronic nature of the child's or adolescent's illness, physical appearance, or stamina, even if he or she has been back at school for a long time.
- The child's or adolescent's healthcare team helps the parents if they report new anxieties or if the child's medical condition changes and affects school performance and peer relationships.
- The child's or adolescent's parents note positive outcomes of school attendance.
- The child's or adolescent's teachers and classmates provide feedback regarding the school-education program. This can be elicited by means of a written evaluation tool that includes basic questions about their level of understanding of the illness before and after the child's or adolescent's return, their comfort level with the student, and classmates' willingness to maintain normal peer relationships with the child or adolescent.
- The child or adolescent, peers, and teachers report feeling able to engage in what they consider to be a normal way of functioning within the school setting; this is a likely indicator of the effectiveness of the school intervention.

### References

Koontz, K., Short, A. D., Kalinyak, K., & Noll, R. B. (2004). A randomized, controlled pilot trial of a school intervention for children with sickle cell anemia, *Journal of Pediatric Psychology, 29,* 7–17.

Shapiro, A. D., Donfield, S. M., Lynn, H. S., Cool, V. A., Stehbens, J. A., Hunsverger, S. L., et al. (2001). Defining the impact of hemophilia: The academic achievement in children with hemophilia study. *Pediatrics, 108,* e105.

United States Department of Health and Human Services. (2008). Your rights under section 504 of the Rehabilitation Act. Retrieved May 25, 2008, from www.hhs.gov/ocr/504.html.

# Professional Nurse-Patient Relationships

*Cynthia Walsh*

## Definitions

Professional boundaries are defined as "the space between the nurse's power and the patient's vulnerability" (National Council of State Boards of Nursing, Inc., 2007, p. 3). The ethic of caring must be considered when discussing professional relationships. A caring relationship involves two members—one caring and the one cared for (Noddings, 2003). In pediatric hematology/oncology nursing, the one caring is the registered nurse and the one cared for is the patient and the family. Mayeroff (1990) defines *caring*: "To care for another person, in the most significant sense, is to help him grow and actualize himself" (p. 1). This definition is the basis of any nurse-patient relationship. It is each nurse's role and responsibility to ensure that the patient and the family become independent from, not dependent on, the healthcare team.

Caring relationships carry risks. The caregiver can feel overwhelmed with the responsibilities, duties, and tasks related to the caring relationship. The nurse has so much information, comfort, and trust from and about the family, he or she may feel extremely burdened. Through their close relationship with the nurse, patients and families may become dependent on him or her, asking opinions about treatment, cure rates, other staff, or their personal life. This overwhelming dependence may result in the nurse ceasing to care for the patient and instead becoming the object of care by the patient and family (Noddings, 2003). In the specialty of hematology/oncology, the continual contact and care the patient and the family receive throughout treatment places the nurse at risk for crossing boundaries that cause families to develop dependence on the healthcare staff rather than to develop independence from them.

## The Nurse-Patient Relationship

The American Nurses Association (2001) position on professional boundaries states, "When acting within one's role as a professional, the nurse recognizes and maintains boundaries that establish appropriate limits to relationships." Boundary-continuum issues can include giving or receiving gifts from patients or families, buying groceries for a hospital-bound family, sharing the details of one's personal life with patients and families, or participating in outside social contacts with former patients or their relatives, among others. Interpretations of boundary issues are expanding in the media, state nursing-practice acts, and in courts of law. Although it is rare, nurses who commit boundary violations may face the loss of licensure or other penalties.

The desire to help others in need paired with the demands of patients and families who require help and caring sets up the entire relationship and situation for complicated problems and potentially harmful boundaries. Nursing education often provides limited opportunities for developing practical skills for dealing with day-to-day situations involving patients and families. Expert nurses must invest their time, talent, and expertise with novice nurses and assist them to become professionals with strong skill sets, which include the nurse-patient-relationship part of nursing. With thorough self-assessment and education, many of these confusing and/or harmful situations can be avoided.

The daily nature of hematology/oncology nursing places nurses in emotional, intimate, stressful, and potentially life-threatening situations. Nurses are caring and compassionate and want to alleviate the suffering that comes with illness. Often in the hematology/oncology nursing specialty, this suffering is not easily avoided or resolved, which is difficult for the patient, family, and professional caregivers. Hematology/oncology diagnoses and the sequelae that accompany them often are the most difficult times of patients' and families' lives. Such situations provide opportunities for professional nurses to have a positive impact on the patient and family. The opportunity lies in empowering the patient and the family to become independent from the healthcare team and not to depend on the nursing and medical staff. This is the primary goal for all professional relationships, regardless of the situation or intent. Again, it is the responsibility of the professional nurse to ensure that the patient and the family feel safe and protected.

## Interpersonal Caring Relationships

Noddings (2003) theorizes that all interpersonal relationships are divided into three different levels that reflect specific degrees of caring for each group. The levels highlight the importance of relationships and the appropriateness of actions taken by each member of the caring relationship.

- First and center level—intimate people in our lives, such as family and friends. We care for this group because we love them. These are the important relationships in our lives.
- Second and middle level—people in our lives for whom we hold personal regard. These relationships are much less intimate and include caring for acquaintances, neighbors, and coworkers.
- Third and outside level—people we have not met before. Ethically and professionally, the nurse is required to care for hospitalized patients and families from this level.

## Key Principles for Protecting the Nurse-Patient/Family Relationship

The College & Association of Registered Nurses of Alberta (2005) identifies key principles involved in nurse-patient/family relationships:

- Patients and families seeking health care are vulnerable.
- The obligation to maintain healthy professional boundaries lies with every registered nurse. Social relationships are not therapeutic ones. Personal, social relationships do not promise healing benefit and are not guided by professional nursing standards or codes of ethics.
- The registered nurse's prior personal relationship with a patient and family or their significant others must not infringe on meeting the patient's therapeutic needs.
- Romantic or sexually intimate relationships are never appropriate during the course of a therapeutic professional relationship with the patient or any of his or her family members.
- Personal relationships with former patients and families must be justified to maintain the public's need for trust in nursing as a profession.

## Nurse's Self-Assessment and Interventions
### Self-Assessment

In the paper *Professional Boundaries for Registered Nurses: Guidelines for the Nurse-Client Relationship*, the College & Association of Registered Nurses of Alberta (2005) discusses the responsibility of the professional nurse to maintain the professional relationship and identified differences between professional and nonprofessional relationships (see **Table 7-3**).

### Table 7-3. Differences Between Professional and Nonprofessional Relationships

| Characteristics of Relationship | Professional Boundaries (nurse-patient) | Nonprofessional (casual, friendship) |
|---|---|---|
| Remuneration | Nurse paid to provide care | No payment for relationship |
| Length of relationship | Time-limited for the length of the patient's need for nursing care | May last a lifetime |
| Location of relationship | Place defined and limited to where nursing care is provided | Place unlimited and undefined |
| Purpose of relationship | Goal-directed to provide care to the patient and family | Pleasing, interest-directed |
| Structure of relationship | For nurse to provide care to the patient and family | Spontaneous, unstructured |
| Power balance | Unequal power—nurse has power due to authority, knowledge, influence, and access to privileged information about the patient and family | Relatively equal |
| Responsibility for the relationship | Nurse is responsible for establishing and maintaining professional relationship, not the patient and family | Equal responsibility to establish and maintain relationship |
| Preparation for the relationship | Nurse is required to have formal knowledge, preparation, orientation, and training | Does not require formal knowledge, preparation, orientation, and training |
| Time spent in relationship | Nurse employed by contractual agreement that outlines hours of work for contact between the nurse and the patient and family | Personal choice for how much time is spent in relationship |

From *Professional Boundaries for Registered Nurses: Guidelines for the Nurse-Client Relationship*, by The College and Association of Registered Nurses of Alberta, 2005, Edmonton, Alberta: Author. Copyright 2005 by The College and Association of Registered Nurses of Alberta. Adapted with permission.

**Self-assessment for boundary crossings and boundary violations:** Boundary crossings are inadvertent actions taken to meet a therapeutic need and result in a return to professional boundaries. Boundary violations cause confusion between the needs of the nurse and those of the patient and the family. The outcome of the violation benefits the nurse at the expense of the patient and the family.

The discussion of nurse-patient, caring, and interpersonal relationships provides a basis for the definition and delineation of professional boundaries. The list that follows allows nurses to examine their day-to-day actions and reflect on the meaning and purpose of their behaviors. If one of these crossings or violations is noted, a high potential exists for other crossings or violations to develop as the nurse becomes more familiar and comfortable with the patients and families with whom he or she works:

- frequently thinking of the patient and the family when away from work
- frequently planning other patients' and families' care around the patient's needs
- spending free time with the patient and the family
- sharing personal information or work concerns with the patient and the family
- feeling responsible if the patient's progress is limited
- engaging in more physical touching than is appropriate
- favoring one patient's care at the expense of another
- keeping secrets with the patient and the family
- selectively reporting the patient's and family's behavior
- swapping patient assignments
- communicating in a guarded and defensive manner when questioned regarding interactions or relationships with a patient and/or family
- receiving gifts from or having continued contact or communication with the patient after discharge
- denying the fact that the patient is a patient
- acting and/or feeling possessive about the patient and or family
- giving attention or treatment to one patient and family that differs from that given to other patients and families
- denying having crossed the boundary from a therapeutic and professional relationship to a nontherapeutic, nonprofessional relationship
- seeing the patient and/or family for an out-of-hospital gathering when no other staff are present
- inappropriately discussing personal problems that should be referred to another health practitioner
- believing that only the nurse understands the patient and/or the family
- the patient and/or family demonstrates an obvious preference for a particular nurse.

Boundary situations are often complex and can be difficult to define, outline, and sometimes maintain on a professional plane. The Registered Nurses' Association of Ontario (2006) outlines five areas in which boundaries may become blurred and cause problems for professional nurses, colleagues, patients, and/or families:

- self-disclosure
- giving or receiving gifts
- dual or overlapping relationships
- developing friendships
- physical contact.

## Types of Boundary Crossings

There are several categories of boundary crossings that are not widely recognized as such but are nevertheless important to consider.

**Self-Disclosure:** Self-disclosure leads to the development of friendships and/or dual relationships with patients and families. These relationships may pressure each person in the relationship to give or receive things such as gifts, money, or physical contact.

**Language:** In the role of caregiver, nurses tend to use terms of endearment with patients and sometimes with families. Terms of endearment may include *dear, sweetheart, honey,* and others. In any nonintimate situation, such terms are demeaning, disrespectful, and potentially offensive. As noted in Table 7-3, there are differences between professional and nonprofessional relationships. The nurse is paid to care for the patient and family. Nonprofessional relationships are clearly social in nature and allow the use of intimate titles and terms of endearment. The nurse is the responsible party in the relationship, even regarding language. Registered nurses must be respectful of each patient and family member and call each one by name. Terms of endearment are reserved for people intimately involved with the patient, not people who are virtual strangers to them.

**Physical touch:** The same concept applies to physical contact with a patient, family member, or visitor. Physical contact includes sitting on a patient's bed, looking at dressings or incisions without first warning the patient, or performing procedures that place the patient in a vulnerable position without appropriate draping. Nurses may be very comfortable in others' space; it is the nature of the job. However, many people are not comfortable with touching, hugging, and other crossings into their personal space, especially when the situation involves strangers. Often there is no knowledge of experiences with physical touch, good or bad. It is important to ask permission before sitting on a patient's bed, giving him or her a hug, or touching him or her.

## Interventions

**Consider factors in self-disclosure:** Because of the intimate degree of care and the time spent with hematology/oncology patients and families, nurses may consider sharing intimate and personal moments of their own lives with patients and families. Nurses who disclose information about their personal lives should consider the following:

- Whose needs does the disclosure meet (i.e., nurse versus patient and/or family)?
- How will the information shared be perceived?
- The purpose or intended impact of the disclosure
- Whether the disclosure could potentially shift the focus from the family to the nurse (focus can include emotions such as sadness, empathy, or anger)
- The impact the disclosure has on the nurse-patient relationship.

**Identify family strengths:** This involves shifting the focus from a family's limitations to its strengths and placing emphasis on the support that exists. The healthcare team often may misunderstand unconventional family situations. Occasionally, the beliefs of the nurse and healthcare team may not agree with or support family systems or circumstances. Each member of the healthcare team must accept living and family situations as they are. The situation is what the patient has, and it is the job of the healthcare team to empower and assist the family in providing the best care possible for the patient.

**Develop neutrality:** Neutrality is the ability to connect with all individuals in an equally caring and professional manner. In nurse-patient relationships, the nurse should aim to meet each individual where he or she is and recognize strengths in an effort to empower each member of the family as well as the family as a whole.

**Think before acting:** Thinking through the larger implications of an action, such as giving or receiving gifts, is a necessary and important component of establishing and maintaining professional relationships.

## Self-Care Interventions for the Nurse

**Be your own best friend:** Do things that nurture your feelings of self-acceptance and improve your self-esteem. The little voice in your head that gives you feedback can be either a cheerleader or your worst critic.

**Find time to be alone:** In a profession defined by doing for others, it is not uncommon to be "othered" out. Schedule a solitary activity or other activities that rejuvenate your mind, body, and soul.

**Take time off:** Time off allows people to renew and strengthen the interpersonal relationships that give life meaning. Leave work at work and embrace the relationships that make you whole and happy.

**Build loving personal relationships:** Talk about and meet your personal-relationship needs outside the work setting, and seek professional help if you feel particularly vulnerable. Nurses who seek a balance between their personal priorities and their professional obligations find their work more satisfying and are more effective on the job.

**Acknowledge your feelings:** Feelings of grief, failure, and disappointment are inevitable in the practice of nursing. Denying these normal human reactions can lead to problems. Find a safe, comfortable way to share your feelings. Professionals who reach out to their colleagues strengthen their own sense of humanness, which helps maintain a healthy bond to the role of caregiver and can stave off burnout.

**Learn to say no and still feel good:** The tendency to please everyone by always saying yes ultimately leads to taking on the impossible. When you say yes and really mean no, anger and resentment can build to self-destructive levels. Return to your life priorities and values and determine whether saying yes really fits. If it does not, saying no can build your sense of self-esteem and sense of personal freedom.

**Avoid overworking, and leave your work at the office, hospital, or clinic:** The nurse's other roles—father, mother, neighbor, community member, friend, significant other, daughter, or son—enhance his or her personal growth and effectiveness. Allowing work to overshadow the other roles can lead to one-dimensional relationships and, ultimately, to becoming an isolated, lonely, incomplete human being. Nurses find great rewards when they learn to delegate appropriately and set limits with patients and colleagues.

**Providing terminal care to a dying child:** As a pediatric hematology/oncology nurse, knowing what to do or say to meet the changing needs of terminally ill patients comes from knowledge of the patient, the family, their experience with cancer, and their needs while approaching death. It involves being fully present as a source of validation, education, comfort, and support during life's most difficult transition.

The death of a child not only affects the nurse's emotions but also can transform his or her practice. Nurses who work with children who die need to find meaning in their work that helps resolve their grief. Self-care on the nurse's part is vital during times when he or she is caring for a dying child.

**Strategies for the nurse dealing with grief issues:**
- Recognize that symbols and rituals surrounding death are important for achieving an understanding and acceptance of death as a part of the life cycle.
- Seek meaning in the circumstance of the death (e.g., the child has been freed from suffering).
- Apply knowledge, particularly that gained through past positive experiences in dealing with death; knowledge of human responses to stressful circumstances also is empowering.
- Recognize personal limits and the need for taking breaks.
- Be honest about the dying process with both the patient and the family.
- Spend time with the patient by listening, educating, and comforting him or her during vulnerable moments.
- Share feelings involving grief with colleagues and healthcare providers.
- Continue to utilize the multidisciplinary specialties of chaplaincy, child life, social work, and psychology.
- Each of the aforementioned specialties has specific training and skills that can help the patient and the family through an emotionally and physically painful process. Good self-care and professional behavior involve all members of the team, not just some.

## Expected Patient and Family Outcomes

- The patient and the family feel empowered when engaged in making healthcare decisions.
- The patient and the family develop a relationship that is independent from the healthcare team.
- The family maintains or builds a connection with the community to further foster its independence, accountability, and overall support and to help to meet its long-term needs.

## Expected Nursing Outcomes

- The nurse has increased confidence in his or her competence, specifically in relation to communication skills and interpersonal relationships.
- The nurse experiences job satisfaction and shows a decreased tendency to burn out.
- The nurse feels empowered by assisting families to become independent and able to handle the complex needs of the patient.

## Examples of Nurse-Patient Relationships

### Crossed Boundary

Lilly, a registered nurse, is caring for Adam, a 14-year-old patient with acute myeloid leukemia. Lilly works the evening shift and arrives at work on a beautiful spring day. Lilly takes care of Adam a lot and is familiar with his care. Walking into his room, Lilly begins to tell Adam and his mom about her day. Having earlier attended her daughter's soccer game, Lilly gives Adam and his mom details of the game. "My daughter scored three goals and was named the most valuable player of the game! My son, who runs track, won three races at his track meet yesterday." Adam and his mom don't ask any more questions, and Lilly goes on with her work.

While this interaction seems relatively benign, it may be tremendously upsetting and discouraging to both Adam and his mom. Lilly doesn't know that Adam is a star soccer player, and he has not been able to practice or play for 3 months. Adam had hoped to play soccer in college, but he now doubts that possibility and starts to grieve the loss of who he used to be and how he had identified himself.

### Gift Giving

Mitch, an experienced nurse, works the night shift on a busy hematology/oncology unit. Toni, a 4-year-old girl with sickle-cell disease, has been hospitalized with pain crises four times during the past 2 months. Toni's home situation is chaotic and busy. She has three older brothers. Between their work schedules and their other children, Toni's parents are not able to be with her in the hospital very often. Each time Toni arrives at the hospital, she does not have a change of clothes or toys. Mitch cares for Toni during most of his shifts and spends a lot of time with her, especially before she goes to sleep at night.

Mitch feels sad for Toni, so he and his wife go shopping for some clothes and toys for Toni to try to make her stay more comfortable. Toni is ready for discharge and her mom comes to pick her up. Toni's mom questions the clothing and toys she has acquired. Toni tells her mom that Mitch brought them for her. The day nurse, Ann, who also cares for Toni a lot, has spent the week feeling left out and unappreciated by Toni, who states "Mitch is my favorite nurse, he brings me all kinds of things and makes me feel special." Toni's mom is clearly upset with Mitch and states, "Don't you think we can provide clothes and toys for our child? I am very upset with this gesture, and I don't want any of these things."

This situation has several elements. Mitch projected onto Toni his ideas of what she needed, discussed her situation with his wife, and insulted Toni's parents by bringing presents and gifts for her. Ann has growing feelings of negativity and dislike for Mitch, as this is not the first time he has crossed this boundary. Giving gifts to patients often "cements" his status as several patients' "favorite nurse."

Regarding the reverse of the aforementioned example, if patients and families feel strongly about giving gifts to individual nurses, it is the nurse's responsibility to suggest that they make a donation to the hospital foundation, for example, so that everyone can benefit from their generosity. In this changing and culturally diverse world, it is often customary for some cultures to show gratitude through gift giving. As long as the gift is nominal, it might be rude or unacceptable to refuse it. In situations such as this, the professional nurse must use his or her best judgment.

### An Unintended Dependent Relationship

Tommy is a 10-year-old patient with hemophilia who is developmentally delayed and has a factor inhibitor. Tommy's dad spends the nights with him but needs to work during the day. Joan is a consistent caregiver for Tommy and they work well together. Joan and Tommy have come up with a "special" way for him to take his oral medications. Tommy takes a bite of chocolate pudding, puts the pills in his mouth, and takes a drink of milk. Joan tells Tommy this is "their" way to take medicine. Joan spends a lot of time with Tommy during her shift, and soon Tommy refuses to take his medications for anyone else. Joan doesn't share information with other staff about his medication-taking style. Two days before discharge, Tommy's dad stays a little later at the hospital before going to work. A different nurse, Amy, takes Tommy's medications to his room. Tommy refuses to take his medications for either his dad or Amy, stating he will only take them for Joan.

The impact of this situation may have a terrible effect on Tommy and his family as well as on Joan. Joan may feel overburdened and overwhelmed by being the only one for whom Tommy will take his medications. Tommy's parents have lost all faith and trust in the hospital and staff and feel as if something happened to steer him away from them and their support.

In this situation, Joan should have put her ideas into Tommy's care plan and ensured that it was easy for everyone to follow. The consistency between the actions and behaviors of the nursing staff would have made for a seamless transition back to home for Tommy and his family.

## References

American Nurses Association. (2001). *Code of ethics for nurses with interpretive statements*. Retrieved May 25, 2008, from http://nursingworld.org/ethics/code/protected_nwcoe813.htm.

College & Association of Registered Nurses of Alberta. (2005). *Professional boundaries for registered nurses: Guidelines for the nurse-client relationship*. Retrieved May 25, 2008, from www.nurses.ab.ca/Carna-Admin/Uploads/Professional%20Boundaries%20Guidelines.pdf.

Mayeroff, M. (1990). *On caring*. New York: Harper Collins.

National Council of State Boards of Nursing, Inc. (2007). *Professional boundaries: A nurse's guide to the importance of appropriate professional boundaries*. Retrieved May 25, 2008, from www.ncsbn.org/ProfessionalBoundariesbrochure.pdf.

Noddings, N. (2003). (2nd Ed.). *Caring: A feminine approach to ethics and moral education*. Berkeley, CA: University of California Press.

Registered Nurses' Association of Ontario. (2006). *Nursing best practice guideline: Establishing therapeutic relationships*. Toronto, Canada: Author.

# Bibliography

**Development of Infants, Toddlers, Preschoolers, School-Age Children, Adolescents, and Young Adults**

Decker, C., Phillips, C. R., & Haase, J. E. (2004). Information needs of adolescents with cancer. *Journal of Pediatric Oncology Nursing, 21*(6), 327–334.

Haluska, H. B., Jessee, P. O., & Nagy, M. C. (2002). Sources of social support: Adolescents with cancer. *Oncology Nursing Forum, 29,* 1317–1324.

Hinds, P. S. (2000). Fostering coping by adolescents with newly diagnosed cancer. *Seminars in Oncology Nursing, 16*(4), 317–327.

Hinds, P. S., Martin, J., & Vogel, R. J. (1987). Nursing strategies to influence adolescent hopefulness during oncologic illness. *Journal of Pediatric Oncology Nursing, 14,* 22.

Lahteenmaki, P. M., Huostila, J., Hinkka, S., & Salmi, T. T. (2002). Childhood cancer patients at school. *European Journal of Cancer, 38,* 1227–1240.

Leondari, A., & Kiosseoglou, G. (2000). The relationship of parental attachment and psychological separation to the psychological functioning of young adults. *The Journal of Social Psychology, 140,* 451–464.

Miles, M. S., & Holditch-Davis, D. (2003). Enhancing nursing research with children and families using a developmental science perspective. *Annual Review of Nursing Research, 2,* 1–20.

Noll, R. B., Reiter-Purtill, J., Vannatta, K., Gerhardt, C. A., & Short, A. (2007). Peer relationships and emotional well-being of children with sickle cell disease: A controlled replication. *Child Neuropsychology, 13*(2), 173–187.

## Family Systems

Hersh, S., & Weimer, L. (2002). Psychiatric and psychological support for the child and family. In P. A. Pizzo & D. G. Poplack (Eds.), *Principles and practice of pediatric oncology* (4th ed., pp. 1365–1391). Philadelphia: Lippincott Williams & Wilkins.

Walker, C. L., Wells, L. M., Heiney, S. P., & Hymovich, D. P. (2007). Family-centered psychosocial care. In C. R. Baggott, K. P. Kelly, D. Fochtman, & G. V. Foley (Eds.), *Nursing care of children and adolescents with cancer* (3rd ed., pp. 365–390). Glenview, IL: Association of Pediatric Hematology/Oncology Nurses.

## Family Resources

Brody, A. C., & Simmons, L. A. (2007). Family resiliency during childhood cancer: The father's perspective. *Journal of Pediatric Oncology Nursing, 24*(3), 152–165.

Clarke, J. N. (2006). Advocacy: Essential work for mothers of children living with cancer. *Journal of Psychosocial Oncology, 24*(2), 31–47.

Clarke, J. N., Fletcher, P. C., & Schneider, M. A. (2005). Mothers' home health care work when their children have cancer. *Journal of Pediatric Oncology Nursing, 22*(6), 365–373.

Frierdich, S., Goes, C., & Dadd, G. (2003). Community and home care services provided to children with cancer: A report from the Children's Oncology Group nursing committee-clinical practice group. *Journal of Pediatric Oncology Nursing, 20*(5), 252–259.

Goodenough, B., Forman, T., Suneson, J., & Cohn, R. J. (2004). Change in family income as a correlate for use of social work services: An Australian study in pediatric oncology. *Journal of Psychosocial Oncology, 22*(2), 57–73.

Labay, L. E., Mayans, S., & Harris, M. B. (2004). Integrating the child into home and community following completion of cancer treatment. *Journal of Pediatric Oncology Nursing, 21*(3), 165–169.

Murray, J. S. (2002). A qualitative exploration of psychosocial support for siblings of children with cancer. *Journal of Pediatric Nursing, 17*(5), 327–337.

Nolbris, M., Enskär, K., & Hellstrom, A. L. (2007). Experience of siblings of children treated for cancer. *European Journal of Oncology Nursing, 11*(2), 106–112.

Stevens, B., Croxford, R., McKeever, P., Yamada, J., Booth, M., Daub, S., et al. (2006). Hospital and home chemotherapy for children with leukemia: A randomized cross-over study. *Pediatric Blood and Cancer, 47*(3), 285–292.

Stevens, B., McKeever, P., Law, M. D., Booth, M., Greenberg, M., Daub, S., et al. (2006). Children receiving chemotherapy at home: Perceptions of children and parents. *Journal of Pediatric Oncology Nursing, 28*(5), 276–285.

Sung, L., Feldman, B. M., Schwamborn, G., Paczesny, D., Cochrane, S., Greenberg, M. L., et al. (2004). Inpatient versus outpatient management of low-risk pediatric febrile neutropenia: Measuring parents' and healthcare professionals' preference. *Journal of Clinical Oncology, 22*(19), 3922–3929.

## Cultural Care

Spector, R. (2004). *Cultural diversity in health and illness.* (4th ed.). Upper Saddle River, NJ: Prentice Hall.

Thibodeaux, A., & Deatrick, J. (2007). Cultural influence on family management of children with cancer. *Journal of Pediatric Oncology Nursing, 24*(4), 227–233.

## School Reentry and Attendance

American Academy of Pediatrics Council on Children with Disabilities. (2007). Provision of educationally related services for children and adolescents with chronic diseases and disabling conditions. *Pediatrics, 119,* 1218–1223.

Cabat, T., & Shafer, K. (2002). Resources for facilitating back to school programs. *Cancer Practice, 10,* 105–108.

Day, S., & Chismark, E. (2006). The cognitive and academic impact of sickle cell disease. *The Journal of School Nursing, 22,* 330–335.

Eiser, C., & Vance, Y. H. (2002). Implications of cancer for school attendance and behavior. *Medical and Pediatric Oncology, 38,* 317–319.

Gradowski, M. (2002). The student with hemophilia. *Hemaware, 7,* 66–68.

Msall, M. E., Avery, R. C., Tremont, M. R., Lima, J. C., Rogers, M. L., & Hogan, D. P. (2003). Functional disability and school activity limitations in 41,300 school-age children: Relationship to medical impairments. *Pediatrics, 111,* 548–553.

Taras, H., & Potts-Datema, W. (2005). Chronic health conditions and student performance at school. *Journal of School Health, 75,* 255–266.

Upton, P., & Eiser, C. (2006). School experiences after treatment for a brain tumour. *Child: Care, Health, and Development, 32,* 9–17.

## Nurse-Patient Relationships

Holder, K., & Schenthal, S. (2007). Watch your step: Nursing and professional boundaries. *Nursing Management, 32*(2) 24–29.

Watson, J. (2006). *Theory of human caring.* Retrieved May 25, 2008, from www2.uchsc.edu/son/caring/content/default.asp.

# Section VIII  Patient and Family Education

Wendy Hobbie

## Section Outline

Teaching by Developmental Level

Family Education

Critical Learning Periods

The Pediatric Hematology/Oncology Nurse As Educator

Bibliography

# Teaching by Developmental Level

*Wendy Landier*

The ability of children to understand a diagnosis of cancer and a required treatment regimen is dependent upon their developmental levels. Nurses, therefore, must use developmentally appropriate teaching strategies to optimize patients' learning experiences (**Table 8-1**). In general, the younger the child, the shorter the attention span and the greater the need for the child's active participation in the learning process (e.g., through medical play). Education about the disease and its treatment should begin during the diagnostic phase and continue through treatment and follow-up. As children grow and enter new developmental phases, more detailed explanations regarding cancer and its treatment are necessary. Siblings also require age-appropriate education about a cancer diagnosis and cancer treatment.

## Developmental Differences According to Age

### Infants
- rely on sensory input and body movement to form concepts (sensorimotor stage)
- require the maintenance of a consistent relationship with a primary caregiver (usually the mother), which is important in establishing a sense of trust
- communicate nonverbally (e.g., cry, smile, coo, laugh)
- develop stranger anxiety between 8 and 12 months of age.

### Table 8-1. Teaching According to a Pediatric Patient's Developmental Level

| Developmental Level | Cognitive Level | Psychosocial Level | Key Teaching Strategies |
|---|---|---|---|
| Infant | Sensorimotor | Trust versus mistrust | Teach parents the importance of having consistent caregivers and maintaining an infant's normal routine within the limits of medical constraints. |
| | | | Encourage parents to use sensory measures, such as cuddling, giving a pacifier, and talking in a soothing voice, to comfort an infant. |
| Toddler | Preoperational-preconceptual | Autonomy versus shame and doubt | Give explanations in terms of the senses—what a toddler will hear, smell, feel, or see. |
| | | | Teach only about external body parts because toddlers cannot conceptualize internal body parts. |
| | | | Limit teaching sessions to 10 minutes or less. |
| | | | Choose words carefully because toddlers interpret words literally. |
| | | | Implement procedural teaching just prior to a procedure. |
| Preschooler | Preoperational-intuitive | Initiative versus guilt | Use simple terms to explain procedures and treatments. |
| | | | Engage in supervised medical play with dolls. |
| | | | Use picture books and body outlines because preschoolers can understand simple explanations about internal body parts. |
| | | | Keep teaching sessions about 10–15 minutes in length. Implement procedural teaching shortly before a procedure. |
| School-age child | Concrete operations | Industry versus inferiority | Use correct medical terminology when teaching. |
| | | | Use concrete terms when giving explanations. |
| | | | Allow child to have hands-on practice with equipment by using a doll and body outline for a younger child and a body outline alone for an older child. |
| | | | Prepare the child for procedures several hours prior to or the day before the procedures are scheduled to occur. |
| | | | Limit teaching sessions to about 20 minutes in length. |
| Adolescent | Formal operations | Identity versus role confusion | Provide explanations using correct medical terminology and detail. |
| | | | Include patients in family conferences and decisions regarding the plan of care. |
| | | | Teach about how treatment will affect body image; describe possible interventions (e.g., wigs and scarves for alopecia). |
| | | | Provide opportunities for teaching patients when their parents are not present. |
| | | | Keep in mind that teaching adolescents with their peer group is effective. |

### Toddlers
- use words in a general fashion, but are unable to form true concepts (preconceptual phase of the preoperational stage)
- often exhibit negativism and ritualistic behavior
- engage in animistic thinking (i.e., the belief that objects can think, feel, and come alive)
- imitate adults
- display a strong desire for independence and mastery of their environment.

### Preschoolers
- use words to represent objects, feelings, and actions (the intuitive phase of the preoperational stage)
- engage in egocentric and magical thinking (at times may have difficulty distinguishing between reality and fantasy)
- often have imaginary playmates
- may view illness and treatment as punishment for perceived misdeeds
- show extreme concern regarding body integrity
- typically are full of enthusiasm (i.e., show initiative) and are eager to learn.

### School-Age Children
- are capable of logical, concrete thought
- are able to comprehend physical causes for phenomena
- invest much energy in mastering cognitive, motor, and social skills and build self-esteem with the mastery of new skills.

### Adolescents
- are capable of abstract, formal operational thought
- are able to imagine possibilities and to think introspectively
- lack breadth of experience; may make unwise choices
- want to establish their own identity and uniqueness.

## Nursing Assessment and Interventions

### Assessment
- Determine the child's developmental and cognitive levels, psychosocial level, language ability, degree of apprehension, and illness state (i.e., his or her physical and emotional readiness to learn).
- Identify appropriate interventions and teaching methods to use with the child.

### Interventions
- Consider a variety of teaching methods, including individual or group instruction, medical play, books and other written materials, audio and/or video recordings, and electronic media.
- Document teaching or other interventions and their outcomes.
- Select an appropriate teaching method on the basis of the child's developmental level (**Table 8-2**).
  
  **Infant:**
  - Focus most instructions on the parents.
  - Inform the parents of the infant's need to maintain a close relationship with the primary caregivers.
  - Encourage parents to room-in (parents may require assistance when planning for the care of their other children).
  - Allow parents to stay with their infant during procedures.
  - Provide comfort measures involving the senses of touch (e.g., cuddling, stroking), motion (e.g., rocking, providing a pacifier), sight (e.g., mirrors, brightly colored toys), and sound (e.g., soft voice, music, audio recordings).
  - For older infants, begin basic teaching by allowing them to explore medical equipment; model the use of the equipment (e.g., stethoscope) first on a doll, then on their parents, and finally on the child.
  
  **Toddler:**
  - Approach the toddler at eye level.
  - Use simple words and short sentences.
  - Do not use words that can be misinterpreted by literal-thinking toddlers (e.g., "a stick in the finger" may be interpreted literally as a tree branch coming out of a finger).
  - Keep explanations brief.
  - Focus on the sensory aspects of experiences, such as what the toddler will feel, hear, taste, or see.
  - Do the teaching in the presence of a parent to prevent the toddler from experiencing separation anxiety.
  - Use transition objects, such as dolls, puppets, and play equipment, for teaching.
  - Do not use body outlines because toddlers are not capable of conceptualizing internal body parts.
  - Emphasize aspects that allow the toddler to preserve his or her autonomy, and allow choices whenever possible (e.g., ask questions, such as "Would you like juice or milk to drink with your medicine?").
  
  **Preschooler:**
  - Emphasize that the preschooler did not do anything to cause the illness and that illness is no one's fault.
  - Use dolls and medical play (e.g., a body outline can be used in conjunction with dolls because a preschooler is capable of understanding simple explanations regarding the internal body).
  - Use picture books and video recordings designed for preschoolers. Discuss issues related to body integrity and emphasize placement of adhesive bandages after a needle stick or surgical procedure.
  - Avoid words that could be misinterpreted by literal-thinking preschoolers.
  - Encourage the preschooler's questions and interactions during teaching sessions.
  
  **School-age child:**
  - Use concrete explanations that emphasize the physical aspects of the disease and treatment.
  - Describe the treatment from the school-age child's experiential viewpoint (e.g., provide information about whether the medication will be given as a pill or a shot, whether the child will receive treatment in the hospital or the clinic, and when the child will be able to return to school).
  - Use analogies to explain complex topics (e.g., "Your white blood cells are like soldiers—they fight the invading germs.").

Table 8-2. Examples of Teaching According to a Pediatric Patient's Developmental Level: Explaining the Diagnosis and Treatment of Leukemia

| Developmental Level | Concept | Explanation |
|---|---|---|
| Infant | Diagnosis | Explanations using adult learning concepts should be given to the infant's parents or other caregivers. |
| | Treatment | |
| Toddler | Diagnosis | "Your blood is sick." |
| | Treatment | "This medicine is to help your blood get better." |
| Preschooler | Diagnosis | "Do you remember how you have been very tired and your nose has been bleeding? You came to the hospital to find out why you were having these troubles. We checked your blood and your bone marrow—the place where your blood is made—and found out what was causing the trouble. Your blood is sick. This sickness is called leukemia." |
| | Treatment | "We will give you some special medicine, called 'chemo,' to help fix your blood." |
| School-age child | Diagnosis | "You know that since you came to the hospital, we have been checking your blood and bone marrow to find out why you have been so tired and pale and having nosebleeds. It is important to find out what is causing these troubles so that we can help you to get well again. We found out that there is a problem in your bone marrow. Your bone marrow is a factory that makes your blood. Your blood is made of cells. Cells are the very smallest parts of you. When you look at blood, it looks red, but there are really three kinds of cells in your blood—red blood cells, white blood cells, and platelets. The red blood cells give your body oxygen for energy. The white blood cells are like soldiers—they fight infection and keep you from getting sick. And the platelets stop the bleeding when you get a cut or nosebleed. Right now there are too many white blood cells in your bone marrow. There are so many white blood cells that they are crowding out your red blood cells and platelets. And all those white blood cells aren't even doing their job of being soldiers to fight infection—they are just causing trouble. This trouble is called leukemia—it is a cancer of the white blood cells." |
| | Treatment | "We need to give you special medicines, called chemotherapy, to help you get well again. The chemotherapy will get rid of the leukemia cells and let your healthy bone marrow cells get back to work. Some of the medicine can be taken by mouth either as a pill or liquid, whichever way is easiest for you. Some of the medicine will be given in shots; we will tell you when you will be getting these shots. Some of the medicine will be given in your lower back; we call this a spinal tap. And some of the medicine needs to go right into your blood and into a vein. The blue lines on your hands and arms are called veins—they are like highways that carry your blood around your body. We will put a tube, called an IV (or a central line [if applicable]) in one of your veins to give you some of your chemotherapy." |
| Adolescent | Diagnosis | Explanations of disease using concepts presented for a school-age child should be given to an adolescent, but scientific terminology should be used. |
| | Treatment | The names, routes of administration, potential side effects, and dosage regimens of chemotherapeutic drugs should be given. The patient should be involved in the consent process. The prognosis and possibility of a fatal outcome should be discussed with patients in their upper teens. |

- If the school-age child is deemed to be too old for dolls, refer to a teaching doll as a "dummy," or use a body outline.
- Provide the school-age child with written materials at his or her reading level, and allow the child to have hands-on experience to increase understanding of the disease and treatment (e.g., arrange for the child to view his or her blood smears under the microscope).
- Use developmentally appropriate audio or video recordings and electronic media.
- Reassure the school-age child that he or she did nothing to cause the illness and that illness is not anyone's fault.

**Adolescent:**
- Give a detailed, scientific explanation of the disease and its treatment.
- Offer to include the adolescent in medical conferences and treatment decisions, if the patient so desires.
- Arrange for teaching sessions with the adolescent, either individually or with his or her peers.
- Use body outlines to clarify information.
- Use developmentally appropriate written materials, audio and/or video recordings, and electronic media.
- Assure the adolescent that he or she did nothing to cause the illness.
- Anticipate concerns regarding the adolescent's changing body image (e.g., give the adolescent an opening to express concerns by saying, "Many teens your age are concerned about losing their hair while on chemotherapy. Are you worried about that?").

## Expected Patient and Family Outcomes

### Infant
- The parents verbalize an understanding of the infant's disease and treatment plan.
- The infant maintains a trusting relationship with the parents.
- The infant begins to adjust to medical equipment that will be used frequently, such as a stethoscope and sphygmomanometer.

### Toddler
- The toddler is able to verbalize a simple explanation of the illness and treatment (e.g., "I go to the hospital because my blood is sick.").
- The toddler is able to cooperate for routine aspects of treatment, accepting the elements of autonomy that are offered (e.g., the toddler takes medicine well when allowed to choose between juice or milk to drink with the medicine).

### Preschooler
- The preschooler is able to describe the basic concepts of the illness (e.g., "I have leukemia; my bone marrow makes blood, and my blood got sick.").
- The preschooler is able to describe the basic aspects of treatment (e.g., "I have to take chemo and come to the clinic so my blood can get better.").
- The preschooler is able to verbalize that illness is not his or her fault and that treatment is not a punishment for anything that he or she did.

### School-Age Child
- The school-age child is able to describe the illness in simple detail (e.g., he or she can describe how blood is produced in the bone marrow, the functions of red blood cells, white blood cells, and platelets, and how leukemia affects healthy blood cells).
- The school-age child is able to name and explain the various modalities of treatment that he or she is receiving.
- The school-age child is able to verbalize that he or she did not do anything to cause the illness.

### Adolescent
- The adolescent is able to use scientific terminology to describe the disease in detail.
- The adolescent participates in treatment conferences and consent decisions.
- The adolescent is able to verbalize that he or she did not do anything to cause the illness.
- The adolescent is able to describe treatment modalities and verbalize an understanding of the treatment schedule and overall plan.

## Family Education

*Judith M. Doell*

Consistent with the nursing process, family education begins with a thorough assessment. Before providing disease- and treatment-related information, nurses must evaluate a family's coping strategies, support systems, self-care practices, educational level, preferred learning strategies, and cultural background. It is also important to establish parental roles early on and determine who will be the primary students of the family's education. Educating the patient and the family in the face of an oncology diagnosis requires constant evaluation of the family members' readiness to learn.

Family education most often refers to adults—parents or guardians—who are the primary caregivers. After the learners have been assessed, these adults are given information about the diagnosis, treatment plan, potential and probable side effects, complications, and stressors. To be most effective, family education should be based on adult learning principles. The family education process is based upon adult learning and teaching principles and consists of a variety of informal and structured learning activities and experiences designed to promote active involvement, application, and learning (**Table 8-3**).

---

**Table 8-3. Benefits of Family Education**

**Education helps the family of a patient with cancer deal with the following stressors:**

- coping with the crisis of a cancer diagnosis
- coping with the stress of assimilating a vast amount of extensive and detailed information
- participating in informed decision making about the child's treatment
- coping with the anxiety related to caring for the child with cancer
- learning how to deal with treatment-related conditions, side effects, and emergency situations
- coping with disruptions in normal individual and family functioning and the psychological distress the patient or other family members may be experiencing
- learning how to use available resources
- learning about possible delayed consequences of the original cancer or its treatment or both.

---

### Principles of Adult Learning

Principles of adult learning furnish the nurse with a series of actions to begin, maintain, and enhance the effectiveness of an educational event (**Table 8-4**). These principles not only highlight the nurse's roles as clarifier, coach, and transmitter of information, but also increase the potential for families of children with cancer, as well as nurses, to learn across the continuum of care. The following are the general principles related to how adults learn:

- Adults are autonomous and generally self-directed.
- Adults attach more meaning to knowledge gained, have accumulated a foundation of experiences, and may have fixed viewpoints.
- Adults become ready to learn when they feel the learning situation is relevant or if they have to cope with an unfamiliar situation.
- They have a practical and problem-centered learning orientation and seek learning opportunities that focus on solutions and increase their competence.
- Adults must apply what they have learned immediately and expect that their new knowledge will be useful immediately.

| Table 8-4. Guidelines for Adult Education |
|---|
| 1. Conduct a comprehensive assessment to determine the adult's learning needs. |
| 2. Create a safe environment conducive to adult learning. |
| 3. Cultivate a positive teacher-learner relationship and dialogue based on mutual trust and respect. |
| 4. Formulate objectives (i.e., the directions of the learning). |
| 5. Incorporate cognitive, psychomotor, and affective aspects of learning in the design and enactment of learning activities and experiences. |
| 6. Determine the proper sequencing of content and effective reinforcement methods. |
| 7. Promote inductive and deductive learning through practice and reflection. |
| 8. Respect the learners as decision makers and subjects of their own learning. |
| 9. Establish learning activities and experiences that allow the learners to see the immediate usefulness of what they have just learned. |
| 10. Measure progress and reassess learning needs (i.e., evaluate the educational process). |

## Nursing Assessment of a Family's Learning Needs

The necessary comprehensive nursing assessment includes the following:

- Investigate the child's medical history, diagnosis, treatment plan, and prognosis.
- Obtain a general sense of what the family and the child currently understand through a dialogue with the primary physician and other healthcare providers on the team.
- Determine the family's current knowledge base (e.g., by asking them to describe, in their own words, the child's disease, treatment plan, and what the child already knows about the disease).
- Assess the child's current health maintenance routines (e.g., hygiene, nutrition).
- Discover the issues and topics that are of immediate concern to the family.
- Determine the family's preferred learning styles (e.g., discussion, reading, practice, or computer-based learning and Internet access).
- Identify situations and conditions that could present barriers to effective learning (e.g., inability to read and comprehend English; physical impairments, such as deafness or blindness; financial constraints, such as unemployment or lack of health insurance; psychosocial stressors, such as a divorce, a recent death in the family, a sibling with a physical or mental disability, or chronic illness; the family's current health status; a limited support system; and religious beliefs).
- Determine how the family's culture may influence the educational process, and plan to include interpreters, appropriate written materials, and social support, as needed.
- Ascertain the family's current coping style(s).
- Recognize that the parental response to a diagnosis and anticipated management of their child with cancer may interfere with their ability to concentrate on and comprehend what is taught.

## Planning and Intervention

The following are the planning and intervention measures that should be taken:

- Determine the outcomes of family education.
  - Family members will possess accurate, current information about the child's cancer and treatment plan.
  - Family members will know when to watch the child closely, how to deal with problems, and when to be more protective.
  - Family members will continue to perceive the child with cancer in a developmentally appropriate way.
- Identify and agree on learning objectives with the family.
- Formulate a teaching plan that includes the characteristics of adult learning and teaching principles (**Table 8-5**); prioritizes the information the family needs to know rather than the information that might be nice to know; and bases the content, teaching methods, sequencing, and resources on identified learning objectives and the family's perceptions, concerns, current knowledge base, and learning styles, as well as on the child's diagnosis and treatment plan.
- Select appropriate teaching strategies. Verbal, along with written, information will usually predominate, but computer-based patient education can effectively improve knowledge outcomes in an increasingly computer-savvy society. Demonstrations and video modules also can effectively involve the learner.
- Introduce educational materials and resources to promote and reinforce learning (e.g., reliable Web sites, books, pamphlets, written guidelines, handbooks, and videotapes, as well as medication and follow-up calendars, to reinforce the cognitive component of learning). Puppets or dolls may be used with parents and children to explain medical procedures. To ensure the health-education materials can be understood by most people, it is recommended that they be presented at a fifth-grade level.
- Teach in an environment conducive to learning; minimize distractions.
- Use clear explanations; avoid medical jargon, or explain medical jargon as you proceed.

| Table 8-5. Characteristics of Adult Learners and Their Educational Implications ||
|---|---|
| Characteristics | Implications for Teachers |
| Learn by their own and others' experiences. | Teach by providing actual experiences. Use simple definitions, analogies, and storytelling. |
| Have mixed motives for learning | Provide support, guidance, feedback, and resources. |
| May need more time to learn | Give learners some control over their pace. Prioritize content from general to specific. Use resources for reinforcement. |
| Are problem-centered learners | Address perceived problems and issues first. |

- Explain and reinforce complex concepts by using analogies and definitions.
- Give parents opportunities to practice with equipment and to demonstrate what has been taught to reinforce the psychomotor component of learning.
- Provide access to interdisciplinary members of the care team, who can instruct and educate in their area of expertise (e.g., child-life specialist, dietitian, discharge planner).
- Use individual and group discussions and support groups as educational opportunities.
- Encourage parents and children to keep a journal to reinforce the effective component of learning.
- Consider alternative approaches, such as using interpreters, foreign-language cards and pamphlets, and assistive equipment, to overcome physical and linguistic barriers to learning.
- Select the appropriate content focus, which may include, but is not limited to, cancer pathophysiology, diagnostic tests and procedures, cancer treatments (e.g., chemotherapy, radiation therapy), basic healthcare habits, bone-marrow suppression, management of general physical side effects (e.g., nausea, vomiting, alopecia), psychosocial care, oncologic emergencies, central venous access devices, discharge planning, home care, and delayed consequences of cancer therapy.
- Use accepted methods to standardize and enhance learning (**Table 8-6**).

## Evaluating the Outcomes of Family Education

- Measure family outcomes by assessing whether family members can do the following:
    – Describe the type of cancer the child has and the treatment plan.
    – Verbalize an understanding of expected and potential, as well as immediate and delayed, treatment-related effects, procedures, and follow-up care.
    – Demonstrate the skills needed to care for the child at home.
    – Verbalize how and when to contact appropriate healthcare team members about problems encountered at home.
    – Discuss the preventive and precautionary measures and symptoms associated with treatment-related effects that can pose an immediate threat to the child's well-being.
- Document the content that has been taught, the learning level the family has attained, any remaining learning gaps, and a recommended plan for addressing the child's and the family's other learning needs. This will be a reference point for continuing evaluation of outcomes.
- Use the following evaluation strategies:
    – family members' verbalization of understanding
    – demonstrations and opportunities for family members to demonstrate what has been taught
    – identification of learning gaps by questioning.

In conclusion, nurses must continually reassess the learning needs of the family and reconsider learning objectives, content focus, and sequencing of information, with ongoing modification and implementation of the teaching plan. Nurses always

---

**Table 8-6. Family Education Checklist: What the Family Should Know**

**Treatment Plan**

The type of chemotherapy the child is receiving and its side effects

The date, time, and location of the next appointment

Important telephone numbers

The days on which blood counts should be done

**Important Signs to Report**

Signs of infection
 - fever (temperatures of 101° F/38.3° C and above)
 - cough or rapid breathing
 - earache
 - sore throat
 - the child's inability to bend his or her neck
 - stomach pain
 - red or irritated skin around the child's bottom
 - blisters, rashes, ulcers on the skin
 - redness, swelling, pus around the central line

Change in behavior or level of consciousness

Break in the central line

Leaking around or from the central line

Bleeding, increased bruising, or petechiae

Difficulty or pain when eating, drinking, or swallowing

Changes in bowel habits (e.g., constipation, diarrhea)

Uncontrolled nausea and vomiting

Paleness, increased fatigue

Inability to drink or eat

Exposure to chicken pox

**Important Precautions**

Do not give the child aspirin (Ecotrin) or products containing aspirin

Do not take the child's temperature rectally or otherwise manipulate that area, and do not give the child suppositories

**Healthcare Habits and Infection Precautions**

Good handwashing

Proper nutrition

Proper mouth care

Avoidance of crowds and contagious persons

Daily bath or shower

Sufficient rest

Knowing the proper way to take a temperature

Proper central line care

**Supportive Medications (including the reasons for their use and information about dosage and administration)**

*Pneumocystis carinii* prophylaxis (TMP-SMZ [Bactrim])

Colony-stimulating factor therapy (G-CSF [Neupogen])

Supplemental or adjuvant medications (e.g., allopurinol [Zyloprim], magnesium, calcium)

Antiemetic, bowel, and/or pain medication regimens

**Miscellaneous**

Nutritional support (e.g., total parenteral nutrition, lipids, supplements)

need to be mindful of stresses that may affect learning, and take advantage of teachable moments as they arise, while consistently documenting the teaching and communication with the patient's healthcare team.

# Critical Learning Periods

*Judith M. Doell*

Critical learning periods for children with cancer and their families are characterized by uncertainty, change, and the need to gain knowledge and control. Common critical learning periods in the care of children with cancer and their families include the time of diagnosis; the beginning of treatment; each new cycle of therapy, relapse or recurrence; relocation to a different healthcare center; completion of treatment; survivorship; and palliative care. Within these critical learning periods, nurses are challenged to find appropriate teaching moments and to teach toward mutually determined goals. Nurses must closely assess family learners for anxiety, as moderate-to-severe anxiety can interfere with their ability to focus and understand new information. The goal should be to inform the family without overwhelming them.

## Educational Priorities for the Newly Diagnosed Patient and Family

Educational priorities are different for each patient, not just because of the diagnosis and treatment, but because of the family's response. The family may define areas of knowledge deficit that they perceive as a priority, and those may not always be the nurse educator's priority. Mutual goals need to be agreed upon and should adhere to theories of adult learning (see the subsection "Family Education").

## An Overview of the Common Concerns About Childhood Cancer

An overview for patients and their families should include information about the pathophysiology of cancer; current theories related to epidemiology; diagnosis and prognosis; diagnostic test results; misconceptions about cancer, remission, and relapse; and stable, progressive, and recurrent disease. The time spent on this content will vary greatly with a newly diagnosed patient, depending on the individual learner's priorities and the patient's anxiety level.

## A Review of Investigational Protocol Issues

It is important to ascertain the parent's knowledge and comprehension of an investigational protocol and to clarify any misconceptions. Issues that should be addressed are the patient's rights, informed consent, and how to read a roadmap (i.e., the outline describing the patient's treatment schedule). Sometimes parents need reassurance that their child will receive widely approved therapy.

## Definition of Childhood Cancer Treatment

Defining childhood cancer treatment includes providing facts about how the proposed therapy works, how treatment is administered, the supportive care measures that the patient will actually or potentially need, and discussion of immediate risks and long-term implications of treatment.

## General Side Effects of Treatment

Patients and families should be informed about bone-marrow suppression, nausea and vomiting, diarrhea, constipation, mucositis, alopecia, risks of sun exposure, altered nutrition, chemotherapy-related precautions, pain, and behavioral changes (see Section V, "Side Effects of Treatment," for more information on side effects).

## Bone-Marrow Suppression

Patients and families need to be informed about blood-cell counts and the different cell functions, so they can better understand neutropenia, thrombocytopenia, anemia, and the signs and symptoms associated with these conditions. The highest priority is to provide information about neutropenia and fever with an explanation of probable hospitalization. The child may require blood-product transfusion secondary to anemia and thrombocytopenia. In addition, parents need to be aware of restrictions on over-the-counter medications and routine immunizations. (For more information, see Section V, "Side Effects of Treatment.")

## Description of Venous Access Devices for Children

This information should include the reasons for venous access, a description and model of the catheter that will be used, and basic information on maintenance of the catheter. The specific care of a central venous line (CVL) needs to be addressed when the family requests the information or upon placement of the CVL. (See Section VI, "Supportive Care," for further discussion on venous access devices.)

## Discussion of the Impact of Treatment on the Child's Activities

This topic is important right away, as it includes restrictions, maintenance of a normal lifestyle, educational services that can be provided while the child is in the hospital, time when the child can return to school, school reentry programs, and how to obtain access to school district services and locate teachers for homebound students (see Section VII, "Psychosocial Issues").

## Discussion of Family Issues

This discussion should focus on the family's existing support systems, coping issues, availability of community and financial resources, applications for assistance, the names of support services and groups, the needs of the patient's siblings, concerns about discipline and child care, issues related to disclosing information to a child with cancer and to the child's siblings, and issues related to the parents' employment (see Section VII, "Psychosocial Issues").

## Educational Priorities for the Patient and Family During Treatment

During treatment, informed consent should be reviewed in conjunction with new cycles and phases. New chemotherapy agents and their side effects must be discussed. Throughout therapy, the patient and the family must learn to plan for anticipated hospital and clinic visits. They also might need help with issues related to day-to-day living, such as maintenance of a normal lifestyle, school versus at-home education for the patient, sibling considerations, discipline, coping, community and financial resources, and the parents' employment.

## Educational Priorities for the Relapsed Patient and Family

### Reinforcement of Treatment-Related Information
The issues for these patients and their families include investigational therapies, new chemotherapy agents and their side effects, new treatment modalities and their side effects, and the addition of biologic-response modifiers and their side effects. Families also must be briefed on the necessity of signing new informed-consent documents.

### Facilitation of Coping Strategies and Communication
The goals are to promote honesty within the family, use age-appropriate information with the child and his or her siblings, listen to the entire family's concerns, and, if needed, utilize interdisciplinary support, such as psychology and social work to help with coping. There may be a greater need to explore community and financial resources.

## Educational Priorities for the Patient and Family Who Move to a Different Geographic Area

### Information to Help Provide a Smooth Transition to a New Cancer Center
The patient and the family may require help establishing a relationship with a new oncologist and staff and obtaining addresses, locations, and telephone numbers of physicians and treatment centers in the city to which they are moving. Nurses should help establish a date for the patient's next clinic or hospital visit and treatment, review the treatment protocol and determine the family's level of understanding of it, and provide a review of the anticipated side effects of ongoing treatment.

## Educational Priorities for the Patient and Family Who Have Completed Therapy

### Help With a Smooth Transition at the Completion of Therapy
This assistance includes acknowledging the positive and negative aspects of completing treatment. It is an ongoing responsibility to discuss the potential late complications of cancer therapy, but it must be a priority at the end of therapy. Patients and families should receive a treatment summary, written information, and a follow-up plan and schedule. They will need information regarding survivorship programs. In addition, they may not have been able to comprehend information regarding late effects until this time, and nurses should provide comprehensive information as needed.

### Discussion of the Patient's and the Family's Fears Regarding a Recurrence
The patient and the family should have opportunities to discuss their concerns about a recurrence and should be given referrals to support groups. Test results should be reported to the patient and the family on a timely basis.

### Discussion of the Importance of Returning to a Normal Life
Assistance in this area includes reviewing the signs that a family is returning to normalcy, discussing school-related concerns, assessing family relationship issues, and fostering the child's needs for greater independence.

### Discussion About the Relationship With Healthcare Providers After Therapy Concludes
This discussion involves the changing relationship with the oncology staff and the role of the primary-care physician.

## Educational Priorities for the Patient and the Family During Palliative Care

### Information About the Palliative-Care Phase of Illness
The concept of palliative care is discussed, with continued emphasis on the importance of quality of life and comfort care. This information includes a review of the options for care, such as phase 1 trials, hospice, home care, and hospital care. The family's ability to provide interventions also must be considered. In addition, healthcare providers should address changes in care, such as a decreased need for blood work and clinic visits, and provide information about the anticipated progression of the child's disease.

### Discussion of Children's Concept of Death
When talking with parents about their children's understanding of death, discussion should center on the developmental age of the child and sibling(s) and how their developmental age affects their ability to conceptualize death. Encourage the parents to explain death to the child and sibling(s) in a developmentally appropriate, honest, caring, and open way.

### Discussion of the Need for Comfort Measures
A discussion of comfort measures includes changes in the child's physical condition and a review of the child's need for supportive measures, such as oxygen, pain medications, and other interventions.

### Discussion of the Importance of Parents' Communication With Their Terminally Ill Child and the Child's Siblings
The goal of this discussion is to promote honesty within the family by teaching the parents about the common responses of children in similar situations so that they can provide age-appropriate information to their terminally ill child and the child's siblings.

### The Family's Need for Awareness of Grief
The family needs assistance with understanding the grieving process as well as with referrals to support groups and to available community resources (see Section IX, "Care for the Terminally Ill Child and the Family").

## Nursing Assessment and Interventions Directed Toward the Patient's and the Family's Learning Needs

### Assessment
- Identify specific learning goals for the patient and the family for their identified critical learning period.
- Assess the patient's and the family's previous experience with cancer and current needs to understand the disease and its treatment, their developmental and educational levels, language and literacy barriers, emotional and physical barriers, cultural and religious beliefs, and the availability of resources or support.

### Interventions
- Select individualized methods and resources for teaching the patient and the family.
- Define methods for evaluating the patient's and the family's achievements, such as direct observation of their behavior, oral questioning, written tests, and self-reports.
- Prioritize goals in collaboration with the patient, the family, and the healthcare team.
- Include the patient and the family in planning and teaching sessions.
- Develop a teaching plan for the patient's and the family's critical learning period.
- Document educational strategies or other interventions and their outcomes.

### Expected Patient and Family Outcomes
- The patient, the family, or both are able to verbalize the information that has been taught.
- The patient, the family, or both are able to demonstrate satisfactorily the skills they have been taught.

The long-term goals should be that the patient and the family are empowered and well armed with knowledge about the diagnosis and treatment, which will facilitate good coping and family function throughout therapy and into survivorship.

## The Pediatric Hematology/Oncology Nurse as Educator

*Judith M. Doell*

Pediatric hematology/oncology nurses today receive specialized training on the job and are frequently involved in the design and implementation of research studies. They are also at the core of communication of the specialized needs of these patients to other healthcare providers, the community, and schools. They are uniquely qualified to educate and empower families with the knowledge to live with their child's cancer.

Pediatric hematology/oncology nurses gain much knowledge in the daily practice of caring for patients and from participating in ongoing, structured, continuing education. Their experience builds on their knowledge, and pediatric oncology nurses become exceptional, knowledgeable resources for other disciplines, students, and one another. They are a resource for other healthcare professionals regarding the care of children with cancer. Teaching strategies should be tailored to each audience based upon individual learning needs.

### Education of New Hematology/Oncology Nurses

Information on disease, treatment, and symptom management should be presented to new hematology/oncology nurses. This information can be presented through in-service sessions, one-on-one teaching segments, self-paced modules, and electronic or Internet offerings. Orientation and mentoring should be provided for all new hematology/oncology nurses. A comprehensive orientation program includes skill validation, review of institutional policies and standards, introduction to available resources, and identification of a preceptor or mentor.

### Education of Nurses in Other Specialties

Nurses in other specialties, such as emergency medicine, intensive care, and community health, often are required to care for children with cancer. The pediatric hematology/oncology nurse should serve as a resource for nurses in other specialties by providing information on disease, treatment, and symptom management and by being available for ongoing consultation. Nursing education should be directed toward specific patient-identified outcomes (e.g., obtaining access to implanted central venous catheters, administering chemotherapy, monitoring for side effects, interpreting laboratory values, and recognizing the signs and symptoms of neutropenia).

### Education of School Nurses and Other School Staff

Issues related to a patient's reentry to school should be addressed with the family, school nurses, and other school staff members (see the discussion on school reentry in Section VII, "Psychosocial Issues"). This information should include input about possible limitations on the patient's physical activities as well as background on the patient's potential or actual learning problems. A well-organized reentry plan helps the child, family, teacher, classmates, and school personnel deal realistically with the special needs of a child with cancer.

### Education of Multidisciplinary Team Members

Multidisciplinary team members should receive basic information on disease, treatment, and symptom management. They also should know about how the side effects of treatment can affect the delivery of discipline-specific care. Their general and specific concerns about patients should be addressed and include ongoing open dialogue with the oncology nurse.

### Individual Continuing Education and Professional Development

Nurses working in the area of pediatric hematology/oncology are responsible for their own ongoing education. The field is changing rapidly, and pediatric hematology/oncology nurses should have the knowledge necessary to maintain state-of-the-art and state-of-the-science nursing skills.

Professional-practice and patient-care skills can be enhanced by becoming a certified pediatric oncology nurse (CPON®). This certification is offered by the Oncology Nursing Certification Corporation (see www.oncc.org for further information). Pursuing a graduate degree in the specialty is another way to obtain clinical and professional advancement. Finally, joining professional organizations such as the Association of Pediatric Hematology/Oncology Nurses (APHON) and the Oncology Nursing Society (ONS) can provide pediatric oncology nurses with peer support as well as clinical and professional advancement opportunities.

## Educational Assessment and Interventions

### Assessment

- The most important (and first) step in assessment is to understand the target audience and what it needs, desires, and expects with respect to education.
- Review the learner's past experiences.
- What is the learner's current knowledge base, and in what context will he or she use the new information?
- Consider the value of the information to be taught.
- Determine the learner's readiness and ability to learn.
- Identify barriers to learning, including language barriers; cultural differences; preconceived notions about cancer and treatments; and the learner's level of education, anxiety, and motivation to learn.
- Identify educational outcomes.

### Interventions

- Review the principles of adult education before the start of a program. If the target audience is a sibling or cohort at school, review teaching according to developmental level.
- Schedule a specific time for disseminating information, but remain flexible.
- Provide an outline or overview of the material that is to be presented.
- Identify available resources, including clinical experts, approved Internet sites, written materials, and audio and visual materials.
- Use computer technology to create storyboards on appropriate topics in pediatric oncology for patients, families, nurses, students, or the general public.
- Provide journal club discussions about new findings in the nursing literature.
- Document the instruction that has been provided.

### Expected Educational Outcomes

- The learner is able to verbalize the information that has been taught.
- Various evaluation methods have been used, including demonstrations, informal observations, tests, structured observations, discussions, and checklists.
- The learner is able to demonstrate satisfactorily the skills that have been taught.
- The patient and the family receive optimal care from members of the multidisciplinary healthcare team.

The goal of the pediatric hematology/oncology nurse as an educator is to create a knowledgeable healthcare team and support system for patients who have been diagnosed with cancer and their families. This goal extends beyond the hematology/oncology nurse, and its realization provides a much larger cushion of knowledgeable providers for this special population.

## Bibliography

### Teaching by Developmental Level

Bukatko, D., & Daehler, M. W. (2001). *Child development: A thematic approach* (4th ed.). Boston: Houghton Mifflin.

Rankin, S. H., Stallings, K. D., & London, F. (2005). *Patient education in health and illness* (5th ed.). Philadelphia: Lippincott Williams & Wilkins.

### Family Education

Cutilli, C. C. (2006). Do your patients understand? Providing culturally congruent patient education. *Orthopaedic Nursing, 25,* 218–224.

Friesen, P., Pepler, C., & Hunter, P. (2002). Interactive family learning following a cancer diagnosis. *Oncology Nursing Forum, 29,* 981–987.

Lewis, D. (2003). Computers in patient education. *CIN: Computers, Informatics, Nursing, 21,* 88–96.

Russell, S. S. (2006). An overview of adult-learning processes. *Urologic Nursing, 26,* 349–352, 370.

### Critical Learning Periods

Bashore, L. (2004). Childhood and adolescent cancer survivors' knowledge of their disease and effects of treatment. *Journal of Pediatric Oncology Nursing, 21,* 98–102.

Stephenson, P. (2006). Before the teaching begins: Managing patient anxiety prior to providing education. *Clinical Journal of Oncology Nursing, 10,* 241–245.

### The Pediatric Hematology/Oncology Nurse as Educator

Agre, P., Dougherty, J., & Pirone, J. (2002). Creating a CD-ROM program for cancer-related patient education. *Oncology Nursing Forum, 29,* 573–580.

Gomez, E., & Clark, P. (2001). The Internet in oncology nursing. *Seminars in Oncology Nursing, 17,* 7–17.

Zisak, A., & Conrad, K. (2004). Using technology to develop and distribute patient education storyboards across a health system. *Oncology Nursing Forum, 31,* 131–135.

# Section IX  Care for the Terminally Ill Child and the Family

Cheryl Rodgers

## Section Outline

Children and Death

Physical Care of the Terminally Ill Child

Psychosocial Care of the Terminally Ill Child

Bereavement

Professionals' Grief, Distress, and Bereavement

Moral Distress

Ethical Dilemmas in Terminal Care

Legal Concerns in Terminal Care

Bibliography

# Children and Death

*Angela M. Ethier*

## General Principles

A diagnosis of cancer is the prelude to the question asked by most children with cancer, "Am I going to die?" When children's questions about dying and death are avoided, their fears are magnified. A child's understanding of death evolves throughout childhood, and it is common for children to repeatedly ask questions about the death of a loved one. Children typically have three questions after the death of a sibling: Why did my sister (or brother) die (and was it my fault)? Will it happen to me? What happens after you die? Discussing death with children in a developmentally appropriate and caring manner can facilitate their understanding of the concept as they mature.

Understanding death is a continuous, lifelong process that begins in childhood and generally follows an individual's cognitive development. Death is a complex and multidimensional concept composed of the following five subconcepts:
- universality—all living things die, and death is unavoidable and unpredictable
- irreversibility—when a person dies, he or she cannot become alive again
- nonfunctionality—functions of the body and mind (e.g., eating, sleeping, seeing) cease
- causality—death is caused by the breakdown of the functions of the body
- noncorporeal continuation—there is some form of personal continuation after death (e.g., in the memories of loved ones, through reincarnation, in the ascension of the soul).

Typically between the ages of 4 and 6 years, children have an understanding of universality and irreversibility, and by age 7, they understand nonfunctionality and causality. Younger children view death as a behavior—as permanently going away or going to sleep—and not as a biological event. A child's concept of death may be influenced by cultural factors and personal experiences.

## Understanding Death and Grief Reactions

### Infants (0–1 year)
It is believed that infants have no concept of death. Infants react to the grief of family members in the home and to changes in their routine.

### Toddlers (1–2 years)
Toddlers perceive death as temporary and reversible. They react to family members' grief responses, separation from caregivers, and alterations in their routine and surroundings. Behavioral responses to loss can include crying; fussiness; clinging; biting; hitting; turning away; withdrawal; regression in speech, toileting, eating, and drinking; and physical illness. The toddler moves between grieving and playing, which can be misunderstood as not experiencing grief.

### Preschool Children (3–5 years)
Preschoolers may continue to perceive death as a state of being less alive (similar to the state of someone who is sleeping or who is away on a trip). Between 4 and 5 years of age, some preschoolers may begin to understand the universality and irreversibility of death. Magical thinking may lead preschoolers to believe that their misdeeds or thoughts have caused their sibling's illness and death, causing feelings of guilt. Preschoolers interpret words literally, so euphemisms regarding death need to be avoided. For example, children at this age who hear of a pet being "put to sleep" may fear going to sleep. Preschoolers' greatest fear about death is being separated from their parents. Because of the preschooler's limited coping strategies for dealing with loss, play often provides relief from intense feelings. This behavior does not indicate indifference or an inability to grieve. Behavioral responses to loss can include regressive behaviors, sleeping and eating disturbances, physical symptoms (e.g., stomachache, headache), intensification of normal fears, emotional outbursts, and irritability.

### School-Age Children (6–11 years)
By the age of 7, most school-age children have an adultlike understanding of death. They ask more questions about life and death than younger children, including asking what happens to the body after death. Remnants of magical thinking may persist and create feelings of guilt and fear. They may personify death as a bogeyman or a ghost. Dying is viewed as a threat to the school-age child's sense of security. School-age children may experience teasing from peers for being different (i.e., having experienced a loss). Behavioral responses to loss can include difficulties with eating and sleeping, physical symptoms (e.g., stomachache, headache), fear of abandonment, worry about the health and safety of other family members, difficulty concentrating, problems in school, and emotional outbursts.

### Adolescents (12–20 years)
In addition to understanding death in much the same way that adults do, adolescents may search for spiritual meaning in the loss and ponder what happens after death. At this stage in life, they are separating from their family and developing their own identity. As death draws near, adolescents may find it difficult to cope with increased isolation from their peers and dependence on their family. Adolescents often display intense emotional reactions toward death. Their behavioral responses can include anger, withdrawal, crying, insomnia, difficulties in school, physical illnesses, and risk-taking behaviors (e.g., reckless driving, drug use, inappropriate sexual activity).

## Grief in Children

### Four Tasks of Grief Work
Children who are grieving should be allowed to complete the process, which includes
- telling the story of their loved one
- identifying their emotions and expressing them
- finding meaning in the experience and the loss
- making the transition from their relationship with the physical presence of the deceased person to a relationship based on history, memories, and the notion of what kind of person the deceased might have become.

### Facilitating the Grieving Process
Children do not grieve in the same way that adults do and are

limited by their verbal ability and coping skills in expressing themselves. Children process their grief over a longer period than adults. Providing a safe and predictable environment with supportive and trusted individuals; providing an atmosphere of open, honest, and developmentally appropriate communication; using concrete terms and avoiding euphemisms; and facilitating children's grief work through play and art activities can give support to grieving children. There is no phenomenon that differs as much from person to person as grief. There is no right way to grieve. The words, actions, and attitudes of healthcare providers can have a long-lasting positive or negative effect on children and their family members. Grief reactions are varied and may include denial, sadness, anger, guilt, blame, weight loss, difficulty sleeping, gastrointestinal (GI) symptoms, anxiety, depression, and acting-out behaviors.

Children may experience complicated grief. The intensity and duration of their grief behaviors may indicate the need for referral to a mental healthcare provider. Warning signs of an intense, possibly destructive response include the absence of grief, persistent blaming or feelings of guilt, suicidal thoughts or actions, serious eating problems, long-standing depression, isolation from friends and family, fighting or criminal behaviors, unwillingness to speak about the deceased or an expression of only positive or only negative feelings about the deceased, failing or overachieving in school, accident proneness, inappropriate sexual behaviors, major personality or attitude changes, and addictive behaviors (e.g., drug use, overeating).

## Nursing Assessment and Interventions

### Assessment

- Assess the family's structure, roles, communication style, coping mechanisms, social support, previous loss history, and cultural and spiritual beliefs related to death and grief.
- Assess the child's and family's grief reactions.
- Use art and play to help the child express himself or herself.
- Identify the child's and family's cultural and spiritual needs related to death and grief.
- Identify the child's and family's current understandings, and clarify misconceptions.

### Interventions

- Inform parents of children's developmental understanding of death and common reactions to death and grief.
- Promote sensitive, honest communication with the child and his or her family, using the words *died* and *dead* and avoiding euphemisms.
- Answer questions and avoid providing unwarranted information.
- Promote the expression of grief emotions (e.g., crying).
- Facilitate uninterrupted opportunities for the child and family members to talk with or without healthcare providers, spiritual counselors, and others as desired.
- Facilitate memory-making opportunities for the child and family before and after the child's death (e.g., creating memory books, videotaping, storytelling, developing family rituals).
- Provide information regarding grief resources (e.g., grief counselors, bereavement support groups, literature).

# Physical Care of the Terminally Ill Child

*Janice Nuuhiwa*

## General Principles

Research related to symptom management in children with terminal illnesses is limited. Formal assessment tools for symptoms other than pain in children are not available. The assessment of symptoms is often a synthesis of the child's own description and the family's observations and opinions.

Approaches to symptom management should include pharmacologic and nonpharmacologic therapy, practical nursing care, and holistic support for the child and the family.

## Dimensions of Terminal Illness

The concepts discussed in this section are described in **Table 9-1**.

### Terminal phase

The terminal phase is usually the last 2–3 months of life, although it can have a longer or shorter duration. Conventional or experimental methods for a cure or remission are no longer feasible at this stage of the illness.

### Terminal period

This period comprises the dying process and usually involves the last 2–3 weeks of life.

### Terminal event

The terminal event is the actual physical dying process, which spans the last days or hours during which death is imminent.

### Bereavement

Bereavement encompasses an indefinite period of mourning the death of the child. In the face of progressive life-threatening illness, this phase can begin before the death and extend up to several years after a child's death (for a more detailed discussion, see the subsection "Bereavement," which appears later in this section).

## Symptom Management for Children Dying of Cancer

### Pain

Most children who are terminally ill and have solid tumors require pain control. These tumors commonly have metastases to the spine and major nerves. Effective pain relief may require aggressive measures.

A minority of children with hematological malignancies experience disease-related pain. The onset of their pain is rapid, so pain management is most crucial during the terminal period.

Pain is a complex sensation influenced not only by the degree of physical damage to tissues but also by the psychological, social, and cultural factors that are unique to each person. Pain management requires a family-centered, interdisciplinary, and collaborative approach. Clinicians must know the principles of childhood development if they are to use appropriate tools when measuring children's pain. Consistent use of a pain-assessment tool is critical. Healthcare providers must have a sound understanding of the anatomic and physiologic bases of pain

### Table 9-1. Signs of Approaching Death

| | 1–3 Months to Weeks Preceding Death | 1–2 Weeks to Days Preceding Death | Hours to Minutes Preceding Death |
|---|---|---|---|
| **Physical changes** | Central nervous system: Children need more sleep.<br><br>Gastrointestinal: Children lower their intake. | Central nervous system: Children have a heightened sensitivity to sight, sound, smell, and activity; increased pain, confusion, and weakness; and varied sleep-and-wake patterns. Children have decreased awareness or a surge of energy.<br><br>Respiratory: There are respiratory irregularities.<br><br>Circulatory: Temperature fluctuates and color changes.<br><br>Gastrointestinal: Intake decreased.<br><br>Genitourinary: Bladder control and the amount of urine decreases. | Respiratory: Breathing will gradually slow and cease.<br><br>Circulatory: Heartbeat and pulse are not present; skin color changes to gray.<br><br>Genitourinary: The child may have an involuntary loss of stool and urine. |
| **Possible support measures related to physical changes** | Provide food and fluids if the child desires them.<br><br>Plan periods of rest and activity according to the child's ability to tolerate these measures. | Give medications to relieve pain, symptoms, and discomfort.<br><br>Provide familiar comfort measures (see **Table 9-2**).<br><br>Provide assistance with the child's physical care needs at night.<br><br>Dress the child in light cotton clothing; provide light bedcovers.<br><br>Anticipate the child's bowel and bladder control needs. | |
| **Emotional and spiritual changes** | The child "cocoons." | The child is afraid of being alone, especially at night.<br><br>There is a diminishing circle of visitors that consists of family only.<br><br>The child is restless, agitated, and anxious.<br><br>The child shows anger or impatience with loved ones.<br><br>The child talks with the unseen or unheard, has out-of-body experiences, and finishes "unfinished" business. | |
| **Possible support measures related to emotional and spiritual changes** | Accept and allow the child to set the pace. | Listen quietly.<br><br>Keep the child in touch with time and place.<br><br>Touch the child gently if it is appropriate.<br><br>Continue to laugh and play with the child.<br><br>Respect the child's privacy.<br><br>Use soft, indirect lighting in the child's room.<br><br>Have someone stay with the child at night.<br><br>Acknowledge the child's experiences. | Say good-bye in whatever way is possible.<br><br>Honor the child's dignity.<br><br>Touch the child gently when cleansing his or her body. |

perception. Knowledge of the underlying pathophysiology of the disease process also is essential (see the discussion of pain in Section V, "Side Effects of Treatment").

**Principles of terminal pain management:** Certain actions must be taken to provide the most effective system for managing the pain of children with terminal illnesses:

- At regular intervals, conduct a thorough but rapid assessment of the child's pain.
- Avoid unnecessary delays in pain treatment.
- Educate the child and the family about pain and pain control and include them in devising and implementing the treatment plan.
- Set the following goals:
  - The child can sleep undisturbed by pain.
  - The child experiences complete relief from pain when resting.
  - The child is free of pain when moving around or being handled.
- Follow a stepwise approach to analgesia that considers the severity of the pain. This model of analgesic prescription, firmly established by the World Health Organization, includes stepwise progression from a nonopioid analgesic (e.g., acetaminophen [Tylenol]) to a weak opioid (e.g., codeine), and, finally, to a strong opioid (e.g., morphine) (see the discussion of pain in Section V, "Side Effects of Treatment").
- Consider adjuvant therapy. These drugs have little or no intrinsic analgesic effects but produce useful pain relief as an adjunct to standard analgesic drugs. They include nonsteroidal antiinflammatory drugs, corticosteroids, antidepressants, anticonvulsants, muscle relaxants, and anxiolytics (see the discussion of pain in Section V, "Side

Effects of Treatment"). The addition of a sedating or hypnotic agent (e.g., propofol) could be considered for pain that is unresponsive to continuous-infusion opioids.

- Administer drugs orally whenever possible.
- Schedule medications to be given around the clock to maintain adequate drug levels. Constant pain requires regular administration of analgesics.
- Develop a plan for treating breakthrough pain.
- Try to prevent side effects associated with analgesic drug therapy whenever possible, and when they occur, treat them aggressively to promote comfort.

## Anemia and Bleeding

Patients may develop anemia and thrombocytopenia during the terminal phase of the disease. These sequelae also may occur in patients who have solid tumors with metastases to the bone marrow. Ongoing discussions regarding how to handle the symptoms associated with underlying bone-marrow failure should be conducted with the child's family.

The patient's ambulatory status can be used as a guide for recommending a transfusion of packed red blood cells (RBCs). For example, if the patient is up and about and is demonstrating symptoms of anemia (e.g., decreased strength, dizziness, shortness of breath, tachycardia) or showing signs of continued blood loss, periodic transfusions of RBCs could be an appropriate course of action. It should not be assumed that transfusion therapy will continue once it has been started, because the patient's clinical situation could change, and eventually transfusions will be unlikely to provide any clinical benefits.

The care provider should consider a patient's clinical status when determining his or her need for platelet transfusions. A platelet transfusion should be considered if a child manifests symptoms of bleeding (e.g., nosebleeds, hematuria, bloody stools). Massive external bleeding is an unusual event in terminally ill pediatric patients. However, as a precaution in the event that an overwhelming hematemesis or hemoptysis occurs, a bleeding kit, along with an appropriate analgesic and sedative, should be readily available.

## Seizures

Seizures are most common in patients with brain tumors or brain metastases. Seizures can occur spontaneously when central nervous system bleeding caused by thrombocytopenia occurs or when the child develops hypocoagulability. Seizures also can occur because of tumor growth that causes increased intracranial pressure.

Medical treatment for seizures is given to prevent or control their occurrence or severity. When seizures occur in a patient who is already on anticonvulsant therapy, they usually can be controlled by increasing the doses of the medications that have already been prescribed. A short-acting benzodiazepine can be used to quickly suppress the seizures. Diazepam (Valium) administered per rectum or intravenously (IV) is the usual first line of treatment. Midazolam (Versed) can be given intranasally to control seizures and may be an option if the per rectum route is not tolerated. A variety of anticonvulsants are available, and the individual agency or institution may have a particular treatment preference. When seizures are a strong possibility, families caring for a child at home should have a supply of diazepam (an IV formulation or a compounded suppository), lorazepam (Ativan) in either tablet or intensol liquid form, or midazolam and should be taught how to administer the drug.

A frequent side effect of anticonvulsant therapy is sedation. An acceptable balance between seizure control and lethargy should be achieved.

## Dyspnea

The development of air hunger and respiratory distress can be one of the most disturbing and difficult symptoms to treat. The etiology of the respiratory distress must be established to determine the most appropriate treatment. Respiratory distress can be caused by pulmonary disease or damage, infection, malignant infiltration, pleural effusion, cardiac failure, obstruction of the superior vena cava or by extrathoracic problems, such as anemia, ascites, or pain in the chest wall.

Although palliative measures such as radiation or drainage of ascites or effusions provide only temporary relief, they still may be worthwhile. Each episode should be considered individually to determine the goal of an invasive procedure. If the underlying cause of dyspnea is not amenable to treatment, the best possible relief may be achieved by combining a variety of pharmacologic methods with supportive measures. Simple, practical measures for relieving respiratory distress, such as using a fan, keeping the windows open in the patient's room, finding the optimal position for the patient, and using progressive relaxation techniques, may be useful.

The sensation of air hunger also can be decreased with opioid drugs. Opiates reduce anxiety and alleviate pain, which itself can lead to dyspnea. In addition, opiates specifically affect the respiratory center by reducing its sensitivity to changes in blood oxygen and carbon dioxide tensions. They can, therefore, produce significant improvement in dyspnea, regardless of the cause. Nebulized opioids provide an additional route for administering site-specific dosing to treat dyspnea, and recent reports about the success of this method have been encouraging.

Oxygen can give some short-term relief to patients suffering from dyspnea; however, some children may have a claustrophobic reaction to the oxygen cannula or mask. Anxiolytic agents (e.g., alprazolam, diazepam) can be helpful in relieving the anxiety associated with dyspnea.

Children with pulmonary metastases are more likely to have greater oxygen requirements. Preparation for meeting the oxygen requirements of a patient being cared for at home usually includes the use of liquid oxygen. Malignancies with no pulmonary involvement usually are managed effectively with either a regular oxygen tank or an oxygen concentrator.

Excessive secretions can be problematic for some children as their disease progresses. For some, this is a chronic problem, whereas for others, excessive secretions are associated with the terminal event. Scopolamine hydrobromide (Isopto-Hyoscine) administered subcutaneously or by patch, is an effective agent for reducing secretions.

## Fever and Infections

Families of children with cancer are reminded repeatedly that fever can signal a life-threatening complication if the child is neutropenic. The shift from curative to palliative care may be difficult for them to understand as they observe their child develop a fever with no emergent action taken. Families should be informed that fever in terminally ill children might not necessarily indicate infection but could instead be related to the disease process.

The decision to treat the fever with antibiotics or antifungals should be made jointly by the family and members of the child's healthcare team. Issues that should be considered are how responsive the infection might be to treatment, whether medications could be administered in the patient's setting of choice, whether either the drugs or their administration could result in significant toxicity, and how uncomfortable the child might be if antibiotics were withheld. Treatment of fever in a child in the terminal stage of disease could include simple measures such as sponging with tepid water or administering acetaminophen (Tylenol) at regular intervals.

### Nausea and Vomiting

The neurophysiology and control of nausea and vomiting are complex and not fully understood. The act of vomiting appears to be coordinated by the vomiting center in the medulla and can be induced by a variety of stimuli. Antiemetic agents may work at either one or a number of sites (e.g., vomiting center, neurotransmitter receptors in the gut wall, vestibular pathways) and can be selected rationally according to the presumed cause.

Persistent nausea and vomiting can be exhausting symptoms to control. The etiology of a patient's nausea should be established to determine the appropriate treatment. The cause of vomiting often can be deduced through knowledge of the disease process, inquiry about the nature of the vomiting and the circumstances in which it occurs, and the presence of associated symptoms, such as headache or constipation. Nausea and vomiting also can be the result of tumor invasion or a consequence of opioid therapy.

Many pharmacologic approaches to the treatment of nausea and vomiting exist, and clinicians must make their decisions on the basis of each patient's previous experience with antiemetic agents and their evaluation of the current problem. Persistent vomiting may require a combination of several drugs that have different mechanisms of action.

### Constipation

Constipation is a common problem that can cause anorexia, nausea, discomfort, and overflow diarrhea. Contributing factors include lack of gastrointestinal motility, a poor or low-fiber diet, low fluid intake, decreased physical activity, weakness and muscle wasting, and medications (e.g., opioids, phenothiazines, anticholinergics). At least one, and often many, of these factors contribute to constipation in terminally ill children.

Prevention is the best course of treatment. Docusate sodium, lactulose, senna, and bisacodyl are common agents used in combination for the treatment and prevention of constipation. Adequate doses and a combination of oral drugs should be tried before resorting to suppositories (bisacodyl) or enemas (sodium citrate or docusate sodium).

### Anorexia

Treatable causes of anorexia (including nausea, vomiting, constipation, mucositis, depression, or excessive portions of food) should be considered. It is natural, however, for children near death to become less interested in food. Severely ill children who have a minimal level of activity can survive comfortably for extended periods with little nutrition. However, a child's failure to eat often is a problem for parents and other family members, because for many families, eating is equated with nurturing and maintaining the child's strength.

Support should be focused on the family. Family members should be helped to accept the child's natural loss of appetite. The family may wish to offer frequent small portions of the child's favorite foods. IV hydration or total parenteral nutrition usually is inappropriate for a child during the terminal period. However, if the family has had previous experiences with IV nutrition for the child, they may insist on this intervention (see the subsection "Ethical Dilemmas in Terminal Care").

### Restlessness and Anxiety

A patient's restlessness can be the result of pain, anxiety, or sleeplessness. Restlessness in a child should be evaluated promptly, and the child's narcotic regimen should be reevaluated. Restlessness and anxiety also can be signs that a child needs communication, reassurance, and emotional support. Pharmacologic agents cannot and should not replace time spent listening to and talking with a child about his or her fears and anxieties.

Medications such as benzodiazepines may be indicated when a child is very close to death, a time when agitation and confusion occur as a result of irreversible organ failure.

## Nursing Assessment and Interventions

### Assessment

- Recognize that management of terminal symptoms is not standardized.
- Explore the child's and the family's fears related to the onset of certain symptoms or the inability to control them.
- Consult with family members and help them care for their child in a manner that is compatible with their wishes.
- Recognize that physiological signs and symptoms tend to develop more quickly in children.
- Recognize that symptoms are rarely simple physical events; they are more likely to be complex experiences with physical, emotional, social, and spiritual components (see the subsection "Psychosocial Care of the Terminally Ill Child").

### Interventions

- Prioritize the patient's comfort as the primary goal. Remember that families vary in their ability and willingness to tolerate symptoms, so the meaning of comfort for individuals and families also varies (Table 9-2).
- Determine the family's preferences for treatment and intervention; a compromise between the family's wishes and the physician's orders may be required.
- Emphasize symptom management that focuses on the uses of noninvasive, palliative approaches.
- Provide a cohesive team approach to determining the strategy of care for the child; team members should contribute their own personal and professional skills.
- Ensure ongoing, direct, and honest communication between team members and the family.

### Table 9-2. Measures that Enhance the Patient's Sense of Comfort and Security

| Measure | Description |
| --- | --- |
| Quiet presence | Sit calmly and quietly, not necessarily touching. |
| Massage | Use oils or lotions that will not irritate the child's skin; play music quietly to help the child relax. |
| Therapeutic touch | This is done only by a person trained in therapeutic touch, a method that works with a person's energy field to bring comfort and relief from physical and emotional pain. |
| Music, videos, toys, blankets | Help to maintain a link with what is familiar from the child's home; children may come to the hospital or hospice with their favorites. |
| Family gatherings | Explore ways to create lasting memories, treasures, and rituals that will keep the child's presence felt after his or her death. |
| Picture board | Have family members and friends gather pictures of times shared together; place them on a bulletin board near the bed where everyone can see them. |
| Room environment | Encourage the family to bring items that will provide comfort from home; modify the child's room according to his or her developmental age and preferences. |
| Books | Engage the child in choosing an appropriate book (many children enjoy having someone read to them). |
| Family, friends, a spiritual support person, pets | Respect and enable the dying child to see people and pets. At times, the child's requests may seem very spontaneous and not practical, but to the child it may be part of finishing unfinished business. |

- Provide anticipatory guidance for the child and the family regarding the course of the child's illness and appropriate teaching to ease their fears and anxiety.
- Understand that the recognition that they have coped with difficulty and provided the best possible care for their child often is comforting for parents.

## Psychosocial Care of the Terminally Ill Child

*Janice Nuuhiwa*

### General Principles

Initiating a plan of care for a terminally ill child requires a multifaceted approach. The healthcare team, along with the child and family, must work together as partners to guide decisions for future interventions. The team can best actuate the goals of care after a complete assessment of the child's and family's values, beliefs, and wishes.

Nurses work with professionals from other healthcare disciplines to facilitate psychosocial care. Nurses play a primary role in helping to present and explain care options, the side effects of interventions, and patients' expected physical changes. These conversations usually raise numerous psychosocial issues for a child and a family. It is during these critical moments that children and families benefit from the therapeutic psychosocial support that nurses offer.

### Goals of Family-Centered Care

Questions that should guide the care of terminally ill children and their families include the following:
- What are the current roles of the family members?
- How will the child's death alter the roles of other family members?
- What is the family's previous history with death or other loss?
- What are the family's coping patterns?
- Are there any rituals in which the child or family would like to engage at this time?
- Are there situations that can cause added stress and loss for the family?

### Attend to the Needs of the Family

The impending death of a child causes trauma and disconnection within a family. Family members can become isolated from each other and their friends. Family members may disagree about the approach to care, and friends may be unable to tolerate the intense pain of the loss when the death finally occurs.

In addition, communication between family members may be strained because of the difficulty they may have in coping with the loss. The child and the family may pretend that everything is all right while knowing that the reality is much different; this protective denial among family members only serves to isolate them more.

The family's feelings of loss of control may have begun at the time of the child's diagnosis. Facing the terminal aspects of the disease can worsen the sense of being out of control. The normalcy that the family needs may be impossible to achieve during this stage of the child's disease.

Financial concerns may increase. Often, one or both parents need to consider taking a leave of absence from their job. In addition, insurance coverage often is limited. Pediatric hospice benefits frequently do not cover what is considered routine pediatric terminal care (e.g., private-duty nursing, at-home blood transfusions). Requests for exceptions or an acknowledgment of necessity must be obtained to provide this essential care.

### Actuate Care Goals

The values and wishes of the child and the family about care at the end stage of the disease should guide medical interventions (e.g., home versus hospital; high-tech versus low-tech interventions). Whenever possible, the child and family should be given options. The family can then carefully weigh the risks and benefits of each option and make an informed decision. The child and family should be informed about current and anticipated physical changes. Most families can cope better if they know what to expect. It is not necessary to go into great detail, however, until the changes are likely to occur.

### Attend to the Needs of the Dying Child

Comfort for a dying child should be the primary concern. Other goals include pain control, expert symptom management, and emotional peace. Dying patients often have a fear of being alone, so loved ones should be encouraged to remain nearby. Terminally ill children also are concerned about the future of their families. The child should be assured that the family will survive the loss.

Communication is critical. A dying child may need "permission" to talk about the dying process. This permission can be given by providing simple, honest, age-appropriate information about what is happening. Family members, nurses, and other healthcare providers should talk about what the child needs to discuss, answer questions, and update information as needed. Explanations may have to be given more than once. The child also may want to talk, not just listen.

The dying child should remain connected with the people in his or her life. This connection can be maintained by having the child spend time with or be involved in activities with siblings, parents, and other people who are important to him or her. Safe and familiar surroundings help to alleviate unnecessary anxieties (see the subsection "Children and Death").

### Attend to the Needs of Siblings

Emotional comfort for siblings is important. A change in the family's routine and the parents' inability to parent are usual occurrences during the terminal stages of a child's illness. The dying child's siblings may witness inconsolable distress in their parents; the anguish this can bring to these children may be difficult for them to bear.

Communication is one of the most important factors in supporting the siblings through this time. Siblings should receive information about what is happening to their dying brother or sister. They should be given simple, honest, age-appropriate information about the situation. They should be allowed to talk about whatever they need to discuss, and their questions should be answered and updates provided as the need arises. Siblings' feelings about the dying child and the dying process should be explored in an age-appropriate manner. Often, they are unsure how to process feelings of guilt, anger, abandonment, and other emotions that arise during this family transition. Parents should acknowledge these emotions and help the siblings process their experience. Sibling support groups, child-life specialists, and social workers may be enlisted to assist them at this time. Siblings often struggle emotionally when contradictory information is disclosed. What they have overheard and what has been told to them may be very different.

Siblings need to spend special time with and be involved in activities with the dying child. Participation, no matter how minor, in the care of the dying child can be crucial to the sibling's ability to cope.

Saying good-bye is very important for siblings. They should be encouraged to view their sibling after he or she has died. Young children usually benefit by seeing that their brother or sister is no longer breathing or moving.

Siblings may fear that life will never be the same after their brother's or sister's death. They also recognize that the parent they view as powerful cannot fix the situation. Furthermore, siblings often are the last family members whose loss is acknowledged. As a result of their brother's or sister's death, siblings may have lost their companion, playmate, rival, idol, or parent substitute. They may fear that they will be expected to fill the dying child's role.

### Attend to the Needs of the Parents

Parents need information about how to care for themselves, their dying child, and their other children. They should be encouraged to spend time with all of their children and to maintain as much normalcy as possible.

Support from a spouse may be difficult at this time. Feelings of helplessness or fear of burdening a spouse may make mutual support impossible. Spouses should be encouraged to maintain a united approach to care, and family members should be encouraged to share their feelings clearly and honestly. Open communication and compromise are the goals. The dying child's parents may need assistance with crucial decisions such as those involving palliative management of pain and other symptoms, hospice and hospital admissions, home-based care, support groups, disclosure of information, and plans for a funeral.

### Attend to the Needs of the Grandparents

Grandparents can experience physical and emotional isolation from the terminally ill child and other family members. This isolation can be self-imposed because of their own intense feelings of grief and loss. Coping with the death of a grandchild is a double loss because the grandparents not only experience the loss of a grandchild but also witness their own child suffer the worst loss imaginable for a parent.

### Respect the Child's and Family's Spiritual Beliefs

It is important to determine families' religious preferences and to respect individual customs. A terminally ill child and his or her family should be encouraged to talk about their beliefs. The child and the family may need to find meaning in the child's suffering. Feelings of guilt and a need for forgiveness and reconciliation should be acknowledged as normal.

The family need to be assured that rituals and traditions (i.e., those related to holidays and celebrations) that normally create special memories and meaning should be continued in the absence of the child. If family members finds solace in prayer, they should be supported. Spiritual beliefs are often challenged during a crisis involving a dying child. Family members' perceptions of the meaning of life can change; they may even question their faith.

### Explore the Child's and Family's Interest in Performing or Creating a Ritual

If the child or family wishes to engage in the dimensions of ritual (i.e., meaning-making, intention, and participation), the nurse can facilitate this process by investigating what the family has done in the past or by sharing rituals that other families have created. Rituals that acknowledge the dying process serve as one way for families to stay connected to the child after his or her. The child's favorite song, a favorite piece of jewelry, or a well-loved stuffed animal can serve as a symbol of the child in future rituals and provide comfort to the bereaved family.

### Facilitate Pediatric-Focused Hospice Care

The parents are the primary caregivers and decision makers and may request palliative care for their child (e.g., IV fluids, antibiotics). Children with cancer are familiar with and may expect a high-tech approach to care. Making the transition to a philosophy of care that offers a number of options for symptom management may be difficult for the child to understand and requires significant flexibility (see the subsection "Ethical Dilemmas in Terminal Care").

Each family may have different reimbursement considerations related to the child's care; therefore, a discussion with the family's insurance case manager may be beneficial for determining the most appropriate payment source. Hospice insurance may not be the most cost-effective option because many hospice programs require a 6-month prognosis. This determination can be difficult to make for children because they often can withstand the excessive stress and strain of progressive tumor growth and live longer than expected. In addition, a prognosis is not always an appropriate guide for making a referral to a hospice. Many children with a prognosis of more than 6 months should be referred to hospices, especially if their disease is incurable. Nurses and other healthcare professionals should check with their local pediatric hospice program for guidance. If hospice care is not obtainable because of clinical limitations or limited insurance coverage, consider partnering with the home-health agency that has been working with the family, if applicable.

Parents may not be able to sign a do-not-resuscitate order, but they might agree to nonaggressive treatment for their child. This fact does not necessarily mean that hospice care is inappropriate. Until the moment of their child's death, many parents sustain the hope that their child will be cured or will not die.

## Nursing Assessment and Interventions

### Assessment
- Evaluate the wishes, beliefs, and values of the child and family for direction concerning the child's terminal care.
- Assess the family members' feelings and concerns.
- Recognize that nurses in this situation share an intimate, personal experience with the child and family.
- Acknowledge that age is not necessarily an accurate predictor of sophistication regarding how children face death. Differences in children's conceptions of death depend upon their life experiences, level of development, intellect, and level of precocity. Their cultural and ethnic backgrounds also are influential. Each child is unique and demands careful consideration, understanding, and compassion.

### Interventions
- Allow the child and the family to maintain control over the direction of care.
- Incorporate the use of rituals, as defined by the child and the family, in the provision of care.
- Respect and support the child's and the family's decisions.
- Develop a multidisciplinary plan of care that addresses the physical, emotional, and spiritual comfort of the child and the family.
- Refer the child and the family to a pediatric hospice program, if they so desire.
- Promote honest, open communication among all family members.
- Share the dying experience with the child and the family:
  - Validate all feelings as normal.
  - Explain to the family that the grieving process is very individualized.
  - Provide emotional support for each issue or crisis as it occurs.
  - Promote a trusting relationship with all healthcare providers.
  - Respond promptly to requests for information.
- Recognize that palliative care includes expert pain and symptom control, recognition of the futility of lifesaving treatment, an emphasis on open communication within the family and between the family and the healthcare team, and support for the bereaved.
- Work with family members to balance their hopes and fears, and help them face death realistically. Emphasize that the parents have done all they could do to save their child.
- Recognize the healing power of listening, touch, books, art, and music.
- Remember that professionals have chosen their roles in this field, but parents of dying children have not chosen this experience.

# Bereavement

Rebecca A. Monroe

## General Principles
Bereavement is the state of having suffered a loss, and grief is the emotional reaction to the loss. The type of grief and bereavement experienced depends upon many factors, including the significance of the survivors' relationship with the deceased person and the circumstances of the death. Bereaved parents have the difficult task of discovering a new life without the physical presence of their child.

The loss of a child is perhaps the most difficult loss to endure because the death of a child seems unnatural. The event represents not only a physical loss but also a loss of the past and an end to parents' future hopes and dreams. Parents lose a part of themselves when their child dies.

## Stages of Bereavement
Elisabeth Kübler-Ross (1993) identified five stages of grief and bereavement that a person goes through when coping with the death of a loved one. The stages are denial, anger, bargaining, depression, and acceptance. A person may experience these stages in any order.

## Tasks of Bereavement
The tasks of bereavement consist of accepting the loss, experiencing the pain, and adjusting to an environment without the deceased person.

## Parental Bereavement Tasks
The parents' bereavement tasks include
- facing the finality of loss
- remembering past events and experiences with their child
- processing the feelings of failure as a parent and of personal diminishment

- building a family life without the child
- discovering healthy ways to continue the relationship with the deceased child on a spiritual and emotional level.

## Unique Features of Parental Bereavement

The death of a child is out of sequence with the natural order of events in a family's life. Fathers' and mothers' grieving styles may be different and may even conflict, so they may be unable to support each other or their surviving children. Parents will experience the grief throughout their lifetime, and significant events may trigger acute grief reactions.

The death of a child is an assault on the parents' sense of identity as parents, protectors, and providers. Feelings of guilt may be related to their perceived failure to protect the child, their past transgressions, and the mere fact of their survival beyond the lifetime of their child.

The second year of grieving may be more difficult than the first. Parents often recall the first year as one in which they "felt numb." Between the second and third years of bereavement, family members may realize that they are forever changed, may feel their grief declining, may feel renewed energy, and may be ready to reinvest themselves in their work and the important relationships in their lives.

## Nursing Assessment and Interventions

### Assessment
- Assess the factors that are unique to parents' bereavement.
- Determine the relationship or role that each family member had with the child (e.g., Was the child an only child? If not, what was his or her birth order? Were siblings of the same sex? Did the family member share similar interests?).
- Determine the family's history of previous losses, and ascertain whether they have any concurrent stresses.
- Evaluate the existing support systems available to each family member.
- Assess family members' anticipatory grieving and involvement with the child prior to the child's death, including their ability to communicate openly about the death, the quality and quantity of the time they spent with the child, and the opportunity they had to say good-bye and to create memories.
- Recognize that grief and bereavement experiences are individual and unique to each person and that the family's culture, community, faith, and support system influence this process significantly.
- Recognize that the degree to which each family member grieves and successfully works through bereavement is related to the extent to which the person allows himself or herself to grieve.

### Interventions
**Prior to the child's death:**
- Establish a primary-care team for inpatient, outpatient, and home care of the child.
- Encourage the family's mutual participation in caring for the child.
- Facilitate communication between the family and the team regarding all healthcare decisions.
- Encourage the family to use its personal support systems, but also offer others (e.g., a social worker, counselor, or chaplain).
- Determine what the child and family envision for the child's environment at the time of death (e.g., location [home or hospital], people present, comfort objects [special blanket or toy]), and assist the child and family in fulfilling their expectations if possible.
- Assist the child and family with saying good-byes, carrying out last wishes, and creating memories.
- Reinforce the family's positive role in the child's life.
- Prepare the child and the family for the physical changes and emotions that might occur near death.

**At the time of the child's death:**
- Be sensitive to the family's cultural and religious preferences.
- Assist with notification of the death and with funeral or memorial arrangements, if such assistance is requested.
- Prepare the child's body with or without the family's assistance; some parents may want to bathe and dress the child themselves.
- Provide compassionate postmortem care.
- Include the child's siblings in the after-death experience; even very young children should be included.

**After the child's death:**
- Provide active listening statements; "I'm sorry" or "I care" can be comforting.
- Comfort with physical touch if appropriate (e.g., hugging, hand-holding).
- Use the words *death* and *died,* because children can be confused by substitute words such as *lost* or *taken.*
- Call or write the family to extend sympathy, or send a card with a written memory of the child.
- Refer the family to other sources of support (see the list of resources for families at the end of this subsection).
- Speak about the child because most parents appreciate that their child is remembered and welcome an opportunity to talk about their grief or share their memories.
- Educate the family about grief and bereavement experiences.
- Effective interventions for families can be simple, or they can be part of a structured bereavement program.
- Implement bereavement rounds during which the care team can discuss the death and identify areas of concern that can be addressed during bereavement follow-up.
- Implement a structured bereavement program, and arrange for bereavement materials to be sent to families at certain intervals (e.g., on the anniversary of the child's death, birthdays, holidays).
- Develop rituals of remembrance within the family or at the institution (e.g., a memorial service).

### Reference
Kübler-Ross, E. (1993). *On death and dying.* New York: Maxwell Macmillan International.

# Section IX Care for the Terminally Ill Child and the Family

> **Resources for Families**
>
> **National Organizations**
>
> **American Cancer Society**
> National Office
> 250 Williams Street NW, Suite 600
> Atlanta, GA 30303
> 800/ACS-2345 (227-2345)
> www.cancer.org
>
> **Candlelighters Childhood Cancer Foundation**
> National Office
> PO Box 498
> Kensington, MD 20895
> 800/366-2223
> www.candlelighters.org
>
> **Centering Corporation**
> 7230 Maple Street
> Omaha, NE 68134
> 866/218-0101
> www.centeringcorp.com
>
> **Children's Hospice International**
> 1101 King Street, Suite 360
> Alexandria, VA 22314
> 800/24-CHILD (242-4453), 703/684-0300
> www.chionline.org
>
> **The Compassionate Friends**
> PO Box 3696
> Oak Brook, IL 60522
> 877/969-0010
> www.compassionatefriends.org
>
> **Rainbows**
> 2100 Golf Road, Suite 370
> Rolling Meadows, IL 60008
> 800/266-3206
> www.rainbows.org

# Professionals' Grief, Distress, and Bereavement

*Cynthia A. Stutzer*

## General Principles

A bereaved person has suffered the loss of a loved one. *Grief* is the emotional reaction to the loss and is a normal, healthy process. It is the "affective and cognitive component of bereavement, involving a wide array of emotions (e.g., sadness, despair, numbness, anger, fear, relief). . . . and cognitive responses (e.g., shock, indecision, denial search for meaning)." (Valente & Saunders, 2002, p. 9). Grief may begin well before a child dies. It can start at the time of the diagnosis, at relapse, or at any time during the treatment or palliative-care phases. Distress occurs when people do not allow themselves to express grief.

## Factors and Situations That Influence Professionals' Grief

### Factors and Situations at the Time of a Child's Death

A number of factors and situations can affect a healthcare professional's experience of grief, including
- the immediate circumstances of the death
- the decision making before, during, and after the death
- a perception that the death was preventable
- a perception that the child suffered
- the suddenness of the death
- the nurse's conception of a "good" death and the family's reaction to the death.

### Environmental Factors

Environmental factors also affect the level of grief that professionals are able to express. These factors include
- the workplace culture (e.g., the notion that "being professional means you don't cry")
- the level of support offered by the healthcare facility (including education support)
- the presence or absence of supportive colleagues and friends
- workplace stress
- the number of concurrent stresses or crises in the nurse's life at the time of the child's death, including other losses (bereavement overload)
- the nurse's level of satisfaction with his or her job
- the time available for emotional support and debriefings
- policies that may conflict with the nurse's values and beliefs
- fear of legal action
- stigma associated with the death, especially if the death was iatrogenic.

### Intrapersonal Factors

Intrapersonal factors that affect the grief experience include the nurse's
- values and beliefs
- work and life experiences
- social, cultural, ethnic, religious, or spiritual background
- previous experiences of grief and loss (including whether he or she is reexperiencing grief over past losses)
- coping patterns and skills
- perception of unfinished business with the deceased child and the child's family
- personal expectations within the situation
- assigned meaning to the death
- need to feel in control of a situation
- level of self-esteem
- self-blame
- experience as a nurse
- professional identity
- ability to deal with his or her emotions and openly express grief.

### Interpersonal Factors

Interpersonal factors include
- the nature of the relationship with the child and the child's family (including the nurse's perception of his or her place in, and contribution to, the child's life)
- the nurse's relationships with other team members, the patient, and the family
- conflict and communication problems among team members and with the family
- fear or criticism
- the level of ability to provide input into the decision-making process regarding the child's care

- the extent to which the nurse incorporates the emotions of the child, the family, and colleagues into his or her own grieving process.

## Responses to Grief

### Physical Symptoms
The physical responses that professionals can experience include insomnia or an increased desire to sleep; nausea; stomach pain; weight loss or gain; fatigue; lack of strength; hyperactivity; restlessness; heart palpitations; sighing; loss of or increase in sexual desire; hair loss; diarrhea; constipation; shortness of breath; crying; nervousness; tension; feelings of emptiness or heaviness; impatience; irritability; and a tightness in the throat.

### Emotional or Psychological Symptoms
Professionals can experience symptoms such as sadness, depression, anger, inability to concentrate, feeling out of control, vulnerability related to their own or their loved ones' mortality, frustration, feelings of inadequacy, a sense of powerlessness related to their inability to change the outcome, doubt about their professional competence, lower self-esteem, loneliness or isolation, feeling overwhelmed by the unfairness of the situation, and guilt.

Professionals might feel some emotional numbness, which is a self-protective reaction that can help them do what needs to be done to care for a dying child and the child's family. However, this reaction can be harmful if it continues to the point where individuals are unable to find an appropriate outlet for their grief. These professionals also might undergo a physical or emotional withdrawal from patients and families whose uncertain futures could eventually cause them pain and grief.

Other reactions include feeling valued, or sometimes devalued, by the child, the family, and other members of the healthcare team. Some professionals feel grateful that they have done everything possible for the patient, that they have been able to facilitate a peaceful and dignified death, that the child has taught them so much, and that they have shared a part of life with the patient and family. In addition, professionals may acquire a renewed appreciation of life, a feeling of relief that the patient's suffering has ended, and a sense of peace.

## Strategies for Professionals Dealing with Grief
- Recognize the inevitability of the death, and revise goals from focusing on cure to ensuring a comfortable and dignified death for the child.
- Find some kind of meaning in the child's death (i.e., What does this child's life and death mean to others? How has life been changed positively by knowing this child and his or her family? What has the experience taught others about life and humanity?).
- Discover or develop a personal sense of spirituality.
- Develop and apply greater personal knowledge about the physical and psychosocial aspects of care during the period of dying, death, and grief to deliver the best possible care to other patients and their families.
- Realize that some situations cannot be changed, no matter how good the care that was delivered. Reflect upon the interventions that worked, and discuss with colleagues those that did not go well. Learn from every experience, both positive and negative; acknowledge feelings about them; and then let those feelings go. Self-blame for situations in which a caregiver has no power or experience with should be avoided. Sometimes the best legacy bequeathed by a child who has died is the increased skill, knowledge, and understanding that the child's caregivers can bring to similar situations in the future.
- Strive to separate work and personal life by developing a ritual or process for leaving work behind when off duty. This should become easier as experience in coping with grief increases.
- Use briefing and debriefing sessions to share experiences with colleagues, and seek support from colleagues, friends, and professional grief counselors. Letting others know what is happening at the time it is happening often helps one prepare for a patient's death.
- Maintain good health by continuing to exercise and eat properly, rest, and get enough sleep. Create a routine that will promote health and prevent illness. Develop a balance between the demands of work, family life, and other individual needs.
- Draw on internal resources.
- Use the expertise of colleagues, and ask questions when trying to find ways to cope with grief. Use others as role models for grieving.
- Plan ahead, anticipate grief, and focus actions and interventions to influence it. For example, being honest and spending time with the child and family may help to avoid regrets later when reflecting on the experience. Conversely, physical or emotional withdrawal might help professionals avoid pain and grief in the short term but could result in feelings of regret at a later time.
- Complete unfinished business by finding a way to say goodbye, either by attending the patient's funeral or by creating a memorial of some type in the child's honor. For example, some facilities have memorial services or "remembrance teas." Many nurses create their own rituals (e.g., lighting a candle, walking on the beach, reading a special poem, or listening to a piece of music) to honor dead patients who have touched their lives. Writing a note to a bereaved family can mean a great deal to them and can help bring closure to the relationship.
- Learn about the normal grieving process. Distinguish between grief reactions and depression, and manage each appropriately.
- Develop an awareness of personal grief reactions and triggers, and identify the characteristics that trigger a more intense grief reaction. For example, a child who is the same age as a nurse's own child or who reminds the nurse of another patient who has died may trigger a grief reaction. Children with certain physical or personality characteristics might also stimulate a more intense grief response.
- Take time to create joy and peace and to affirm life. Learn to self-nurture. Recognize the need to laugh and have fun even in the midst of sorrow.
- Seek professional help, if necessary, to work through personal feelings of grief.

Management has a role to play in helping professionals deal with grief. Managers need to identify the ways in which the workplace affects grief. For example, if a nurse wants to be informed when a child has died, provisions should be made for making the notification and giving the nurse the option of remaining home from work to avoid facing the patient's empty bed.

Facilitating or providing educational opportunities for staff to learn about grief and bereavement, developing policies that acknowledge and support professionals' grief, changing assignments, giving professionals time off, changing their work schedules, providing mentoring opportunities, forming stress management teams for critical incidents, instituting "bereavement rounds," and holding multidisciplinary team debriefings are ways in which an institution can help professionals deal with grief. Debriefing can take place in an individual or a group meeting, but it is important to have a skilled facilitator who will not become caught up in the emotions of the situation. Skilled facilitators can lead a discussion as participants discuss the death, its meaning, their emotions, and the impact of the death on themselves, the work group, and others.

## Proposed Models for Professionals' Grief and Bereavement

Most traditional models that describe the experience of those who have lost a loved one do not accurately describe the grief and bereavement that healthcare professionals experience. Although no well-tested models for professionals' grief and bereavement exist, reviewing the following models may help nurses explore their own grief reactions and lead to self-understanding.

Kaplan (2000) proposes a model with three interactive and integrated components. These dynamic, nonlinear components are

- "emotional tension," that is, managing strong feelings while maintaining professional caregiving
- personal grief
- physical and emotional symptoms.

Influencing factors may help or inhibit this process. Papadatou (2000) describes factors that affect the grieving process and its outcomes. She states that grieving is an individual and social process with interaction between an individual's lifestyle (e.g., beliefs, values, and assumptions) and his or her "work style," which includes the work environment and workplace "rules" (formal and informal, written and unwritten). This interaction affects the normal, healthy fluctuation between avoiding or repressing grief and experiencing grief.

Tasks that must be undertaken (Papadatou, 2000) include "making meaning" and "loss transcendence." Making meaning—that is, interpreting events and representing the situation in symbolic terms—allows individuals and teams to gain a sense of mastery and integration and to overcome confusion and doubt. Loss transcendence involves discovering behaviors, thoughts, and emotions that allow reinvestment in life and in oneself.

Tasks for the bereaved professional are further described by Saunders and Valente (1994; Valente & Saunders, 2002). They are

- finding meaning—emotionally and cognitively processing the death
- restoring or maintaining personal and professional integrity and self-esteem and eliminating self-blame
- responding to and managing feelings
- realigning relationships with family, colleagues, and patients and their families.

### References

Kaplan, L. J. (2000). Toward a model of caregiver grief: Nurses' experiences of treating dying children. *Omega, 41,* 187–206.

Papadatou, D. (2000). A proposed model of health professionals' grieving process. *Omega, 41,* 59–77.

Saunders, J. M., & Valente, S. M. (1994). Nurses' grief. *Cancer Nursing, 17,* 318–325.

Valente, S. M., & Saunders, J. M. (2002). Nurses' grief reactions to a patient's suicide. *Perspectives in Psychiatric Care, 39,* 5–14.

# Moral Distress

Cynthia A. Stutzer

## General Principles

"Moral distress occurs when one knows the right thing to do, but institutional or other constraints make it difficult to pursue the desired course of action" (Raines, 2000, p. 30). Moral distress also can occur in situations of "internal constraints, such as . . . being socialized to follow orders, [feeling] the futility of past actions, fear of losing . . . jobs, self doubts and lack of courage" (Wilkinson, 1987–1988, p. 21). There may be initial distress, which occurs when the distressing event or issues are first perceived, followed by reactive moral distress, which occurs when the precipitating obstacles, stressors, or dilemmas cannot be acted upon or resolved. The very nature of nursing and how we define ourselves within the nurse-patient relationship may contribute to increased moral distress.

Corley (2002) proposes a theory of moral distress that demonstrates the impact on the

- patient—increased discomfort or suffering
- nurse—resignation, burnout, decision to leave the profession
- organization—high nurse turnover, decreased quality of care, low patient satisfaction.

Moral distress has not been well addressed in nursing education. Exploring the interrelationships among moral concepts (e.g., moral integrity, sensitivity, commitment) can lead to better understanding of moral distress and how to address it. Moral residue results from the "cumulative effects of unresolved moral distress" (Corley, Minick, Elswick, & Jacobs, 2005, p. 386).

## Factors and Situations That Can Produce Moral Distress

The degree of moral distress that a healthcare professional experiences depends upon the following areas of potential conflicts and their resolution:

- the process of making the shift from cure to comfort (e.g., when there is no hope for a cure, goals are changed and redefined to include a peaceful, dignified death)
- aggressive treatment that prevents palliative care in the face of perceived medically futile treatment
- decision making and communication (e.g., not having input into decisions about patients and their families,

implementing decisions with which the healthcare professional might not agree, carrying on treatment that is unwarranted or painful, having a child participate in research when he or she is dying, deciding what to tell the child and the family or how to tell them)
- conflicting priorities (e.g., quality-of-life needs and societal, cultural, and ethnic mores) and determination of the "right" thing to do for the child, the family, the staff, and the workplace
- the professional's own values, beliefs, morals, and religious or spiritual beliefs
- disagreements with physicians and other colleagues on the healthcare team
- the recognition that family members may have different opinions about what is happening and may base their decisions relating to care on those opinions
- the inability to keep promises made to the child or the family
- the nature, intensity, and assigned meaning of relationships between the nurse, child, and family
- the inability to find meaning in suffering while also being unable to influence the situation producing the suffering
- difficult workplace issues (e.g., staffing, work hours, and workload, as well as cumulative stressors such as newly diagnosed patients, relapses, deaths, and organizational stresses)
- differing coping styles.

Moral distress also can arise when the healthcare professional
- is caring for patients and families in a research-oriented milieu
- is unable to articulate his or her own moral stance
- is responsible for the care of a patient but does not have the authority to make decisions
- perceives that a patient's suffering, pain, or symptoms are not being adequately relieved
- perceives that he or she lacks influence in the workplace
- perceives that the institution's ethical decision-making process is unclear or inadequate.

## Responses to Moral Distress

Individuals' responses to moral distress include anger, frustration, resentment, exhaustion, or sorrow; feelings of helplessness or powerlessness; a sense of erosion of personal integrity and self-esteem; feelings of passivity, uncertainty, and personal and professional disillusionment; physical or emotional withdrawal; a sense of failure; a feeling of being undervalued; and guilt. Some professionals might use sarcasm, cry, or leave their current work assignment; others might manipulate situational constraints to gain control, provide comfort to the patient, and advocate for the patient and family; still others might avoid certain patients, families, or situations or refuse certain assignments, thus compromising patient safety. Healthcare professionals might experience a level of stress that leads to quiet suffering, diminished self-worth, or burnout. Personal and professional relationships can be affected. Moral outrage can occur when there is a "perceived inability to stop/prevent the immoral actions of others" (Wilkinson, 1987–1988, p. 25). Positive effects may increase personal and professional growth or prompt the professional to acquire the skills to work through difficult situations.

## Strategies for Dealing with Moral Distress

- Increase knowledge regarding clinical situations and the influence of ethnicity and culture.
- Clarify personal beliefs, values, and principles, and determine how these guide individual nursing practice and influence care decisions.
- Communicate clearly and discuss issues with others.
  - Assess the patient's and the family's understanding of the situation.
  - Clarify the implications of the patient's and the family's decisions.
  - Provide additional information or education to help the patient and family make decisions.
  - Determine how decisions are communicated because eliciting different points of view can help people clarify their own beliefs, and talking with others can help them resolve issues and decide on a course of action. Sharing concerns with others and offering explanations are ways of providing support.
- Recognize moral dilemmas.
  - Identify situations that conflict with one's own moral principles and those that cause moral distress. Individuals who are able to recognize such triggers take action to reduce moral distress.
  - Ascertain whether decisions made by the patient, family, and other members of the team are consistent with the nurse's personal beliefs, values, and principles. The best way for professionals to recognize a moral dilemma is to acknowledge their own discomfort with a situation. Identify feelings as "moral distress."
- Discover resources, both personal and professional.
- Identify how an institution can help healthcare professionals resolve their ethical dilemmas (e.g., by instituting ethics rounds or ethics committees, providing education and mentorship about ethical decision making, and developing policies and procedures for identifying and working through ethical dilemmas).
- Develop a plan of action for dealing with ethical dilemmas. As situations arise, decide on a moral course of action after compiling background information and data pertaining to the situation and identifying all the people involved in the dilemma who might be affected by the decisions.
- Plan how to advocate for the child and the family.
- Consider different courses of action and identify potential obstacles and consequences of each action on the patient, the patient's family, colleagues, the workplace, and the nurse.
- Prepare to defend actions. There may be times when the wishes of a patient or a family cannot be carried out. For example, there would be legal ramifications if a child asked for help in taking his or her life and the nurse complied with that request.
- Discuss moral and ethical issues with colleagues. Decide how to work together to create an ethical environment.
- Recognize the negative impact of moral distress on patient safety and on the moral climate of the workplace (i.e., it may lead either to avoiding patients or families because of guilt or to being overly solicitous).

- Increase nursing leaders' and other organizational leaders' awareness of the impact of moral distress on patients, families, and employees. Nursing managers, in particular, can offer support and guidance to employees.
- Educators can develop formal education programs that address legal, ethical, and moral issues.

**References**

Corley, M. C. (2002). Nurse moral distress: A proposed theory and research agenda. *Nursing Ethics, 9*, 636–650.

Corley, M. C., Minick, P., Elswick, R. K., & Jacobs, M. (2005). Nurse moral distress and ethical work enviroment. *Nursing Ethics, 12*, 381–390.

Raines, M. L. (2000). Ethical decision making in nurses: Relationships among moral reasoning, coping style, and ethics stress. *JONA's Healthcare Law, Ethics, and Regulation, 2*, 29–41.

Wilkinson, J. M. (1987–1988). Moral distress in nursing practice: Experience and effect. *Nursing Forum, 23*(1), 16–29.

# Ethical Dilemmas in Terminal Care

*Kristin Stegenga*

## General Principles

Despite significant advances in treatment and supportive care for children with cancer and blood disorders, some children will die from their disease or associated sequelae. Providing appropriate care to the terminally ill child and his or her family can be one of the most challenging aspects of nursing care in pediatric hematology and oncology. Gaining insight into the needs and dilemmas that may arise during this life stage often requires nurses to consider issues within an ethical framework. Many of the traditional ethics-related concepts are important in the consideration of issues related to the care of terminally ill children.

## Autonomy

The principle of *autonomy* involves the patient's and family's right to make choices regarding medical and supportive care. Children and adolescents should be involved in decisions to the extent that they are developmentally able. Patients older than 18 years can refuse treatment or aspects of treatment.

## Beneficence

The principle of *beneficence* means "to do good." Nursing care should involve decisions or actions that promote the best interests of patients. An example of this principle might be ensuring adequate pain relief for a dying child.

## Nonmaleficence

The principle of *nonmaleficence* means "to do no harm." Nursing care should include an examination of how interventions may place a burden on a patient and the family. An example might be avoiding a treatment in which the burden on the child outweighs the benefits.

## Justice

The principle of *justice* includes the fair allocation of resources and avoidance of discrimination in care provision. Examples include providing care to an individual regardless of ability to pay or seeking out resources for a family who needs services not covered by a third-party payer.

## Double Effect

The concept of *double effect* applies to situations in which producing the desired outcome for a patient has the risk of a negative effect. An example of this concept would be the administration of palliative chemotherapy because it may extend the patient's life but also may cause significant negative side effects.

## Fidelity

The concept of *fidelity* implies that medical professionals place their patient's best interests first when considering options. Doing this can be considerably more complicated within the realm of pediatric hematology/oncology because the patient and family may be viewed as a collective unit, but the needs and desires of one may conflict with the other.

## Nursing Assessment and Interventions

### Assessment

- Recognize situations that create ethical dilemmas (see **Table 9-3**).
- Examine the risks and benefits inherent in potential interventions from the perspective of the patient, family, and healthcare team.
- Explore the values and needs of the patient and family. Facilitate discussions as appropriate to determine the course of action that is in the patient's best interest.
- Assess the patient and family for potentially conflicting desires (e.g., parent-parent or parent-child, especially adolescents, who may have their own views of their situation and needs). Promote an open dialogue between conflicting family members or consult with the medical team to help mediate the situation.
- Examine potential ethical dilemmas within an ethical framework.
- Continually assess the needs of the patient and family as their needs change along the terminal-care trajectory.

### Interventions

- Maintain expert knowledge related to the symptoms and needs of the patient and family at the end of life to optimize quality of life.
- Consult with other healthcare team members as needed to provide the best management of the symptoms and needs of the patient and family.
- Maintain open communication with the patient and family.
- Minimize avoidable conflict; partner with families to determine family culture, values, communication patterns, and decision-making approaches so that care and communication can be tailored specifically to the patient's and family's needs.
- Provide anticipatory guidance wherever possible to prepare the patient and family.
- Educate the patient and family regarding options for treatment and support, and explain the potential benefits and sequelae of those options.
- Provide support for the decisions of the patient and family regardless of one's personal philosophy or values.

Table 9-3. Common Ethical Dilemmas Encountered When Caring for Terminally Ill Children

| Dilemma | Rationale for Providing Life-Prolonging Measures to the Patient | Rationale for Withholding Life-Prolonging Measures or Other Measures from the Patient |
| --- | --- | --- |
| Medications for pain control | Comfort is the primary goal.<br>The quality of the child's life will improve.<br>The dying process will be easier if the child is free from pain. | Opioid narcotics may cause a decreased level of cognition.<br>Depending on the child's level of pain and stage of illness, pain medications may shorten life (see the brief discussion of double effect in this section).<br>Taking narcotics can result in addiction (this fear in relation to terminally ill patients is unfounded). |
| Chemotherapy or experimental therapy | These therapies can prolong the patient's life span.<br>The patient may possibly have an increase in the quality of life.<br>Providing these therapies conveys the message that the family has done everything it could have to save the child. | These therapies decrease the child's blood counts and increase the risk of infection.<br>The side effects of treatment may be painful or uncomfortable. |
| Supplemental nutrition and hydration (intravenous, nasogastric, g-tube) | The child may be hungry or thirsty.<br>The child cannot and will not eat.<br>These measures alleviate the fear that the child will starve to death.<br>The primary role of parents is to feed and nourish their child.<br>These measures relieve parental guilt feelings. | Supplemental oral feedings beyond what a child can ingest may actually cause nausea and vomiting.<br>These measures can cause an increase in the tumor's growth (i.e., they feed the tumor).<br>An increase in fluid volume can result in congestive heart failure, increased respiratory secretions, and/or pulmonary congestion, which leads to the question of whether to administer a diuretic and have the child endure its side effects.<br>Increased urine output can lead to increased risk of skin breakdown if the child is incontinent.<br>There is a risk of ascites.<br>Withholding IV fluids decreases nausea and vomiting, shortness of breath, and incontinence.<br>Death is more comfortable and natural when supplemental nutrition is not provided.<br>Ice chips are effective in managing a dry mouth.<br>Complaints of being thirsty are associated with the dying process, not the patient's level of hydration (Zerwekh, 1997). |
| Families that resist do-not-resuscitate orders | The family believes they are giving up.<br>This directive conflicts with the family's cultural or religious beliefs.<br>The family is in denial about the fact that the child is actually going to die.<br>The family cannot assume responsibility for stopping interventions that might prolong the child's life. | The directive allows nature to take its course.<br>The family believes the child has suffered enough. |
| Autopsy | An autopsy will aid in research that may help other children.<br>An autopsy may be able to establish or determine if the disease has a genetic link. | The child and family have endured enough.<br>The autopsy will not provide valuable medical information. |

# Section IX  Care for the Terminally Ill Child and the Family

## Legal Concerns in Terminal Care

*Kristin Stegenga*

### General Principles
It is important that nurses who provide care to terminally ill children understand the legal implications of aspects of this type of care. Each state has its own laws and enforcement practices related to terminal-care issues and death at home. In addition, individual institutions and agencies have their own policies governing these practices. Nurses can educate families and assist them in navigating these policies and laws so that issues do not arise during this already challenging time.

### Legal Considerations
Many legal issues surrounding the end of life can arise for the family and medical team. Laws governing do-not-resuscitate (DNR) orders vary from state to state. They also vary with respect to which agencies are bound by DNR orders; for example, whether paramedics or schools are required to recognize DNR status when a child is in their care. In addition, each state has laws regarding pronouncement of death (including who is authorized to make that pronouncement), transportation of corpses, and notifications required when a child dies at home. In some states, autopsies are mandatory in the case of home deaths.

Narcotic pain medications are also regulated by state and national laws. Prescriptive authority, transmission of changes in prescription, and the amount of pain medication prescribed at any given time may vary by state. Parents may find that these legal issues present barriers to their child's adequate pain relief, which can add to their distress at this difficult time.

Nurses, too, may encounter legal issues surrounding decisions at the end of life. Disagreements may occur between the parent and the patient as well as between the parent and the medical team regarding end-of-life care. Most of these disagreements can be resolved informally without legal intervention. Open dialogue is especially important in meeting the needs of the patient and family without having to resort to legal intervention.

### Nursing Assessment and Interventions

#### Assessments
* Become aware of the laws and statutes in your state governing the provision of care at the end of life.
* Determine the criteria for DNR status, both in the hospital and in the community.
* Promote open and clear communication between all involved parties to avoid misunderstanding.

#### Interventions
* Follow existing laws and procedures for your area regarding DNR, narcotics usage, and hospice care.
* Provide anticipatory guidance to families regarding these laws and procedures so that they are prepared and able to make the decisions they deem most appropriate for themselves and the patient.

## Bibliography

### Children and Death
Kirwin, K. M., & Hamrin, V. (2005). Decreasing the risk of complicated bereavement and future psychiatric disorders in children. *Journal of Child and Adolescent Psychiatric Nursing, 18*(1), 62–78.

Slaughter, V. (2005). Young children's understanding of death. *Australian Psychologist, 40*(3), 179–186.

### Physical Care of the Terminally Ill Child
Brown, M., Hockenberry-Eaton, M., Lamb, D., Chordas, C., Kline, N., & Bottomley, S. (2000). *End of life care for children.* Austin, TX: Texas Cancer Council.

Casey, M., Grund, E., Quammen, H., Miller, B., McCormick, P., & Bostrom, B. (2007). Propofol use in pediatric patients with severe cancer pain at the end of life. *Journal of Pediatric Oncology Nursing, 24*(1), 29–34.

Cohen, S. P., & Dawson, T. C. (2002). Nebulized morphine as a treatment for dyspnea in a child with cystic fibrosis. *Pediatrics, 110,* e38.

Dougherty, M., & Debaun, M. R. (2003). Rapid increase of morphine and benzodiazepine usage in the last three days of life in children with cancer is related to neuropathic pain. *Journal of Pediatrics, 142,* 373–376.

Harbord, M. G., Kyrkou, N. E., Kyrkou, M. R., Kay, D., & Coulthard, K. P. (2004). Use of intranasal midazolam to treat acute seizures in paediatric community settings. *Journal of Paediatrics and Child Health, 40*(9–10), 556–558.

Hockenberry-Eaton, M., Barrera, P., Brown, M., Bottomley, S., & O'Neill, J. (1999). *Pain management in children with cancer.* Austin, TX: Texas Cancer Council.

Kane, J., & Primono, M. (2001). Alleviating the suffering of seriously ill children. *The American Journal of Hospice and Palliative Care, 18,* 161–169.

Mitchell, A. M., Gale, D. D., Matzo, M. L., McDonald, M. C., & Gadmer, N. (2002). Critique of transcultural practices in end-of-life clinical nursing practice. *Nursing Forum, 37*(4), 24–31.

### Psychosocial Care of the Terminally Ill Child
Contro, N., Larson, J., Scofield, S., Sourkes, B., & Cohen, H. (2002). Family perspectives on the quality of pediatric palliative care. *Archives of Pediatric and Adolescent Medicine, 156,* 14–19.

Hongo, T., Watanabe, C., Okada, S., Inoue, N., Yajima, S., Fujii, Y., et al. (2003). Analysis of the circumstances at the end of life in children with cancer: Symptoms, suffering, and acceptance. *Pediatrics International, 45,* 60–64.

Kobler, K., Limbo, R., & Kavanaugh, K. (2007). Meaningful moments: The use of ritual in perinatal and pediatric death. *Maternal Child Nursing, 32,* 288–295.

Wilkins, K., & Woodgate, R. (2005). A review of qualitative research on the childhood cancer experience from the perspective of siblings: A need to give them a voice. *Journal of Pediatric Oncology Nursing, 22,* 305–319.

Zwerdling, T., Davies, S., Lazar, L., Crawford, B., Tucker, L., Boughner, A., et al. (2000). Unique aspects of caring for dying children and their families. *The American Journal of Hospice and Palliative Care, 17,* 305–311.

## Bereavement

Field, M. J., & Behrman, R. E. (Eds.). (2003). *When children die: Improving palliative and end-of-life care for children and their families.* Washington, DC: The National Academies Press.

Fletcher, P. N. (2002). Experiences in family bereavement. *Family and Community Health, 25*(1), 57–70.

Fochtman, D. (2007). Palliative care. In C. R. Baggott, K. P. Kelly, D. Fochtman, & G. V. Foley (Eds.), *Nursing care of children and adolescents with cancer* (3rd ed., pp. 400–425). Glenview, IL: Association of Pediatric Hematology/Oncology Nurses.

Goodenough, B., Drew, D., Higgins, S., & Trethewie, S. (2004). Bereavement outcomes for parents who lose a child to cancer: Are place of death and sex of parent associated with differences in psychological functioning? *Psycho-Oncology, 13*(11), 779–791.

Hilden, J., & Tobin, D. R. (2003). *Shelter from the storm: Caring for a child with a life-threatening condition.* Cambridge, MA: Perseus Publishing.

Kushner, H. S. (2001). *When bad things happen to good people.* New York: Schocken Books.

Steeves, R. H. (2002). The rhythms of bereavement. *Family and Community Health, 25*(1), 1–10.

## Professionals' Grief, Distress, and Bereavement

International Work Group on Death, Dying and Bereavement. (2006). Caregivers in death, dying, and bereavement situations. *Death Studies, 30,* 649–663.

Papadatou, D., Bellali, T., Papazoglou, I., & Petraki, D. (2002). Greek nurse and physician grief as a result of caring for children dying of cancer. *Pediatric Nursing, 28,* 345–353.

Rich, S. (2002). Caregiver grief: Taking care of ourselves and our patients. *International Journal of Trauma Nursing, 8,* 24–28.

Rushton, C. H., Reder, E., Hall, B., Comello, K., Sellers, D. E., & Hutton, N. (2006). Interdisciplinary interventions to improve pediatric palliative care and reduce health care professional suffering. *Journal of Palliative Medicine, 9*(4), 922–933.

## Moral Distress

Corley, M. C., Elswich, R. K., Gorman, M., & Clor, T. (2001). Development and evaluation of a moral distress scale. *Journal of Advanced Nursing, 33,* 250–256.

Erlen, J. A. (2001). Moral distress: A pervasive problem. *Orthopaedic Nursing, 20,* 76–80.

Georges, J. J., & Grypdonck, M. (2002). Moral problems experienced by nurses when caring for terminally ill people: A literature review. *Nursing Ethics, 9,* 155–178.

Nathaniel, A. K. (2006). Moral reckoning in nursing. *Western Journal of Nursing Research, 28*(4), 419–438.

Rodney, P., Varcoe, C., Storch, J. L., McPherson, G., Mahoney, K., Brown, H., et al. (2002). Navigating towards a moral horizon: A multisite qualitative study of ethical practice in nursing. *Canadian Journal of Nursing Research, 34,* 75–102.

Storch, J., Rodney, P., & Starzomski R. (2004). *Toward a moral horizon; Nursing ethics for leadership and practice.* Toronto, Canada: Pearson Education Canada.

## Ethical Dilemmas in Terminal Care

Brown, R. T. (Ed.). (2006). *Comprehensive handbook of childhood cancer and sickle cell disease: A biopsychosocial approach.* New York: Oxford University Press.

Field, M. J., & Behrman, R. E. (Eds.). (2003). *When children die: Improving palliative and end-of-life care for children.* Washington, DC: The National Academies Press.

Rushton, C. H. (2005). A framework for integrated pediatric palliative care: Being with dying. *Journal of Pediatric Nursing, 20,* 311–325.

Truog, R. D., Meyer, E. C., & Burns, J. P. (2006). Toward interventions to improve end-of-life care in the pediatric intensive care unit. *Critical Care Medicine, 34,* S373–S379.

Wainwright, P., & Gallagher, A. (2007). Ethical aspects of withdrawing and withholding treatment. *Nursing Standard, 21,* 46–50.

## Legal Concerns in Terminal Care

Brown, R. T. (2006). *Comprehensive handbook of childhood cancer and sickle cell disease: A biopsychosocial approach.* New York: Oxford University Press.

Field, M. J., & Behrman, R. E. (Eds.) (2003). *When children die: Improving palliative and end-of-life care for children.* Washington, DC: The National Academies Press.

Rushton, C. H. (2005). A framework for integrated pediatric palliative care: Being with dying. *Journal of Pediatric Nursing, 20,* 311–325.

# Section X  Late Effects of Childhood Cancer

Wendy L. Hobbie

## Section Outline

Definition and Overview

Central Nervous System

Hypothalamic-Pituitary Axis

Thyroid Function

Vision and Hearing

Head and Neck

Cardiovascular System

Respiratory System

Gastrointestinal and Hepatic Systems

Genitourinary System

Reproductive System: Testes

Reproductive System: Ovaries

Musculoskeletal System

Hematopoietic System

Immune System

Second Malignant Neoplasms

Psychosocial Effects: Personal-Emotional

Psychosocial Effects: Political-Social

Psychosocial Effects: Educational Issues

Promoting Health After Childhood Cancer

Bibliography

# Definition and Overview

*Wendy L. Hobbie*

## Definition

The late effects of childhood cancer and its treatment can be defined as a broad range of persistent adverse effects that are related to the disease process, its therapy, or a combination of the two. The onset of late effects can occur months to years after therapy is completed. Early recognition and prompt management of these sequelae can, in some cases, lessen the severity of the residual problems.

In addition, health maintenance and promotion regarding modifiable risk factors may improve overall health and quality of life.

## Overview

### Epidemiology

Approximately 9,500 new cases of cancer occur annually in children younger than 15 years of age. Nearly 80% of these children can expect to be cured. In the United States, current estimates indicate that 1 in 900 people age 15 to 45 years is a survivor of childhood cancer. That number is expected to increase to 1 in 250 people by 2010. Significant disabilities affect the quality of life of almost half of long-term cancer survivors. In a recent questionnaire study, Oeffinger and colleagues (2006) evaluated survivors treated between 1970 and 1986 for chronic illnesses. Sixty-two percent of childhood-cancer survivors suffered from at least one chronic health condition and 27.5% had a life-threatening effect from cancer therapy.

### Causes

Late effects can be caused by treatment, the disease process, or a combination of the two (**Table 10-1**). Treatments that can cause late effects include surgery, radiation therapy, chemotherapy, effects of infection, or other events that occur during treatment and supportive care (e.g., administration of aminoglycosides or immunosuppressives).

### Factors Associated With the Development of Late Effects:

- initial diagnosis—location and extent of the primary disease
- type and intensity of treatment
- age and developmental stage at time of diagnosis and treatment
- genetic or familial predisposition that may interact with treatment-related injuries.

### Categories of Late Effects

Late-effects categories include physical, psychological, cognitive, economic, and social/emotional. With physical late effects, any organ system can be affected. Effects range from mild to severe. Second malignant neoplasm can occur and often has devastating effects. Emotional late effects can include psychological and social adjustments. Cognitive effects can have the most profound effect on quality of life and achievement of life goals. Social/economic late effects include concerns about finances and insurability. Other late effects can include difficulties in academic achievement and employment issues such as job discrimination.

### Reference

Oeffinger, K. C., Mertens, A. C., Sklar, C. A., Kawashima, T., Hudson, M. M., Meadows, A. T., et al. (2006). Childhood cancer survivor study: Chronic health conditions in adult survivors of childhood cancer *New England Journal of Medicine, 355,* 1572–1582.

# Central Nervous System

*Joanne Quillen*

## Definition

Neuropsychological deficits and neurologic abnormalities are significant late effects of cancer for many long-term survivors. Their incidence is variable and depends upon the type and location of the original disease, the timing and method of central nervous system (CNS) treatment, and the patient's age at diagnosis. CNS changes can occur as a result of irradiation of the whole brain, surgery, corticosteroids, or intravenous chemotherapy or intrathecal chemotherapy. Neuropsychological deficits typically manifest as a significant decline in a person's intelligence quotient (IQ) (i.e., by 10 to 20 points) and in academic achievement scores. Other manifestations include specific deficits in integration of visual and motor functions, memory, attention, processing speed, and motor skills. The most common neurologic abnormalities include atrophy and decreased subcortical white matter. Calcifications and leukoencephalopathy are less common.

## Risk Factors

### Radiation Therapy

Radiation therapy is the treatment most commonly associated with late CNS toxicities. Irradiation of the whole brain produces structural changes such as dystrophic calcification, mineralizing microangiopathy, and cerebral atrophy. Children treated before the age of 6 years usually have more serious toxicities than children who were older when they received treatment. Children who are younger than 2 years are most vulnerable to CNS-radiation-related toxicity.

Leukoencephalopathy is associated with irradiation of the whole brain at a dose greater than 1,800 centigrays (cGy). There is a noted synergy between radiation therapy and drugs such as methotrexate (Mexate). Radiation therapy disrupts the blood-brain barrier, which leads to increased levels of methotrexate in the CNS, which in turn increases the risk of producing leukoencephalopathy. Hyperfractionated radiotherapy may be less damaging to a normal CNS.

### Neurocognitive Deficits

Learning disabilities are dependent upon the cumulative radiation dosage and age of the patient. Neurocognitive deficits are more severe and frequent in children who were younger than 5 years when they received cranial radiation therapy. However, cranial radiation at any age may affect cognitive functioning. Subtle neurocognitive deficits may become apparent only when the individual is learning new concepts and with increased academic challenges.

### Table 10-1. Late Effects Associated with Childhood Cancer Treatments

| Organ System | Risk Factors | Potential Late Effects | Evaluation/Interventions |
|---|---|---|---|
| **Central nervous system—cognitive** | Radiation therapy to brain > 1,800 cGy<br>Methotrexate (Mexate; high-dose intravenous or intrathecal)<br>Resection of a CNS tumor<br>ARA = C (intrathecal or high-dose intervention) | Learning disabilities<br>Leukoencephalopathy<br>Mineralizing microangiopathy<br>Cerebral atrophy | Arrange for the following:<br>– neurocognitive testing<br>– psychoeducational assistance<br>– a CT or an MRI scan (at baseline and when there are symptoms)<br>– an EEG<br>– an audiogram<br>– vision screening<br>– a neurological consultation, as indicated<br>– educational or vocational testing<br>– referral to school liaison program. |
| **Central nervous system—peripheral neuropathy** | Vincristine (Oncovin)<br>Vinblastine (Velban)<br>Etoposide (VP-16)<br>Cisplatin (Platinol) | Generalized weakness<br>Tingling and numbness<br>Foot drop<br>Paresthesias<br>Areflexia | Arrange for a thorough neurological examination on an annual basis.<br>Encourage the patient to protect the affected area from exposure to extreme temperatures.<br>Arrange for physical and occupational therapy.<br>Referral to pain team (for neuropathic pain management). |
| **Endocrine—hypothalamic-pituitary axis (HPA)** | Radiation therapy to HPA >1,800 cGy<br>Resection of tumor in HPA region<br>Radiation therapy to HPA of >3,000 to 4,000 cGy<br>Resection of tumor in HPA region | Growth hormone deficiency<br>TSH deficiency<br>Adrenocorticotropic hormone (ACTH) deficiency<br>Gonadotropin deficiency<br>Hyperprolactinemia<br>Obesity | Obtain the patient's height, weight, and sitting height measurement annually (every 6 months at ages 9–12 years).<br>Chart measurements on a growth curve.<br>Obtain a bone age film, as clinically indicated.<br>Assess Tanner stage during a physical exam.<br>Ensure that appropriate hormone testing is done.<br>Consult an endocrinologist if growth hormone therapy is indicated.<br>Delay puberty with GnRH therapy.<br>Ensure that thyroid studies are done at baseline and every 3–5 years or as directed by an endocrinologist.<br>Check cortisol level to assess for ACTH deficiency.<br>Measure LH, FSH, estradiol, or testosterone levels to assess for gonadotropin deficiency.<br>Obtain prolactin levels to assess for hyperprolactinemia.<br>Ensure that the patient is on appropriate hormone replacement for the specific deficiency.<br>Provide anticipatory guidance on symptoms related to the specific deficiency. |
| | Radiation therapy to the HPA >2,000 cGy, effects may be seen at doses as low as 1,000 cGy<br>Resection of tumor in the HPA region | Precocious puberty | Obtain height and plot it on a growth curve annually.<br>Determine bone age every 2 years until growth is complete.<br>Measure LH, FSH, estradiol, or testosterone levels.<br>Consult an endocrinologist, as needed.<br>Obtain a pelvic ultrasound and GnRH stimulation testing, as needed.<br>Ensure that patient is on appropriate hormone therapy, as indicated.<br>Delay puberty with GnRH therapy. |

*(continued)*

## Chemotherapy

High doses of methotrexate, given intravenously or intrathecally, are associated with neuroanatomic pathology and neurocognitive deficits. Vinca alkaloids (e.g., vincristine [Oncovin], vinblastine [Velban], etoposide [VP-16], cisplatin [Platinol]) are associated with peripheral neuropathy. Platinum-based chemotherapy has been associated with hearing loss, which can contribute to learning problems. Intrathecal or intravenous (IV) methotrexate and IV cytarabine (Cytosine Arabinoside) are associated with leukoencephalopathy.

Table 10-1. Late Effects Associated with Childhood Cancer Treatments (continued)

| Organ System | Risk Factors | Potential Late Effects | Evaluation/Interventions |
|---|---|---|---|
| Thyroid | Radiation therapy to the neck or cervical spine >2,000 cGy<br>Total body irradiation >750 cGy<br>Partial or complete thyroidectomy<br>Prior lymphangiogram<br>Total body irradiation >1,000 cGy | Hypothyroidism<br>Overt (elevated TSH, decreased T4)<br>Compensated (elevated TSH, normal T4)<br>Thyroid nodules<br>Hyperthyroidism (Graves' disease) (decreased TSH, elevated T4)<br>Thyroiditis<br>Benign or malignant tumors | Obtain at least annual thyroid studies, usually thyroxine and TSH (may include free T4).<br>Refer patient to an endocrinologist.<br>Patient may require thyroxine replacement.<br>Provide anticipatory guidance on symptoms related to hyperthyroidism or hypothyroidism. |
| Ophthalmology | Steroids<br>Radiation >800 cGy TBI | Cataracts | Recommend an annual ophthalmoscopic exam.<br>Assess for a decreased red reflex.<br>Patient may require cataract extraction. |
| | Radiation >4,500 cGy | Decreased tear production (lacrimal gland)<br>Fibrosis of the lacrimal duct<br>Ulcerations or telangiectasis of the eyelids<br>Decreased visual acuity/vision loss<br>Conjunctive necrosis or scarring<br>Thinning of the sclera<br>Ulceration of the cornea (radiation retinopathy, optic atrophy, xeropthalmia) | Recommend an annual ophthalmologic examination and appropriate follow-up for identified problems. (Patient may require cataract extraction.)<br>Recommend tear replacement, as needed.<br>Provide education regarding proper eye care. |
| Ears/Hearing | Aminoglycosides<br>Recurrent otitis media<br>Carboplatin<br>Cisplatin (platinol)—cumulative dose ≥360 mg/m$^2$<br>CNS neoplasm<br>Age <3 years at treatment<br>Loop diuretics<br>Radiation to the head/neck/cranial radiation | Sensorineural high-frequency hearing loss<br>Tinnitus<br>Vertigo<br>Abnormal speech development<br>Otosclerosis, chronic otitis media<br>Cerumen impaction | Perform baseline audiogram brainstem auditory evoked response (BAER) and then perform one every 2–3 years and at every 3 and 5 years if abnormal; follow every year until stable, then every 3 years.<br>Examine the canal.<br>Recommend preferential seating in school, amplification, and hearing aids, as indicated.<br>May require speech therapy, as indicated.<br>Consult with an ENT, an audiologist, and a neurologist, as indicated. |
| Head and Neck | Radiation >4,000 cGy | Xerostomia<br>Intranasal scarring<br>Epilation, alopecia<br>Fibrosis<br>Hypoplasia, bony deformity<br>Decreased salivary function<br>Muscle hypoplasia, constricting fibrosis<br>Osteoradionecrosis<br>Chronic sinusitis<br>Dysphagia | Inspect the mucosa.<br>Recommend dental examination every 6 months.<br>Encourage behaviors that promote dental, head, and neck health: meticulous oral hygiene, no tobacco use, stretching exercises, physical therapy as indicated, and a diet low in concentrated sugars.<br>Provide resource information on wigs and alternative hairstyles.<br>Patient may require saliva substitutes.<br>Sinus CT and otolaryngology consult as needed (refer to gastroenterology with dysphagia and obtain endoscopy). |
| | Radiation ≥1,000 cGy | Thyroid nodules/cancer<br>Thyroid dysfunction (hypo or hyper)<br>Dysphagia | Annual physical examination.<br>Annual thyroid ultrasound.<br>Obtain endoscopy with dysphagia and refer to gastroenterology. |

(continued)

# Section X  Late Effects of Childhood Cancer

**Table 10-1. Late Effects Associated with Childhood Cancer Treatments** (continued)

| Organ System | Risk Factors | Potential Late Effects | Evaluation/Interventions |
|---|---|---|---|
| Dental | Radiation >100 cGy given when the patient is <5 years old<br><br>Chemotherapy: vincristine (Oncovin), dactinomycin (Actinomycin-D), methotrexate (Mexate), mercaptopurine (Purinethol), cyclophosphamide (Cytoxan), procarbazine (Matulane), mechlorethamine (nitrogen mustard) | Abnormal tooth and root development, thinning or shortening<br>Dental caries<br>Enamel dysplasia<br>Periodontal disease<br>Tooth decay<br>Malocclusion<br>Craniofacial abnormalities | Recommend orthodontic evaluations, as indicated.<br>Provide periodontal prophylaxis.<br>Obtain radiographic studies of irradiated bone every 3–5 years.<br>Dental examination and hygiene every 6 months<br>Regular fluoride applications |
| Cardiovascular | Anthracyclines<br>>300 mg/m$^2$<br>>200 mg/m$^2$ with radiation therapy to the thorax (including chest, mantle, mediastinal, whole lung, spinal)<br>Other chemotherapy, primarily high-dose cyclophosphamide (Cytoxan) | Arrhythmias<br>Cardiomyopathy<br>Pericardial damage | Obtain MUGA/echo, EKG, and chest X ray (baseline and then <300 mg/m$^2$—every 5 years; <300 mg/m$^2$ and radiation to the heart—every 2 years; ≥300–400 mg/m$^2$—every 2 years; ≥300 mg/m$^2$ and radiation to heart—yearly; ≥400 mg/m$^2$—yearly.<br>Refer to a cardiologist, as indicated.<br>Use Holter monitor and have exercise testing done as clinically indicated. |
| | Radiation >3,000 cGy to mediastinum, or whole lung or mantle >2,500 cGy when given with anthracyclines >3,000 cGy to spine<br>Total body irradiation<br>Female gender<br>Black race<br><5 years old at treatment | | Patient may require cardiac medication.<br>Provide anticipatory guidance for symptoms of cardiac dysfunction and the side effects of cardiac medications.<br>End-stage cardiomyopathy may require a heart transplant.<br>Additional evaluation recommendation for patients who receive >300 mg/m$^2$ in the following situations:<br>– pregnancy<br>– prior to initiation of exercise (especially isometric programs). |
| | Radiation >4,000 cGy | Valvular damage | Obtain echocardiogram and chest X ray (baseline, then every 3–5 years if normal or if the patient is symptomatic).<br>Patient will require penicillin prophylaxis when having surgery or dental procedures. |
| | Radiation >3,000 cGy | Coronary artery disease | Obtain an EKG (baseline, then every 2–3 years if normal, or if the patient is symptomatic).<br>Obtain a stress test (baseline, then every 3–5 years if normal, or if the patient is symptomatic).<br>Arrange for a consultation with a cardiologist, as indicated.<br>Provide education on the importance of a physical conditioning program and a low-sodium, low-fat diet. |
| Respiratory | Radiation >1,000 cGy to the pulmonary field<br>Chemotherapy: (bleomycin (Blenoxane), busulfan (Leukeran), mitomycin (Mutamycin), methotrexate (Mexate), cytarabine (Cytosine Arabinoside), carmustine (BCNU), lomustine (CCNU), vinca alkaloids, alkylating agents<br>Increased risk with radiation dose ≥4,000 cGy radiation field<br>Large lung volume in radiation field<br>Combination of radiation and radiation-sensitizing chemotherapy | Pneumonitis fibrosis | Obtain a chest X ray (baseline, then every 2–5 years if normal).<br>Perform pulmonary function tests, including diffusion capacity (baseline, then every 3–5 years if normal and prior to anesthesia).<br>Perform a CT, which may help define lung volumes.<br>Perform a ventilation quotient scan, as indicated.<br>Prescribe pneumococcal (Pneumovax) and influenza virus vaccines (Fluogen) annually.<br>Refer patient to a pulmonologist, as needed.<br>Provide education regarding healthy behaviors, avoidance or cessation of smoking, and maintaining physical conditioning.<br>Treat the patient's symptoms with corticosteroids, bronchodilators, expectorants, antibiotics, oxygen, and bed rest, as needed.<br>Provide anticipatory guidance for those who have received bleomycin (Blenoxane) regarding the risk of respiratory failure with high levels of oxygen (avoid scuba diving). |

(continued)

### Table 10-1. Late Effects Associated with Childhood Cancer Treatments (continued)

| Organ System | Risk Factors | Potential Late Effects | Evaluation/Interventions |
|---|---|---|---|
| Gastrointestinal | Radiation >4,000 cGy<br><br>Chemotherapy: doxorubicin (Adriamycin) and dactinomycin (Actinomycin-D); radiation therapy enhances methotrexate (Mexate) and 6-mercaptopurine (Purinethol)<br><br>Surgery, which may enhance radiation therapy and is also associated with obstruction<br><br>Bone marrow transplant | Fibrosis, strictures, obstruction<br><br>Enteritis<br><br>Adhesions<br><br>Ulcers<br><br>Malabsorption<br><br>Splenomegaly and thrombocytopenia, which can occur after radiation therapy<br><br>Graft-versus-host disease leading to GI tract strictures, fibrosis<br><br>GI malignancy | Obtain height and weight on an annual basis.<br><br>Obtain stool guaiac on an annual basis, and annual rectal examination after the age of 40 years. Obtain a CBC with mean corpuscular value on an annual basis.<br><br>Obtain blood chemistries on an annual basis.<br><br>Provide anticipatory guidance regarding dietary modification as needed.<br><br>Refer to or consult a gastroenterologist, as needed.<br><br>Dilate the fibrotic or obstructed area.<br><br>Obtain radiographic studies, as indicated.<br><br>Educate the patient regarding medication administration and side effects, as indicated.<br><br>Educate the patient regarding a high fiber diet. |
| Hepatic | Radiation >2,600 cGy<br><br>Chemotherapy: dactinomycin (Actinomycin-D) radiotherapy enhancer, methotrexate (Mexate), 6-mercaptopurine (Purinethol)<br><br>Surgery (a hepatic resection can enhance the development of sequelae)<br><br>Blood transfusions (especially prior to 1992) | Fibrosis<br>Cirrhosis<br>Hepatitis<br>–radiation-induced hepatitis<br>–transfusion-mediated viral hepatitis, which may include hepatitis B, C, or cytomegalovirus | Refer to or consult a gastroenterologist, as needed.<br>Obtain the following:<br>–chemistry panel on an annual basis<br>–baseline hepatitis panel<br>–abdominal ultrasound or liver biopsy, as indicated, to assess for hepatitis.<br><br>Patient may require dietary management for fibrosis.<br><br>Hepatitis may require treatment with interferon.<br><br>End-stage liver disease may require a liver transplant.<br><br>Educate patient about healthy behaviors as well as avoiding alcohol or other hepatotoxic drugs.<br><br>Educate the patient regarding medication administration and side effects, as indicated. |
| Genitourinary | Radiation<br>–kidney >2,000–2,500 cGy<br>–bladder >3,000 cGy (before puberty)<br>–bladder >5,000 cGy (after puberty)<br>–prostate >4,000–6,000 cGy<br>–vagina >4,000 cGy<br>–uterus >2,000 cGy (before puberty)<br>–uterus >4,000–5,000 cGy (after puberty)<br>–ureter/urethra >5,000 cGy<br>–pelvic >5,000 cGy | Hypoplastic kidney<br>Nephrotic syndrome<br>Bladder fibrosis or hypoplasia<br>Decreased volume of seminal fluid<br>Hypoplastic or atrophied prostate<br>Fibrosis (vaginal, uterine, ureter)<br>Stricture of urethra | Perform an annual examination with close attention to the patient's blood pressure, height, and weight.<br><br>Obtain a urinalysis, BUN, creatinine, hemoglobin/hematocrit, and creatinine clearance or GFR (yearly).<br><br>Consult a nephrologist or urologist as indicated, for patients with hypertension, proteinuira, culture-negative hematuria, or progressive renal insufficiency.<br><br>Patient may require low-protein, low-salt dietary modifications.<br><br>Serum sodium, potassium chloride, carbon dioxide, calcium, magnesium phosphorus (for those at risk for tubular dysfunctions (baseline; if normal repeat every 5 years). |
| | Chemotherapy<br>–cisplatin (Platinol)<br>–ifosfamide (Ifex)<br>–cyclophosphamide (Cytoxan)<br><br>Supportive therapies<br>–aminoglycosides<br>–cyclosporine [Sandimmune]<br>–amphotericin | Glomerular dysfunction (cisplatin)<br>Tubular dysfunction (cisplatin and ifosfamide)<br>Fibrosis, hypoplasia, or secondary malignancy of bladder (cyclophosphamide, ifosfamide)<br>Hemorrhagic cystitis (cyclophosphamide, ifosfamide) | Supplement magnesium and phosphorus, as indicated.<br>End-stage kidney disease may require dialysis or a kidney transplant.<br>Patient may require medication for hypertension, as indicated. |
| | Surgery<br>–nephrectomy<br>–removal of other genitourinary organs<br>–damage to nerves<br><br>Age (young children may experience increased effects, which may not become apparent until the child reaches an age when the organ is unable to compensate) | Incontinence<br>Infertility | Educate the patient regarding kidney health after a nephrectomy, recommend that the patient avoid contact sports and maintain hydration, and encourage the patient to wear a Medic-Alert bracelet.<br><br>Provide anticipatory guidance related to potential problems with incontinence and infertility, as needed.<br><br>Counsel and educate patient regarding prompt reporting of dysuria or gross hematuria. |

(continued)

## Table 10-1. Late Effects Associated with Childhood Cancer Treatments (continued)

| Organ System | Risk Factors | Potential Late Effects | Evaluation/Interventions |
|---|---|---|---|
| Reproductive–Testes | Radiation >100–600 cGy to testes<br>Radiation to the hypothalamic-pituitary axis<br>Total body irradiation | Testicular atrophy<br>Delayed or arrested pubertal development<br>Infertility | Assess pubertal history.<br>Assess Tanner stage annually.<br>Determine testicular size (volume and turgor).<br>Obtain LH, FSH, and testosterone levels for delayed pubertal development and when it is clinically indicated.<br>Obtain thyroxine and TSH levels.<br>Refer to or consult with an endocrinologist when necessary.<br>Semen analysis, as needed |
| | Chemotherapy: alkylating agents (procarbazine [Matulane], cisplatin [Platinol], cyclophosphamide [Cytoxan], ifosfamide [Ifex]), nitrosoureas (carmustine [BCNU], lomustine [CCNU])<br>Busulfan (mylgran)<br>Mechlorethamine (mustargen)<br>Melphalan (Alkeran)<br>Chlorambucil (Leukeran)<br>Surgery (orchiectomy, or peritoneal node dissection)<br>Age (pubertal males have the highest risk for toxicity)<br>Thyroid dysfunction | Oligospermia or azospermia<br>Ejaculatory or other dysfunction<br>Infertility<br>Hypogonadism | Obtain a bone age film, as indicated.<br>Obtain analysis of sperm at maturity and when clinically indicated.<br>Provide anticipatory guidance regarding symptoms of testosterone deficiency or germ cell damage.<br>Consult an endocrinologist when it is indicated.<br>Provide fertility counseling.<br>Educate the patient regarding performing testicular exams on himself.<br>Provide education regarding hormone replacement therapy and side effects if it is indicated.<br>Prevention of osteoporosis and atherosclerosis. |
| Reproductive–Ovaries | Radiation >400 cGy to ovaries<br>Radiation to the hypothalamic-pituitary axis<br>Total body irradiation<br>Chemotherapy alkylating agents; procarbazine (Matulane), nitrosoureas; carmustine (BCNU), lomustine (CCNU)<br>Busulfan (mylgran)<br>Ifosfamide (Ifex)<br>Cyclophosphamide (Cytoxan)<br>Mechlorethamine (mustargen)<br>Melphalan (Alkeran)<br>Chlorambucil (Leukeran)<br>Surgery (oophorectomy, oophoropexy)<br>Age (older females are at greater risk of ovarian failure) | Delayed menarche<br>Delayed or arrested pubertal development<br>Oligomenorrhea or amenorrhea after puberty<br>Infertility<br>Early menopause | Assess pubertal history.<br>Assess Tanner stage annually.<br>Obtain LH, FSH, and estradiol levels for delayed pubertal development and when it is clinically indicated.<br>Obtain thyroxine and TSH levels.<br>Obtain menstrual and pregnancy history.<br>Obtain a bone age film, as indicated.<br>Obtain an ultrasound of the ovaries, as indicated.<br>Recommend measurement of basal body temperature.<br>Consult with an endocrinologist when indicated.<br>Provide anticipatory guidance regarding the symptoms of estrogen deficiency and early menopause.<br>Provide fertility counseling and education regarding alternate strategies for parenting.<br>Patient may require hormone replacement.<br>Provide education regarding hormone replacement therapy and prevention of osteoporosis and atherosclerosis.<br>Counsel women at risk of early menopause regarding fertility options. |

*(continued)*

## Corticosteriods

Oral prednisone/dexamethasone and intrathecal hydrocortisone may be associated with long-term neurocognitive impairment.

## Surgery

Resection of a CNS tumor places a patient at risk for developing neurocognitive deficits, which are related to the location and the extent of the surgery required to remove the tumor.

## Clinical Presentation

### Neurocognitive Deficits

Neurocognitive deficits can present as difficulties with reading, verbal and nonverbal memory, arithmetic, receptive and expressive language, and speed of mental processing. Other negative effects include attention deficits, decreased IQ, behavioral problems, poor school attendance, poor hand-eye coordination, or personality changes.

Table 10-1. Late Effects Associated with Childhood Cancer Treatments (continued)

| Organ System | Risk Factors | Potential Late Effects | Evaluation/Interventions |
|---|---|---|---|
| Musculoskeletal/ growth | Radiation >1,000–2,000 cGy<br>Surgery<br>– muscle loss or resection<br>– amputation<br>– limb salvage<br>– laminectomy<br>Younger age at the time of treatment<br>Chemotherapy<br>– steroids<br>– vinca alkaloids<br>– methotrexate<br>Hypogonadism<br>GH deficiency | Partial or complete arrest of the growth of epiphysis<br>Spinal abnormalities<br>Muscle hypoplasia<br>Asymmetry of muscles<br>Decreased range of motion<br>Gait abnormalities<br>Discrepancy in the length of an extremity<br>Osteonecrosis (AVN)<br>Slipped capitofemoral epiphysis<br>Pathological fracture<br>Osteoporosis<br>Osteopenia | Make a careful comparison and measurement of irradiated and nonirradiated areas.<br>Obtain a bone age film, as indicated.<br>Obtain and plot on growth chart the patient's height, weight, and sitting-height measurements annually.<br>Perform radiographic studies of the irradiated area (baseline, yearly during rapid growth, and if normal, then every 5 years).<br>Refer to or consult an orthopedist, as clinically indicated.<br>Encourage a routine physical exercise program for both range of motion and strengthening.<br>Educate the patient about the importance of weight control and exercise.<br>Provide anticipatory guidance regarding realistic expectations about potential growth and function of the affected area and educate regarding osteoporosis prevention with calcium and vitamin D.<br>Treat exacerbating or predisposing conditions (i.e., hypogonadism). |
| Hematopoietic and immunologic | Radiation<br>– marrow-containing bones<br>– total body irradiation<br>– asplenia, if spleen was in radiation field<br>Blood transfusion(s) (prior to 1985)<br>Splenectomy<br>Chemotherapy<br>– high doses for extended periods<br>– etoposide (VP–16)<br>– tenopside (VM–26)<br>– alkylators: melphalan or nitrogen mustard | Hypoplastic or aplastic bone<br>Frequent, recurrent infection<br>Decreased immunoglobulin levels<br>Overwhelming bacterial infection<br>Acute myeloid leukemia<br>Human Immunodeficiency Virus (HIV) | Obtain a CBC with differential.<br>Perform a bone marrow aspiration, as clinically indicated.<br>Obtain immunoglobulin levels, as indicated.<br>Obtain T-cell studies, as indicated.<br>Consult with an immunologist when it is indicated.<br>Encourage annual evaluations.<br>Recommendations for asplenic individuals:<br>– prophylactic penicillin<br>– pneumococcal vaccine, meningococcal, H. influenza<br>– prompt treatment with symptoms of fever, chills, or infection<br>Medic-Alert bracelet noting asplenia<br>Test for HIV |
| All Systems (including skin/dermatologic) | Radiation<br>– higher daily fractions or cumulative treatment dose<br>– extended treatment volumes<br>Chemotherapy<br>– alkylators | Secondary benign or malignant neoplasm in radiation field | Perform annual physical exam with inspection of skin and soft tissues in radiation treatment field(s).<br>Refer to oncology, as indicated.<br>Refer to dermatology, as indicated. |

## Leukoencephalopathy

Leukoencephalopathy can present as dementia, dysarthria, dysphagia, ataxia, spasticity, seizures, or coma. In some cases, blindness also can occur.

## Peripheral Neuropathy

Peripheral neuropathy can present as foot drop, paresthesias, or numbness of the hands or feet.

## Diagnostic Workup

A diagnostic workup consists of a comprehensive yearly history and physical examination. The patient should receive a baseline computed tomography (CT) scan of the head to evaluate for calcifications. Follow-up CT scans of the head should be obtained if clinically indicated. Magnetic resonance imaging should be done, if clinically indicated, to provide greater anatomic detail and better detection of white-matter changes and leptomeningeal and spinal disease. Neuropsychological testing should be done when the patient has completed therapy to establish a baseline, and then routinely (i.e., every 2 to 3 years) during the hallmark stages of academic advancement. In addition, a patient's school performance should be monitored.

## Medical Treatment

Medical treatment involves neurocognitive and behavioral rehabilitation, including appropriate school placement, provision of community and school resources to meet the patient's special needs, counseling, and training in behavior management. Psychopharmocological intervention can include administration of methylphenidate (Ritalin) or other psychotropic drugs to manage symptoms such as poor concentration.

## Nursing Assessment and Interventions

### Assessment
- Review the survivor's academic performance, including parents' and teachers' appraisals of performance, grade level in school, conduct or behavioral problems, and attention problems, as well as strengths and weaknesses in school and attendance.
- Make an assessment of additional available resources as well as those already being used by the child.

### Interventions
- Reinforce the importance of having lifelong follow-up assessments annually with a healthcare provider who is familiar with the survivor's cancer history, treatment, and risks for developing late effects.
- Review neuropsychological results with the family and school staff as necessary.
- Encourage early intervention with specialized educational programs, tutoring, and resource classes.
- Educate teachers about the child's previous cancer history and the potential for long-term side effects.
- Encourage parents to advocate for their child's educational needs.
- Advocate for occupational and physical therapies when they are needed.
- Educate the child about peripheral neuropathy, and caution that affected areas should be protected from exposure to excessive heat or cold.
- Provide the survivor or parents with the Children's Oncology Group (COG) Internet link, www.survivorshipguidelines.com, for information regarding educational issues, hearing loss, and peripheral neuropathy. Also, educate the survivor to share the COG link with his or her primary-care provider.

### Expected Patient Outcomes
- The survivor is knowledgeable about the risks for neuropsychological and neurologic toxicities.
- The survivor has annual follow-up visits.
- The survivor has access to and uses resources in the school and the community to help achieve academic goals.
- The survivor's teachers are knowledgeable about his or her previous treatment and late effects and provide appropriate intervention.
- The survivor or the family can advocate for the child's needs.

# Hypothalamic-Pituitary Axis

*Deborah Diotallevi and Elaine Pottenger*

## Definition
The hypothalamus and the pituitary gland work synergistically to maintain homeostasis of the endocrine system and are connected by the pituitary stalk. Abnormalities of the hypothalamic-pituitary axis (HPA) are commonly seen after a patient has received radiation for tumors of the head, neck, and face. Low-dose cranial irradiation employed in central-nervous-system prophylaxis and cytoreductive total body irradiation may also cause neuroendocrine damage. Surgical trauma and tumor location near the HPA also may contribute to neuroendocrinopathies. Hypothalamic-pituitary injury can cause alterations in levels of growth hormone (GH), thyrotropin, gonadotropin, adrenocorticotropin hormone (ACTH), prolactin, antidiuretic hormone (ADH), or vasopressin.

## Risk Factors

### Radiation Therapy
Injuries from radiation therapy can result from doses that range from 1,800 to 5,000 cGy and include
- growth abnormalities: doses equal to or greater than 1,800–2,000 cGy
- precocious puberty: doses greater than 1,800–2,000 cGy
- gonadotropin deficiency: doses greater than 3,000–4,000 cGy
- thyroid-stimulating hormone (TSH) deficiency: doses greater than 3,000 cGy
- ACTH deficiency: doses greater than 3,000–4,000 cGy
- hyperprolactinemia: doses greater than 4,000–5,000 cGy.

Higher doses of radiation are associated with greater risk of developing a hormone deficiency. Abnormalities of the neuroendocrine system can become evident soon after completion of therapy but may also take several years to develop. Growing children are most profoundly affected.

### Surgery
The HPA is vulnerable to damage by surgical trauma.

### Tumor Location
Children with tumors in the HPA (i.e., craniopharyngioma or hypthalamic-chiasmatic tumor) region have a 30% chance of developing an ADH deficiency before surgery and a 16% chance after surgery.

## Clinical Presentation

### Growth Hormone Deficiency (GHD)
GHD is the most common, and generally the first, abnormality noted after a patient has had radiation to the HPA. GHD can result in a reduction in growth velocity that is inappropriate for a child's age and stage of puberty. Postpubertal patients may note a decrease in relative muscle mass and an increase in adipose tissue. Furthermore, there is new evidence of a relation between GH deficiency and a metabolic syndrome, which includes increased amount of adipose tissue, high cholesterol levels, hypertension, and early-onset atherosclerosis.

### Precocious Puberty
Precocious puberty is manifested by breast development before the age of 8 years in girls and signs of genital development and testicular enlargement in boys younger than 9 years. Additional manifestations include accelerated bone maturation, premature epiphyseal fusion, and reduced final height.

### Gonadotropin Deficiency
Gonadotropin deficiency is the failure to progress through puberty, arrested puberty, or amenorrhea. In girls, the influence of adrenal androgen on pubic and axillary hair development without corresponding breast development must be distinguished

from true puberty. Breasts that have been irradiated might not grow during puberty. In boys, testicular enlargement may be delayed. Primary gonadal failure occurs in boys who have received testicular irradiation (see the discussions in the subsections "Reproductive System: Testes" and "Reproductive System: Ovaries").

### ACTH Deficiency
ACTH deficiency presents as decreased stamina, lethargy, fasting hypoglycemia, and dilutional hyponatremia similar to inappropriate vasopressin secretion.

### Hyperprolactinemia
Hyperprolactinemia (noted most commonly in females) is failure to proceed through puberty, arrested puberty, galactorrhea or amenorrhea, decreased libido, and, in males, impotence.

### Diabetes Insipidus
Deficiency of ADH secretion presents with obvious symptoms of excessive thirst and urination with nocturia or enuresis.

## Diagnostic Workup
A diagnostic workup includes an annual comprehensive history and physical examination. Specific assessments include the following.

### GHD
Assessment includes a determination of the patient's growth velocity, bone age, and Tanner stage. Assessment of thyroid function and routine blood studies to exclude other systemic illnesses that can affect growth (e.g., renal dysfunction) should be completed. Measurement of insulin-like growth factor 1 (IGF1) and insulin-like growth factor-binding protein 3 (IGFBP3) should be obtained. Low plasma levels of IGF1 and IGFBP3 are highly suggestive of GHD in a high-risk population. Formal GH-stimulation testing using two different provocative agents is done because standard testing may not uncover a GHD. False negatives are common in this test. If testing is normal and growth continues to be abnormal, a physiological assessment, with frequent serum sampling of growth hormone over a period of 12–24 hours, may be warranted.

### Gonadotropin Deficiency
Luteinizing hormone and follicle-stimulating hormone levels are obtained before puberty and then periodically throughout puberty if there are delays or arrests in pubertal progression. In addition, testosterone levels are obtained in males and estradiol levels usually are obtained in females. Gonadotropin-releasing hormone (GnRh) stimulation testing may provide additional clinical information.

### Precocious Puberty
Careful assessment of sexual development using Tanner staging is done. Diagnostic tests to assess for precocious puberty include determining the patient's bone age and testing for GnRh. GH testing may be indicated, given that the patients with precocious puberty also may be GH deficient.

### TSH Deficiency
To assess for TSH deficiency, basal plasma concentrations of thyroxine and TSH level should be obtained.

### ACTH Deficiency
To assess for ACTH deficiency, a random serum-cortisol level should be obtained first thing in the morning. If this level is abnormal, 1-hour ACTH stimulation testing should be done.

### Hyperprolactinemia
To assess for hyperprolactinemia, random samples of serum plasma prolactin should be obtained. This testing should be directed by an endocrinologist.

### Diabetes Insipidus
To assess for an ADH deficiency, a urinalysis, with specific gravity, serum and urine electrolytes, and osmolarity, should be obtained.

## Medical Treatment

### GHD
It is recommended that GH therapy not be given for at least 1 year after completion of cancer treatment. Ongoing studies are investigating whether a correlation exists between GH replacement and secondary malignancies. However, there is currently no evidence that children treated with GH are at increased risk of experiencing a relapse of their primary tumor.

### Precocious Puberty
A gonadotropin-releasing hormone analog is used to suppress pubertal development. Preliminary data show that treating a patient with GH while he or she is being treated with gonadotropin-releasing hormone increases the patient's overall height.

### Gonadotropin Deficiency
Gonadotropin deficiency is treated primarily by replacing the appropriate hormones—estrogen for females and testosterone for males. Care for this condition should be directed by an endocrinologist (see the discussion of reproductive systems in the subsections "Reproductive System: Testes" and "Reproductive System: Ovaries").

### TSH Deficiency
Treatment consists of thyroxine replacement therapy with medications such as levothyroxine (Synthroid). Care of survivors with TSH deficiency should be directed by an endocrinologist.

### Adrenocorticotropin Deficiency
Hydrocortisone is used to treat adrenocorticotropin deficiency. A low dose, given twice a day, usually is sufficient. During times of stress (e.g., a febrile illness), an increased dose is required. Mineralocorticoids also may have to be replaced. Care of survivors with adrenocorticotropin deficiency should be directed by an endocrinologist.

### Hyperprolactinemia
Hyperprolactinemia is treated with bromocriptine or related dopaminergic agents. Care of survivors with hyperprolactinemia should be directed by an endocrinologist.

### Diabetes Insipidus
Desmopressin is used to treat an antidiuretic hormone deficiency. Care of survivors with ADH deficiency should be directed by an endocrinologist.

## Nursing Assessment and Interventions

### Assessment
- Review the patient's history for
  - poor linear growth
  - halted, absent, or early pubertal development
  - symptoms of hypothyroidism
  - symptoms of antidiuretic hormone deficiency
  - symptoms of hyperprolactinemia, including menstrual or pregnancy history or both, and history of sexual function.
- A physical examination should include
  - patient's height and weight plotted on a growth chart that notes the growth velocity over time as well as parental heights
  - patient's sitting height (if the spine has been irradiated, subtract the standing height from the sitting height to assess the amount of leg growth)
  - Tanner stage of development.

### Interventions
- Reinforce the importance of having lifelong, annual, follow-up assessments with a healthcare provider familiar with the survivor's cancer history and treatment and with the risks of developing late effects.
- Obtain accurate measurements of the patient's height and weight and plot them on a growth curve.
- Educate the survivor about the particular endocrine dysfunction that he or she is at risk for developing and the corresponding signs and symptoms.
- Educate the survivor taking replacement hormones about proper administration.

### Expected Patient Outcomes
- The survivor knows about his or her risks for developing endocrine dysfunction.
- The survivor continues to have annual follow-up visits.
- The survivor complies with the medication regimen.
- The survivor is asymptomatic while on replacement medication and reports abnormal symptoms if or when they occur.
- The survivor maintains appropriate serum levels and growth indices.

## Thyroid Function

*Deborah Diotallevi and Elaine Pottenger*

### Definition
Thyroid abnormalities can occur after radiation therapy to the thyroid gland or the hypothalamic-pituitary axis (see the subsection "Hypothalamic-Pituitary Axis"), after surgical removal of the thyroid, or after precondition therapy for allogeneic transplants (busulfan/cyclophosphamide). The most common effect is hypothyroidism that can be either overt or compensated. Other abnormalities include Graves disease (hyperthyroidism), thyroiditis, and benign or malignant tumors (see the subsection "Second Malignant Neoplasms"). The peak incidence of thyroid abnormalities occurs 2–5 years after treatment, although the risk continues for many years.

### Risk Factors
The risk factors for thyroid abnormalities include
- radiation therapy greater than 1,000 cGy to the head, neck, chest, or spinal axis
- single-dose or total-body irradiation equal to or greater than 750 cGy
- busulfan/cyclophosphamide used for cytoreduction for bone-marrow transplantation
- patients who are pubertal while receiving treatment may be at greater risk for thyroid late effects.
- lymphangiograms done at the time of diagnosis have been associated with the development of thyroid late effects; however, lymphangiograms are not currently the standard of care. In addition, a thyroid malignancy is associated with thyroid dysfunction and is a rationale for treating patients with subclinical hypothyroidism.
- thyroidectomy (see the subsection "Second Malignant Neoplasms")
- radiolabeled antibodies used in the diagnosis and treatment of neuroblastoma (i.e., MIBG)
- allogeneic bone-marrow transplantation (i.e, autoimmune hyperthyroidism from adoptive transfer of abnormal clones of T or B cells).

### Clinical Presentation

#### Hypothyroidism
The symptoms of hypothyroidism are intolerance of cold; constipation; weight gain; dry skin; generalized muscle weakness; muscle and joint aches; fatigue; lethargy; hoarseness; bradycardia; hypotension; puffy, round face; brittle hair; alopecia; periorbital edema; poor linear growth; amenorrhea; problems concentrating; depression; high cholesterol level; arrested pubertal development; and an elevated serum thyroid-stimulating hormone (TSH) level with a corresponding decrease in serum thyroxine (T-4).

#### Compensated Hypothyroidism
This type of hypothyroidism generally is asymptomatic, but testing reveals an abnormal thyroid profile suggesting impending thyroid failure (i.e., elevated TSH and normal T-4).

#### Graves Disease (hyperthyroidism)
The symptoms of Graves disease are tachycardia; excitability; anxiety; nervousness; problems concentrating; intolerance of heat; increased sweating; weight loss; increased appetite; muscle weakness; fatigue; diarrhea; moist skin; tremors of the hand; irregular menstrual periods; and exophthalmos. Serum-blood studies reveal a decrease in TSH and an elevation of T-4.

#### Thyroiditis
Thyroiditis presents with the signs and symptoms of hypothyroidism and an elevation in serum-thyroid antibodies.

#### Benign or Malignant Tumor
Presentation may vary. Any palpable nodule or enlargement of the thyroid should be evaluated by an endocrinologist.

### Mixed Hypothyroidism
Evidence of central hypothyroidism (see the subsection "Hypothalamic-Pituitary Axis") plus mildly elevated TSH level.

## Diagnostic Workup
An annual examination should include careful palpation of the patient's thyroid gland. Serum TSH and thyroxine (usually free T-4, but may vary depending upon the institution) and other thyroid studies are done as directed by an endocrinologist. Survivors who have received cranial or craniospinal radiation and/or women taking birth control pills should be evaluated for thyroid function based on free T-4 rather than T-4.

## Medical Treatment

### Hypothyroidism
Patients are given replacement levothyroxine (Synthroid).

### Compensatory Hypothyroidism
Most centers treat this condition with levothyroxine, but treatment decisions are based on the potential of increased risk of tumor development.

### Graves Disease (hyperthyroidism)
Graves disease is treated with surgical removal of part or all of the thyroid gland, thyroid ablation with radioactive iodine, or antithyroid drugs.

### Thyroiditis
Thyroiditis may be self-limiting and may require no intervention except for periodic serum-thyroid studies to monitor levels. Treatment for persistent or symptomatic thyroiditis usually consists of hormone replacement.

### Benign or Malignant Tumor
Tumors are surgically resected. If they are benign, no further treatment is necessary. A differentiated carcinoma may require additional therapy. These conditions should be monitored by an endocrinologist.

## Nursing Assessment and Interventions

### Assessment
- Review the patient's history for any signs or symptoms of thyroid abnormalities.
- Perform a physical examination that includes careful palpation of the patient's thyroid gland.

### Interventions
- Reinforce the importance of having lifelong, annual, follow-up assessments with a healthcare provider who is familiar with the survivor's cancer history, treatment, and risk of developing late effects.
- Order appropriate follow-up studies.
- Inform the survivor about the risk of developing thyroid abnormalities and corresponding signs and symptoms.
- Inform the survivor about the importance and benefits of hormone-replacement therapy.
- Inform the survivor about the potential side effects of hormone-replacement therapy.

## Expected Patient Outcomes
- The survivor is knowledgeable about the potential for thyroid dysfunction.
- The survivor complies with recommendations for follow-up evaluations.
- The survivor is asymptomatic while on replacement medication and reports abnormal symptoms to medical providers if or when they occur.
- The survivor maintains appropriate serum levels of thyroid hormones.

# Vision and Hearing

*Debra A. Eshelman-Kent*

## Definition
Visual late effects can result from neoplastic involvement of the optic tracts, high-dose steroids, radiation injury, surgery (e.g., enucleation), or as a consequence of chronic graft-versus-host disease after stem-cell transplantation. Hearing deficits can result from neoplastic involvement of the ear as well as from chemotherapy, radiation therapy, or prolonged use of antimicrobials.

## Risk Factors

### Abnormalities of the Ear
**Radiation:** In general, risk factors include radiation doses greater than 30 Gy, alone or in combination with host factors, such as central-nervous-system tumors, nasopharyngeal tumors, younger age at treatment, and concurrent medical conditions (e.g., otitis media and chronic cerumen impaction). Radiation administered prior to platinum chemotherapy (e.g., cisplatin [Platinol]) or combined with other ototoxic agents (e.g., aminoglycosides) can result in hearing problems such as sensorineural hearing loss or tinnitus. High doses of radiation (i.e., >50 Gy) alone or in combination with host factors, such as younger age at treatment, can result in tympanosclerosis, otosclerosis, conductive hearing loss, or eustachian-tube dysfunction.

**Chemotherapy:** Platinum derivatives have known ototoxic effects that may be potentiated by radiation or ototoxic drugs (i.e., aminoglycosides). Generally, cumulative cisplatin doses greater than or equal to 360 mg/m$^2$ result in hearing problems. Additional studies to determine ototoxic dose/effects relationships for carboplatin are warranted.

### Abnormalities of the Eye
**Radiation:** Radiation-induced ocular complications are generally associated with direct orbital/eye radiation or higher-dose cranial radiation. Late effects vary, depending on the radiation dosage and eye structure involved.
- Reduced visual acuity and orbital hypoplasia generally are caused by doses greater than 30 Gy.
- Cataracts generally are caused by doses greater than 10 Gy, total body irradiation (TBI) greater than or equal to 2 Gy in a single fraction, or TBI greater than or equal to 5 Gy fractionated. Radiation combined with steroids and busulfan increases the risk for cataract development.

- Lacrimal-duct atrophy generally is caused by doses greater than or equal to 30 Gy.
- Xerophthalmia (severe) generally is caused by doses greater than or equal to 30 Gy.
- Keratitis and keratoconjunctivitis generally are caused by doses greater than 50 Gy.
- Retinopathy generally is caused by doses greater than 30 Gy.
- Optic chiasm neuropathy generally is caused by doses of 50 to 65 Gy, with exacerbation caused by other comorbid conditions, such as diabetes mellitus or hypertension.

**Chemotherapy:** Corticosteroids most commonly are associated with the development of cataracts. Busulfan has also been associated with the development of cataracts. Steroids are a known risk factor for cataracts, glaucoma, and uveitis.

**Surgery:** Enucleation (e.g., retinoblastoma) may increase the risk for alteration in body image secondary to impaired cosmesis, contribute to orbital hypoplasia, and impact potential fit or function of prosthesis, especially if concurrent radiation is used.

**Stem-cell transplantation:** Chronic graft-versus-host disease may result in xerophthalmia.

## Clinical Presentation

### Abnormalities of the Ear

The signs and symptoms of ear problems include hearing abnormalities (e.g., high-frequency [sensorineural] hearing loss or permanent hearing loss) indicated by abnormal speech development. Other hearing problems include tinnitus; vertigo; structural alterations caused by radiation and leading to fibrosis, which causes an inability to visualize ear landmarks; or abnormal production of cerumen.

### Abnormalities of the Eye

The signs and symptoms of ocular late effects include decreased visual acuity, vision loss, blurred vision, or cataract. Additional symptoms may include lachrymal-duct atrophy, severe xerophthalmia with graft-versus-host disease, keratitis, keratoconjunctivitis, telangiectasias, retinopathy, optic chiasm neuropathy, enophthalmos, painful eye, and ocular hypoplasia secondary to radiation. Glaucoma presents with eye pain, headache, nausea, vomiting, and decreased peripheral vision.

## Diagnostic Workup

### Ears

An otoscopic examination should be done at least annually to visualize the tympanic membranes and ear structures. A baseline audiogram or brainstem auditory-evoked response should be performed and repeated periodically as clinically indicated. An evaluation for hearing aids should be made as appropriate. Refer patients with chronic cerumen or hearing deficits secondary to postradiation changes to an otorhinolaryngologist or to a neurologist when clinically indicated.

### Eyes

Evaluation depends on the structure of the eye that is affected. Evaluation may include slit-lamp examination, fundoscopic examination, testing for visual acuity, or measurement of ocular pressure. Referral to an ophthalmologist should be made as appropriate.

## Medical Treatment

### Ears

Treatment consists of an audiologic consultation when clinically indicated; amplification (e.g., placement of a frequency modulated system in the patient's school); hearing aids; and removal of impacted cerumen to aid tympanic-membrane motility. For some patients with vertigo, referral to a neurologist may be warranted.

### Eyes

Treatment consists of extraction of any cataract if it interferes with a survivor's activities of daily living; steroid eye drops for iritis; tear replacement, as needed, for abnormalities of the lachrymal gland; photocoagulation to prevent progression of neovascularization and retinopathy; corneal transplants; medications for lowering intraocular pressure if the patient has glaucoma; and dilation of the tear duct if a patient has fibrosis.

## Nursing Assessment and Interventions

### Assessment

- Review the survivor's history to determine whether any previous speech, hearing, or visual problems predated treatment for malignancy.
- Assess for existing speech, hearing, or visual problems.
- Assess for poor school performance or problems in school.
- Assess for headaches, blurred vision, lazy eye, squinting, pain, double vision, myopia, tinnitus, and current speech problems.
- Assess for speech discernment during the physical examination.
- Assess for red reflex during the physical examination.

### Interventions

- Reinforce the importance of having lifelong, annual, follow-up assessments with a healthcare provider who is familiar with the survivor's cancer and treatment history.
- Ensure that the survivor obtains appropriate diagnostic tests.
- Educate the survivor about the potential long-term effects of previous therapy on vision and hearing.
- Educate school personnel about the survivor's special needs; ensure that the child has preferential seating in school if he or she has hearing or visual problems; recommend that the school offer amplification devices as well as adequate access to educational resources to maximize the survivor's learning.
- Reinforce the need for protective ultraviolet sunglasses and other methods to preserve vision (e.g., tear replacement products).
- Reinforce the need for hearing conservation as appropriate (i.e., avoid environments with very loud noises).

## Expected Patient Outcomes

- The survivor is knowledgeable about the risk factors for developing visual or hearing impairments.
- The survivor continues to have recommended ophthalmic examinations and audiograms as determined by the Children's Oncology Group *Late Effects Guidelines*.
- The survivor has access to hearing amplification and correction of visual problems when they are needed.

# Head and Neck

*Maureen M. Reilly and Claire A. Carlson*

## Definition

The head-and-neck region may be affected by tumors or treatments that include surgery, radiation, or chemotherapy. Late effects of treatment can include bone hypoplasia, deformity, dental abnormalities, vasculature damage, and changes in the skin and mucous membranes.

## Risk Factors

### Vasculature Changes

**Radiation therapy:** Radiation doses to the cranium, nasopharynx, oropharynx, cervical spine, supraclavicular region, or mantle can cause vascular injury that leads to fibrosis in vessel walls and the perivascular interstitial spaces. At doses greater than 4,000 cGy, fibrosis and resultant thinning can occur in the carotid and subclavian arteries. Studies show that there is an increased risk for stroke in these patients, particularly when prior radiation therapy is combined with a family history of stroke or a history of smoking. Cranial radiation at doses greater than 30 cGy is associated with an increased risk for vasculopathies in the larger vessels of the brain. This damage can lead to transient ischemic attacks, strokes, and focal seizures. The cause for late-occurring stroke appears to be accelerated atherosclerosis in the area of prior radiotherapy. Although rare, cranial radiation may also weaken the walls of cerebral vessels and cause hemorrhage.

**Chemotherapy:** Currently there is little evidence that links chemotherapy exposure to vasculature changes in the head and neck.

### Skin and Mucous Membranes

**Radiation therapy:** Radiation-induced vascular injury and fibrosis in the nasal mucosa can alter sinus drainage, resulting in chronic sinusitis, particularly with doses to the cranium, orbit, ear, and nasopharynx that are greater than or equal to 3,000 cGy. Fibrosis and thinning of the vessels can lead to telangiectasia and atrophy of the skin and membranes. Radiation can stimulate the production of melanin, leading to permanent darkening of irradiated areas, and can affect hair follicles, which may cause permanent alopecia. In general, the aging process of skin is accelerated by radiation therapy. Secondary skin cancers and an increased risk for developing malignant melanoma later in life have been associated with radiation therapy.

**Chemotherapy:** Available data linking chronic changes of the mucosa in children with chemotherapy exposures are limited. However, late skin changes are associated with certain cytotoxic drugs. Bleomycin may cause skin changes that are related to an increase in the size of melanocytes. Permanent alopecia of the scalp has been associated with busulfan in high doses, particularly when combined with cyclophosphamide, as is common in bone-marrow-transplant conditioning regimens.

### Bone and Connective Tissue

**Radiation therapy:** Radiation, especially when given in doses greater than 3,000 cGy to the head or neck, can cause hypoplasia, craniofacial abnormalities, fractures, necrosis, and poor healing related to a decreased blood supply to bone. Connective tissue may exhibit fibrosis and hypoplasia. Patients younger than 5 years of age at the time of radiation are at higher risk.

**Chemotherapy:** There are no documented late effects.

### Salivary Glands and Taste Buds

**Radiation therapy:** If the field of radiation included the major salivary glands (i.e., parotid, submandibular, and sublingual), decreased salivation may occur because of atrophy of the secretory cells. This effect usually is seen in patients who have had doses greater than 5,000 cGy; with doses less than 4,000 cGy, the salivary glands and taste buds appear to retain their ability to secrete saliva.

**Chemotherapy:** There is little evidence of long-term effects.

### Dental

The pathophysiology of treatment-induced damage to dentition is related to the cytotoxic effect of radiation or chemotherapy or both to the developing tooth buds. Damage to the salivary gland causes dental damage indirectly by altering the flora of the mouth, thereby promoting tooth decay.

**Radiation therapy:** Radiotherapy is associated with the most severe dental defects, particularly when administered at doses greater than 1,000 cGy to children younger than 5 years of age. Children who have received total body irradiation (TBI) are reported to have significantly more teeth with altered root development compared with children who received chemotherapy alone. Dental abnormalities include tooth and root agenesis, enamel dysplasias, caries, malocclusion, microdontia, arrested and altered root development, and periodontal disease.

**Chemotherapy:** Patients who receive chemotherapy over extended periods are at more risk for dental abnormalities due to the prolonged nature of tooth development during childhood. Abnormalities include malocclusion; enamel hypoplasia and opacities; hypodontia; microdontia; supernumerary teeth; enlarged pulp chambers; altered root development; and marked shortening of premolar root, as well as thinning and constriction of the roots. Although exposure to any chemotherapy may affect dental development, cyclophosphamide, vincristine, and vinblastine are specific agents known to disrupt tooth growth and affect enamel and root formation.

**Bone-marrow transplant:** Young children who have received a bone-marrow transplant with TBI as a conditioning regimen are at particular risk for disturbances in dental development. The most common disturbances are arrested root development with v-shaped roots, premature apical closure, microdontia, enamel disturbances, and aplasia.

## Clinical Presentation

### Vasculature Changes

Patients should be assessed for cerebrovascular complications such as stroke, premature carotid artery disease, Moyamoya disease, and occlusive-cerebral vasculopathy. Presenting symptoms may include mental-status changes, headache, weakness, hemiparesis, numbness or tingling, or aphasia. Symptoms of subclavian-artery disease may include diminished brachial and radial pulses, pallor of upper extremities, and coolness of the skin or unequal blood-pressure measurements.

## Skin and Mucous Membranes

The skin may be pale, and there may be thinning of the epithelium, loss of pliability, submucosal induration, and chronic ulcerations. Patients also may have intranasal scarring, along with changes in normal production of mucus and sinus drainage. These conditions may lead to chronic sinusitis, chronic nasal discharge, postnasal drip, nasal obstruction, facial pain, and headache. Other late effects include hyperpigmentation or hypopigmentation, telangiectasias, atrophy, dryness, trismus (i.e., lockjaw), and xerostomia. Hair color and texture changes may occur at the radiation site. Patients can experience permanent hair loss with doses of 4,500–5,000 cGy.

## Bone and Connective Tissue

Patients may present with bony deformities, muscle hypoplasia, loss of elasticity, constricting fibrosis, osteoradionecrosis, and necrosis or ulcers of the soft tissue.

## Salivary Glands and Taste Buds

The signs and symptoms include xerostomia, dental caries, and decay that can lead to osteoradionecrosis and changes in the ability to taste.

## Dental

Patients can have root and crown abnormalities, root agenesis, premature apical closure, enamel hypoplasia, and microdontia, as well as foreshortening or agenesis of their developing teeth, and gingival hyperplasia.

## Diagnostic Workup

A diagnostic workup includes the following elements:
- inspection of the oral mucosa, nares, and the skin and soft tissue of the neck
- assessment of neck and jaw mobility for trismus, crepitus, limited mandibular movement, and abnormal growth
- radiographic studies of irradiated bone every 3–5 years and as indicated
- salivary flow rate and appropriate dental prophylaxis for high-risk patients
- periodontal prophylaxis, including a thorough dental and radiologic examination
- computed tomography scan of sinus and otolaryngology consultation as needed
- yearly neurologic exam, including assessment of memory impairment, paresthesias, extremity weakness, aphasia, vision changes, and carotid pulses or bruits
- doppler carotid ultrasound or brain magnetic resonance imaging with diffusion-weighted imaging and magnetic resonance angiography as clinically indicated for patients with potential for cerebrovascular complications; consult with neurology/neurosurgery specialists and follow up as needed.

## Medical Treatment

### Vasculature Changes

Treatment may include revascularizaton surgery in cases where risk for stroke is high. Management of hyperlipidemia with diet or lipid-lowering agents to mediate the development of atherosclerosis in the carotid and cerebral arteries should be considered. Other treatments may include pharmacologic intervention with antiplatelet agents. The efficacy of these strategies is not known.

### Skin and Mucous Membranes

Treatment includes dermatologic consultation and removal of suspicious moles and dysplastic nevi. For chronic sinusitis, treatment should include aggressive management of infections with the guidance of an ear, nose, and throat specialist.

### Bone and Connective Tissue

Treatment includes orthopedic and plastic surgery, as well as dental and orthodontic follow-up care when needed; physical therapy when needed for maintaining the mobility of the oral cavity, head, and neck; and stretching exercises for the oral cavity to minimize microstomia.

### Oral Cavity

Treatment consists of a periodontal consultation, a professional cleaning every 6 months, and prophylactic fluoride treatment, as well as an orthodontic consultation when needed and a saliva substitute if needed.

## Nursing Assessment and Interventions

### Assessment

- Review the survivor's history for dental problems, neck and jaw mobility, and skin problems.
- Inspect the patient's oral mucosa and teeth, neck mobility, skin appearance, and distribution of hair.
- Determine the patient's level of participation in prophylactic measures, such as dental cleaning, daily oral care, skin care, and physical activity.

### Interventions

- Reinforce the importance of having lifelong, annual follow-up assessments with a healthcare provider who is familiar with the survivor's cancer history, treatment, and risk for developing late effects.
- Educate the survivor about the long-term effects of cancer therapy on the oral cavity, bones, and connective tissues.
- Educate the survivor, especially one who has altered taste ability and who may have a tendency to consume increased amounts of sweets, regarding dietary controls to decrease the potential for developing caries.
- Educate the survivor regarding the importance of maintaining mobility of the jaw and neck.
- Encourage the survivor to follow up with subspecialists as indicated.
- Provide psychosocial support to patients with altered body image related to craniofacial abnormalities/hypoplasia; make referrals to counseling as needed.
- Educate the survivor on lifestyle behaviors that promote dental health and maintain adequate head and neck mobility.
  - Discourage the survivor from using tobacco products.
  - Encourage daily oral care, including brushing, flossing, and use of a mouth rinse.
  - Encourage the survivor to maintain a diet low in concentrated sugars.
  - Encourage the survivor to do stretching and other exercises to maintain head and neck mobility as needed.

- Provide education with regard to neurologic symptoms and a heart-healthy, low-cholesterol diet.
- Educate the patient about the importance of avoiding sun exposure and tanning and using sunblock.
- Educate the patient about assessing moles using the ABCD method (i.e., **a**symmetry, **b**order, **c**olor, and **d**iameter).

## Expected Patient Outcomes
- The survivor is knowledgeable about the potential long-term effects of therapy to the oral cavity, bones, connective tissues, skin, and vasculature.
- The survivor adopts healthy lifestyle behaviors.
- The survivor complies with recommendations for follow-up care.

# Cardiovascular System

*Joanne Quillen*

## Definition
Cardiac toxicity can result from both chemotherapy and radiation therapy. It most commonly takes the form of cardiomyopathy, pericarditis, and valvular or coronary artery disease and can occur within months to years after the exposure.

## Risk Factors
Females and young children have a higher incidence of late cardiovascular effects. Myocardial impairment increases as the survivor ages.

## Anthracyclines
The incidence of cardiomyopathy is related to the total cumulative dosage of anthracycline (e.g., doxorubicin [Adriamycin], daunomycin [Cerubidine], idarubicin [Zavedos], mitoxantrone [Novatrone], epirubicin [Pharmorubicin]). A cumulative dosage greater than $300mg/m^2$ places the childhood cancer survivor at greatest risk for cardiac abnormalities. The schedule under which anthracycline is administered also is a factor; there is less toxicity with continuous infusion or weekly doses compared with the administration of a bolus on a schedule of every 3 weeks. Although anthracyclines pose the greatest threat for cardiomyopathies, exposure to other chemotherapeutic agents have been shown to cause cardiovascular changes. These include cyclophosphamide (Cytoxan), dactinomycin (Actinomycin-D), mitomycin (Mutamycin), dacarbazine (DTIC), vincristine (Oncovin), bleomycin (Blenoxane), and methotrexate (Mexate).

## Radiation
Mediastinal radiation enhances anthracycline toxicities. A dose of 4,000 cGy is the usual radiation threshold. Total body irradiation—mantle, whole lung, whole abdomen, left flank, and spine—may enhance anthracycline toxicity or may be a risk factor alone.

Other factors that enhance the possibility of myocardial toxicity include an underlying cardiac abnormality, primary tumor in the chest, pregnancy, recreational drug use, health behaviors (e.g., diet, exercise), and uncontrolled hypertension.

## Clinical Presentation

### Pericarditis
The signs and symptoms of pericarditis include fatigue, cyanosis, ascites, peripheral edema, hypotension, chest pain, dyspnea, fever, venous distention, pulsus paradoxus, muffled heart sounds, effusion, and friction rub.

### Cardiomyopathy
The signs and symptoms of cardiomyopathy include tachycardia, tachypnea, shortness of breath, dyspnea, edema, hepatomegaly, fatigue, cough, hypertension, syncope, arrhythmias, cardiomegaly, gallop rhythms, palpitations, congestive heart failure, or pleural effusion.

### Valvular Damage
The signs and symptoms of valvular damage include weakness, cough, dyspnea, new murmur, and pulsating liver.

### Coronary Artery Disease
The signs and symptoms of coronary artery disease include chest pain on exertion, dyspnea, diaphoresis, pallor, hypotension, or arrhythmias.

## Diagnostic Workup
A diagnostic workup consists of the following:
- baseline studies at entry to long-term follow-up; then follow-up studies based on age at diagnosis and initiation of treatment, cumulative anthracycline dose, or cumulative radiation dosage exposure; and results of all follow-up studies
- a comprehensive annual history and physical examination
- echocardiogram and electrocardiogram
- chest X rays
- holter monitor and other cardiac studies performed as indicated
- a cardiology consultation for survivors with cardiac symptoms or abnormal screening studies. This is especially important during pregnancy for those who received the higher doses of anthracyclines or who have abnormal screening studies and before receiving general anesthesia.

## Medical Treatment

### Pericarditis
If tamponade develops, a patient may require pericardiocentesis. Effusion usually is resolved in 1–10 months but can persist for years. If effusion becomes chronic, a patient may require a pericardiectomy.

### Cardiomyopathy
Treatment may include afterload-reducing agents, digoxin, and diuretics. Cardiac transplantation may be a consideration for the most extreme cases that do not respond to medical therapy.

### Valvular Damage
Depending on the degree of dysfunction, penicillin prophylaxis may be given when a patient is scheduled for surgery or dental procedures. A patient may require surgical replacement of the damaged valve.

## Coronary Artery Disease
Treatment includes diuretics and other cardiac medications. Dietary restrictions may include low-sodium, low-fat foods. A patient may require balloon-dilatation angioplasty or coronary artery bypass surgery.

## Nursing Assessment and Interventions
### Assessment
- Review the survivor's history for exercise tolerance, fatigue, chest pain, dizziness, dyspnea, cough, shortness of breath, palpitations, fever, and lifestyle behaviors (e.g., smoking, drugs, activity level).
- Ensure that a physical examination assesses for
  - abnormal vital signs (e.g., blood pressure, pulse, respiration)
  - abnormal heart-sound (e.g., murmurs, rubs, thrills, gallops)
  - edema
  - venous distention
  - hepatomegaly
  - perfusion (i.e., capillary refill).

### Interventions
- Reinforce the importance of having lifelong, annual follow-up assessments with a healthcare provider who is familiar with the survivor's cancer history, treatment, and risk for developing late effects.
- Ensure that appropriate diagnostic tests are obtained.
- Educate the survivor about lifestyle behaviors that limit cardiac compromise.
  - Encourage close supervision of a survivor's cardiac function during pregnancy.
  - Discourage the use of tobacco products and alcohol.
  - Reinforce healthy dietary habits, including a low-fat, low-sodium, high-fiber diet to prevent obesity and hyperlipidemia.
  - Encourage routine aerobic activity; instruct the patient to avoid isometric exercise.
- Ensure that adequate information is available to survivors who are treated for cardiomyopathy.
  - Encourage the patient to follow up with a cardiologist as needed.
  - Provide anticipatory guidance regarding symptoms of cardiac dysfunction and the side effects of cardiac medications.
  - Educate a survivor with valvular damage about the need for prophylactic penicillin before having surgery or dental procedures.
  - Provide education on the side effects of specific cardiac medications.
  - Provide the survivor with the Internet link to the Children's Oncology Group survivorship guidelines pertaining to heart health.
- Educate survivors diagnosed with prolonged QT interval about medications that may exacerbate the problem.

## Expected Patient Outcomes
- The survivor is knowledgeable about the risk of cardiac toxicity.
- The survivor has adopted healthy lifestyle behaviors.
- The survivor complies with recommendations for follow-up care.

# Respiratory System
Claire A. Carlson and Maureen M. Reilly

## Definition
Radiation therapy to the lungs or systemic chemotherapy may result in acute or chronic impairment of respiratory function. Changes can be seen in both the lung parenchyma and the musculoskeletal components of the thoracic cage. Decreases in lung volumes and compliance as well as perfusion of gases can occur. Chronic changes may occur even if the acute course of treatment has proven to be asymptomatic.

## Risk Factors
### General Considerations
Combinations of therapies, younger age at exposure, higher cumulative doses, concurrent infection, and baseline dysfunction (due to effects of asthma or smoking) increase the risk for toxic effects of therapy on lung function.

### Chemotherapy
Bleomycin (Blenoxane) is the chemotherapeutic agent most commonly associated with pulmonary toxicity, particularly pulmonary fibrosis. Dose-related effects are seen with bleomycin with doses greater than 400 u/m$^2$; in children, injury has been seen at doses between 60 and 100 units/m$^2$.

Exposure to alkylating agents such as nitrosureas (e.g., carmustine [BCNU], lomustine [CCNU]), and busulfan is linked with fibrosis and pneumonitis. With nitrosureas, damage is dose dependent; doses of BCNU greater than 600 mg/m$^2$ are at highest risk. Transplant doses of busulfan greater than 500 mg/m$^2$ appear to present greater risk, although a clear dose-dependent relationship has not been established.

Other agents, including cyclophosphamide, methotrexate, and cytosine arabinoside, are also associated with pulmonary damage.

### Radiation Therapy
Radiation to the thorax, mediastinum, whole lung, mantle, or total body irradiation (TBI) is associated with both acute and chronic pulmonary toxicity. The extent of damage depends on the total dose, volume of tissue irradiated, and how the dose is fractionated. Smaller doses delivered in multiple fractions rather than larger, single doses to lung tissue are less damaging. Cumulative doses to lung tissue greater than 10–15 Gy, TBI greater than 6 Gy in a single fraction, or fractionated TBI greater than 12 Gy present the highest risk. Potential for damage is increased when radiation is combined with the administration of known pulmonary toxic chemotherapy such as bleomycin, busulfan, BCNU, and CCNU, as well as with radiomimetic agents such as doxorubicin and dactinomycin.

### Age
Young children (especially those younger than 3 years at the time of treatment) are at greatest risk, because, in addition to the direct effects of treatment on their lungs, radiation also can impair normal growth and development of the thoracic cage, airways, and lung parenchyma.

### Surgery
Surgical interventions to the lung or surrounding tissue (e.g., lobectomy, wedge resection, rib resection) may cause acute or chronic pulmonary dysfunction.

## Clinical Presentation
The pathophysiology of treatment-induced lung damage is likely related to several factors, including DNA damage, free radical formation, and allergic or inflammatory response to the chemotherapy or radiation exposure. The degree of symptoms of pulmonary dysfunction is variable. Some survivors may be completely asymptomatic even with an abnormal finding on the pulmonary-function test; others may have more severe impairments with symptoms that interfere with daily activities and may require medical intervention.

### Pulmonary Edema
Noncardiac pulmonary edema involving endothelial inflammation and vascular leak within the lung tissue is an acute reaction associated with the administration of agents such as cytosine arabinoside and interleukin-2. The condition responds to oxygen therapy and diuresis; generally, even in severe reactions, a return to baseline lung function occurs.

### Pneumonitis
Pneumonitis can occur 1–3 months after radiation therapy or chemotherapy. Symptoms include low-grade fever, congestion, cough, and fullness in the chest. Severe pneumonitis can result in dyspnea, nonproductive cough or a cough productive of small amounts of pinkish sputum, and pleuritic chest pain. Acute pnuemonitis may resolve completely but can often lead to the gradual development of pulmonary fibrosis.

### Fibrosis
Fibrosis can occur months or even years after treatment; changes are gradual and progressive but tend to stabilize after 1 to 2 years. Many patients are asymptomatic. There are minimal symptoms if fibrosis occurs in only one lung and if less than 50% of that lung is affected. Patients with severe fibrosis may have chronic respiratory failure and dyspnea on exertion, fatigue, cough, decreased exercise tolerance, orthopnea, cyanosis, oxygen dependence, and chronic cor pulmonale. Pulmonary function testing often demonstrates a pattern of restrictive lung disease. Oxygen therapy for patients who have received bleomycin should be carefully monitored throughout their lifetime. The use of supplemental oxygen at high concentrations in these patients has been associated with the development of respiratory failure and pulmonary fibrosis, even years after the administration of this agent.

## Diagnostic Workup
A diagnostic workup consists of the following:
- a comprehensive annual history and physical exam
- baseline radiography (i.e., anteroposterior and lateral chest films); if normal, repeat every 2–5 years and before the patient receives general anesthesia
- baseline pulmonary function tests (including DLco and spirometry) repeated every 2–3 years, before general anesthesia, and if the patient is symptomatic or has evidence of pulmonary dysfunction or progression; obtain tests as needed.

## Medical Treatment
### Prevention
Preventive measures consist of monitoring a patient's pulmonary function and obtaining chest X rays during treatment. Early detection of changes may allow for tailoring of therapy to minimize further pulmonary injury. Pneumococcal vaccine (Pneumovax) and influenza virus vaccines (Fluogen) should be given to treated patients to prevent infections that can exacerbate symptoms. Avoidance or cessation of smoking should be emphasized.

### Treatment
Corticosteroids, bronchodilators, expectorants, antibiotics, oxygen, and bed rest may be needed to relieve symptoms.

## Nursing Assessment and Interventions
### Assessment
- Review the survivor's treatment history to determine his or her risk factors.
- Review the survivor's medical history for symptoms of respiratory compromise, including fatigue, intolerance or change in tolerance to activity, chronic cough with or without fever, orthopnea, and dyspnea.
- Determine oxygen saturation via pulse oximetry.
- Ensure that the survivor's physical examination includes assessment for
  - abnormalities in vital signs (heart rate or respiratory rate)
  - color of skin or nails or both for evidence of pallor, jaundice, or cyanosis
  - respiratory effort and use of accessory muscles or nasal flaring
  - abnormal or decreased breath sounds (e.g., rales, crackles).

### Interventions
- Reinforce the importance of having lifelong, annual follow-up assessments with a healthcare provider who is familiar with the survivor's cancer history, treatment, and risks for developing late effects.
- Ensure that the survivor obtains appropriate diagnostic tests.
- Educate the survivor about behaviors that limit respiratory compromise:
  - avoid smoking, recreational drugs, secondhand smoke, and strong odors and chemicals
  - receive vaccinations to prevent respiratory infection, including pneumococcal vaccine (Pneumovax) and influenza virus vaccine (Fluogen).
- Educate the survivor who has received bleomycin and other pulmonary-toxic therapy about the need to inform healthcare providers about his or her treatment history before receiving anesthesia because of the risk of respiratory failure with high levels of oxygen (i.e., the patient should avoid $FiO_2$ of more than 30% intraoperatively and postoperatively).
- Avoid scuba diving due to potential barotraumas and exacerbation of pulmonary fibrosis with high oxygen concentration. Patients who desire to scuba dive should be advised to obtain medical clearance before diving.
- Ensure that the survivor has adequate information regarding the respiratory diagnosis when he or she is treated for respiratory dysfunction.

- Encourage the survivor to have a follow-up visit with a pulmonologist.
- Review the instructions for administering medications for symptom relief and discuss their potential side effects.

## Expected Patient Outcomes
- The survivor is knowledgeable about the risks for pulmonary toxicity.
- The survivor adopts healthy lifestyle behaviors and is knowledgeable about health behaviors that may cause pulmonary injury or increase his or her risk for a second cancer.
- The survivor complies with recommendations for follow-up care.
- The survivor uses medications correctly for symptom relief.

# Gastrointestinal and Hepatic Systems

*Claire A. Carlson and Maureen M. Reilly*

## Definition

Gastrointestinal (GI) and hepatic late effects are relatively uncommon. When they do occur, they can be life threatening and may have a significant impact on the survivor's quality of life. Improvements in contemporary treatment approaches for pediatric malignancies, particularly with regard to the elimination or reduction of radiation doses, may lessen the likelihood that future long-term survivors will develop severe or debilitating GI/hepatic effects. However, the long-term impact of problems such as chronic graft-versus-host disease (GVHD), veno-occlusive disease, and transfusion-acquired hepatitis may continue to be problematic as survivors age.

Fibrosis and enteritis are the most common pathological abnormalities of the GI tract in long-term survivors of cancer, and they can arise at any site from the esophagus to the rectum. Strictures, adhesions, obstruction, ulcers, and malabsorption also can occur. Fibrosis and cirrhosis are the most common pathological abnormalities of the liver in long-term survivors. Hepatitis also can occur and can be symptomatic or subclinical.

## Risk Factors

### GI Late Effects

**Radiation therapy:** Persistent or chronic GI late effects are most often associated with radiation therapy. Problems result from inflammation of the mucosa, which impairs the digestion and absorption of nutrients (i.e., enteritis/malabsorption), scars the tissue (i.e., fibrosis), or narrows the luminal opening of the GI tract (i.e., stricture). Incidence is related to the total dose, volume, and site of radiation. Parts of the small intestine (e.g., the duodenum or ileum) appear to be more sensitive to radiation than the esophagus or colon. Patients who are treated with total body irradiation, abdominal or pelvic radiation greater than 25–30 Gy, or spinal radiation greater than 20–30 Gy are at risk for developing bowel obstruction, chronic enterocolitis, or fistula or intestinal strictures. Risk is increased with doses greater than 45 Gy or when combined with abdominal surgery. Bowel obstruction is rarely seen in those who have had abdominal radiation but not abdominal surgery.

Treatment with total body irradiation, abdominal or pelvic radiation greater than 25 Gy, or spinal radiation greater than 25 Gy is associated with increased risk for the development of secondary GI malignancies, such as colorectal cancer. Risk is highest with doses greater than 25 Gy, particularly when given in higher daily fractions or when combined with chemotherapy (especially alkylators). Screening should begin 10 years after radiation exposure or at age 35, whichever occurs later.

Radiation to the neck, thoracic/cervical spine, mantle, mediastinum, chest, or upper-abdominal fields at doses greater than 30 Gy or total body irradiation predisposes to the development of esophageal strictures; doses greater than 40 Gy present the highest risk. The development of acute radiation esophagitis or recurrent candidal esophagitis also increases the risk of this complication. Esophageal strictures can have a significant impact on quality of life and may require multiple dilatation procedures as the survivor ages.

**Chemotherapy:** The development of chemotherapy-related GI complications typically are acute reactions, such as mucositis, and complete resolution usually occurs after the chemotherapy is stopped. Anthracyclines and dactinomycin have radiomimetic effects that may enhance acute GI toxicity and contribute to late-onset, radiation-related toxicity. Vinblastine, dactinomycin, doxorubicin, 5-fluorouracil, and methotrexate have been shown to cause esophageal ulcerations, fibrosis, and strictures.

**Surgery:** Laparotomy for staging or for surgical removal of tumor has been associated with the development of intestinal obstruction. Adhesions also may develop after abdominal surgery. Risk is increased when radiation is used in combination with surgery.

**Bone-marrow transplantation:** The development of transplant-related GI effects depends on the total radiation dose used for the transplant-conditioning regimen, the presence of GVHD, or a combination of both factors. GVHD can lead to strictures of the GI tract or perimuscular fibrosis. GVHD of the small bowel may lead to chronic diarrhea and impaired absorption.

### Hepatic Late Effects

**Radiation:** Irradiation of the liver can cause varying degrees of hepatic damage, including hepatic fibrosis and cirrhosis. The incidence is difficult to estimate because the damage often is subclinical and unreported. Children's livers are more sensitive than adults. Radiation to the whole or upper abdomen greater than or equal to 30 Gy or total body irradiation can cause liver damage. It is possible to irradiate smaller portions of the liver at higher doses without long-term complications. Doses greater than 40 Gy to at least one third of the liver volume or 20–30 Gy to the entire liver increase the risk for hepatic injury. History of hepatic-resection veno-occlusive disease, chronic hepatitis, or chronic alcohol use in conjunction with exposure to radiation therapy increases the risk for development of hepatic damage. Splenomegaly and thrombocytopenia may develop as a consequence of portal hypertension and hypersplenism after a patient has had radiation to the abdomen.

**Chemotherapy:** Most children recover completely from the hepatotoxic effects of chemotherapy. Dactinomycin (Actinomycin-D) and doxorubicin (Adriamycin) can enhance the hepatic effects of radiation. Although the two are normally excreted through the biliary system, their toxicity may be exaggerated when the patient has hepatic fibrosis. Methotrexate (Mexate) is associated with the development of hepatic dysfunction, fibrosis, and cirrhosis. The incidence of these conditions can be as high as 80% for those treated for more than 2.5 years with daily administrations of low-dose methotrexate; however, these conditions usually are stabilized or resolved after therapy is completed. Daily oral methotrexate therapy is associated with a higher incidence of fibrosis and cirrhosis than intermittent parenteral dosing. The agent 6-mercaptopurine (Purinethol) has been associated with liver damage; however, it has not been well studied. Thioguanine (6TG) has been associated with acute hepatotoxicity, specifically veno-occlusive disease; this may be followed by chronic dysfunction, including portal hypertension, nodular hyperplasia, fibrosis, and siderosis (i.e., iron deposits in the liver).

**Bone-marrow transplantation:** Long-term liver injury from allogeneic bone-marrow transplantation is related to chronic GVHD, chronic infections (usually chronic hepatitis C), and drug-related toxicity. Approximately 80% of patients with chronic GVHD have liver involvement. Chronic liver toxicity associated with cirrhosis and hepatic failure can lead to early death in allogeneic-transplant survivors.

**Transfusions:** The screening of blood products for the hepatitis B virus did not begin until 1972; similarly, hepatitis C screening was not refined until the early 1990s. Therefore, patients who were exposed to blood products before 1972 are at risk for transfusion-mediated hepatitis B, and those exposed before 1993 are at risk for hepatitis C. The risk includes exposures to red cells, platelets, fresh frozen plasma, whole blood, granulocytes, cryoprecipitate, intravenous immunoglobulin, varicella zoster globulin, factor concentrates, allogeneic marrow, cord blood, or stem cells. Transfusion-mediated hepatitis B or hepatitis C can be symptomatic or subclinical and may cause chronic liver damage.

Patients who have received multiple blood transfusions may experience an overload of iron stored in the liver that can cause chronic hepatic damage. Chelation may be required in severe cases.

## Clinical Presentation

Presenting signs depend upon the degree of injury. If the injury is mild, patients may be asymptomatic, and the abnormalities may be detected incidentally.

### Intestinal Fibrosis and Enteritis

The signs and symptoms of intestinal fibrosis and enteritis are severe, intermittent abdominal pain; dysphagia; vomiting; diarrhea; constipation; bleeding with or without anemia; weight loss; poor linear growth; fatigue; obstruction; or rectal pain. Enteritis, ulceration, and bowel resection can lead to malabsorption, perforation, or fistulization.

### Adhesions and Strictures

The signs and symptoms of adhesions and strictures are abdominal pain, bilious vomiting, hyperactive bowel sounds, or dysphagia. A young child with an upper-GI obstruction may present with reflux and aspiration pneumonia.

### Cholelithiasis

Symptoms include colicky abdominal pain that is often related to intake of fatty foods and excessive flatulence. There may also be upper-right-sided abdominal tenderness or positive Murphy's sign on palpation.

### Hepatic Fibrosis

Transaminase levels may or may not be elevated. Other signs and symptoms can include elevated bilirubin, hepatomegaly, icterus/jaundice (often not present until fibrosis and cirrhosis develop), itching, bruising, portal hypertension, and encephalopathy.

### Hepatitis

Many patients with chronic hepatitis have no signs or symptoms. Chronic infection over a long period may cause significant liver damage, cirrhosis, and, in rare cases, liver cancer. The signs and symptoms of hepatitis can include elevation of transaminase and bilirubin levels, anorexia, malaise, nausea, vomiting, abdominal pain, arthralgia, jaundice, hepatomegaly, hepatic fibrosis, positive hepatitis screens for hepatitis B surface antigen, antihepatitis B core, antihepatitis C virus, or hepatitis C virus by polymerase chain reaction.

## Diagnostic Workup

A diagnostic workup consists of the following:

- comprehensive annual history and physical that includes an evaluation for signs of hepatic dysfunction (e.g., hepatomegaly, splenomegaly, icterus, pruritis, spider angioma, palmar erythema, ascites) and GI dysfunction (e.g., abdominal pain, bloating, dysphagia, bowel changes, bloody or tarry stools, weight loss, nausea/vomiting)
- annual measurements of the survivor's height and weight as a screen for malabsorption
- chemistry panel that includes alanine aminotransferase, aspartate aminotransferase, albumin, gamma-glutamyl transferase, electrolytes, calcium, phosphorus, magnesium, uric acid, amylase, cholesterol, total protein, bilirubin, and alkaline phosphatase obtained at baseline and then as clinically indicated
- complete blood count on an annual basis
- stool guaiac every year (for those who have had abdominal irradiation or surgery, or for those older than 50 years); add flexible sigmoidoscopy or double-contrast barium enema every 5 years or colonoscopy every 10 years
- serum total protein and albumin levels yearly in patients with chronic diarrhea or fistula. For patients at risk for enteritis, serum total protein and albumin levels at baseline and then as clinically indicated.
- serology studies for hepatitis A, B, and C if the survivor has had previous blood transfusions or if the survivor's chemistry panel is elevated
- serum ferritin to assess for iron overload in survivors who have had multiple transfusions
- prothrombin time to assess for disruption of the liver's ability to generate clotting proteins in patients with abnormal liver function or known hepatic dysfunction
- abdominal ultrasound and liver biopsy if the survivor has persistent elevations of transaminase or bilirubin levels or if hepatitis B or C has been detected

radiograph of any symptomatic area to assess for adhesions or an obstruction.

## Medical Treatment

Suspected late GI and hepatic effects should be evaluated in collaboration with a gastroenterologist or hepatologist. Surgical consultation may be needed for management of obstruction or stricture or for symptomatic cholelithiasis.

- Intestinal Fibrosis—Management consists of dilatation of the affected area and dietary management.
- Enteritis—Dietary management is the treatment for enteritis.
- Bowel Obstruction—A bowel obstruction is evaluated with abdominal radiographs, decompression (if needed), and appropriate contrast studies. The survivor may require surgical resection or balloon dilatation to alleviate an obstruction.
- GI Strictures—Assessment includes a barium test followed by an endoscopy. Treatment may include dilatation of the affected area.
- Esophagitis—Esophagitis can be managed with pharmacological agents.
- Cholelithiasis—Dietary avoidance of fatty foods may control symptoms. Cholecystectomy may be needed to treat refractory pain or biliary obstruction.
- Hepatic Fibrosis or Cirrhosis—Hepatic fibrosis or cirrhosis can be treated by administering diuretics or managing a patient's diet. End-stage hepatic disease may require a liver transplant.
- Hepatitis—Viral hepatitis can be treated with interferon or antiviral agents or both; if a patient develops end-stage cirrhosis, a liver transplant may be required. The goal of treatment often is to control or suppress the virus rather than cure the infection. Patients who do not have hepatitis and do not demonstrate immunity should be given immunizations for both hepatitis A and B. Currently, no vaccine is available for hepatitis C.

## Nursing Assessment and Interventions

### Assessment

- Review the history of the survivor's GI symptoms, including any difficulty swallowing, heartburn, loss of appetite, nausea, vomiting, indigestion, constipation, diarrhea, change in bowel habits, rectal bleeding, bloody or tarry stools, abdominal pain, food intolerance, or hemorrhoids; review symptoms that may suggest hepatic dysfunction, such as jaundice, pruritus, hepatosplenomegaly, ascites, spider angiomas, or palmar erythema.
- Assess the amount of the survivor's consumption of alcohol and hepatotoxic over-the-counter or prescription medications. Include assessment for use of herbal supplements.
- Ensure that the survivor is carefully assessed for
  - abnormalities in blood pressure
  - hepatomegaly
  - jaundice.

### Interventions

- Reinforce the importance of having lifelong, annual follow-up assessments with a healthcare provider who is familiar with the survivor's cancer history, treatment, and risk for developing late effects.
- Ensure that the survivor obtains appropriate diagnostic tests.
- Educate the survivor about the importance of avoiding alcohol or other hepatotoxic drugs, especially if he or she has a history of liver dysfunction.
- Educate the survivor about dietary management; chronic malabsorption and malnutrition may require strict dietary management. Low-fat, low-residue, gluten-free, and lactose-free diets can help control the symptoms associated with GI dysfunction. Intestinal fibrosis may require the patient to maintain a high-fiber diet; intestinal enteritis may require a modification in the survivor's diet to control symptoms.
- Encourage vaccination against hepatitis A and B for survivors who do not demonstrate immunity.
- Emphasize the importance of early colorectal cancer screening for at-risk patients.
- Counsel those with known chronic hepatitis B on ways to avoid spreading the infection to others, such as using barrier protection if sexually active. Even if the survivor has no symptoms, those with chronic infection can spread the virus to others.
- Educate the survivor about taking medication when it is necessary.

## Expected Patient Outcomes

- The survivor is knowledgeable about the risks for GI and hepatic toxicities.
- The survivor adopts healthy lifestyle behaviors.
- The survivor complies with recommendations for follow-up care.
- The survivor complies with dietary and pharmacologic recommendations.

# Genitourinary System

*Debra A. Eshelman-Kent*

## Definition

Late genitourinary complications can involve the kidneys, bladder, uterus, vagina, ureters, prostate, testes, and ovaries. Effects on the ovaries and testes are discussed in the subsections "Reproductive System: Testes" and "Reproductive System: Ovaries." Damage usually occurs as a result of treatments that can compromise the growth, development, or integrity of the genitourinary structures. Abnormalities take the form of structural and functional impairment of the involved organ(s).

## Risk Factors

### Radiation therapy

Whole abdominal, para-aortic/splenic, spinal, pelvic, and total body irradiation include structures of the genitourinary system in the radiation portal and may cause subsequent dysfunction (e.g., renal insufficiency, fibrosis, difficulty voiding, hypertension, and hydronephrosis).

**Kidney:** Renal insufficiency and hypertension usually are associated with doses greater than or equal to 10 Gy.

**Bladder:** Dysfunctional voiding, fibrosis, vesicouretral reflux, hemorrhagic cystitis, and hydronephrosis are associated with doses greater than 30 Gy and may be exacerbated by concomitant use of cyclophosphamide or ifosfamide. Bladder malignancies have also been reported.

**Ureter, urethra:** Risk of late effects generally is associated with doses greater than 5,000 cGy.

**Pelvis (female):** Radiation to the pelvis can result in vaginal fibrosis/stenosis and, at doses greater than 20 Gy in a prepubertal female, uterine-growth retardation. Ovarian dysfunction is seen following pelvic radiation. (This topic is covered in depth in the subsection "Reproductive System: Ovaries.")

**Pelvis (male):** Pelvic and testicular radiation may result in Leydig-cell and germ-cell functioning. (This topic is discussed in greater detail in the subsection "Reproductive System: Testes.") Decreased functioning of the prostate gland is noted in moderate-to-high doses of radiation, resulting in decreased seminal fluid.

### Radiation Therapy and Chemotherapy Used in Combination

Lower doses of radiation (e.g., <15 Gy) coupled with certain chemotherapeutic agents, such as cisplatin (Platinol), cyclophosphamide (Cytoxan), methotrexate (Mexate), dactinomycin (Actinomycin D), nitrosoureas, and anthracyclines, have been associated with exacerbation of genitourinary late effects. A monomephric patient may be at additional risk.

### Chemotherapy

Cisplatin (Platinol), carboplatin, ifosfamide (Ifex), and cyclophosphamide (Cytoxan) can cause glomerular dysfunction, hemorrhagic cystitis, fibrosis of the bladder, dysfunctional voiding, and atypical bladder epithelium. With methotrexate, acute toxicities predominate; the majority of patients recover from them without late sequelae. The effects of cyclophosphamide on urinary structures are generally reported at doses greater than 3 gm/m$^2$ and can be lessened with the concurrent administration of mesna. Ifosfamide generally is associated with renal toxicity at high doses—the greatest risk seems to exist in survivors who received 60 g/m$^2$—or when used in combination with other nephrotoxic agents (e.g., cisplatin, aminoglycosides, amphotericin B, immunosuppressants), and in younger children (<5 years at treatment).

Alkylating agents (e.g., busulfan, carmustine, procarbazine, cyclophosphamide), cisplatin, and carboplatin have been linked to gonadal dysfunction in males and females. Males seem to be at greater risk than females. Both sexes are at greatest risk if they have received mechlorethamine, Oncovin, prednisone, and procarbazine (i.e., MOPP) in more than 3 cycles, busulfan (greater than 600 mg/m$^2$), cyclophosphamide (greater than 7.5 g/m$^2$), or alkylators combined with radiation to the genitourinary structures.

### Surgery

Removal of a paired organ usually is not associated with increased risk of late effects unless there is underlying damage to the remaining organ, whereas removal of a nonpaired organ (e.g., prostate, uterus, or bladder) can lead to infertility and incontinence. Retroperitoneal lymph-node dissection may be associated with parasympathetic dysfunction and lead to retrograde ejaculation or impotence.

### Age

Renal and bladder dysfunction might not become apparent until a survivor grows to a size that exceeds the ability of the affected organ to compensate. Children younger than age 5 who receive radiation may experience greater radiation toxicities at lower dosages.

### Supportive Therapies

Therapies include antimicrobials and graft-versus-host-disease prophylactic medications (e.g., cyclosporine [Sandimmune]); with prolonged use, they may result in kidney damage.

## Clinical Presentation

### Renal Insufficiency

The signs and symptoms can include either tubular dysfunction or nephritis presenting with hematuria, fatigue, hypertension, hypomagnesemia, Fanconi syndrome, proteinuria, anemia, or growth abnormalities.

### Bladder Dysfunction

The signs and symptoms can include mucosal irritation, microscopic or macroscopic hematuria, urgency, frequency, dysuria, hemorrhagic cystitis, incontinence, pain, and fibrosis.

### Prostate

A patient may have the inability to achieve an erection and diminished ejaculum.

### Vagina, Uterus

A patient can present with alteration in sexual function, uterine vascular insufficiency (resulting in adverse pregnancy outcomes such as miscarriage, low-birth weight, or premature labor), or altered gonadal function (i.e., delayed or arrested puberty).

### Ureter, Urethra

There are limited data on late effects in children.

## Diagnostic Workup

A diagnostic workup consists of the following:
- annual comprehensive history and physical examination and a blood pressure reading
- annual urinalysis and assessment of serum blood urea nitrogen, creatinine, electrolytes, and magnesium levels
- baseline creatinine clearance test (if any abnormalities are noted in the blood studies listed above), glomerular filtration rate, and organ-specific tests based on toxicity (e.g., cystoscopy, voiding cystourethrogram, intravenous pyelogram, computed tomography, or magnetic resonance imaging of the affected area, or glomerular filtration rate)
- an infertility evaluation.

# Section X  Late Effects of Childhood Cancer

## Medical Treatment

### Cystitis
Treatment can include hydration, instillation of alum solutions, cauterization of bleeding sites, sometimes a partial or total cystectomy, bladder augmentation, and urological follow-up care.

### Kidney Dysfunction
The survivor should be evaluated by a nephrologist as clinically indicated for treatment of hypertension, progressive proteinuria, progressive renal insufficiency or hematuria or both. Antihypertensives or electrolyte supplementation may be indicated.

### Strictures
Treatment involves dilatation or placement of stents; urinary diversion is sometimes necessary.

### Damage to Reproductive Organs
Treatment for damage to the reproductive organs usually involves surgical revisions or corrections.

## Nursing Assessment and Interventions

### Assessment
- Review the survivor's history for urinary-tract infections, hematuria, polyuria, dysuria, urgency, frequency, enuresis, and alteration in sexual function.
- Ensure that a physical examination includes an assessment of vital signs (especially blood pressure) and appropriate blood work, such as kidney function tests, electrolytes, calcium, phosphorus and magnesium, and urinalysis.
- Assess the skin, organs, and structures in the radiation field.

### Interventions
- Educate the survivor about long-term effects of treatment to the genitourinary system.
- Reinforce the importance of having lifelong, annual follow-up assessments with a healthcare provider who is familiar with the survivor's cancer history, treatment, and risk for developing late effects.
- Ensure that appropriate diagnostic tests are performed.
- Caution the survivor against engaging in contact sports, and explain the need to protect the remaining kidney if he or she has had a nephrectomy.
- Ensure that appropriate referrals to a nephrologist or urologist have been made.
- Emphasize that the survivor should have prompt treatment when he or she has symptoms related to a urinary-tract infection.
- If renal late effects are evident, caution against chronic use of nonsteroidal antiinflammatory agents (e.g., aspirin, ibuprofen, and naproxen). Caution against taking any new medications (prescription or over-the-counter) without checking with a healthcare provider.
- If patients have salt-wasting tubular dysfunction, advise them that low magnesium levels may bring on coronary atherosclerosis.

## Expected Patient Outcomes
- The survivor is knowledgeable about his or her individual risk factors.
- The survivor seeks prompt attention for urinary-tract infections or symptoms or both.
- The survivor complies with recommendations for follow-up care.

# Reproductive System: Testes

*Susan K. Ogle and Wendy L. Hobbie*

## Definition
Primary testicular failure may occur after chemotherapy, after radiation to the pelvis or testes, or after surgical removal of the testes. The germinal cells that produce sperm are more sensitive to the toxic effects of therapy than the Leydig's cells that produce testosterone. Therefore, for the majority of males, normal pubertal development and adult sexual function usually are preserved, however fertility may be affected. It is important to note that recovery of spermatogenesis can occur 3–5 years after the use of some chemotherapeutic agents has ceased.

## Risk Factors

### Chemotherapy
Males are at increased risk of infertility if given more than three cycles of nitrogen mustard, vincristine, procarbazine, and prednisone; combination therapy for Hodgkin's disease; or higher cumulative doses of chemotherapy, including transplant condition regimes such as busulfan and cyclophosphamide. In addition, any alkylating agent combined with testicular or pelvic radiation or total body irradiation increases the risks. Alkylating agents also can affect the function of the Leydig's cells in pubertal or postpubertal males when cumulative doses are high or used in combination with another agent. These survivors may need hormone replacement.

### Radiation Therapy
Radiation to the testes, whether direct or scattered, can cause azoospermia. Low doses (e.g., 10 cGy) can cause temporary azoospermia, while dosages of 200 cGy or greater are likely to result in permanent azoospermia. Leydig's cells that produce testosterone are damaged by doses greater than 2,000 cGy.

### Surgery
Retroperitoneal lymph-node dissection, which is done for staging of germ-cell or testicular tumors, can damage ejaculatory function. Orchiectomy (i.e., removal of a testicle) decreases testosterone and sperm production, but normal function may be maintained if the remaining testicle is unaffected.

### Age
Pubertal and prepubertal males are at risk of infertility. Prepubertal males are not as resistant to treatment effects as once believed. Secondary testicular failure is a result of damage to the hypothalamic-pituitary axis caused by radiation therapy (see the subsection "Hypothalamic-Pituitary Axis"). Thyroid dysfunction and chronic illness also may affect reproductive function and should be taken into consideration during an evaluation of gonadal dysfunction.

## Clinical Presentation

The signs and symptoms of primary testicular dysfunction can include delayed or arrested pubertal development, testicles that are small for the patient's Tanner stage, oligospermia or azoospermia, elevated gonadotropin levels, and Leydig's cells dysfunction. Leydig's cells dysfunction is manifested by decreased testosterone production, increased follicle-stimulating hormone (FSH), and luteinizing hormone (LH) levels, as well as by germinal-cell dysfunction that is associated with increased FSH and normal LH and testosterone levels.

## Diagnostic Workup

A diagnostic workup consists of the following:
- comprehensive history and physical examination including height, weight, and Tanner staging, including testicular volume measured by Prader orchiometry
- comprehensive history, including sexual function, erection, nocturnal emissions, libido, and medicinal or recreational drug use
- laboratory tests, including serum FSH, LH, and testosterone levels; T-4 and thyroid-stimulating hormone levels at age 11 years or older and for children with signs of delayed puberty or testosterone deficiency
- semen analysis, as requested by the patient, if age-appropriate and a sufficient length of time has passed since treatment ended
- bone-age radiological study.

## Medical Treatment

Before receiving treatment, pubertal males (Tanner 3 and greater) should be offered the option of semen analysis and banking. This preserves reproductive potential in the face of dysfunction caused by gonadotoxic therapy. Treatment of gonadal failure includes hormone replacement with testosterone supplementation during the patient's pubertal development. Also, testosterone may be given to enhance the patient's well-being and decrease the risk of osteoporosis in postpubertal males who have low levels of testosterone.

## Nursing Assessment and Interventions

### Assessment
- Review the survivor's treatment history to determine his risk factors.
- Review the survivor's medical history for symptoms of testosterone deficiency, which can include decreased testicular volume, poor erectile function, and decreased libido.
- Perform a complete annual physical examination and ensure that Tanner staging has been assessed.

### Interventions
- Reinforce the importance of lifelong, annual follow-up assessments with a healthcare provider who is familiar with the survivor's cancer history, treatment, and risk for developing late effects.
- Educate the survivor about the use of contraceptives to avoid an unwanted pregnancy, because testicular dysfunction may not be permanent.
- Ensure that adequate information is available for survivors who are treated for reproductive dysfunction.
  – Follow up with an endocrinologist or urologist or both.
  – Review with the patient instructions for the proper administration of medications.
- Make referrals for survivors who need counseling on fertility or alternative options for parenting.

## Expected Patient Outcomes
- Survivor is knowledgeable about the risk for reproductive failure and available interventions.
- Survivor is knowledgeable about his contraceptive options.
- Survivor complies with recommendations for follow-up care.
- Survivor is knowledgeable about his alternative options for parenting.

# Reproductive System: Ovaries

*Susan K. Ogle and Wendy L. Hobbie*

## Definition

Primary, secondary, or premature ovarian failure is defined as elevated serum gonadotropins, low or undetectable estrogen levels, and, in the postpubertal female, failure to progress through puberty or amenorrhea. These effects can occur after chemotherapy, abdominal or pelvic irradiation, or surgical removal of the ovaries. Normal pubertal development, postpubertal production of estrogen, and production of mature ova for fertilization can be affected. Treatment can cause depletion of oocytes, but the results might not be immediately evident.

## Risk Factors

### Chemotherapy
Higher cumulative doses of alkylating agents, or combinations of alkylating agents with or without radiation below the diaphragm, and total body irradiation all can damage the ovaries. In addition, female survivors may be at increased risk of developing premature menopause based on their treatment protocol.

### Radiation
Direct, scattered, or transmitted radiation to the ovaries in doses of 400 to 1,200 cGy can result in ovarian failure. In addition, radiation to the head, neck, or central nervous system in doses greater than 4,000 cGy may cause secondary ovarian failure (see the subsection "Hypothalamic-Pituitary Axis").

### Surgery
If one ovary is removed and if the second ovary has been unaffected by treatment, normal function can be maintained.

### Age
The number of oocytes remaining in the ovaries is proportional to a female's age; older females have fewer eggs and therefore are at greater risk of failure. Secondary ovarian failure is a result of damage to the hypothalamic-pituitary axis caused by radiation (see the subsection "Hypothalamic-Pituitary Axis"). Thyroid dysfunction and chronic illness can also affect reproductive function and should be part of a thorough evaluation.

## Clinical Presentation
Clinical presentation depends on pubertal status. In the prepubertal female, no breast buds by age 12 or no progression beyond a Tanner II stage by age 14 is highly suggestive of ovarian dysfunction. In the postpubertal female, irregular menses or amenorrhea in addition to symptoms of menopause (e.g., hot flashes, mood swings, headache, vaginal dryness, dyspareunia, and low libido) may be evident.

## Diagnostic Workup
A diagnostic workup consists of the following:
- a comprehensive annual history, including menstrual and pregnancy history (if applicable) is necessary.
- referral to a reproductive endocrinologist or fertility specialist when initial laboratory results and symptoms suggest ovarian dysfunction.
- laboratory tests for measuring follicle-stimulating hormone, luteinizing hormone, and estradiol levels, as well as free T-4 and thyroid-stimulating hormone. Other studies should be done as directed by an endocrinologist or reproductive endocrinologist.
- Radiological studies, including a bone-age film and an ultrasound of the survivor's ovaries, may be useful.

## Medical Treatment
### Prevention
Preventive measures include oophoropexy or shielding the ovaries from radiation. Currently, the standard of care for females pretransplant is to preserve ovarian tissue, either in the form of an embryo or an ova. In addition, for women who are survivors at significant risk for premature ovarian failure, some centers offer ova preservation.

### Hormone-Replacement Therapy
In prepubertal females, hormone replacement therapy (HRT) may be given to stimulate development of the gonadal organs if primary ovarian failure has been established. HRT might be given with growth hormone to maximize the survivor's growth potential. Hormone replacements can be given after puberty to decrease menopausal symptoms as well as to prevent osteoporosis and heart disease.

## Nursing Assessment and Interventions
### Assessment
- Review the survivor's treatment history to determine her risk factors.
- Review the survivor's history for symptoms of estrogen deficiency, including primary or secondary amenorrhea, menstrual changes, decreasing size of breasts, breast discharge, hot flashes, mood swings, headache, vaginal dryness, dyspareunia, and low libido.
- Perform a complete physical examination including Tanner staging.
- Review and interpret the patient's laboratory results.

### Interventions
- Reinforce the importance of having annual, lifelong follow-up examinations with a healthcare provider familiar with her cancer history, treatment, and risk for developing late effects.
- Educate the survivor about the use of contraceptive methods to prevent unwanted pregnancy if the status of her fertility is uncertain.
- Ensure that adequate information is provided to a survivor who is treated for ovarian failure.
- Ensure that the survivor visits an endocrinologist and gynecologist for an annual Pap test and pelvic examination.
- Ensure that medications are properly administered.
- Encourage the survivor at risk for early menopause not to postpone pregnancy if she wants to have children or to consider ova/embryo cryopreservation.
- Provide a referral for a survivor who needs counseling on fertility or seeks alternative options for parenting.

## Expected Patient Outcomes
- Survivor is knowledgeable about her risk for ovarian failure and the interventions that are available.
- Survivor complies with recommendations for follow-up care.
- Survivor is knowledgeable about contraceptive options.
- Survivor is knowledgeable regarding alternative options for parenting.

# Musculoskeletal System
*Debra A. Eshelman-Kent*

## Definition
Damage to the musculoskeletal system is most often caused by radiation that disrupts the cytoarchitecture and damages small vessels, thus preventing full muscle development because of ischemia. Damage also can be the result of surgical removal of a portion of the musculoskeletal system. Surgery, radiation, chemotherapy, and steroids can result in a variety of musculoskeletal late effects, including weakness, alteration or loss of function, osteopathy (such as osteopenia and osteoporosis), or fracture. Survivors may experience an altered body image and self-concept after amputation, limb-salvage, or poor development of a specific body part. The survivor's quality of life and overall functional status may be impaired.

## Risk Factors
### Radiation Therapy
In general, the higher the cumulative radiation dose and the younger the age at treatment, the greater the potential deficits. Second neoplasms (malignant or benign) may occur in radiated areas.

**Quantity of radiation:** Generally a dose of less than 1,000 cGy causes minimal changes; a dose of 1,000 to 2,000 cGy produces partial arrest of the growth of the epiphysis and muscle hypoplasia. Doses greater than 2,000 cGy usually result in complete arrest of the epiphysis. Fractionated doses of radiation decrease the risk of late effects when compared with a single-dose schedule. Historically, orthovoltage radiation (used more commonly before 1970; e.g., cobalt) results in more musculoskeletal damage than does megavoltage because of increased absorption by bone and skin. Total body irradiation has been associated with the development of exostoses in the transplant population.

**Field size and location:** Larger fields can produce greater deficits. Modern radiation techniques have improved the control of field size by permitting more symmetrical delivery of radiation, but it is important to recognize that there is scatter radiation to surrounding tissues no matter the energy source that is used. An example of the significance of field size can be found in the past, when flank radiation (e.g., Wilms' tumor) resulted in scoliosis, but the incidence of scoliosis has decreased with the use of modern technology and the port being changed to include the entire vertebral body in the field of radiation. The growth of the tissue is impacted symmetrically, thereby decreasing scoliosis. An example of the significance of scatter radiation can be found in radiation to soft tissues of the cheek (such as may be done to treat rhabdomyosarcoma), which may result in cosmetic changes, dental abnormalities, or potentially alter the function of the hypothalamus-pituitary axis.

**Age at the time of treatment:** Radiation therapy produces greater effects on the bones, muscles, and soft tissues of younger children. The epiphyseal plate of the bone may be damaged, causing slower or halted growth of bones. Hypoplasia of the irradiated developing muscle tissue also can occur.

### Chemotherapy

Prolonged use of steroids can result in avascular necrosis of the femoral heads, osteopenia, or osteoporosis. Both genders are at risk. Risk may be increased in patients with comorbid conditions, such as hyperthyroidism, growth hormone deficiency, or hypogonadism. Family history or predisposition to osteopenia or osteoporosis is relevant when assessing risk. Corticosteroid-associated bone morbidity has been linked with the treatment of leukemia. Acute vincristine-related neuropathy can predispose a patient to chronic foot drop, resulting in gait abnormalities. Antimetabolite therapy, especially methotrexate, has been implicated in the development of osteopathy.

### Surgery

The loss of muscle groups, especially in the lower extremities, can result in gait disturbances and weakness. Effects of limb-sparing procedures include functional deficits, limb-length discrepancies, problems with internal hardware, pain (phantom and neuropathic), chronic infection, increased energy expenditure, and contractures. Amputation of either a part of or an entire extremity also may result in muscle imbalance or functional deficits that require rehabilitation. Laminectomies may contribute to chronic back pain and have the potential to restrict mobility of the spine.

## Clinical Presentation

### Effects on Bone

Patients may experience the following effects on bone as a result of radiation: spinal abnormalities (e.g., kyphosis, lordosis, loss of stature), discrepancies in limb length, exostoses, slipped capitofemoral epiphysis, pathologic fracture, and delayed or arrested tooth development. Osteonecrosis/avascular necrosis of the femoral head, which typically develops during the acute treatment phase, may be problematic because of persistent residual effects. Multifocal osteonecrosis is more common than unifocal osteonecrosis. The effects on bone from surgery may include alterations in gait or functional impairment of the affected part. The effects on bone from chemotherapy (e.g., methotrexate) and steroids include increased risk for osteopenia or osteoporosis. Survivors may present with a history of bone fracture.

### Effects on Muscle and Soft Tissue

The effects on muscle and soft tissue due to radiation include hypoplasia and muscle asymmetry because of reduced or uneven growth. This includes breast tissue, especially in the prepubertal female.

## Diagnostic Workup

A diagnostic workup consists of the following:
- careful inspection and palpation of structures in irradiated fields
- comprehensive annual history and physical exam
- X rays of the affected or irradiated area (the frequency is determined by the type and degree of deficit)
- serial measurements of the survivor's standing and sitting height and weight
- observation of the survivor's gait, posture, muscle tone, size, and strength
- measurement of the circumference of the involved part or extremity and comparison with nonradiated areas
- bone-density evaluation
- an orthopedic consultation; prosthetist and physical-therapy referral as indicated.

## Medical Treatment

### Limb-Length Discrepancies

Treatment includes using a shoe lift, contralateral epiphysiodesis to arrest growth in the nonaffected limb, and contralateral limb shortening or ipsilateral lengthening procedures.

### Slipped Capitofemoral Epiphysis

This condition is a medical emergency that requires fixation.

### Pathological Fractures

This type of fracture can require internal fixation, immobilization, and bone grafting; if it recurs, it may require amputation.

### Scoliosis

Bracing is indicated in the growing patient who has curves greater than 20 degrees that are rapidly progressing or curves greater than 30 degrees. Curves greater than 45 degrees, although rarely seen with contemporary therapy, usually require fusion.

### Exostosis

Treatment depends on the site and the size and symptoms associated with the exostosis.

### Amputation

Treatment consists of monitoring the functional capability and condition of the stump and the functioning of the adaptive prosthesis.

### Osteopenia and Osteoporosis

Treatment normally is patient-specific and usually includes calcium supplementation, bisphosphonates, and treatment of exacerbating conditions (e.g., hormone replacement for hypogonadism). Scans to evaluate bone-mineral density should be done as clinically indicated.

### Avascular Necrosis and Osteonecrosis
Treatment is patient dependent, and orthopedic follow-up is indicated.

### Psychological and Psychosocial Concerns
Referrals should be made to appropriate healthcare providers and resources.

## Nursing Assessment and Interventions
### Assessment
- Review the patient's history for reports of pain, as well as for alterations in growth, functional status, and activities of daily living.
- Assess the survivor for alterations in self-esteem and body image.
- Ensure that a physical examination assesses for the following:
  – abnormalities in the skin or structures in the irradiated fields, with prompt evaluation of bony growths or suspicious skin lesions
  – gait changes, posture, and functional deficits
  – muscle growth, symmetry, tone, size, and strength
  – scoliosis
  – active and passive range of motion of all joints that were in the radiation field.
- Assess the fit and function of the prosthesis or orthotic device in collaboration with a prosthetist, orthopedist, and physical therapist.

### Interventions
- Reinforce the importance of lifelong, annual follow-up assessments with a healthcare provider who is familiar with the survivor's cancer history, treatment, and risk for developing musculoskeletal late effects.
- Ensure that proper diagnostic tests are done.
- Assist with strategies to help the survivor adapt to changes in body image (e.g., support groups, psychological counseling, or therapy) or changes in function (e.g., occupational therapy, physical therapy, modifications to automobiles and workspace).
- Educate the survivor and the family about precautions and potential late effects, including
  – preventive measures, such as calcium supplementation and overall good nutrition to reduce the risk for potential fracture
  – realistic expectations about growth and function
  – avoiding excessive weight gain
  – the impact of nutrition on growth
  – necessary restrictions on involvement in contact sports (if clinically indicated)
  – the risk for second malignant neoplasms.
- Stress the importance of having ongoing orthopedic, orthotic, and physical-therapy evaluations.

## Expected Patient Outcomes
- The survivor is knowledgeable about the risk for musculoskeletal late effects and second malignant neoplasms (especially if radiation was received).
- The survivor is functional in activities of daily living.
- The survivor has a positive self-concept and complies with follow-up visits.

# Hematopoietic System
*Jill E. Brace O'Neill*

## Definition
Compromised bone-marrow function, or myelosuppression, secondary to radiation therapy or chemotherapy is the primary hematopoietic late effect. To date, only limited research exists on the late-developing hematologic effects of cancer treatment. The hematopoietic symptoms of the long-term effects of radiation therapy and chemotherapy can include hypoplastic or aplastic bone-marrow aspirates or myelosuppression (including neutropenia and thrombocytopenia).

## Risk Factors
### Chemotherapy
The degree of marrow damage depends upon the age of the patient at the time of treatment (e.g., older patients who often experience delayed recovery of T-cell function are at higher risk). Increasing doses of alkylating agents and topoisomerase II inhibitors also can predispose a patient to develop therapy-related myelodysplasia.

### Radiation Therapy
The degree of marrow damage depends upon the radiation dosage and volume the patient received. The chronic-radiation injury particularly damages the bone-marrow stroma (or microvasculature), accounting for marrow dysfunction. When a small field with less than 10%–15% of the bone-marrow organ is irradiated beyond fractionated doses of 30 Gy or single doses of 20 Gy, permanent ablation or hypoplasia occurs. A 4,000-cGy dose of total nodal irradiation can impair bone-marrow reserve for up to 7 years after completion of therapy. Recovery from 4,000–5,000 cGy given over 4–6 weeks can take more than 2 years. Twenty-five percent of patients who have received 850–1,000 cGy (as a single-dose total body irradiation) have platelet counts below 100,000 for more than 4 months.

### Chemotherapy Used in Conjunction With Radiation Therapy
Chemotherapy used in conjunction with radiation therapy may have a synergistic effect and therefore may increase the overall risk of hematopoietic late effects (i.e., permanent damage to primitive stem cells or to the marrow microenvironment). Therefore, hematopoietic stem-cell transplantation places the survivor at the highest risk for hematopoietic disorders.

## Clinical Presentation
A survivor can present with hypoplastic or aplastic bone marrow and, less commonly, peripheral cytopenia.

## Diagnostic Workup
A diagnostic workup consists of
- a detailed history and physical examination
- laboratory studies including a CBC with differential
- bone-marrow aspirate as indicated.

## Medical Treatment

Treatment is based upon the survivor's presenting symptoms and clinical findings. Measures are supportive and rarely corrective and include administration of blood and blood products, administration of hematopoietic growth factors, or hematopoietic stem-cell transplantation.

## Nursing Assessment and Interventions

### Assessment

- Obtain a detailed medical history, paying particular attention to recurring infections, symptoms of anemia, or a tendency for bleeding.
- Examine the patient for symptoms of anemia or bleeding diathesis.
- Obtain annual complete blood counts with differential for 15 years after exposure to alkylating chemotherapy.
- Identify the factors and characteristics of the survivor that are associated with specific, adverse, hematologic sequelae (e.g., older age at time of treatment and escalating doses of alkylating agents).

### Interventions

- Reinforce the importance of lifelong, annual follow-up assessments with a healthcare provider who is familiar with the survivor's cancer history, treatment, and risk for developing late effects.
- Encourage ongoing surveillance to identify and treat late hematologic effects resulting from therapy.
- Educate the survivor about the need for regular medical evaluations and laboratory testing.

## Expected Patient Outcomes

- The survivor and the family understand any late-developing symptoms of the hematologic system related to cancer treatment.
- The survivor and the family understand the importance of maintaining long-term follow-up contact with a pediatric oncology center so that potential hematologic late effects of treatment can be evaluated and managed.

# Immune System

*Jill E. Brace O'Neill*

## Definition

Immune function may be compromised because of surgery, chemotherapy, or radiation therapy, or a combination of these cancer treatments.

## Risk Factors

### Radiation Therapy

Total body irradiation of 1,000 cGy can impair cell-mediated immunity; incomplete T-cell reconstitution has been reported up to 4 years after a bone-marrow transplantation. The effects of radiation involving smaller nodal or marrow fields on the immune system vary. The function of the spleen may be partially or completely compromised by radiation of the spleen with doses of 4,000 cGy or more.

### Surgery

Infection is the major risk after a splenectomy, particularly the risk of sudden and overwhelming infection from encapsulated organisms (i.e., pneumococci, *Haemophilus influenzae*, *Neisseria meningococcus*). One function of the spleen is to filter out substances, such as waste and infectious organisms. It also is responsible for early antibody response. Without the spleen, the immune response is decreased.

### Chemotherapy

The long-term effects of chemotherapeutic agents on the immune system have not been well documented.

## Clinical Presentation

A survivor may have frequent recurring infections and a decrease in immunoglobulin levels.

## Diagnostic Workup

A diagnostic workup consists of

- a detailed history and physical examination, with particular attention given to infections
- tests to determine immunoglobulin levels (i.e., IgG, IgM, IgA, and IgE levels)
- T-cell studies and T-4 and T-8 subsets studies
- consultation with an immunologist as necessary.

## Medical Treatment

Treatment depends upon the diagnosis. There should be a follow-up with an immunologist when warranted.

## Nursing Assessment and Interventions

### Assessment

- Obtain a detailed patient history and evaluate for any recurrent infections.
- Assess the results of the survivor's physical examination.

### Interventions

- Reinforce the importance of lifelong, annual follow-up assessments with a healthcare provider familiar with the survivor's cancer history, treatment, and risk for developing late effects.
- Educate the survivor and the family about potential immunological late effects and their presenting symptoms.
- Educate the survivor and the family about potential complications associated with having asplenia (caused by either radiation to the spleen or splenectomy).
  - Asplenic patients have a 10% or less risk of developing an overwhelming bacterial infection. *Streptococcus pneumoniae* is the most common pathogen that causes bacteremia in children with asplenia. Less common causes of bacteremia include Hib, *N meningitidis*, other streptococci, *Escherichia coli*, *Staphylococcus aureus*, and gram-negative bacilli, such as *Salmonella* species, *Klebsiella* species, and *Pseudomonas aeruginosa*. People with functional or anatomic asplenia also are at increased risk of fatal malaria and severe babesiosis.

- Thus, immunization with pneumococcal conjugate and/or polysaccharide vaccine and Hib vaccine according to age-specific guidelines are recommended. Emphasize the importance of having a pneumococcal vaccination, *Haemophilus b* conjugate vaccine, meningococcal vaccine (according to the American Academy of Pediatrics), and annual influenza vaccine.
- In general, antimicrobial prophylaxis (in addition to immunization) should be considered for all children with asplenia younger than 5 years of age and for at least 1 year after splenectomy.
- A daily prophylactic dose of penicillin (e.g., Pen-Vee-K) or erythromycin (i.e., erythromycin ethyl succinate) (for those with penicillin allergies) is strongly recommended. Young-adult survivors can be given a prescription for penicillin or erythromycin to keep at home in case they develop a fever of 101 °F or higher, but they also should be instructed to seek medical attention from a primary-care provider at the time the fever occurs.

## Expected Patient Outcomes
- The survivor and the family understand the importance of early intervention in the event of fever or other signs and symptoms of infection if he or she has had a splenectomy.
- The survivor and the family understand and can identify late-developing symptoms of the immunologic system related to cancer treatment.
- The survivor and the family understand the importance of and compliance with long-term follow-up care, including evaluation and management of potential late effects of treatment on the immune system, at a clinic that specializes in treating cancer survivors.

# Second Malignant Neoplasms

*Elizabeth H. Whittam*

## Definition
Second (and subsequent) malignant neoplasms can result either from exposure to previous cancer therapy or from genetic determinants that caused the initial childhood cancer. The cumulative risk of developing a second cancer 20 years after having a childhood cancer is estimated to be 3%–5%.

## Risk Factors

### Chemotherapeutic Agents
Exposure to chemotherapeutic agents (e.g., alkylating agents, epipodophyllotoxins) is a risk factor for the subsequent development of acute myelogenous leukemia; peak incidence occurs 4–6 years after initial therapy ceases.

### Therapeutic Radiation
Exposure to therapeutic radiation is associated with an increased incidence of a variety of second and subsequent cancers, including carcinomas (e.g., breast, thyroid, colorectal, gastric), sarcomas (e.g., soft tissue and bone), central-nervous-system tumors, and skin cancer (i.e., melanoma and nonmelanoma skin cancer). In general, the risk for radiation-related second cancers begins to increase 8–10 years after completion of the radiation therapy. Risk is associated with dose, type, and field of radiation.

### Genetic Mutations
Certain familial genetic mutations predispose family members to specific cancers, including Von Recklinghausen neurofibromatosis or Li-Fraumeni family cancer syndrome. In addition, genetic predispositions may further increase the risk for some radiation-related cancers.

## Surveillance for Second Cancers
Survivors should have an annual evaluation that consists of a history and physical examination, counseling about risk reduction, and discussion of second-cancer surveillance based on the treatment exposures, lifestyle behaviors, and family history. **Table 10-2** provides an overview of recommended screening tests for second-cancer surveillance. For more detail, refer to the Children's Oncology Group's *Long-term Follow-up Guidelines for Survivors of Childhood, Adolescent, and Young Adult Cancers* (available at www.survivorshipguidelines.org).

## Clinical Presentation

### Leukemia
The symptoms include fatigue, anemia, thrombocytopenia, granulocytopenia, bone pain, bleeding, fevers, and frequent infections.

### Solid Tumors
The symptoms include fatigue, anorexia, palpable mass, bloody stools or melena, anemia, or pain.

### Central Nervous System
The symptoms include seizures, headaches, altered mental states, visual changes, nausea, and vomiting.

## Diagnostic Workup and Medical Treatment
For a survivor presenting with the symptoms discussed above, the diagnostic workup consists of a history and physical exam, followed by testing as warranted by the findings. Medical treatment depends on the diagnosis of the second malignancy, previous treatment for the primary malignancy, and current available therapies.

## Nursing Assessment and Interventions

### Assessment
- Review the survivor's interval medical history for reports of recent weight loss, fatigue, malaise, pain, bleeding abnormalities, persistent fevers, recurrent infections, and hematochezia.
- Review the family's medical history for malignancies and hematological and genetic disorders.
- Perform a physical examination. The following components should be included, with particular attention given to therapeutic exposures listed parenthetically:
  - complete vital signs, with attention to weight changes
  - skin assessment for evidence of bleeding (epipodophyllotoxins, alkylating agents)
  - skin assessment for change in pigmentation, atypical skin lesions, or suspicious nevi (within radiation field)

### Table 10-2. Surveillance for Second (or Subsequent) Malignant Neoplasms Based on Treatment Exposures

| Treatment Exposure | Second/Subsequent Cancer | Screening Test |
|---|---|---|
| **Chemotherapy** | | |
| Epipodophyllotoxins | Acute myeloid leukemia | Complete blood count with differential |
| Alkylating agents | Myelodysplasia | Interval: yearly up to 10 years after exposure |
| Heavy metals | | |
| Nonclassical alkylators | | |
| Anthracyclines | | |
| Hematopoietic cell transplant | | |
| Cyclophosphamide | Bladder cancer | Urinalysis<br>Interval: yearly |
| **Radiation** | | |
| Cranial, head and neck, mantle, or total body irradiation | Thyroid cancer | Thyroid exam<br>Interval: yearly |
| Chest, mantle, mediastinal, lung irradiation ≥20 Gy | Breast cancer | Clinical breast exam<br>Interval: yearly beginning at puberty until age 25 and then every 6 months |
| | | Annual mammogram and adjunct breast magnetic resonance imaging<br>Interval: yearly beginning 8 years after radiation or at age 25, whichever occurs last |
| Whole abdomen, upper abdominal fields, pelvic, or spinal (thoracic, lumbar, sacral) ≥30 Gy | Colorectal cancer | Colonoscopy<br>Interval: every 5 years (minimum) beginning at age 35 |
| Whole abdomen or pelvic irradiation | Bladder cancer | Urinalysis<br>Interval: yearly |
| Any radiation | Melanoma and nonmelanoma skin cancer | Dermatologic exam of irradiated fields<br>Interval: yearly |

Adapted from *Long-Term Follow-Up Guidelines for Survivors of Childhood, Adolescent, and Young Adult Cancers*, by Children's Oncology Group, 2006, Arcadia, CA: Author.

- oropharyngeal examination for ulcerations or masses (head, neck, or mantle radiation)
- thyroid examination for enlargement or thyroid nodules (head, neck, or mantle radiation)
- breast examination, both females and males (chest or mantle radiation)
- palpation of the abdomen for hepatosplenomegaly
- evaluation of palpable lymph nodes
- palpation of soft tissue (within radiation field).

### Interventions
- Reinforce the importance of lifelong, annual follow-up assessments with a healthcare provider familiar with the survivor's cancer history, treatment, and risk for developing late effects.
- Educate the survivor and the family about the early warning signs of cancer.
- Educate the survivor about the benefits of having routine cancer screenings and the appropriate interval between such screenings.
- Ensure that appropriate diagnostic tests are ordered and that the patient receives the results as appropriate.
- Perform an assessment of the patient that ensures early identification of second malignant neoplasms.
- Educate the survivor about healthy lifestyle behaviors that can reduce his or her risk of second malignant neoplasms (e.g., dietary recommendations; avoiding tobacco products, tanning beds, and excessive alcohol consumption; using sunscreen).

### Expected Patient Outcomes
- The survivor and the family know the risk factors for developing second malignant neoplasms and can identify their signs and symptoms early enough to seek medical intervention if it is needed.
- The survivor returns for follow-up examinations, as recommended, and obtains yearly evaluations at a clinic for long-term cancer survivors.

# Psychosocial Effects: Personal-Emotional

*Branlyn E. Werba*

## Definition
Survivors of childhood cancer are resilient emotionally and typically grow up to lead productive lives. Still, living with a diagnosis and history of cancer can be associated with emotional challenges that vary through development and can persist long after treatment ends. Survivors and their family members often report that they feel changed by the experience of cancer, both for the better and the worse. They may feel different from others their age, experience uncertainty about the future, and feel vulnerable regarding the possibility of future health problems. They may continue to experience medical late effects from cancer treatment, which can be frustrating and limit their ability to achieve life goals. All of these challenges can affect long-term survivors' self-esteem, body image, and other aspects of their personal and emotional lives. Additionally, posttraumatic stress disorder (PTSD) has been identified recently as a significant problem in as many as 20% of the young-adult survivor population.

## Risk Factors

### Age
A cancer diagnosis can be traumatic for any child; however, the age of the child and his or her developmental level influence the cancer experience. As survivors become young adults, they may be at greater risk for experiencing distress due to increasing awareness of the ongoing impact of cancer.

### Family Support and Communication
The emotional adaptation by the family to cancer over time contributes to a child's overall adjustment. For example, if parents experience ongoing anxiety or posttraumatic stress related to their child's cancer experience, it can affect their parenting style. In addition, the family's ways of communicating about cancer and life issues in general influence how well a survivor communicates.

### Medical Problems
The number and severity of continuing medical problems, including beliefs about how medical problems will impact their life, can influence survivors' emotions and adjustment. For example, it is common for survivors to experience grief and loss if they learn that they are infertile as a result of their cancer treatment.

### Coping
The coping style of a survivor and a family affects their ability to adjust and assimilate the experience into their lives. Coping with their cancer histories and with the reactions of their peers and society in general are major challenges for survivors of childhood cancer.

### Education
Successfully reintegrating into school after cancer, identifying new abilities or learning challenges, and addressing social issues are important components for academic success. Anxiety and embarrassment about educational abilities, physical limitations, or differences can contribute to school avoidance or poor academic performance.

### Preexisting Emotional Problems or Life Stressors
A survivor is more likely to experience emotional distress related to cancer if he or she has preexisting mental-health difficulties, a history of other traumatic events, or other stressful life circumstances.

## Clinical Presentation
When a survivor experiences emotional distress, he or she can have one or more of the following complaints: sleep disturbances, flat or depressed affect, mood swings, feelings of helplessness or hopelessness, inability to concentrate, weight loss, change in appetite, anxiety related to returning to the clinic or school, fear of recurrence of the disease, poor self-esteem or body image, and school- or work-related problems. Specific symptoms associated with PTSD include reexperiencing the cancer event (through nightmares or flashbacks), feeling psychologically numb, displaying avoidance behaviors (such as not wanting to return to the clinic or address health issues), and experiencing a heightened sense of arousal (such as panic when a new health symptom arises or when there is a subtle reminder of the cancer experience).

## Nursing Assessment and Interventions

### Assessment
- Assess for adequate sleep, weight, and nutrition.
  - Inquire about sleep patterns and note any changes.
  - Plot height and weight on a growth chart.
  - Obtain a dietary history and note any changes in appetite.
- Assess general mood and note any wide variations in affect.
- Inquire about anxiety related to returning to the clinic, a previous diagnosis, or other concerns.
- Assess social adjustment, including the following:
  - involvement in age-appropriate activities at school or work
  - ability to relate to peers and develop friendships outside the family
- Consider the survivor's comfort level with his or her physical appearance (i.e., body image) after treatment.
- Assess for pain symptoms and consider the impact of pain on mood.
- Assess school or work performance, including progress and attendance patterns or rehabilitation needs.
- Consider the parent's expectations of the survivor's physical and cognitive abilities and whether they are consistent with the survivor's actual functional abilities.
- Assess the family's readiness for making the transition to adulthood:
  - Have the parents been able to encourage the survivor's independence?
  - Is the survivor being given increasingly greater amounts of age-appropriate information about his or her medical needs and care?
  - Do the survivors or parents have any misconceptions about their child's health that could limit the survivor's confidence about leaving home or attending college?

### Interventions
- Provide anticipatory guidance about cancer and its impact, including information about the disease process, treatment, and potential late effects.
- Educate the survivor about lifestyle behaviors that promote good health and adjustment.
- Educate the survivor about available resources that can provide information and support regarding survivorship issues (e.g., the Candlelighters Childhood Cancer Foundation, the American Cancer Society, the National Coalition for Cancer Survivorship, the Leukemia Society, the Lance Armstrong Foundation, and the National Cancer Institute).
- Provide information about counseling services and local support groups
- Provide referrals to a psychologist or a psychiatrist if issues interfere with medical care or impair other aspects of daily functioning (e.g., work, school, relationships).

### Expected Patient Outcomes
- The survivor is able to identify emotional issues related to survivorship.
- The survivor verbalizes an understanding of available community and counseling resources.

## Psychosocial Effects: Political-Social

*Branlyn E. Werba and Wendy L. Hobbie*

### Definition
Even in the 21st century, a history of cancer may lead to discrimination in several aspects of the survivor's life. Discrimination most often occurs in the form of education-related issues, difficulty in obtaining health and life insurance, and employment problems, any of which may require legal action for resolution. Survivors can advocate for their rights by being aware of laws that protect against discrimination and resources for navigating these complex systems.

### Risk Factors

#### Employment Problems
The employment problems of cancer survivors can take many forms. Childhood-cancer survivors experience discrimination that is based primarily on the survivor's history of cancer. Employers may have misconceptions about cancer, its prognosis, or its impact on job performance. These misconceptions may lead to survivors having difficulties getting a job, securing full-time employment with benefits, being denied promotions, being denied insurance or other benefits, receiving lower salaries, being rejected for military service, and experiencing job lock.

#### Insurance Problems
Attempting to secure adequate insurance (health, life, or disability) can create frustration. Policy cancellations, increased premiums, preexisting-condition clauses, extended waiting periods, and denial of benefits exemplify types of discrimination.

#### Education-Related Issues
(See the subsection "Psychosocial Effects: Educational Issues.")

#### Legal Issues
Legal issues relate to employment and education-related discrimination (see the discussions of these topics later in this subsection).

### Clinical Presentation
Survivors may report having experienced discrimination at school or at work. They also may have insurance or legal problems related to denial of insurance coverage, high premiums, or denial of supplemental security income. Such problems may increase when survivors become young adults and must obtain insurance and income independently from their parents.

### Nursing Assessment and Interventions

#### Assessment
- Assess the survivor's educational abilities, progress, and goals.
- Assess the survivor's employment status.
- Assess the survivor's insurance status.
- Assess the survivor's understanding of his or her legal rights.

#### Interventions
**Employment:**
- Provide the survivor with information about federal and state laws that protect him or her from discrimination:
  - The Americans with Disabilities Act (ADA) of 1990 prohibits discrimination in employment on the basis of a disability and provides for equal access to public facilities. The ADA protects survivors from inquiries by potential employers about their disability or medical history before a job offer is made. This law applies to companies with 15 or more employees and is enforced by the U.S. Equal Employment Opportunity Commission. Anyone who has specific questions regarding the ADA can contact the agency at 800/669-6820 or 202/663-4900, or visit the agency's Web site at www.eeoc.gov.
  - The Family and Medical Leave Act of 1993 mandates job security for workers in companies with 50 or more employees who must take a leave of absence of up to 12 weeks to care for a seriously ill child, spouse, parent, or themselves. The law requires an employer to continue to provide benefits, including health insurance, during the leave period.
  - The Employee Retirement and Income Security Act is a federal law that protects workers from being fired because of their cancer history.
  - Military-service applications are considered on a case-by-case basis. The U.S. Department of Defense, under Directive No. 6130 (March 31, 1986), provides a means for cancer survivors to be considered for military service. Survivors who have not required any cancer-related surgical or medical treatment for 5 years and who are considered free of cancer can be granted a medical waiver and be considered fit for military service. However, a survivor must meet the physical requirements of the position for which he or she has applied. Military

# Section X Late Effects of Childhood Cancer

recruiters may be unfamiliar with the directive, and survivors are encouraged to read the directive and self-advocate.
- Educate the survivor about ways to avoid discrimination. The survivor should
  - apply for positions for which he or she is qualified
  - avoid volunteering information regarding cancer history unless it might directly affect the ability to perform a job or participate in an educational program
  - be truthful about his or her medical history on either a job or an insurance application
  - answer questions truthfully when asked about cancer history and be prepared to explain current health status and prognosis
  - provide a letter from the treating healthcare facility that addresses his or her current health status, prognosis, and ability to work
  - avoid asking about health-insurance benefits during the interview process. After a job offer has been made, review the benefits package before accepting the position
  - seek employment in larger companies (those with more than 300 employees), because smaller companies may be exempt from meeting certain provisions of the aforementioned laws
  - consider assistance from a job or school counselor.

**Education-related issues:** (See the subsection "Psychosocial Effects: Educational Issues" for more information.)

**Self-Advocacy and Education:**
- Educate survivors about the importance of self-advocacy.
- Provide resource information on organizations that can assist with advocacy efforts.
  - Candlelighters Childhood Cancer Foundation is a nonprofit organization that provides information about the legal rights of cancer survivors. This organization provides assistance in resolving problems with health-insurance claims, employment discrimination, waivers into military service, and access to equal education. The organization can be contacted at 800/366-2223, or visit its Web site at www.candlelighters.org.
  - The National Coalition for Cancer Survivorship is a nonprofit organization that provides information about legal rights and advocacy services. It publishes two free brochures that are available online ("Working it Out: Your Employment Rights As A Cancer Survivor" and "What Cancer Survivors Need to Know About Health Insurance"). The organization can be reached at 877/622-7937, or visit the Web site at www.canceradvocacy.org.
  - The American Cancer Society is a nonprofit organization that provides information and publications on cancer and insurance issues. This organization can be contacted at 800/ACS-2345, or visit its Web site at www.cancer.org.
  - The Job Accommodation Network is a free consulting service designed to increase the employability of people with disabilities. Additional information is available at 800/526-7234 or http://janweb.icdi.wvu.edu.

**Legal Counsel:**
- Provide survivors with information about cancer organizations that can help them obtain appropriate legal counsel. Such organizations include Candlelighters Childhood Cancer Foundation (800/366-2223), the National Coalition for Cancer Survivorship (301/650-9127), some units of the American Cancer Society, and the Cancer Legal Resource Center (866/843-2572).

**Health Insurance:**
- Provide survivors with information about their rights and resources in obtaining health insurance.
  - Most states sponsor a comprehensive health insurance plan, also called a "high-risk pool." This plan helps people obtain health insurance regardless of their physical condition or medical history. To obtain information about services available in a specific state, survivors can contact their state's office of the insurance commissioner, or find the information online using Georgetown University Health Policy Institute's "Consumer Guide for Getting and Keeping Health Insurance" (www.healthinsuranceinfo.net).
  - Some insurance companies and employers offer an open-enrollment period each year, during which time coverage usually can be obtained regardless of a person's medical history. Survivors should be directed to contact the office of the insurance commissioner of their state.
  - The Comprehensive Omnibus Budget Reconciliation Act requires employers to offer group medical coverage to employees and their dependents who otherwise would lose their group coverage due to individual circumstances.
  - The Health Insurance Portability and Accountability Act of 1996 allows individuals to change jobs without losing coverage if they have been insured for at least 12 months.
  - The Medical Information Bureau is a health data bank that provides information for insurance companies. Survivors can contact this organization to find out the information that healthcare plans use for their eligibility criteria.
- Encourage the survivor and the family to be persistent in pursuing coverage.
- Encourage the survivor to consider political advocacy to promote changes in health-insurance laws.

## Expected Patient Outcomes
- The survivor understands that resources are available.
- The survivor is knowledgeable about the issues that have been discussed and about recommended interventions.

# Psychosocial Effects: Educational Issues

*Branlyn E. Werba*

## Definition
School attendance, academic performance, and career achievement may be challenged by a diagnosis and treatment of childhood cancer. Survivors can be further challenged by possible late effects of treatment, including neurocognitive deficits, hearing and visual impairments, physical limitations, and missed educational opportunities (see the subsection "School Reentry and Attendance" in Section VII, "Psychosocial Issues").

## Risk Factors

### High Rate of Absenteeism

Absenteeism often occurs during cancer treatment but may continue into survivorship because of frequent medical appointments, hospitalizations, or the severity of the child's ongoing medical problems. Families may keep children away from school due to concerns about health risks of attendance, potential for stress on the child, or the child's own school avoidance. Such absenteeism can have a long-term negative impact on educational achievement and the development of age-appropriate social skills and friendships.

### Type of Diagnosis and Treatment

Survivors of acute lymphoblastic leukemia and brain tumors are at greatest risk for developing learning problems associated with cancer treatment. Survivors of acute myelogenous leukemia, Non-Hodgkin's lymphoma, or those who were treated with radiation of the head and neck are also at higher risk. Other aspects of treatment associated with learning problems include stem-cell transplantation and treatment at a younger age (particularly younger than age 3). In addition to radiation, intrathecal chemotherapy and high-dose methotrexate are associated with learning difficulties.

## Clinical Presentation

A survivor can present with a variety of learning problems that impact school performance, such as impairments in attention and concentration, overactivity, slower processing speed, and impaired memory and organizational skills (neurocognitive problems). These problems are often subtle but can increase as a child becomes older. Other circumstances may add to educational difficulties, including numerous school absences, inadequate classroom placements, or inappropriate parent and teacher expectations. Finally, the child may have medical problems and physical impairments that impede full participation in school.

## Nursing Assessment and Interventions

### Assessment

- Assess the survivor's school attendance record and academic performance.
- Assess for risk factors for learning problems and indications for neuropsychological testing.
- Assess for additional physical problems that may impact learning, including visual, hearing, or motor impairments.
- Consider ways in which the family, medical team, and the school communicate about learning needs.
- Assess the parents' expectations about the survivor's abilities and progress in school.

### Interventions

- Provide necessary information to the school about the child's cancer history (see the subsection "School Reentry and Attendance" in Section VII, "Psychosocial Issues").
- Educate parents about the importance of maintaining normalcy in their child's life and the benefits of school attendance.
- Reinforce recommendations for curriculum modifications and accommodations when they are indicated.
- Refer the survivor for neuropsychological testing if risk factors are present; this testing provides a detailed assessment of the child's cognitive strengths and weaknesses. Follow-up testing may be helpful to monitor changes over time.
- Inform the survivor and his or her parents about organizations that provide school resources and advocacy information:
  - Candlelighters Childhood Cancer Foundation (800/366-2223; www.candlelighters.org) publishes the book *Educating the Child with Cancer: A Guide for Parents and Teachers.*
  - National Children's Cancer Society (301/650-9127; www.beyondthecure.org)
- Educate the survivor and his or her family about the three federal laws that ensure equal access to education:
  1. The Individuals with Disabilities Education Act of 1990 requires states to provide free and appropriate education to all children ages 3–21 years.
  2. The Americans with Disabilities Act prohibits discrimination against people with an actual disability, perceived disability, and history of a disability. This law is enforced by the U.S. Equal Employment Opportunity Commission (800/669-6820; 202/663-4900).
  3. Section 504 of the Rehabilitation Act of 1973 prohibits schools that receive federal funding from discriminating against qualified students because of their cancer history.

## Expected Patient Outcomes

- The survivor is knowledgeable about late effects of cancer treatment that can negatively impact educational achievement.
- The survivor and the family demonstrate their understanding of available resources, including written materials, community organizations, and academic-testing opportunities.

# Promoting Health After Childhood Cancer

*Roseann Tucci*

Health promotion and health maintenance are the foundations of cancer-survivorship care. As the focus of follow-up care shifts from the primary cancer diagnosis to the potential late effects of therapy, healthcare providers must emphasize the importance of modifiable risk factors. Through education about potential risks and necessary follow-up care, the survivor can recognize modifiable risk factors and the role they can play in his or her future health and quality of life. What follows are several recommendations that were compiled from COG's survivorship guidelines (2006).

- Educate the survivor about his or her cancer diagnosis, treatment, and potential risks for health problems related to past treatment, and provide him or her with a written, individualized summary of the diagnosis and treatment.
- Encourage the survivor to take responsibility by making sure he or she has annual, lifelong follow-up assessments, ideally at a survivorship clinic or from a knowledgeable and attentive healthcare provider who is familiar with his or her cancer history, treatment, and potential health risks related to treatment.

- Educate a female survivor on the importance of having the following routine screenings for cancer:
  - breast self-examinations every month for those who have begun to have menstrual cycles
  - mammography every year beginning at age 40. For female patients who have received irradiation to the chest area, annual mammography and breast magnetic resonance imaging (an ACS recommendation from 2007) should begin 8 years after irradiation or at age 25, whichever occurs later. Those who have a family history of breast cancer ideally should be seen by a geneticist to determine an imaging schedule.
  - a pelvic examination with a Pap smear every year beginning at age 18 or earlier if the patient is sexually active.
- Educate all survivors on the importance of
  - checking serum lipid panel beginning at age 25 and then on a yearly basis
  - a rectal examination starting at age 45 and then on a yearly basis
  - stool testing for occult blood starting at age 50 (ACS recommendation)
  - sigmoidoscopy starting at age 50 (ACS recommendation).
- Educate the survivor on the importance of engaging in the following healthy lifestyle behaviors:
  - using sunscreen with a sun-protection factor of 30 or more and avoiding tanning beds
  - maintaining a well-balanced diet that is low in fat and high in fiber (e.g., fruits, vegetables, whole grains), eating foods rich in vitamin C (e.g., dark-green, leafy vegetables, citrus fruits, orange or yellow vegetables), and avoiding excessive intake of salt
  - ensuring adequate daily calcium intake
  - maintaining an ideal body weight
  - engaging in moderate-to-vigorous activity for 30 minutes 5 times a week
  - avoiding all tobacco products
  - limiting the amount of alcoholic beverages
  - avoiding the use of controlled substances and street drugs
  - practicing safe sex
  - allowing adequate time for rest
  - avoiding prolonged stress.

## Reference

Children's Oncology Group. (2006). *Long-term follow-up guidelines for survivors of childhood, adolescent, and young adult cancers (Version 2.0)*. Retrieved May 26, 2008, from www.survivorshipguidelines.org/pdf/LTFUGuidelines.pdf.

---

### Survivorship Web Resources

**www.acor.org**
The Association of Cancer Online Resources (ACOR) provides a comprehensive list of follow-up survivorship clinics in the United States, in addition to other resources, on its site.

**www.beyondthecure.org**
The mission of Beyond the Cure is to help childhood cancer survivors integrate the cancer experience into their new lives as survivors and successfully handle the challenges that are ahead of them, as well as to celebrate survivorship.

**www.cancer.umn.edu/ltfu**
The Childhood Cancer Survivor Study (CCSS) is a component of St. Jude Children's Research Hospital's Long-Term Follow-Up Study. A collaborative, multi-institutional study funded by the National Cancer Institute, CCSS is composed of individuals who survived 5 or more years after treatment for cancer, leukemia, a tumor, or a similar illness diagnosed during childhood or adolescence. CCSS, which includes all participants in the Long-Term Follow-Up Study with a confirmed diagnosis of cancer, is a retrospectively established cohort of 20,346 childhood cancer survivors diagnosed between 1970 and 1986. It also includes approximately 4,000 siblings of survivors who serve as the comparison group for the study.

**www.childrenscause.org**
The Children's Cause for Cancer Advocacy (CCCA) is an organization that works as a national catalyst to stimulate drug discovery and development for childhood cancers, expand resources for research and treatment, and address the needs and concerns of survivors.

**www.fertilehope.org**
Fertile Hope is a national, nonprofit organization dedicated to providing reproductive information, support, and hope to cancer patients whose medical treatments present the risk of infertility.

**www.livestrong.com**
The Lance Armstrong Foundation/LIVESTRONG™ Web site covers a wide range of topics of interest to cancer survivors, from practical advice to survivorship stories.

**www.planetcancer.org**
The Planet Cancer Web site provides a unique voice for young adults who have been affected by cancer. The Web site offers information, connections, entertainment, and support. The heart of Planet Cancer's Web site is its forum, a thriving online community where users find and communicate with other young adults with cancer from around the world.

**www.survivorshipguidelines.org**
The *Long Term Follow-Up Guidelines for Survivors of Childhood, Adolescent, and Young Adult Cancers* provides recommendations for screening and management of late effects that may potentially arise as a result of therapeutic exposures used during oncology treatment. These guidelines represent a statement of consensus from a panel of experts in the late effects of pediatric cancer treatment.

**www.theSAMFund.org**
The broad mission of Surviving And Moving Forward: The SAMFund for Young Adult Survivors of Cancer is to assist U.S. cancer survivors who are between the ages of 17 and 35 with their transition into a successful posttreatment life. The foundation will distribute grants and scholarships to enable survivors to pursue their educational or professional goals and offer outreach and information about the postrecovery transition to young adults approaching the end of treatment.

# Bibliography

## Definition and Overview

American Cancer Society. (2006). *Cancer facts & figures 2006* (No. 5008.01, pp. 11–12). New York: American Cancer Society (National Media Office).

Bottomley, S. J., & Kassner, E. (2003). Late effects of childhood cancer therapy. *Journal of Pediatric Nursing, 18,* 126–132.

Ganz, P. A. (2001). Late effects of cancer and its treatment. *Seminars in Oncology Nursing, 17*(4), 241–248.

Hobbie, W., Ruccione, K., Harvey, J., & Moore, I. M. (2007). Care of survivors. In C. R. Baggott, K. P. Kelly, D. Fochtman, & G. V. Foley (Eds.), *Nursing care of children and adolescents with cancer* (3rd ed., pp. 426–464). Glenview, IL: Association of Pediatric Hematology/Oncology Nurses.

Keene, N., Hobbie, W., & Ruccione, K. (2006). *Childhood cancer survivors: A practice guide to your future.* (2nd ed.). Sebastopol, CA: O'Reilly.

Parisi, M. T., Fahmy, J. L., Kaminsky, C. K., & Malogolowkin, M. H. (1999). Complications of cancer therapy in children: A radiologist's guide. *Radiographics, 9,* 283–297.

Ries, L. A. G., Smith, M. A., Gurney, J. G., Linet, M., Tamra, T., Young, J. L., et al. (Eds.). (1999). *Cancer incidence and survival among children and adolescents: United States SEER Program 1975–1995* (NIH Publication No. 99-4649). Bethesda, MD: National Cancer Institute.

Schwartz, C. L., Hobbie, W. L., Constine, L. S., & Ruccione, K. S. (2005). *Survivors of childhood and adolescent cancer: A multidisciplinary approach.* Berlin, Germany: Springer-Verlag.

## Central Nervous System

Butler, R. W., & Mulhern, R. K. (2005). Neurocognitive interventions for children and adolescents surviving cancer. *Journal of Pediatric Psychology, 30*(1), 65–78.

Challinor, J., Miaskowski, C., Moore, I., Slaughter, R., & Franck, L. (2000). Review of research studies that evaluated the impact of treatment for childhood cancers on neurocognition and behavioral and social competence: Nursing implications. *Journal of the Society of Pediatric Nursing, 5,* 57–74.

Moleski, M. (2000). Neuropsychological, neuroanatomical, and neurophysiological consequences of CNS chemotherapy for acute lymphoblastic leukemia. *Archives of Clinical Neuropsychology, 15,* 603–630.

Nathan, P. C., Patel, S. K., Dilley, K., Goldsby, R., Harvey, J., Jacobsen, C., et al. (2007). Guidelines for identification of, advocacy for, and intervention in neurocognitive problems in survivors of childhood cancer. *Archives of Pediatric Adolescent Medicine, 161*(8), 798–806.

## Hypothalamic-Pituitary Axis

Cohen, L. E. (2003). Endocrine late effects of cancer treatment. *Current Opinion in Pediatrics, 15,* 3–9.

Leung, W., Rose, S. R., & Merchant T. E. (2005). Neuroendocrine complications of cancer therapy. In C. L. Schwartz, W. L. Hobbie, L. C. Constine, & K. S. Ruccione (Eds.), *Survivors of childhood and adolescent cancer: A multidisciplinary approach* (2nd ed., pp. 161–180). Heidelberg, Germany: Springer-Verlag.

## Thyroid Function

Cohen, L. E. (2002). Endocrine late effects of cancer treatment. *Current Opinions in Pediatrics, 15,* 3–9.

Sklar, C., Boulad, F., Small, T., & Kernan, N. (2001). Endocrine complications of pediatric stem-cell transplantation. *Frontiers in Bioscience 6,* 17–22.

## Vision and Hearing

Bertolini, P., Lassalle, M., Mercier, G., Raquin, M. A., Izzi, G., Corradini, N., et al. (2004). Platinum compound related ototoxicity in children: Long term follow-up reveals continuous worsening of hearing loss. *Journal of Pediatric Hematology Oncology, 26*(10), 649–655.

Gurney, J. G., Ness, K. K., Rosenthal, J., Forman, S. J., Bhatia, S., & Baker, K. S. (2006). Visual, auditory, sensory, and motor impairments in long-term survivors of hematopoietic stem cell transplantation performed in childhood: Results from the Bone Marrow Transplant Survivor Study. *Cancer, 106,* 1402–1408.

Holstrom, G., Borgstrom, B., & Callissendorff, B. (2002). Cataract in children after bone marrow transplantation: Relation to conditioning regime. *Acta Ophthalmologica Scandinavica, 80,* 211–215.

Landier, W., & Merchant, T. (2005). Adverse effects of cancer treatment on hearing. In C. L. Schwartz, W. L. Hobbie, L. S. Constine, & K. S. Ruccione (Eds.), *Survivors of childhood and adolescent cancer: A multidisciplinary approach* (2nd ed., pp. 109–123). Heidelberg, Germany: Springer-Verlag.

Oberlin, O., Rey, A., Anderson, J., Carli, M., Raney, R. B., Treuner, J., et al. (2001). Treatment of orbital rhabdomyosarcoma: Survival and late effects of treatment. Results of an international workshop. *Journal of Clinical Oncology, 19,* 197–204.

Packer, R. J., Gurney, J. G., Punyko, J. A., Donaldson, S. S., Inskip, P. D., Stovall, M., et al. (2003). Long-term neurologic and neurosensory sequelae in adult survivors of a childhood brain tumor: Childhood cancer survivor study. *Journal of Clinical Oncology, 21,* 3255–3261.

Paulino, A. C., Simon, J. H., Zhen, W., & Wen, B. (2000). Long-term effects in children treated with radiotherapy for head and neck rhabdomyosarcoma. *International Journal of Radiation, Oncology, Biology, Physics, 48,* 1489–1495.

## Head and Neck

Bowers, D. C., Liu, Y., Leisenring, W., McNeil, E., Stoval, M., Gurney, J. G., et al. (2006). Late occurring stroke among long-term survivors of childhood leukemia and brain tumor survivors: A report from the childhood cancer survivor study. *Journal of Clinical Oncology, 33,* 5277–5282.

Bowers, D. C., McNeil, E., Liu, Y. ,Yasui, Y., Stoval, M., Gurney, J. G., et al. (2005). Stroke as a late treatment effect of Hodgkin's Disease: A report from the Childhood Cancer Survivor Study. *Journal of Clinical Oncology, 23,* 6508–6515.

Children's Oncology Group Late Effects Committee and Nursing Discipline. (2006, March). *Long-term follow-up guidelines for survivors of childhood, adolescent and young adult cancers.* (Version 2.0). Retrieved May 26, 2008, from www.survivorshipguidelines.org.

Dahllof, G., Jonsson, A., Ulmner, M., & Huggare, J. (2001). Orthodontic treatment in long-term survivors after pediatric bone marrow transplantation. *American Journal of Orthodontic Dentofacial Orthopedics, 120,* 459–465.

Duggal, M. S. (2003). Root surface areas in long-term survivors of childhood cancer. *Oral Oncology, 39,* 178–183.

Estilo, C. L., Huryn, J. M., Kraus, D. H., Sklar, C., Wexler, L. H., Wolden, S. L., et al. (2003). Effects of therapy on dentofacial development in long-term survivors of head and neck rhabdomyosarcoma: The Memorial Sloan-Kettering Cancer Center experience. *Journal of Pediatric Hematology/Oncology, 25*(3), 215–222.

Handschel, J., Sunderkotter, C., Kruse-Losler, B., & Prott, F. J. (2001). Late effects of radiotherapy on oral mucosa in humans. *European Journal of Oral Science, 109,* 95–102.

Holtta, P., Alaluusua, S., Saarinen-Pihkala, U. M., Wolf, J., Nystrom, M., & Hovi, L. (2002). Post-transplant complications. Long-term adverse effects on dentition in children with poor-risk neuroblastoma treated with high-dose chemotherapy and autologous stem cell transplantation with or without total body irradiation. *Bone Marrow Transplantation, 29,* 121–127.

Hull, M. C., Morris, C. G., Pepine, C. J., & Mendenhall, N. P. (2003). Valvular dysfunction and carotid, subclavian, and coronary artery disease in survivors of Hodgkin's lymphoma treated with radiation therapy. *Journal of the American Medical Association, 290,* 2831–2837.

Karsila-Tenovuo, S., Jahnukainene, K., Peltomaki, T., Minn, H., & Kulmala, J. (2001). Disturbances in craniofacial morphology in children treated for solid tumors. *Oral Oncology, 37,* 586–592.

Meeske, K. A., Nelson, M. D., Lavey, R. S., Gee, S., Nelson, M. B., Bernstein, L., et al. (2007). Premature carotid artery disease in long-term survivors of childhood cancer treated with neck irradiation: A series of 5 cases. *Journal of Pediatric Hematology/Oncology, 29*(7), 480–484.

Minicucci, E. M., Lopes, L. F., & Crocci, A. J. (2003). Dental abnormalities in children after chemotherapy treatment for acute lymphoid leukemia. *Leukemia Research, 27,* 45–50.

Oguz, A., Cetiner, S., Karadeniz, C., Alpaslan, G., Alpaslan, C., & Pinarli, G. (2004). Long-term effects of chemotherapy on orodental structures in children with non-Hodgkin's lymphoma. *European Journal of Oral Sciences, 112,* 8–11.

Paulino, A. C., Koshy, M., & Howell, D. (2005). Head and neck. In C. L. Schwartz, W. L. Hobbie, L. C. Constine, & K. S. Ruccione (Eds.), *Survivors of childhood and adolescent cancer: A multidisciplinary approach* (2nd ed., pp. 95–107). Heidelberg, Germany: Springer-Verlag.

Paulino, A. C., Simon, J. H., Zhen, W., & Wen, B. C. (2000). Long-term effects in children treated with radiotherapy for head and neck rhabdomyosarcoma. *International Journal of Radiation, Oncology, Biology, Physics, 48,* 1489–1495.

Sims, S. A., Barker, G. J., & Gilman, A. (2002). Oral complications associated with the treatment of pediatric neuroblastoma case study. *Journal of Clinical Dentistry, 26,* 401–404.

## Cardiovascular System

Adams, M. J., & Lipshultz, S. E. (2005). Review pathophysiology of anthracycline- and radiation-associated cardiomyopathies: Implications for screening and prevention. *Pediatric Blood Cancer, 44,* 600–606.

Bossi, G., Lanzarini, L., Laudisa, M. L., Klersy, C., Raisaro, A., & Arico, M. (2001). Echocardiographic evaluation of patients cured of childhood cancer: A single center study of 117 subjects who received anthracyclines. *Medical and Pediatric Oncology, 36,* 593–600.

Gupta, M., Steinherz, P. G., Cheung, N. K., & Steinherz, L. (2003). Late cardiotoxicity after bolus versus infusion anthracycline therapy for childhood cancers. *Medical Pediatric Oncology, 40,* 343–347.

Heidenreich, P. A., Schnittger, I., Strauss, H. W., Vagelos, R. H., Lee, B. K., Mariscal, C. S., et al. (2007). Screening for coronary artery disease after mediastinal irradiation for Hodgkin's disease. *Journal of Clinical Oncology, 25,* 43–49.

Hudson, M. M., Rai, S. N., Nunez, C., Merchant, T. E., Marina, N. M., Zalamea, N., et al. (2007). Noninvasive evaluation of late anthracycline cardiac toxicity in childhood cancer survivors. *Journal of Clinical Oncology, 25,* 3635–3642.

Kremer, L. C., van Dalen, E. C., Offringa, M., Ottenkamp, J., & Voute, P. A. (2001). Anthracycline-induced clinical heart failure in a cohort of 607 children: Long-term follow-up study. *Journal of Clinical Oncology, 19,* 191–196.

Postma, A., Elzenga, N. J., Haaksma, J., Schasfoort-Van Leeuwen, M. J. M., Kamps, W. A., & Bink-Boelkens, M. T. E. (2002). Cardiac status in bone tumor survivors up to nearly 19 years after treatment with doxorubicin: A longitudinal study. *Medical Pediatric Oncology, 39,* 86–92.

## Respiratory System

Abid, S. H., Malhotra, V., & Perry, M. C. (2001). Radiation-induced and chemotherapy-induced pulmonary injury. *Current Opinion in Oncology, 13,* 242–248.

Children's Oncology Group Late Effects Committee and Nursing Discipline. (2006, March). *Long-term follow-up guidelines for survivors of childhood, adolescent and young adult cancers* (Version 2.0). Retrieved May 26, 2008, from www.survivorshipguidelines.org.

Hinkle, A. S., Proukou, C., & Chen, Y. (2005). Pulmonary effects of antineoplastic therapy. In C. L. Schwartz, W. L. Hobbie, L. C. Constine, & K. S. Ruccione (Eds.), *Survivors of childhood and adolescent cancer: A multidisciplinary approach* (2nd ed., pp. 161–180). Heidelberg, Germany: Springer-Verlag.

Mertens, A. C., Yasui, Y., Liu, Y., Stoval, M., Hutchinson, R., Ginsberg, J., et al. (2002). Pulmonary complications in survivors of childhood and adolescent cancer: A report from the Childhood Cancer Survivor Study. *Cancer, 95,* 2431–2441.

## Gastrointestinal and Hepatic Systems

Andreyev, H. J. (2007). Gastrointestinal problems after pelvic radiotherapy: The past, the present and the future. *Clinical Oncology, 19*(10), 790–799.

Bhatia, S. Yasui, Y., Robison, L. L., Birch, J. M., Bogue, M. K., Diller, L., et al. (2003). High risk of subsequent neoplasms continues with extended follow-up of childhood Hodgkin's disease: Report from the Late Effects Study Group. *Journal of Clinical Oncology, 21,* 4386–4394.

Bismar, M. M., & Sinicrope, F. A. (2002). Radiation enteritis. *Current Gastroenterology Report, 4,* 361–365.

Castellino, S., Lensing, S., Riely, C. A., Rai, S. N., Davila, R., Hayden, R. T., et al. (2004). The epidemiology of chronic hepatitis C infection in survivors of childhood cancer: An update of the St. Jude Children's Research Hospital Hepatitis C Seropositive Cohort. *Blood, 103,* 2460–2466.

Children's Oncology Group Late Effects Committee and Nursing Discipline. (2006, March). *Long-term follow-up guidelines for survivors of childhood, adolescent and young adult cancers* (Version 2.0). Retrieved May 26, 2008, from www.survivorshipguidelines.org.

De Bruyne, R., Portmann, B., Samyn, M., Bansal, S., Knisely, A., Mieli-Vergani, G., et al. (2006). Chronic liver disease related to 6-thioguanine in children with acute lymphoblastic leukaemia. *Journal of Hepatology, 44,* 407–410.

Halonen, P., Mattila, J., Ruuska, T., Salo, M. K., & Makipernaa, A. (2003). Liver histology after current intensified therapy for childhood acute lymphoblastic leukemia: Microvesicular fatty change and siderosis are the main findings. *Medical Pediatric Oncology, 40,* 148–154.

Hudson, M. M. (2005). Late gastrointestinal and hepatic effects. In C. L. Schwartz, W. L. Hobbie, L. C. Constine, & K. S. Ruccione (Eds.), *Survivors of childhood and adolescent cancer: A multidisciplinary approach* (2nd ed., pp. 161–180). Heidelberg, Germany: Springer-Verlag.

Lal, D. R., Foroutan, H. R., Su, W. T., Wolden, S. L., Boulad, F., & La Quaglia, M. P. (2006). The management of treatment related esophageal complications in children and adolescents with cancer. *Journal of Pediatric Surgery, 41,* 495–499.

Nguyen, N. P., Antoine, J. E., Dutta, S., Karlsson, U., & Sallah, S. (2002). Current concepts in radiation enteritis and implications for future clinical trials. *Cancer, 95,* 1151–1163.

Piel, B., Vaidya, S., Lancaster, D., Taj, M., & Pritchard-Jones, K. (2004). Chronic hepatotoxicity following 6-thioguanine therapy for childhood acute lymphoblastic leukaemia. *British Journal of Haematology, 125,* 410–411.

Ravikumara, M., Hill, F. G., Wilson, D. C., Gillett, P. M., Thomas, A., Brown, R., et al. (2006). 6-Thioguanine-related chronic hepatotoxicity and variceal haemorrhage in children treated for acute lymphoblastic leukaemia: A dual-centre experience. *Journal of Pediatric Gastroenterology and Nutrition, 42,* 535–538.

Regimbeau, J. M., Panis, Y., Gouzi, J. L., Fagniez, P. L., & French University Association of Surgical Research. (2001). Operative and long term results after surgery for chronic radiation enteritis. *The American Journal of Surgery, 182,* 237–242.

Strickland, D. K., Jenkins, J. J., & Hudson, M. M. (2001). Hepatitis C infection and hepatocellular carcinoma after treatment of childhood cancer. *Journal of Pediatric Hematology/Oncology, 23,* 527–529.

## Genitourinary System

Bath, L. E., Wallace, W. H., & Critchley, H. O. (2002). Late effects of treatment of childhood cancer on the female reproductive system and the potential for fertility preservation. *British Journal of Gynecology, 109*(2), 107–114.

Ceremuzynski, L., Gebalska, J., Wolk, R., & Makowska, E. (2000). Hypomagnesmia in heart failure with ventricular arrhythmias. *Journal of Internal Medicine, 247,* 78–86.

Marks, L., & Larrier, N. (2005). Genitourinary. In C. L. Schwartz, W. L. Hobbie, L. C. Constine, & K. S. Ruccione (Eds.), *Survivors of childhood and adolescent cancer: A multidisciplinary approach* (2nd ed., pp. 231–240). Heidelberg, Germany: Springer-Verlag.

Muller, J. (2002). Disturbances of pubertal development after cancer treatment. *Best Practice Research Clinical Endocrinology and Metabolism, 16*(1), 91–103.

Ritchey, M. L., Green, D. M., Thomas, P. R., Smith, G. R., Hasse, G., Shochat, S., et al. (1996). Renal failure in Wilms' tumor patients: A report from the National Wilms' Tumor Study Group. *Medical and Pediatric Oncology, 26,* 75–80.

Skinner, R. (2003). Chronic ifosfamide nephrotoxicity in children. *Medical Pediatric Oncology, 41*(3), 190–197.

## Reproductive System: Testes

Ginsberg, J. P., & Maity, A. (2005). The testes. In C. L. Schwartz, W. L. Hobbie, L. C. Constine, & K. S. Ruccione (Eds.), *Survivors of childhood and adolescent cancer: A multidisciplinary approach* (2nd ed., pp. 215–228). Heidelberg, Germany: Springer-Verlag.

Ginsberg, J. P., Ogle, S. K., Tuchman L. K., Carlson, C. A., Reilly, M. M., Hobbie, W. L., et al. (2007). Sperm banking for adolescent and young adult cancer patients: Sperm quality, patient, and parent perspectives. *Pediatric Blood and Cancer, 50*(3), 594–598.

Hobbie, W. L., Ginsberg, J. P., Ogle, S. K., Carlson, C., & Meadows, A. T. (2005). Fertility in males treated for Hodgkin's disease with COPP/ABV hybrid. *Pediatric Blood and Cancer, 44*(2), 193–196.

Houell, S. J., & Shalet, S. M. (2001). Testicular function following chemotherapy. *Human Reproduction Update, 7,* 363–369.

Kenney, L. B., Laufer, M. R., Grant, F. D., Grier, H., & Diller, L. (2001). High risk of infertility and long-term gonadal damage in males treated with high dose cyclophosphamide for sarcoma during childhood. *Cancer, 91,* 613–620.

## Reproductive System: Ovaries

Friedman, D. L. (2005). The ovary. In C. L. Schwartz, W. L. Hobbie, L. C. Constine, & K. S. Ruccione (Eds.), *Survivors of childhood and adolescent cancer: A multidisciplinary approach* (2nd ed., pp. 203–214). Heidelberg, Germany: Springer-Verlag.

Oktay, K., & Sonmezer, M. (2004). Ovarian tissue banking for cancer patients: Fertility preservation, not just ovarian cryopreservation. *Human Reproduction, 19*(3), 477–480.

The Practice Committee of the American Society for Reproductive Medicine. (2004). Practice Committee, position paper: Ovarian tissue and oocyte cryopreservation. *Fertility and Sterility, 82*(4), 993–998.

## Musculoskeletal System

Ginsberg, J. P., Rai, S. N., Carlson, C. A., Meadows, A. T., Hinds, P. S., Spearing, E. M., et al. (2007). Functional outcomes: A comparative analysis of adolescents and young adults with lower-extremity sarcoma. *Pediatric Blood and Cancer, 49,* 964–969.

Kaste, S. C., Jones-Wallace, D., Rose, S. R., Boyett, J. M., Lustig, R. H., Rivera, G. K., et al. (2001). Bone mineral decrements in survivors of childhood acute lymphoblastic leukemia: Frequency of occurrence and risk factors for their development. *Leukemia, 15,* 728–734.

Mattano, L. A., Sather, H. N., Trigg, M. E., & Nachman, J. B. (2000). Osteonecrosis as a complication of treating acute lymphoblastic leukemia in children: A report from the Children's Cancer Group. *Journal of Clinical Oncology, 18,* 3262–3272.

Nagarajan, R., Clohisy, D. R., Negia, J. P., Yasui, Y., Mitby, P. A., Sklar, C., et al. (2004). Function and quality of life of survivors of pelvic and lower extremity osteosarcoma and Ewing's sarcoma: The Childhood Cancer Survivor Study. *British Journal of Cancer, 91,* 1858–1865.

Nagarajan, R., Neglia, J. P., Clohisy, D. R., & Robison, L. L. (2002). Limb salvage and amputation in survivors of pediatric lower extremity bone tumors: What are the long-term implications? *Journal of Clinical Oncology, 20,* 4493–4501.

Paulino, A. C., Simon, J. H., Zhen, W., & Wen, B. (2000). Long term effects in children treated with radiotherapy for head and neck rhabdomyosarcoma. *International Journal of Radiation, Oncology, Biology, Physics, 48,* 1489–1495.

Pfeilschifter, J., & Diel, I. J. (2000). Osteoporosis due to cancer treatment: Pathogenesis and management. *Journal of Clinical Oncology, 18,* 1570–1593.

Raney, R. B., Asmar, L., Vassilopoulou-Sellin, R., Klein, M. J., Donaldson, S. S., Green, J., et al. (1999). Late complications of therapy of 213 children with localized nonorbital soft-tissue sarcoma of the head and neck: A descriptive report from the Intergroup Rhabdomyosarcoma Studies (IRS)-II and III. *Medical and Pediatric Oncology, 33,* 362–371.

Strauss, A. J., Su, J. T., Dalton, V. M., Gelber, R. D., Sallen, S. E., & Silverman, L. B. (2001). Bony morbidity in children treated for acute lymphoblastic leukemia. *Journal of Clinical Oncology, 19,* 3066–3072.

**Hematopoietic System**
Bhatia, S., Blatt, J., & Meadows, A. T. (2006). Late effects of childhood cancer and its treatment. In P. A. Pizzo & D. G. Poplack (Eds.), *Principles and practice of pediatric oncology* (5th ed., pp. 1490–1514). Philadelphia: Lippincott Williams & Wilkins.

**Immune System**
Bhatia, S., Blatt, J., & Meadows, A. T. (2006). Late effects of childhood cancer and its treatment. In P. A. Pizzo & D. G. Poplack (Eds.), *Principles and practice of pediatric oncology* (5th ed., pp. 1490–1514). Philadelphia: Lippincott Williams & Wilkins.
Pickering, L. K., Committee on Infectious Diseases, & American Academy of Pediatrics (Eds.). *Red book: 2006 report of the Committee on Infectious Diseases* (27th ed.). Section 1, Active and passive immunization (p. 83). Retrieved May 26, 2008, from www.aap.org.

**Second Malignant Neoplasms**
Bassal, M., Mertens, A. C., Taylor. L., Neglia, J. P., Greffe, B. S., Hammond, S., et al. (2006). Risk of selected subsequent carcinomas in survivors of childhood cancer: A report from the Childhood Cancer Survivor Study. *Journal of Clinical Oncology, 24,* 476–483.
Cardous-Ubbink, M. C., Heinen, R. C., Bakker. P. J. M., van den Berg, H., Oldenburger, H., Caron, H. N., et al. (2007). Risk of second malignancies in long-term survivors of childhood cancer. *European Journal of Cancer, 43,* 351–362.
Hobbie, W., Ruccione, K., Harvey, J., & Moore, I. M. (2007). Care of survivors. In C. R. Baggott, K. P. Kelly, D. Fochtman, & G. V. Foley (Eds.), *Nursing care of children and adolescents with cancer* (3rd ed., pp. 426–464). Glenview, IL: Association of Pediatric Hematology/Oncology Nurses.
Landier, W., Bhatia, S., Eshelman, D. A., Forte, K. J., Sweeney, T., Hester, A. L., et al. (2004). Development of risk-based guidelines for pediatric cancer survivors: The Children's Oncology Group: Long-Term Follow-Up Guidelines from the Children's Oncology Group Late Effects Committee and Nursing Discipline. *Journal of Clinical Oncology, 22,* 4979–4990.
Maule, M., Scelo, G., Pastore G., Brennan, P., Hemminki, K., Tracey, E., et al. (2007). Risk of second malignant neoplasms after childhood leukemia and lymphoma: An international study. *Journal of the National Cancer Institute, 99,* 790–800.
Neglia, J. P., Friedman, D. L., Yasui, Y., Mertens, A. C., Hammond, S., Stovall, M., et al. (2001). Second malignant neoplasms in five-year survivors of childhood cancer: Childhood cancer survivor study. *Journal of the National Cancer Institute, 93,* 618–629.

**Psychosocial Effects**
Bhatia, S., Jenney, M. E. M., Bogue, M. K., Rockwood, T. H., Feusner, J. H., Friedman, D. L., et al. (2002). The Minneapolis-Manchester quality of life instrument: Reliability and validity of the adolescent form. *Journal of Clinical Oncology, 20,* 2692–2698.
Eiser, C., Hill, J. J., & Blackay, A. (2000). Surviving cancer: What does it mean for you? An evaluation of a clinic based intervention for survivors of childhood cancer. *PsychoOncology, 9,* 214–220.
Hobbie, W. L., Stuber, M., Meeske, K., Wissler, K., Rourke, M. T., Ruccione, K., et al. (2000). Symptoms of posttraumatic stress in young adult survivors of childhood cancer. *Journal of Clinical Oncology, 18,* 4060–4066.
Hoffman, B. (1999). Cancer survivors' employment and insurance rights: A primer for oncologists. *Oncology, 13,* 841–852.
Hoffman, B. (2004). *A cancer survivor's almanac: Charting your journey.* Hoboken, NJ: John Wiley & Sons.
Keene, N., Hobbie, W., & Ruccione, K. (2006). *Childhood cancer survivors: A practical guide to your future* (2nd ed.). Sebastopol, CA: O'Reilly.
Langeveld, N. E., Stam, H., Grootenhuis, M. A., & Last, B. F. (2002). Quality of life in young adult survivors of childhood cancer. *Support Care Cancer, 10,* 579–600.
Langeveld, N. E., Ubbink, M. C., Last, B. F., Grootenhuis, M. A., Voute, P. A., & De Haan, R. J. (2003). Educational achievement, employment, and living situation in long-term young adult survivors of childhood cancer in the Netherlands. *Psycho-Oncology, 12,* 213–225.
Mitby, P. A., Robison, L. L., Whitton, J. A., Zevon, M. A., Gibbs, I. C., Tersak, J. M., et al. (2003). Utilization of special education services and educational attainment among long-term survivors of childhood cancer. A report from the Childhood Cancer Survivor Study. *Cancer, 97,* 1115–1126.
Nathan, P. C., Patel, S. K., Dilley, K., Goldsby, R., Harvey, J., Jacobsen, C., et al. (2007). Guidelines for identification of, advocacy for, and intervention in neurocognitive problems in survivors of childhood cancer: A report from the Children's Oncology Group. *Archives of Pediatrics and Adolescent Medicine, 161,* 798–806.
Schwartz, L., & Drotar, D. (2006). Posttraumatic stress and related impairment in survivors of childhood cancer in early adulthood compared to healthy peers. *Journal of Pediatric Psychology, 31,* 356–366.
Van Dongen-Melman, J. E. W. M. (2000). Developing psychosocial aftercare for children surviving cancer and their families. *ACTA Oncologica, 39,* 23–31.
Zebrack, B. J., Zeltzer, L. K., Whitton, J., Mertens, A. C., Odom, L., Berkow, R., et al. (2002). Psychological outcomes in long-term survivors of childhood leukemia, Hodgkin's disease, and non-Hodgkin's lymphoma: A report from the Childhood Cancer Survivor Study. *Pediatrics, 110,* 42–52.

**Promoting Health After Childhood Cancer**
Keene, N., Hobbie, W. L., & Ruccione, K. (2006). *Childhood cancer survivors: A practical guide to your future.* Sebastopol, CA: O'Reilly.

# Section XI  Hematology

Joan O'Brien-Shea

## Section Outline

Autoimmune Hemolytic Anemia

Sickle-Cell Disease

Thalassemia

Glucose-6-Phosphate Dehydrogenase Deficiency

Hereditary Spherocytosis

Bone-Marrow-Failure Syndromes

Shwachman-Diamond Syndrome

Chronic Neutropenia

Immune Thrombocytopenic Purpura

Evans Syndrome

Thrombosis and Thrombophilia

Hemolytic-Uremic Syndrome

Paroxysmal Nocturnal Hemoglobinuria

Hemophilia

Von Willebrand Disease

Bibliography

# Autoimmune Hemolytic Anemia

*Karyn J. Brundige*

## Definition

*Autoimmune hemolytic anemia* (AIHA) is a group of disorders characterized by a malfunction of the immune system whereby antibodies are produced against antigens (proteins) on the surface of the RBCs (RBCs), resulting in premature erythrocyte destruction (hemolysis).

## Pathophysiology

RBCs normally survive in the peripheral circulation for 100–120 days. RBC production in the bone marrow (erythropoesis) usually compensates for normal RBC destruction. In AIHA, the body's immune system produces antibodies against its own RBCs. RBC survival is proportional to the amount of antibody on the RBC surface; therefore, the greater the amount of antibody, the more rapidly the RBC is destroyed. Anemia develops when hemolysis occurs at a faster rate than RBC production.

Hemolysis in AIHA can be intravascular or extravascular. In intravascular hemolysis, RBC lysis occurs in the circulation. Antibodies (immunoglobulins) bind to the RBC membrane, activating the complement cascade. The membrane of the RBC is damaged, allowing excessive osmosis, or movement of water, toward the inside of the RBC. The cell membrane cannot withstand the osmotic pressure and bursts. If complement fixation to the RBC membrane is not high enough to activate the complement cascade, extravascular hemolysis occurs. The complement on the RBC surface interacts with receptors on macrophages in the lungs, liver, and spleen, resulting in RBC phagocytosis.

Although there are many causes of AIHA, more than 50% of the cases are idiopathic (i.e., have no identified cause). AIHA can be caused by other autoimmune conditions, such as systemic lupus erythematosus (SLE); certain types of infections, such as hepatitis, Epstein-Barr virus (EBV), and mycoplasma pneumonia; medications, such as penicillin and quinine; and by hematologic disorders, such as Evans' syndrome and paroxysmal nocturnal hemoglobinuria.

## Incidence

The annual incidence of AIHA is approximately 1 case per 80,000 persons.

## Clinical Presentation

RBC hemolysis due to autoantibodies may occur acutely or develop gradually and become chronic. Symptoms depend on the extent of RBC destruction and ability of the bone marrow to increase the rate of RBC production. If hemolysis is severe or rapid, symptoms of acute anemia including pallor, jaundice (i.e., yellowish tinge to the skin or sclera due to accumulation of circulating bilirubin in subcutaneous fat), fatigue, and tachycardia appear. Severe anemia can result in hypoxia in vital organs such as the heart and lead to cardiovascular failure. Splenomegaly, due to trapping of RBCs in the spleen, can present with abdominal fullness or discomfort.

A complete review of the following systems should focus on signs and symptoms of anemia and hemolysis:

- General—behavior changes, fatigability, inactivity, malaise
- Skin—pallor, jaundice
- Cardiopulmonary—palpitations, dyspnea, dizziness
- Genitourinary—hemoglobinuria (dark or tea-colored urine)
- Nervous system—headaches, dizziness, change in level of consciousness.

A physical examination should evaluate for presence of the following:

- Skin—pinkness of nail beds, conjunctiva, mucous membranes, and lips
- Eyes—scleral jaundice
- Heart—tachycardia, cardiac flow murmurs, hypotension
- Lungs—tachypnea, adventitious breath sounds, hypoxia (i.e., low oxygen saturation)
- Abdomen—splenomegaly, hepatomegaly
- Nervous system—paresthesia, impaired mental activity, and poor concentration.

## Diagnosis

An evaluation of AIHA includes a comprehensive history and physical examination as outlined. Children with anemia should have a complete blood cell count, reticulocyte count, review of peripheral smear, and Coombs test, as well as measurement of bilirubin, lactate dehydrogenase (LDH), and haptoglobin. All values must be compared with age-matched normal values.

Findings consistent with but not necessarily diagnostic of AIHA include:

- Positive direct Coombs test (also known as direct antiglobulin test [DAT])—RBCs are washed to remove the serum and then incubated with antihuman globulin (i.e., Coombs' reagent). If immunoglobulin or complement factors have become fixed or attached to the RBC surface, the antihuman globulin will clump or agglutinate the RBCs, a positive test indicating antibodies against the RBCs. The Coombs test was first described in 1945 by Dr. Robin Coombs, a British immunologist.
- Low hemoglobin—Anemia may be mild or severe depending on the ability of the bone marrow to compensate for RBC hemolysis.
- Increased reticulocyte count—With increased erythropoesis in response to anemia, reticulocytes may be released into the bloodstream. Reticulocytes are immature RBCs that still contain nuclear ribonucleic acid and stain differently than fully mature RBCs that have extruded their nucleus. The number of reticulocytes in the blood indicates how quickly they are being produced and released by the bone marrow. Reticulocytes normally make up ~1% of the total RBC count, but they may exceed 4% when compensating for anemia.
- Spherocytes, schistocytes, or erythrocyte agglutination that show on a blood smear.
- Increased unconjugated bilirubin, increased LDH, decreased haptoglobin levels, hemoglobinuria—As RBCs hemolyze, LDH and hemoglobin are released into circulation. The hemoglobin is converted to unconjugated bilirubin in the spleen or binds to haptoglobin and is removed by the liver. In severe intravascular hemolysis, free hemoglobin is filtered by the kidney, resulting in dark-red or tea-colored urine.

## Treatment

Treatment for AIHA depends on the specific disease process. Medications or foods that may have caused immune hemolysis (e.g., penicillin, sulfa drugs) should be discontinued if possible.

The following therapies may be used to treat AIHA:
- Corticosteroids—High-dose prednisone therapy (2–4 mg/kg/day) often is initiated if hemolysis is severe or worsening. After it is stabilized, doses may be weaned over several weeks or months.
- Intravenous immunoglobulin (IVIG)—High-dose IVIG (5 gm/kg) may be used to treat AIHA that is not responsive to steroids. The benefit is usually transient (1–3 weeks) due to the continued production of antibodies.
- Splenectomy—May be indicated for severe AIHA that is not responsive to medical therapies.

Supportive care includes:
- Packed RBC (pRBC) transfusion—If the bone marrow is functioning normally, the reticulocyte count will increase within 3 to 5 days of a sudden drop in hemoglobin. Transfusion, which does not treat the cause of the anemia and may pose increased risk for transfusion reaction, is reserved for acute severe hemolysis.
- Folic-acid (folate) supplementation—Folic acid is required for the production of RBCs. In chronic hemolysis, folic-acid supplementation is necessary to prevent megaloblastic (folate-deficient) anemia.

The following therapies may be used for refractory disease:
- Plasmapheresis—Because immunoglobulin M (IgM) is confined to the intravascular space, filtering blood to remove antibodies can temporarily reduce the autoantibody level. Response is generally transient due to continued production of autoantibodies.
- Cytotoxic agents—Antimetabolites (e.g., 6-mecaptopurine, azathioprine), alkylating agents (e.g., cyclophosphamide), mitotic agents (e.g., vincristine, vinblastine)
- Immunosuppressive therapy (e.g., cyclosporine)
- Hormonal therapy (e.g., danazol).

## Prognostic Considerations

Most cases of AIHA in children are transient, last less than 3 months, and are self-limiting. AIHA has a mortality rate of approximately 10%.

## Warm and Cold Antibody AIHA

Warm antibody AIHA is the most common type of AIHA, accounting for approximately 75% of cases. Autoantibodies attach to and destroy RBCs at temperatures equal to or in excess of normal body temperature (37º C). With cold antibody AIHA, the autoantibodies become most active and attack RBCs usually at temperatures well below normal body temperature.

### Warm Antibody AIHA

**Pathophysiology:** Immunoglobulin G (IgG) is the most common antibody involved in warm antibody AIHA. The cause of the autoantibody formation is unknown. The IgG antibodies attach to the RBCs and are recognized by monocytes and macrophages in the spleen, which destroy portions of the RBC membrane, creating schistocytes (RBC fragments). The loss of the membrane causes the RBCs to change from flexible biconcave discs to spherocytes, which, along with other portions of the reticuloendothelial system, are singled out for destruction in the spleen. The RBCs trapped in the spleen result in splenomegaly. Some drugs, such as penicillin and cephalosporins, can bind directly to the RBC membrane. Antibodies are then created against this RBC-drug complex.

About 50% of the cases of warm antibody AIHA are idiopathic and considered (primary). Secondary causes include chronic disease, such as SLE, acute infection, or medication.

**Clinical Presentation:** Warm antibody AIHA can be severe and life threatening. Children may present with acute onset of pallor, jaundice, and dark urine. The spleen is usually palpable.

**Treatment:** If symptoms are mild, no treatment is required. Rapid hemolysis may be treated with steroids (more than an 80% response rate) or IVIG; transfusion is reserved for life-threatening anemia.

**Prognostic Considerations:** Most cases of warm antibody AIHA in children are transient, last less than 3 months, and resolve spontaneously.

### Cold Antibody AIHA

**Definition:** Cold agglutinin disease is a form of AIHA that is caused by cold-reacting autoantibodies.

**Pathophysiology:** Cold agglutinins, or cold antibodies, occur naturally at low titers (levels) and have no activity at higher temperatures. Cold-agglutinin-mediated AIHA most commonly develops in children secondary to an infection, when IgM or IgG cold-reacting antibodies that cross-react with the ABO antigens on the surface of RBCs are produced. These autoantibodies attach to the RBC membrane in the cooler peripheral circulation. If complement fixation to the RBC membrane is high enough, the complement cascade is activated, resulting in lysis of the RBC in the circulation (intravascular hemolysis). If complement fixation to the RBC membrane is not high enough to activate the complement cascade, extravascular hemolysis occurs. The complement on the RBC surface interacts with receptors in the phagocytes of the lungs, liver, and spleen, and the RBC is phagocytized. Unlike other forms of hemolytic anemia, the liver is the main site of hemolysis in cold antibody AIHA.

Cold agglutinin disease is classified as primary or secondary. Primary cold agglutinin disease is chronic and usually occurs after the 5th decade of life. Secondary cold agglutinin disease in children and young adults is usually transient and is caused by infection, most commonly *Mycoplasma pneumoniae*. Viral infections associated with cold antibody AIHA include measles, mumps, influenza, infectious mononucleosis (i.e., Epstein-Barr virus), adenovirus, varicella (i.e., chicken pox), and cytomegalovirus (CMV). Bacterial infections associated with cold antibody AIHA include syphilis and *Haemophilus influenzae*.

**Treatment:** In children, cold antibody AIHA is usually mild and self-limited and rarely requires medical intervention. One supportive-care measure is to avoid exposure to cold. If pRBC transfusion is required, RBCs should be washed and warmed prior to transfusion. Viral infections, such as EBV, CMV, and the mumps, are usually self-limited. Mycoplasma infection, systemic autoimmune disease (e.g., Systemic lupus eruthematosus [SLE]), or lymphoproliferative disease should be treated.

Prednisone therapy is seldom effective. Splenectomy is ineffective because the liver is the predominant site of hemolysis.

**Prognostic Considerations:** In children and young adults, cold agglutinin disease is usually self-limited, with acute hemolysis lasting 1–3 weeks and evidence of cold agglutinins disappearing within 6 months. More chronic cases are less responsive to medical therapies than warm antibody AIHA.

## Nursing Assessment and Interventions

### Assessment
The nurse must be knowledgeable about the signs and symptoms of anemia and be able to perform a comprehensive history and assessment focusing on signs of anemia and hemolysis (see "Clinical Presentation").

### Interventions
Nursing interventions for a child with AIHA depend upon the severity of anemia and the medical intervention plan and including the following:
- Observe laboratory data for evidence of a decrease in hemoglobin and notify the healthcare team.
- Monitor for complications related to anemia.
  - Assess skin for pallor or decreased capillary refill.
  - Assess for decreased energy or fatigue, lethargy, or irritability.
  - Assess for tachycardia, tachypnea, and dyspnea.
  - Assess for headache, hypotension, or syncope.
  - Assess level of consciousness.
- Monitor patient for transfusion complications, including transfusion reactions and volume overload (pulmonary edema).
- Maximize the child's physical tolerance.
  - Provide oxygen, as ordered, when decreased oxygen causes difficulty breathing.
  - Provide quiet play activities that promote physical and intellectual development.
  - Promote times for rest and sleep.
- Teach the family about hemolytic anemia.
  - Explain the signs and symptoms of worsening anemia, such as increased heart rate and respirations, dyspnea, pallor, excessive sleepiness or irritability, headaches, dizziness when standing abruptly, and poor suckling in infants.
  - Review ways to conserve energy and decrease fatigue.
  - Explain the signs and symptoms of worsening hemolysis: abdominal pain, enlarging abdomen, red or dark urine, and jaundice.
  - Discuss medical therapies, rationale for use, potential side effects, and, if parents will administer medications, what to do if a dose is missed.
- Teach the family about postsplenectomy care.
  - Advise that the child wear a medical-alert bracelet.
  - Educate about the risks for sepsis and proper response to fever or infection.

### Expected Patient and Family Outcomes
- Parents and child are able to report the signs and symptoms of anemia and hemolysis.
- The child has minimal complications related to anemia.

## Sickle-Cell Disease

*Beth Savage*

### Definition
First described in 1904 by physician James Herrick, *sickle-cell disease* (SCD) is a hemoglobinopathy, a genetic condition caused by a mutation in the normal dexoyribonuckic acid (DNA) that determines hemoglobin production. Normal hemoglobin, or hemoglobin A, is absent, but hemoglobin S is present, either alone or in combination with another form of abnormal hemoglobin.

### Pathophysiology
Hemoglobin contains two pairs of polypeptide chains, the alpha (α) chain and the beta (β) chain. The sixth position on the β chain in hemoglobin A, normal hemoglobin, is occupied by glutamic acid, an amino acid. However, in a person affected by SCD, this glutamic acid has been replaced by valine.

Normal RBCs (RBCs) containing hemoglobin A are pliable biconcave discs that live for approximately 120 days. However, the RBCs of a person affected by SCD will polymerize and form microtubules, or stiff rods, that cause the cells to change into the characteristic sickle shape (i.e., crescent-moon or banana shape). Certain conditions that result in hypoxia or acidosis are responsible for this polymerization and include infection, fever, exposure to extremes in temperature, and dehydration.

Once RBCs have sickled, they become inflexible and tend to "clog" the vasculature, causing ischemia in the tissue that is served by the affected vessels. Additionally, RBCs that have transformed into the sickle shape are very friable and tend to break open easily, resulting in a shortened life span of only 10 to 20 days. The result is a chronic state of anemia.

### Incidence and Etiology
It is a widely accepted theory that the sickle-cell trait evolved in Western Africa as a genetic mutation in response to malaria. Carriers and those with SCD remain susceptible to malaria, but morbidity and mortality are decreased as compared to those who are not affected. As a result, SCD is most prevalent in areas where malaria is endemic or in places from which carriers historically have emigrated, including Africa, the Mediterranean, India, Pakistan, the Caribbean, South America, and North America.

SCD is the most common inherited disorder in the United States, affecting 72,000 people, with 8,000 new cases annually. Most of these cases are identified through universal screening, which is performed on newborns in almost every state. One in every 500 African Americans has been diagnosed with the disease, and one in every 1,000 to 1,400 Hispanic Americans is affected by it.

## Genetic Implications

SCD has an autosomal-recessive inheritance pattern. With each pregnancy, there is a 25% chance that the baby will inherit two genes for sickle cell or two genes for normal hemoglobin A. There is also a 50% chance the baby will inherit one gene for sickle cell and one normal gene, resulting in a carrier state (**Figure 11-1**).

## Clinical Presentation

Complications of SCD may first be seen between age 6 months and 12 months, as fetal hemoglobin is being replaced by hemoglobin S. There are two characteristics of SCD that determine its presentation. The first is its tendency to be a chronic disease with acute exacerbations. The second is that it is a condition that affects RBCs, which supply oxygen to all of the body. Therefore, SCD can affect any part of the body. Both of these characteristics must be taken into consideration when assessing a patient with SCD.

### Acute Complications

**Fever and Infection:** People with SCD are at a higher risk for pneumonia, bacteremia, and osteomyelitis. The spleen normally serves a role in preventing overwhelming infection. However, because of its low-oxygen environment, the spleen suffers massive infarction during the first 6 to 12 months of life, leaving the child functionally asplenic. Additionally, there is a failure to produce specific IgG antibodies to the polysaccharide encapsulated organisms, especially the *Streptococcus pneumococcus* species. In fact, *Streptococcus pneumonia* sepsis is the leading cause of death in these children. Fever represents a medical emergency and requires immediate evaluation and administration of a broad spectrum antibiotic.

**Pain Crisis:** Vaso-occlusive crisis, or pain crisis, is the hallmark of SCD and the most common reason patients seek medical care. Pain is the result of three factors: (a) ischemia secondary to the occlusion of blood vessels by sickled RBCs, (b) damage to the vascular endothelium, and (c) inflammation. Dactylitis, or hand and foot syndrome, is a vaso-occlusive crisis that occurs in the hands and feet of babies and toddlers and is often the earliest presentation in a patient with SCD.

Pain crisis is treated with increased fluids and analgesics, usually an opioid paired with a nonsteroidal antiinflammatory drug. Assessment of pain and the efficacy of the treatment plan must be ongoing, consistent, and developmentally appropriate. Other factors to consider are family coping styles, cultural practices, past experiences with pain, and efficacy of prior pain management.

**Acute Chest Syndrome:** Responsible for 25% of all deaths in sickle-cell patients, acute chest syndrome is the rapid deterioration in respiratory function. It is caused by the occlusion of the vessels of the lungs with sickled cells. The cardinal signs of acute chest syndrome are fever, increased oxygen demand, and a new infiltrate on chest X ray.

Both pneumonia and pain crisis render the child vulnerable to the development of acute chest syndrome. Therefore, nursing interventions should include frequently evaluating respiratory status, monitoring pulse oximetry, and encouraging incentive spirometry and ambulation in these patients.

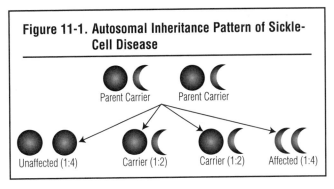

**Figure 11-1. Autosomal Inheritance Pattern of Sickle-Cell Disease**

Acute chest syndrome is treated with antibiotics, pain management, increased oxygenation, and transfusion. The recognition of acute chest syndrome in its early stages may determine whether a simple RBC transfusion or an exchange transfusion is required. In very serious cases, worsening cardiopulmonary status may require mechanical ventilation.

**Splenic Sequestration:** Splenic sequestration is the result of the trapping of sickled RBCs in the spleen. The consequence is an enlarged spleen and a rapid, severe drop in hemoglobin with a compensatory rise in the reticulocyte count. The platelet count drops sharply as platelets become trapped in the spleen as well.

In most cases, splenic sequestration is treated with hydration and transfusion. However, transfusion should be done conservatively to avoid autotransfusion. Autotransfusion occurs when the transfused RBCs cause the spleen to release the trapped RBCs back into circulation, potentially increasing the blood's viscosity. Splenic sequestration is likely to recur, and splenectomy is often necessary. Splenic sequestration is often associated with fever and infection.

**Aplastic Crisis:** Aplastic crisis occurs as the result of a viral infection, almost always parvovirus B19 infection, the virus responsible for the common childhood infection known as fifth disease. The virus causes a temporary shutdown of RBC production in the bone marrow, or reticulocytosis. Yet, the hemolysis that is a component of SCD continues. The outcome is a severe drop in hemoglobin with an extremely low reticulocyte count.

The treatment of aplastic crisis often requires the slow and careful transfusion of RBCs, with close monitoring for volume overload in the child who has compensated for the extreme anemia.

**Cerebral Vascular Accident or Stroke:** Although stroke is an acute complication of SCD, its consequences are lifelong. In SCD, a cerebral vascular accident is caused by sickled RBCs that obstruct blood flow in the vessels of the brain. This obstruction results in ischemia, or infarction of the brain tissue, leading to permanent brain damage.

The first goal of treatment is to stabilize the patient and prevent further brain damage. Exchange transfusion should not be delayed if stroke is suspected. Radiological assessment may be postponed until the patient is stable. Circulation and oxygenation should be supported as needed.

**Priapism:** When sickled RBCs obstruct the venous drainage of the penis, the result is a prolonged, unwanted, and painful erection known as priapism. Priapism, if not treated, can lead to impotence.

Aggressive hydration, vasodilators, and pain management are the treatment of choice. However, simple or exchange transfusion or surgical intervention by a urologist may be necessary.

## Chronic Complications

**Retinopathy:** Retinopathy is seen most often in patients with hemoglobin SC and in adolescent and adult patients. Sickled RBCs block and damage the small vessels of the retina. Collateral circulation develops, but these vessels are fragile and tend to break open, causing hemorrhage and retinal detachment. Some retinopathy may require intervention with laser surgery.

**Cardiac and Pulmonary Changes:** The burden of chronic anemia on the heart often results in cardiomegaly and electrocardiographic (EKG) changes. If left unchecked, the risk of congestive heart disease exists. Pulmonary hypertension has come to light as an increased cause of mortality in adults with SCD. Even that which is considered to be a mildly to moderately increased tricuspid regurgitation jet velocity in the general population has been linked to a tenfold increase in sudden cardiac death in patients diagnosed with SCD. Multiple clinical trials using medications such as sildenafil (Viagra) for the treatment of pulmonary hypertension are under way. Decreased pulmonary function and restrictive airway disease can result from repeated or severe episodes of acute chest syndrome.

**Cholelithiasis (Gallstones):** RBCs contain bilirubin, which is released by hemolysis. Bilirubin is a precursor of bile, which aids in the digestion of fats and is stored in the gallbladder. The hemolysis associated with SCD results in an increase of bilirubin that can cause the formation of stones in the gallbladder. Gallstones can be painful and cause the gallbladder to become inflamed, a condition called cholecystitis. Cholecystectomy (i.e., removal of the gallbladder) is often required to treat this condition.

**Avascular Necrosis:** Sickled RBCs can repeatedly occlude the sole artery that supplies blood to the ball-and-socket joints of the shoulders and hips. Over time, this blockage and the ischemia that results, can cause the "ball" part of the joint to become rough and jagged and may even lead to collapse of the joint.

In younger people, rest and physical therapy may allow for bone remodeling and improvement in the joints. Adolescents and older adults may progress to the point where surgical joint replacement is the only treatment option.

**Renal Impairment:** The environment in the kidneys is quite acidic and hypoxic. As a result, there is considerable sickling in the kidneys, which can damage the glomeruli. The earliest manifestation of SCD in the kidney is hyposthenuria, or the inability to concentrate urine. In the pediatric population, hyposthenuria often results in nocturnal enuresis (i.e., bed-wetting) and contributes to dehydration. Behavioral and medical interventions, used when nocturnal enuresis has other causes, have been helpful in this population as well. Extensive damage to the glomeruli results in nephropathy that may progress to renal failure; dialysis and transplantation are often inevitable.

**Leg Ulcers:** Difficult-to-treat leg ulcers occur in 10%–15% of young adults diagnosed with SCD and are the result of poor perfusion to the skin. They occur most often on the lower leg and begin with a trauma to the skin. Regular transfusion with RBCs is often used to dilute the sickle cells and promote healing. Patient teaching should include proper skin care and prompt reporting of poor wound healing.

**Delayed Growth and Maturation:** Chronic anemia caused by SCD and the ensuing high caloric needs often result in delayed physical growth. Frequently, the start of puberty is delayed as well. These children should be reassured that puberty will start, but at a later age. However, frequent assessments of growth parameters should be made, and early intervention with an endocrinologist and nutritionist is warranted.

**Impaired Cognition:** The impact of SCD on cognitive development is not entirely clear. It is known, however, that there may be "silent" infarcts to the brain tissue that impair cognition. These infarctions most likely play a part in a multifactorial cause of cognitive loss in pediatric patients. Other factors may include missed school days and chronic anemia. An annual transcranial doppler should be performed to assess for increased risk of stroke. Neurocognition should be evaluated by trained neuropsychologists, with accommodations made in the educational plan as needed.

## Diagnostic Workup

Hemoglobin electrophoresis is necessary for making a definitive diagnosis of SCD and for determining the subtype. Frequently performed diagnostic tests include:

- complete blood count (CBC) with reticulocyte count, comprehensive chemistry panel, lactate dehydrogenase (LDH), ferritin, urinalysis with protein/creatinine ratio and micoralbuminuria, and blood cultures
- chest X ray in the presence of respiratory symptoms or fever or both
- abdominal ultrasound if gallstones are suspected
- transcranial doppler to assess increased risk of stroke
- echocardiogram and EKG
- magnetic resonance imaging of joints if avascular necrosis is suspected
- pulmonary function testing
- neuropsychological testing
- ophthalmologic evaluation.

## Treatment

With the implementation of comprehensive care centers for these children, much of the focus has shifted from managing acute and chronic complications to preventing them. At the root of this health maintenance care is newborn screening. This screening has allowed for referrals to comprehensive centers during the first weeks of life and has had a tremendous positive impact on outcomes. The use of prophylactic penicillin, immunization with the 23-valent-pneumococcal vaccine, and family education have all had an extraordinary impact by preventing early death from sepsis.

In some cases, when the child shows a tendency toward a more severe course of the disease, prevention may include the use of hydroxyurea. Through clinical trials, this chemotherapeutic agent has proven to increase overall well-being by raising the fetal hemoglobin level and decreasing leukocytosis, and platelet and reticulocyte counts. However, because of its myelosuppressive potential, its use must be closely monitored.

In extreme cases in which there is a history of stroke, debilitating pain, severe and multiple episodes of acute chest syndrome, or recurrent priapism, regular RBC transfusions may also be used as a preventive measure.

### Future Therapy
Bone-marrow transplantation is the only known cure for SCD. Until recently, this therapy was reserved for only the sickest children who had entirely human leukocyte-, antigen-matched donors. Current research is exploring the use of unrelated donors. Also, many studies are using nonmyeloablative preparatory regimens with the goals of creating a curative chimerism and decreasing toxicity. Gene therapy research is ongoing as well. Finally, there is increased interest in finding ways of increasing fetal hemoglobin and manipulating the RBCs to prevent the damage caused by their sickling.

### Prognostic Factors
The average life span for people living with SCD is 45–65 years. Three findings have been associated with a more severe course of the disease: dactylitis before age 1, a consistently elevated white blood cell count, and a baseline hemoglobin of 7 gm/dL or less. The severity of the disease depends on the subtype inherited, as described in **Table 11-1**. The concurrent inheritance of persistent fetal hemoglobin, which inhibits polymerization in the cells, or α-thalassemia trait, which may raise hematocrit, may contribute to a more favorable outcome for some children.

## Nursing Assessment and Interventions
### Goal
In an acute exacerbation of SCD, the patient experiences minimal complications and returns to a state of wellness as quickly as possible.

**Assessment:**
- Assess the presenting symptoms and obtain a complete history, including documenting fever; pain (location, onset, duration, aggravating and alleviating interventions, and past pain experience); respiratory symptoms; neurological changes; splenic enlargement; anemia (presenting symptoms include headache, fatigue, shortness of breath, and palpitations); priapism; jaundice; medications; allergies; surgical history; and concurrent illnesses.
- Perform a complete physical examination to determine possible source of infection, neurological status, respiratory compromise, presence of murmur, splenic enlargement, and decreased range of motion in joints.
- Review laboratory findings and radiological imaging studies.

**Interventions:**
- Administer antibiotics without delay if patient is febrile.
- Administer aggressive intravenous hydration, pain medications, and RBC transfusions as ordered
- Monitor complete blood cell count (CBCC) and reticulocyte count, take chest X ray, blood and other cultures, vitals, and pulse oximetry readings.
- Monitor frequently for development of new complications, such as neurological changes, respiratory deterioration, ineffective pain management, fever, and splenic sequestration.

### Goal
Chronic complications are avoided or minimized through regular maintenance care.

**Assessment:**
- Review routine laboratory work (e.g., CBC, reticulocyte count, chemistries, LDH, ferritin, urinalysis).
- Review routine screening tests (e.g., transcranial doppler, echocardiogram, radiological studies of joints, abdominal ultrasound, ophthalmologic assessment, pulmonary functions, and neurocognitive assessment).

**Interventions:**
- Early subspecialty referral for abnormal findings
- Consider hydroxyurea therapy, or even chronic transfusion therapy, in the event that complications, or predisposition to complications, are a concern.

### Goal
The patient and family are adequately informed regarding diagnosis, disease, and treatment.

**Assessment:**
- Determine the child's and the family's learning styles.
- Assess the level of knowledge the family has about the diagnosis, inheritance pattern, complications, interventions and treatment, and prognosis.
- Assess the family's knowledge and understanding of the multidisciplinary team's members and roles in treating the child.

**Interventions:**
- Use effective communication tools.
- Provide ongoing instruction and reinforcement of instruction to the patient and the family.

### Table 11-1. Clinical Outcome Based on Disease Subtype

| Subtype | Anticipated Clinical Course |
| --- | --- |
| Hb AS (Trait) | Carrier state, no clinical implications |
| Hb SS | Usually severe |
| Hb SS with ↑ Hgb F | Moderate to severe |
| Hb SC | Moderate to severe |
| Hb Sβ⁰ -Thalassemia | Usually severe |
| Hb Sβ⁺ -Thalassemia | Usually mild to moderate |
| Hb SO-Arab, SD (Punjab), SE | Usually mild to moderate but may be severe |

- Include all caregivers in teaching.
- Transition focus of instruction from parents and caregivers to child when developmentally appropriate.

## Expected Patient and Family Outcomes

The child and the family can do the following:
- Describe SCD and its inheritance pattern.
- List the possible acute and chronic complications that may occur.
- Outline methods to prevent these complications.
- Recognize the onset of complications and develop skills to assess and care for the child at home.
- Understand when and how to seek medical attention.
- Identify community resources.
- Transition to adult hematologic care when appropriate.

# Thalassemia

*Beth Ann Savage*

## Definition

*Thalassemia* is a group of inherited disorders that affect the RBCs. A gene, or genes, required for the synthesis of normal hemoglobin (hemoglobin A) is abnormal. Depending on the type and number of abnormal genes, thalassemia may range from a carrier state to a lethal form.

## Pathophysiology

Hemoglobin is made up of iron and a protein called globin. Four alpha (α)-globin genes and two beta (β)-globin genes are necessary for the synthesis of normal hemoglobin A. Thalassemia is the result of a mutation in any of the four α-globin genes or two β-globin genes. There are two types of thalassemia: alpha thalassemia and beta thalassemia, depending on which type of genes are affected. The severity of the disease depends on the number of genes affected.

## Incidence and Etiology

Thalassemia is found in people from Africa, Southeast Asia, China, India, Pakistan, the Middle East, Greece, Italy, and the places from which these people have emigrated. It is estimated that more than 2 million Americans carry the thalassemia trait but only 1,000 are affected by the most severe form, known as β-thalassemia major.

## Genetic Implications

### Alpha Thalassemia

The four α-globin genes are found on chromosome 16, two on each strand. If one α-globin gene is missing, a carrier state, which has no clinical significance and often goes undetected, results.

When two genes are abnormal the result is α-thalassemia trait. A mild microcytic and hypochromic anemia, which is often mistaken for iron deficiency, may result, but iron supplementation does not correct the anemia. Each strand of chromosome 16 may be missing an α-globin gene or one strand may be missing both. The location of the affected α-globin genes does not have a clinical impact on the affected carrier; however, it may be very significant when passed to offspring.

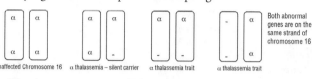

If each parent carries α-thalassemia trait with one abnormal α-globin gene on each strand of chromosome 16, all of their offspring will inherit α-thalassemia trait with the same mutation pattern.

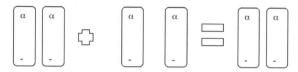

If the mutations are located on the same strand of chromosome 16 in one parent and the other is a silent carrier, there is a one in four chance their offspring will inherit both of their mutations. The result is a condition called hemoglobin H disease, which may present in any form from mild to severe; the severe form requires transfusion support.

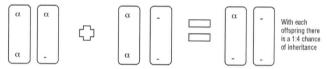

Of greatest clinical concern is the scenario in which two parents have α-thalassemia trait with both abnormal genes on the same strand. There is a one in four chance that their offspring will inherit one affected strand from each parent or have a complete absence of α-globin genes. This creates a condition known as hydrops fetalis and is incompatible with life. If diagnosed prenatally, in-vitro transfusions are begun and lifelong transfusion support is necessary.

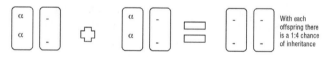

### Beta Thalassemia

Normally, there is one β-globin gene located on each strand of chromosome 11. In β-thalassemia, one or both of these β-globin genes are abnormal; this determines whether the presentation is that of a mild carrier trait (i.e., β-thalassemia minor) or a severe disease (i.e., β-thalassemia major). If both parents carry the trait, there is a 25% chance that their offspring will inherit the disease; β-thalassemia is an autosomal-recessive pattern.

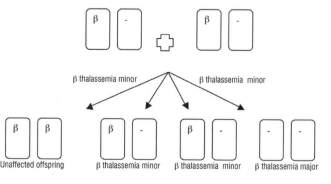

Hundreds of mutations may occur that affect different stages of hemoglobin synthesis. These mutations usually depend on the family's geographic origin. Because of these different mutations, there is a great deal of variability in the presentation of β-thalassemia, and it may result in a condition known as β-thalassemia intermedia. Children with this condition have a milder form of the disease than those diagnosed with β-thalassemia major and may only require support with occasional blood transfusions.

## Clinical Presentation

### Alpha Thalassemia

The anemia associated with α-thalassemia may be absent or range from mild to severe, depending on the number of α-globin genes affected. As previously mentioned, a one-gene deletion (i.e., the silent-carrier state) is of no clinical significance. A two-gene deletion, or trait, may be associated with asymptomatic mild anemia. It is a microcytic anemia (decreased MCV) and the cells are hypochromic. Hemoglobin H disease, or a three-gene deletion, may present with a moderate-to-severe anemia that requires regular transfusions. Finally, a four-gene deletion, hydrops fetalis, is not compatible with postnatal life unless diagnosis is made early in the pregnancy and interventions are taken.

### Beta Thalassemia

Many cases of β-thalassemia are identified through prenatal testing based on family history or ethnic background or through newborn screening programs just after birth. If the diagnosis is not made in one of these ways, babies usually present with a significant anemia and failure to thrive by the age of 6 months. In cases of β-thalassemia intermedia, symptoms may not appear until detected in routine laboratory work or during a period of physiological stress. Those with mild carrier trait, or β-thalassemia minor, may, during a routine assessment of blood work, be found to be only mildly anemic incidentally.

If transfusion needs are not met, children may develop bone changes because of an expanding marrow that is trying to meet the body's needs. These changes include bossing of the skull and cheeks, malocclusion of the teeth, and paraspinal deformities.

Extramedullary erythropoesis is a process whereby blood is produced outside of the marrow to compensate for severe anemia. Such is the case with the spleen in patients with β-thalassemia major and possibly those with β-thalassemia intermedia that is not adequately transfused, which causes the spleen to enlarge. Normally the spleen can hold 20–30 ml of blood. But in β-thalassemia, the spleen can become engorged with as much as a liter of blood. The development of hypersplenism causes the spleen to begin to destroy the RBCs the child receives from the transfusions, thus increasing transfusion needs. Once it develops, hypersplenism is difficult to correct, and a splenectomy is often required.

People living with β-thalassemia intermedia and major are at risk for iron overload. The obvious cause is transfusion-related iron overload. However, even in a patient who is minimally transfused, intermedia iron overload may occur as a result of increased absorption of dietary iron as the body tries to compensate for ineffective RBC production.

### Variant Hemoglobins

Hemoglobin E trait, another hemoglobinopathy, is common in Southeast Asia, where 1 in 12 people are carriers. When a parent carries hemoglobin E trait and β-thalassemia trait, there is a one in four chance that their offspring will inherit the hemoglobin E-b-thalassemia syndrome. Anemia can vary from mild to severe. Likewise, the offspring of parents carrying sickle-cell trait and β-thalassemia trait may inherit a form of sickle-cell disease, hemoglobin S-β-thalassemia.

## Diagnostic

- Complete blood count and reticulocyte count
- Hemoglobin electrophoresis is used to identify Bart's hemoglobin in the neonatal period. In patients with β-thalassemia intermedia and major, there is a compensatory rise in fetal hemoglobin and hemoglobin A2 to compensate for the decrease in or absence of hemoglobin A, a normal hemoglobin.
- Gene mapping is used to identify the actual mutation of the α or β genes and is helpful in genetic counseling.
- Chemistry panel, including ferritin
- Endocrine function tests include thyroid studies, glucose tolerance, and parathyroid, because iron overload affects this system.
- EKG, echocardiogram
- Bone-density testing
- Liver biopsy, superconducting quantum interference device (SQUID), or T2-star (T2*) MRI to assess iron overload quantitatively
- Human leukocyte antigen typing of patient and full siblings
- Audiogram and ophthalmic exam, due to the potential toxicity of chelation agents.

## Treatment

- Patients with thalassemia major cannot survive without transfusion therapy. The goal of such transfusions is to suppress hyperactive erythropoesis and inhibit excessive gastrointestinal iron absorption. It is desirable to maintain pretransfusion hemoglobin levels of at least 10 gm/dL. To meet this goal, patients must be transfused regularly at 2- to 4-week intervals.
- Folic-acid supplementation is used to assist in RBC formation.
- Iron overload is addressed with chelation therapy, either in the form of subcutaneous or intravenous (IV) deferoxiamine or oral deferasirox. Complications of iron overload must be screened for regularly and interventions taken early, even in the well-transfused patient.
- Splenectomy may be necessary if hypersplenism occurs.
- Bone-marrow, cord-blood, and stem-cell transplantation are currently the only cures for thalassemia.
- Hydroxyurea, which can stimulate the production of fetal hemoglobin, may reduce the need for transfusions but does not improve the ineffective RBC production.

## Future Therapy

Ongoing research is examining gene therapy; the manipulation of fetal hemoglobin, either at the genetic level or with the use of medications; and the measurement and treatment of iron overload and other long-term effects of thalassemia.

## Prognostic Factors
The most significant prognostic factor in this population is the degree of iron overload. Systemic iron overload is the most significant cause of mortality in thalassemia patients. Cardiac disease as a result of iron overload is responsible for 70% of all deaths.

## Nursing Assessment and Interventions
### Goal
Chronic complications of extramedullary erythropoesis are avoided through regular transfusion of RBCs.
- **Assessment:**
- Review routine laboratory work (e.g., complete blood count, reticulocyte count).
- Monitor for signs of extramedullary erythropoesis (e.g., facial and other skeletal changes secondary to marrow expansion, splenomegaly).
- **Interventions:**
- Transfuse with RBCs at intervals frequent enough to maintain pretransfusion hemoglobin of 9–10 gm/dL.
- Splenectomy, if indicated, following vaccination with pnemococcal and meningicoccal vaccines.

### Goal
Complications of iron overload and chelation are minimized.
- **Assessment:**
- Review routine laboratory work (e.g., serum ferritin, endocrine function tests, and chemistries).
- Monitor for signs of growth and pubertal delay.
- Assess cardiac function using electrocardiogram, echocardiogram, or stress test.
- Monitor iron-overload level through a liver biopsy SQUID, and T2 MRI.
- Schedule audiogram.
- **Interventions:**
- Refer patients with abnormal findings to subspecialty practitioners as early as possible.
- Administer chelation therapy with subcutaneous or IV deferoxiamine or oral deferasirox.
- Minimize dietary iron intake.

### Goal
The patient and the family are adequately informed about the diagnosis, disease, and treatment.
- **Assessment:**
- Determine the patient's and the family's learning styles.
- Assess the patient's and the family's level of knowledge about the diagnosis, inheritance pattern, complications, interventions and treatment, and prognosis.
- Assess the patient's and the family's knowledge and understanding of the multidisciplinary team's members and their roles in treating the child.
- **Interventions:**
- Use effective communication tools.
- Provide ongoing instruction and reinforcement of instruction to the patient and the family.
- Include all caregivers in teaching.
- Transition focus of teaching from parents and caregivers to the child when developmentally appropriate.

## Expected Patient and Family Outcomes
The child and the family can do the following:
- Describe thalassemia and its inheritance pattern.
- List the possible complications that may occur.
- Outline methods of preventing complications.
- Understand when and how to seek medical attention.
- Identify community resources.
- Transition to adult hematology care when appropriate.

# Glucose-6-Phosphate Dehydrogenase Deficiency

*Deborah L. Robinson*

## Definition
*Glucose-6-phosphate dehydrogenase deficiency* (G6PDD) is an inherited, sex-linked, metabolic disorder of RBCs. It is characterized by an enzyme defect that causes hemolysis of RBCs upon exposure to various exogenous agents.

## Pathophysiology
Glucose-6-phosphate dehydrogenase (G6PD) is an enzyme found in all organisms, including plants, animals, yeasts, and protozoa. G6PD is the first enzyme in the pentose phosphate pathway of glucose metabolism. The main role of the pentose phosphate pathway is to produce nicotinamide adenine dinucleotide phosphate, which, in turn, metabolizes glutathione. Glutathione is an antioxidant crucial for protection of the red cell's hemoglobin and the red-cell membrane. Mutations in the G6PD gene cause a deficiency of the enzyme that results in an interruption of the phosphate pathway and reduction in the availability of glutathione for the cells. If the level of glutathione is too low, the cell's hemoglobin will not bind oxygen, and the cell wall will break down, resulting in hemolysis.

## Incidence and Etiology
G6PDD is the most common metabolic disorder of the RBCs, affecting 35 million people worldwide. It is most common in tropical and subtropical areas of the Eastern Hemisphere, where the prevalence can reach 35% in some areas. G6PDD is inherited as an X-linked trait and is an inborn error of metabolism in humans. More than 300 variants of the disorder have been identified. The majority of persons affected by G6PDD in the United States are of African and Mediterranean ancestry.

## Genetics
G6PDD is a genetic disorder, in that it is sex-linked and inherited in a recessive mode by a gene located on the X chromosome (band Xq28). The disease is fully expressed in males who are hemizygous and females who are homozygous. More than 98% of individuals with this disorder are male. It can occur in females with an extreme phenotype, although this is rare. Deletions of the G6PD gene are incompatible with life and result in the death of the embryo. Point mutations of the gene are responsible for G6PDD. Sporadic mutations are not specific to any geographic area and are the most severe form of deficiency, with only 2% of

normal enzyme activity. Polymorphic mutations have resulted from malaria selection and correlate with specific regions where malaria is endemic (the deficiency provides protection from severe malaria). In the Mediterranean region, polymorphic mutations can result in severe deficiency, with only 3% of normal enzyme activity. In other regions, the polymorphic mutations can be mild to severe, with ranges of 10%–60% of normal enzyme activity. Five classes represent the wide genetic variation of G6PDD. Class I is associated with chronic nonspherocytic hemolytic anemia and severe clinical expression. Classes II and III are usually associated with mild clinical expression. Classes IV and V usually have no clinical problems.

## Clinical Presentation

The most classic manifestation of G6PDD is acute hemolytic anemia. A child with G6PDD is clinically well most of the time and has normal hemoglobin. After exposure to an exogenous agent, such as a medication or a food (e.g., fava beans), the child can experience acute hemolysis. Within 24–48 hours, the child can become lethargic, pale, and experience symptoms of abdominal pain, nausea and vomiting, and diarrhea. The telltale sign of hemolysis becomes apparent during the first 24 hours, with reports of dark-red, brown, or black urine.

On physical exam, the child appears jaundiced and has marked pallor. There may be significant tachycardia and enlargement of the liver and spleen, and heart failure may follow if the hemolysis is severe.

Laboratory findings include
- moderate-to-severe anemia (i.e., RBC levels as low as 2.5 g/dL have been reported)
- RBCs are distorted with a wide RBC distribution width.
- reticulocyte count is elevated by as much as 30%.
- white blood cell count can be elevated, with a predominance of granulocytes.
- Unconjugated bilirubin is elevated.

## Diagnosis

Diagnosis is made by obtaining a sample of blood and performing a qualitative G6PDD test, which measures the decreased activity of the enzyme in red cells.

## Treatment

In the majority of cases, the hemolytic attack associated with a G6PDD is self-limiting and tends to resolve spontaneously. In the absence of additional or preexisting pathology, the bone-marrow response is prompt and effective at replacing the RBCs. Depending on the severity of the hemolysis, it may take 3–6 weeks for the hemoglobin to return to baseline. The criterion for an RBC transfusion is hemoglobin less than 7 gm/dL or a hemoglobin less than 9 gm/dL with persistent brisk hemolysis.

The majority of treatment is aimed at prevention, with the priority being to identify those who have G6PDD. Screening for G6PDD is done in some high-risk areas such as Thailand and Malaysia. Currently there is no routine newborn screening for G6PDD in the United States. After the deficiency is identified, the individual should be instructed to avoid medications that are associated with hemolysis.

Medications reported to cause hemolysis include
- antimalarials
- analgesics
- aulfonamides
- aulfones
- anthelminthics
- aitrofurans
- miscellaneous agents, such as probenecid, dimercaprol, vitamin K analogues, and rasburicase.

In addition to medications, dietary restrictions are required for persons with G6PDD. Ingestion of fava beans has been associated with severe hemolysis.

There are also reports of bacterial infection, especially pneumococcus-causing hemolysis, with G6PDD.

## Nursing Assessment and Interventions

### Assessment

The nurse must be knowledgeable about the pathophysiology of hemolytic anemia secondary to G6PDD and must recognize the signs and symptoms of anemia.

### Interventions

- Monitor laboratory data and report a decrease in hemoglobin to the healthcare team.
- Monitor for signs or symptoms of anemia, including pallor, decreased capillary refill, fatigue, lethargy, headache, hypotension, syncope, tachycardia, tachypnea, dyspnea, and decreased level of consciousness.
- Administer RBC transfusions as ordered with appropriate monitoring of vital signs and assessment for transfusion reaction.
- Assess patient for volume overload.
- Maintain adequate hydration, which is essential because of the brisk hemolysis and risk of renal complications.
- Monitor electrolytes and renal function, especially with ongoing hemolysis.
- Provide patient with adequate rest and limit activities to tolerance.
- Provide additional oxygen if indicated.
- Instruct the patient and family about the signs and symptoms of anemia and indications for transfusion.
- Discuss mechanism of hemolysis related to G6PDD and possible triggers with the patient and the family.
- Provide the patient and the family with information regarding G6PDD and agents that cause red-cell hemolysis, including a detailed list of known medications that should be avoided.
- Explain to the patient and the family that new medications may not have any reported contraindications but should be taken cautiously, with attention given to any signs and symptoms of hemolysis and anemia.
- Review dietary restrictions (e.g., fava beans) and the potential for bacterial infection to cause hemolysis and anemia.
- Ensure that the patient and the family are monitored by a healthcare provider, and provide contact numbers for quickly notifying the healthcare team of any changes in the patient's status.

### Expected Patient and Family Outcomes
- The patient has minimal complications of anemia related to hemolysis.
- The patient or the family can verbalize an understanding of hemolytic anemia related to G6PDD.
- The patient or the family is able to recognize the signs and symptoms of hemolysis and anemia and seek medical attention quickly.
- The patient or the family is knowledgeable about exogenous agents that can cause hemolysis with G6PDD, including medications, food, and infection.

## Hereditary Spherocytosis

*Susanne Rosenberg*

### Definition
*Hereditary spherocytosis* (HS) is a common, inherited, hemolytic anemia involving cell-membrane alterations that result in fragile red cells becoming trapped in the spleen, causing a shortened RBC (RBC) life span.

### Pathophysiology
HS occurs as a result of a defect in the red-cell membrane. Normal RBCs are shaped like a disc. In HS, the RBCs are shaped like a sphere, smaller in diameter, and more rigid than normal RBCs. This leads to increased fragility and the cells' inability to change their shape to pass through certain organs as other RBCs would do. Consequently, these RBCs (i.e., spherocytes) stay in the spleen longer than normal RBCs, thus destroying the membrane surrounding the cell. After circulating through the spleen multiple times, the cell becomes damaged and is eventually destroyed by the spleen. This leads to an extremely shortened RBC life span of about 10–30 days, as opposed to the normal life span of roughly 120 days.

### Incidence and Etiology
HS is one of the most common causes of inherited hemolytic anemia in northern Europe and the United States. The incidence is about 1 in 5,000 births.

### Genetics
HS is autosomal dominant in 60%–70% of cases, recessive in 10%–15% of cases, and involves sporadic mutations in the remaining 20% of cases. The defect is a deficiency in spectrin or ankyrin that leads to alteration in the cell structure, resulting in microspherocytes.

### Clinical Presentation
The classic presenting signs of HS are anemia, jaundice, and splenomegaly. Anemia may be mild or even absent in some cases, depending on whether the hemolysis is well compensated. In such cases, the bone marrow increases the red-cell output with an elevated reticulocyte count. Splenomegaly is usually mild. Patients with a family history of the disease (about 75%) are more likely to be diagnosed early in life. Patients with a new mutation (i.e., with no family history; <25%) are more likely to present later in childhood, often when complications of anemia arise due to parvovirus or other infections.

HS can present at any age from the neonatal period until older adulthood. More severe types of HS present with signs of hemolytic anemia and hyperbilirubinemia during the newborn period. Infants with HS often encounter problems with severe anemia during the physiologic nadir. In general, the hemoglobin is high at birth and falls during the initial 6–8 weeks of life to a physiologic nadir before it gradually increases to childhood levels. Children with HS may have hemoglobin values that are considerably lower than those of children who do not have HS, and may also have life-threatening anemia with various clinical symptoms, including difficulty tolerating feeding, circumoral pallor, tachycardia, nasal flaring, diaphoretic episodes, and lethargy. The process of breaking down the RBCs and thereby increasing the bilirubin in their blood leads to a jaundiced appearance (i.e., yellow skin and eyes). These children are also at increased risk for gallstones because their bodies make extra bile pigment. Infection (specifically parvovirus), fever, and stress can stimulate the spleen to destroy more RBCs than usual, leading to a more severe anemia in an already baseline-anemic child. Such situations require prompt medical attention.

### Diagnosis
Diagnosis is made by examining the family for HS and by laboratory-based findings that include spherocytes on the blood smear, an elevated reticulocyte count with or without anemia, an indirect hyperbilirubinemia, and a positive osmotic fragility test. An osmotic fragility test is performed by placing the individual's RBCs in a saline solution for 24 hours. As a result, the cells will absorb water until the cell membrane bursts. Spherocytes have a cell membrane with a smaller surface area and will burst more readily than normal cells.

### Treatment
Treatment of HS is based on the severity of the disease. Occasionally, Epogen, a synthetic form of a protein that helps the body produce healthy RBCs, may be required. Children often require three subcutaneous shots of Epogen weekly to help sustain a healthy RBC count. Although some children with severe HS develop severe anemia, blood transfusions are rarely required. The decision to transfuse should not be based on the hemoglobin level alone but also on the clinical appearance. After the baseline severity of HS is established, repeat blood counts and other laboratory parameters are measured regularly at hematology visits and as needed if symptoms of anemia or worsening jaundice develop. Treatment before the age of 5 consists of daily folic-acid supplementation to help with the production of healthy RBCs.

In the past, splenectomy was the first line of treatment. However, splenectomy is now recommended only for individuals older than age 6 who have severe disease or for those who develop symptomatic gallstones. The risk of postsplenectomy sepsis should be discussed fully with patients and their families. In addition, partial splenectomy, in which only a portion of the spleen is removed, is now performed on HS patients in an attempt to decrease the risk of postsplenectomy complications.

Removing the spleen does not cure the disease, but it does allow RBCs to live longer so that the child no longer develops severe anemia during periods of stress or infection.

## Prognostic Indications
The majority of individuals with HS have a mild disease course and a normal life span.

## Nursing Assessment and Interventions
### Goal
The patient experiences minimal complications related to HS.
**Assessment:**
- Assess signs and symptoms of anemia (e.g., pallor, tachycardia, energy level, difficulty tolerating feeds).
- Perform a complete physical exam to determine the presence of splenomegaly.
- Review laboratory findings.
- Assess the child's level of pain.

**Interventions:**
- Monitor vital signs frequently.
- Monitor for pallor or increasing jaundice.

### Goal
The patient and the family understand the potential complications of HS.
**Assessment:**
- Assess the patient's and the family's style of communication.
- Assess the patient's and the family's previous experience with and understanding of these complications.

**Interventions:**
- Discuss the possibility of gallstones (from the breakdown of RBCs) in the context of abdominal pain.
- Discuss the risk of aplastic crisis with parvovirus infection.
- Discuss the risk of hemolytic crisis in the context of febrile illnesses and viral infections.
- Instruct the family that the healthcare team must be called if there are indications of
  - increased pallor or jaundice
  - decreased activity level or energy
  - increased spleen size
  - fever (only if patient has had a splenectomy).

### Goal
The patient and the family understand postsplenectomy guidelines for HS.
**Assessment:**
- Assess the patient's and the family's style of communication.
- Assess the patient's and the family's previous experience with splenectomy.
- Assess what the patient and the family have been taught.

**Interventions:**
- Discuss the importance of fever management and prophylactic antibiotics.
- Discuss the importance of up-to-date immunizations.
- Provide the family with the latest information on immunizations for splenectomy patients.

## Expected Patient and Family Outcomes
The patient and the family can do the following:
- Describe HS and the treatment options.
- Describe worsening symptoms that may occur at home and know whom they should notify.
- Describe the symptoms of the most common complications of HS.
- Demonstrate skills and knowledge needed for caring for the child at home.

# Bone-Marrow-Failure Syndromes

*Joan O'Brien Shea*

## Definition
The bone-marrow-failure syndromes are a group of congenital or acquired disorders that result in the inability of the bone marrow to produce one or more cell lines. Aplastic anemia is the complete arrest of bone marrow. Cytopenia occurs when one cell line fails to produce, such as red cells in Diamond-Blackfan anemia and transient erythroblastopenia of childhood. Pancytopenia involves more than one cell line, which is the case in Fanconi anemia and dyskeratosis congenita.

## Pathophysiology
Bone-marrow failure can be inherited or acquired and can involve just one cell line or all three cell lines. The pathophysiology of these defects includes the following mechanisms of action: (a) a decrease in or damage to the hematopoietic stem cells and their microenvironment, resulting in hypoplastic or aplastic bone marrow; (b) maturation defects, such as vitamin B 12 or folate deficiency; and (c) differentiation defects, such as myelodysplasia.

This subsection discusses acquired aplastic anemia, inherited aplastic anemias, and red-cell aplasias.

## Aplastic Anemia
### Definition
*Aplastic anemia* is defined as peripheral blood pancytopenia and hypocellular bone marrow and is either acquired or inherited. Inherited forms of aplastic anemia include Fanconi anemia and dyskeratosis congenita.

### Acquired Aplastic Anemia
**Incidence and Etiology:** Acquired aplastic anemia is not associated with any one geographic area or ethnic background. It has two peak age distributions, ages 15–25 and older than 60 years, but it can affect people of any age. It affects males and females equally and occurs in approximately 2 people per million per year.

Aplastic anemia in childhood is most often idiopathic, or unknown. The literature on adult aplastic anemia discusses multiple chemical and environmental factors associated with prolonged exposure. However, the fact that the incidence of aplastic anemia has not lessened with the decreased use of associated chemicals raises questions about the results of previous reports linking chemical and environmental exposure to aplastic anemia. Some researchers believe that a genetic predisposition to aplastic anemia related to exposure involves cells that may absorb and process the chemicals differently, resulting in a genetic event that leads to marrow failure.

The chemical benzene has the strongest link to aplastic anemia, and is a known carcinogen used widely in rubber factories but is no longer permitted for use in the United States. Multiple medications, including nonsteroidal antiinflammatory drugs, neuroleptics, sulfonamides, corticosteriods, psychotropics, and those containing gold salts, among others, have been associated with acquired aplastic anemia. Exposure to high levels of radiation, such as those resulting from nuclear accidents, also has been linked to acquired aplastic anemia. Several viruses are also known to precipitate aplastic anemia. Parvovirus is the most common link, along with hepatitis, human immunodeficiency virus, and Epstein-Barr virus.

Patients diagnosed with paroxysmal nocturnal hemoglobinuria are known to have a predisposition to aplastic anemia.

**Clinical Presentation:** The clinical presentation of aplastic anemia is directly related to its severity at the time of diagnosis. Signs of thrombocytopenia, such as petechia and ecchymosis in various stages, are the most common presenting symptoms secondary to the short life span of platelets. Signs of anemia, such as pallor and fatigue, occur later. Fever in the absence of obvious infection may occur secondary to neutropenia but is less common.

**Diagnosis:** The diagnosis of aplastic anemia is based on careful examination of the peripheral blood smear and bone-marrow aspirate and biopsy. A complete blood count (CBC) shows a significant decrease in one or more cell lines, resulting in neutropenia, thrombocytopenia, or anemia. Examination of the peripheral smear shows normal RBC morphology. Reticulocyte count is also low, demonstrating the lack of cell production. Bone-marrow aspirate and biopsy in aplastic anemia demonstrates the absence of hematopoiesis. The marrow often is replaced by fatty cells.

After careful examination of the peripheral blood sample and results of the bone-marrow aspirate and biopsy, the disease is classified as either moderate or severe (**Table 11-2**). Disease severity at the time of presentation is directly correlated to prognosis. Very severe aplastic anemia is diagnosed when the absolute neutrophil cell count (ANC) is less than 200 cells/mm$^3$. The diagnosis of aplastic anemia is made when all other causes of pancytopenia are ruled out. Hepatosplenomegaly and lymphedema are often evidence of an underlying malignancy. Young children who present with aplastic anemia should be carefully evaluated for congenital causes of marrow hypoplasia.

**Treatment:** A hematopoietic marrow transplant from a sibling with matching human leukocyte antigens (HLAs) is the treatment of choice in pediatric aplastic anemia and has the highest rate for cure.

When an HLA match is unavailable, immunosuppression with antithymocyte globulin and cyclosporine is the preferred treatment. Immunosuppressive protocols now include the use of corticosteroids and growth factors and may promote an increased survival rate.

**Supportive Care:** Symptom control is essential when treating a patient with aplastic anemia. Fevers should be treated immediately with broad spectrum antibiotics. Unlike children treated with chemotherapy, children with aplastic anemia suffer from prolonged periods of neutropenia without recovery. Usually, if blood cultures remain negative for 48 hours, the empiric treatment and observation can be discontinued. A concurrent rising ANC is not a necessary discharge criterion for a child with aplastic anemia. Transfusion therapy should be limited to symptom control to decrease the possibility of sensitization.

**Prognostic Considerations:** Prognosis is directly linked to the severity at the time of diagnosis. Treatment of severe bleeding and intravenous antibiotics can prevent devastating complications. Reports of cure after hematopoietic stem-cell transplantation (HSCT) range from 75%–90%. Unsuccessful cure of aplastic anemia after HSCT is directly related to graft-versus-host disease and infectious complications. Reports of successful treatment of aplastic anemia with immunosuppressive agents or medications vary, but the national average appears to be about 50%. Bacterial and fungal infections are associated with immunosuppressive treatment.

## Congenital Aplastic Anemia

Congenital aplastic anemias are a group of inherited disorders associated with the combination of congenital physical anomalies and bone-marrow failure. Bone-marrow failure may be present at birth but more often presents later in life.

**Fanconi Anemia:** Fanconi anemia (FA) was first described by Dr. Guido Fanconi in 1927 after observing physical anomalies and pancytopenia in brothers. It is the most common congenital bone-marrow failure syndrome.

*Incidence and Etiology.* Although FA is present at birth, the age at diagnosis ranges from 2 years to 15 years, and, rarely, into adulthood. It is an autosomal-recessive disorder. FA occurs in approximately 1 in every 5 million births and affects all races and males and females equally. The frequency of the carrier gene is about 1 in 300. Fanconi anemia

*Genetics.* FA is an autosomal-recessive disease; both parents must carry the gene. Recent research has identified 11 genes associated with Fanconi anemia. (i.e., A, B, C, D1 [BRCA2], D2, E, F, G, I, J, and L) The genes identified have been associated with cell apoptosis, interference with tumor necrosis factor, and

### Table 11-2. Classification of Acquired Aplastic Anemia

| Moderate | Severe |
| --- | --- |
| ANC <1,200 | ANC <500 |
| Platelet count <80,000 | Platelet count <20,000 |
| Anemia with reticulocyte <1.5% | Reticulocyte <1% |
| Bone-marrow cellularity <50% | Bone-marrow cellularity <25% |
| Two or three cell lines decreased for more than 6 weeks | At least two cell lines are severely depressed |

propensity to malignancy. The BRCA2 gene, which has been well publicized because of its connection with breast cancer, is identical to FA-D1. With the identification of these genes, studies are now examining their link to clinical manifestation and survival.

*Clinical Presentation.* Although the disease is present at birth, clinical presentation varies with age and symptomatology. Pancytopenia often presents at around age 7, and physical anomalies occur in 80% of the cases but may not be obvious initially. Classic symptoms and physical abnormalities of FA may include the following:
- Skin pigment change: darkened areas of the skin, café-au-lait spots, vitiligo
- Short stature
- Upper-limb anomalies: missing, extra, or misshapen thumbs; underdeveloped or absent radius; anomalies of the hands; abnormalities of the ulna
- Small testicles, genital changes
- Skeletal anomalies: congenital hip abnormality, scoliosis, spinal or rib malformations
- Microcephaly
- Eye or eyelid anomalies: small eyes, stabismus
- Ear anomalies: small or low-set ears; or deafness
- Broadened nose
- Kidney malformations: may be absent or are horseshoe shaped or hypoplastic
- Hip, leg, and toe abnormalities
- Gastrointestinal or cardiopulmonary malformations. Other potential findings
- Mental retardation/learning disability
- Low birth weight/failure to thrive
- An affected sibling.

*Diagnosis.* The degree of physical anomalies varies in FA and often diagnosis is not made until bone-marrow failure is apparent. Laboratory findings include macrocytic anemia that develops with decreased red-cell production. Thrombocytopenia is often an early sign, and as the disease progresses, neutropenia occurs. Bone marrow is hypocellular and fatty. Some patients develop myelodysplastic syndrome (MDS) or acute myeloid leukemia (AML). The standard diagnostic test for FA is chromosome breakage analysis using diepoxybutane (DEB) or mitomycin-C (MMC). A blood sample is plated and sprinkled with either DEB or MMC and matched with a healthy control. After 48–72 hours the chromosomes of FA patients break because of exposure to the chemical, as seen in **Figure 11-2.** Children should be tested for FA if they present with aplastic anemia, MDS, or AML with any one of the previously mentioned physical anomalies or a family history of leukemia, MDS, or aplastic anemia.

*Treatment.* HSCT is the only curative treatment for FA. Conditioning regimens for patients with FA use lower-dose cyclophosphamide and little, if any, radiation secondary to the increased sensitivity to toxicities.

Androgen therapy (i.e., artificial male hormone therapy) with either oxymetholone or nandrolone decanoate, in combination with steroids, produces an increase in blood counts. The response does not always include all cell lines; most often only RBCs respond, and the results are not always long lasting. Androgen therapy has been used to treat patients with FA since the 1950s,

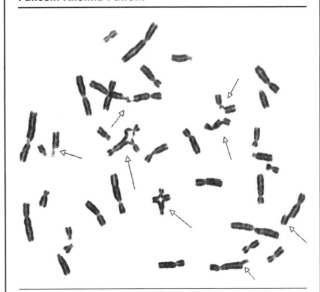

**Figure 11-2. Chromosome Breakage with DEB in a Fanconi Anemia Patient**

Image courtesy of Lisa Moreau, Comprehensive Center for Fanconi Anemia, Dana-Farber Cancer Institute, Boston, MA.

and some patients can be maintained for years with this treatment, but it is not curative.

Growth factors, such as G-CSF and GM-CSF, increase neutrophil counts in most patients with FA. Some patients have also experienced an increase in platelet count; fewer have experienced an increase in hemoglobin. The use of growth factors for patients with FA has increased in recent years.

With the identification of many of the FA genes, new therapies involving gene transfer are being explored and likely represent the future of treatment for FA. Information on clinical trials can be found on the National Institutes for Health Web site (www.nih.gov) or from the Fanconi Anemia Foundation.

*Prognosis.* HLA-matched, sibling-allogeneic HSCT provides the best potential survival, with an average survival rate near 66%. Cord, haplo, and unrelated or mismatched transplants are performed as a last resort and have about a 29% overall survival rate. Platelet count and age at time of transplant are also directly related to outcome. HSCT performed at the earliest sign of marrow failure has the best outcome. Approximately 50% of patients respond to androgen therapy. Patients with FA are at a higher risk for developing malignancies, most often head and neck and gynecological. Fifty percent of patients may develop myelodysplastic syndrome or leukemia with advancing age.

*Nursing Considerations.* Several nursing considerations unique to the patient with FA, along with those associated with all bone-marrow-failure syndromes, are significant. Patients with FA are more sensitive to carcinogens, so these should be avoided. Carcinogens include tobacco smoke, paint thinners, gasoline, pesticides, and formaldehyde. Also, even low doses of radiation have been shown to increase chromosome breakage in children with FA; X rays and computed tomography (CT) scans should be done only when absolutely clinically necessary. Magnetic resonance imaging is recommended over X rays and CT scans for evaluation.

**Dyskeratosis Congenita:** *Dyskeratosis congenita* (DKC), also known as Zinsser-Engman-Cole syndrome, is a rare inherited disorder. It is associated with progressive bone-marrow failure characterized by a triad of dermatologic symptoms, which include reticulated skin hyperpigmentation, nail dystrophy, and leukoplakia. On the cellular level, there is telomerase dysfunction, ribosome deficiency, and protein-synthesis dysfunction.

*Incidence and Etiology.* DKC is rare, in that to date slightly more than 200 cases have been reported in the world. It affects all races and ethnic groups. DKC is X linked and therefore primarily affects males.

*Genetics.* The DKC gene has been identified as DKC1 at chromosome Xq28. The cells have decreased telomerase activity and therefore affect rapidly growing cells, such as those of the skin, mucosa, and bone marrow, which require telomerase for proliferation. Telomeres are repeat structures found at the ends of chromosomes, whose function is to stabilize chromosomes. With each cycle of cell division, the length of telomeres is shortened, and the enzyme telomerase compensates by maintaining telomere length in germ line and stem cells. Because telomeres' function is to maintain chromosomal stability, they play a critical role in preventing cellular division and cancer progression. Rapidly proliferating tissues with the greatest need for telomere maintenance (e.g., bone marrow) are at greatest risk for failure.

A few cases in both males and females have been found to be autosomal recessive and autosomal dominant in origin. Females tend to have less severe symptoms because of skewed X-chromosome patterns.

*Clinical Presentation.* Physical findings of DKC, which usually present in the first decade of life, include hyperpigmented skin areas that most often involve the face, neck, shoulders, and trunk. Nail dystrophy affecting hands and feet, distinctive ridges, and small nail plates are present. Other physical signs may include abnormalities of the eyes, such as conjunctivitis, cataracts, glaucoma, and strabismus. Abnormal dentition and multiple dental caries, osteoporosis, short stature, urethral stenosis, hypospadias, and hypoplastic testes are among other findings.

Leukoplakia of the mucosal lining and bone-marrow failure most often present in the second decade of life. Transformation to leukemia may occur at the time of bone-marrow failure.

Thrombocytopenia is often the first sign of bone-marrow failure; progression to complete marrow failure always occurs. Symptoms of DKC are often similar to those of FA, and the differential diagnosis is made by chromosome-breakage analysis.

*Diagnosis.* Diagnosis of DKC most often is made during the patient's second or third decade of life, when a history of nail and skin symptoms is combined with marrow failure or malignancy. Definitive diagnosis is made by the absence of chromosomal breakage with DEB testing and the identification of the DKC1 gene on chromosome Xq28.

*Treatment.* HSCT is the only known treatment for DKC. Approximately 20% of patients develop pulmonary complications; therefore, patients undergoing HSCT should not receive busulfan and their lungs must be shielded during radiation. Androgen therapy and splenectomy have been shown to prolong survival, but only by a small margin.

*Prognosis.* DKC survival rates are poor even after HSCT is performed. Death most often occurs because of bone-marrow failure or secondary malignancy when patients are in their twenties. Patients with DKC have a higher incidence of squamous-cell carcinomas and leukemia.

## Pure Red-Cell Aplasia
### Definition
*Pure red-cell aplasia* is the inability of the bone marrow to produce red cells. It is either inherited or acquired. Diamond-Blackfan anemia (DBA) is the inherited form of red-cell aplasia.

There are several acquired forms of red-cell aplasia that are either acute or chronic; some stem from immune-mediated diseases such as lupus and rheumatoid arthritis; viruses such as parvovirus B19, hepatitis, and Epstein-Barr; and drugs such as antiepileptics and sulfonamides. Malignancies and pregnancy also have been associated with red-cell aplasia. The majority of acquired red-cell aplasias occur in adults and are almost always chronic. Acquired red-cell aplasia in children is known as transient erythroblastopenia of childhood (TEC), and it is acute and self-limiting.

### Diamond-Blackfan Anemia
DBA is a rare, chronic, pure red-cell aplasia that usually presents during the first few months of life; 90% of patients with DBA are diagnosed by 9 months of age. Patients with DBA have a cell defect that leads to early cell death of erythroid (RBC) precursors, resulting in severe anemia.

**Incidence and Etiology:** Worldwide, approximately 400 cases of DBA are reported per year. DBA affects all races, but there is a higher incidence in Caucasians. The male-to-female ratio is equal in dominant and sporadic patterns of inheritance but higher in males in the recessive pattern.

**Genetics:** The inheritance pattern of DBA is unclear. In autosomal-dominant DBA cases, males and females are affected equally. Families with recessive inheritance tend to have a greater number of males, suggesting an X-linked pattern, but because this is not true in all cases, the inheritance pattern is not well defined. A large number of patients with DBA have no clear family history, a fact that suggests the presence of a new mutation. Such cases are considered to be sporadic.

A defect in the ribosomal protein gene RPS19 has been implicated in some, but not all, patients with DBA, suggesting that other unidentified genetic mutations are present. The RPS19 gene is located on chromosome 19q13.2. Currently, patients diagnosed with DBA are tested for the presence of an RPS19 mutation, but because the mutation is not present in all cases, it is not considered a diagnostic criterion.

**Clinical Presentation:** Pallor, lethargy, and other signs of anemia in infancy are the most common presenting symptoms of DBA. Anemia may be the only presenting symptom.

Distinct physical anomalies are present in fewer than 50% of patients diagnosed with DBA and include the following:
- Head and neck abnormalities known as "Cathie face," which includes very light blonde hair, snub nose, wide-set eyes, thick upper lip and an "intelligent expression." Other craniofacial abnormalities include cleft lip or palate.
- Hand abnormalities that usually involve the thumbs, which can be triphalangeal, bifid, accessory, absent, or hypoplastic.

These abnormalities can be either unilateral or bilateral.
- Short stature and low birth weight are common findings in patients with DBA.
- Cardiac defects such as aortic stenosis, patent ductus arteriosus, and atrial septal defects have been reported in a small number of cases.
- Genitourinary abnormalities including hypoplastic genitalia, duplicate ureters, and horseshoe kidney.

Although these physical anomalies are distinct and, when combined with anemia, lead to a diagnosis of DBA, more than 50% of patients with DBA still have no physical symptoms.

Laboratory findings include macrocytic (large-cell) anemia in the majority of patients at presentation; however, RBCs may be normal in the early stage of the disease. The median level of hemoglobin at the time of diagnosis is <7 gm/dL. The absence or decreased number of reticulocytes indicates poor RBC production. Many patients with DBA have an increased platelet count (i.e., >400,000/mm$^3$) but platelet size and function are normal. Occasionally mild neutropenia is present. The majority of patients have an increase in fetal hemoglobin, which is a characteristic of "stress erythropoiesis." Bone-marrow aspirate and biopsy shows erythroid hypoplasia or aplasia (absence of RBC precursors).

**Diagnosis:** The majority of patients are diagnosed by the age of 9 months. Diagnosis is made by examination of the peripheral smear, bone-marrow aspirate, and biopsy. The presence of anemia and reticulocytopenia and the absence of erythroid precursors in an otherwise normal bone marrow confirm the diagnosis.

**Treatment:** A large number of patients with DBA respond to steroids; Prednisone is the steroid of choice. A small number of patients have had remission with a short course of steroids but most require chronic steroid use. A slow taper of steroids after response is necessary. Many patients can be maintained on low-dose steroids. HSCT from an HLA-matched sibling is used only after attempts to control DBA with steroids have failed. Chronic RBC transfusions are the mainstay of treatment for many patients with DBA. Chronic transfusion therapy eventually results in iron overload; therefore, chelation therapy is necessary.

**Prognostic Considerations:** HSCT is the only cure for DBA. With advances in transfusion therapy and the use of low-dose steroids, patients can live into their third and fourth decade of life. Death is often the result of complications of iron overload from chronic transfusion therapy or complications of HSCT. There is a higher incidence of leukemia and myelodysplastic syndrome in DBA patients.

## Transient Erythroblastopenia of Childhood

*Transient erythroblastopenia of childhood* (TEC) is an acute, self-limiting anemia caused by decreased erythroid production of the bone marrow that is usually preceded by a viral illness and affects previously healthy children. There is a temporary peripheral reticulocytopenia and anemia with normal white blood cells and platelet lines. The presenting Hgb is usually about 6, reticulocytes are about 1%, and there is a normal MCV.

**Incidence and Etiology:** Because of its transient nature, the true incidence of TEC is unclear, and those who have mild symptoms often are not diagnosed. There are no gender or racial differences. The majority of cases occur in children between ages 1–3 (80%), with the highest incidence at around 23 months; only 10% present after age 3. Most patients (approximately 50%) have a history of a viral illness or have had a vaccination 1–2 months prior to diagnosis. A history of a viral illness suggests an immune-mediated response, but a clear connection has yet to be made. There is no genetic predisposition to TEC.

**Clinical Presentation:** The classic signs of anemia, such as pallor, fatigue, murmur, and tachycardia, are the presenting symptoms. Anemia is usually severe at the time of diagnosis because of the child's ability to compensate for very low levels of hemoglobin. A history taken on presentation often reveals that the child had a respiratory or gastrointestinal virus within the past 1–2 months.

Laboratory findings usually show normocytic anemia with an average hemoglobin of 6.8 gm/dL but the level can range from 2 to 10 gm/dL. RBCs are normal in shape and size, and a reticulocyte count of less than 1% is often present. Bone-marrow aspirates have demonstrated the absence of erythroid precursors, but bone-marrow aspirate and biopsy are not always necessary for diagnosis in the absence of other signs of pancytopenia, physical anomalies, or family history of anemia. Bone-marrow aspirates should be performed only if the anemia persists for more than 2 months.

**Diagnosis:** Diagnosis of TEC is made by the presence of normocytic anemia and the absence of other cytopenias or familial history of anemia.

**Treatment:** Many children who require medical attention for TEC are in the recovery phase at the time of diagnosis, are not experiencing physical distress from anemia, and need only to be observed. The average length of time that anemia persists is 4 weeks. Transfusion therapy is indicated for patients with physical signs of anemia, such as a flow murmur or tachycardia. A single transfusion is often sufficient to relieve symptoms while the disease runs its course.

**Prognosis:** Prognosis for TEC is excellent; TEC resolves spontaneously in about 4–6 weeks without relapse. Although extremely rare, complications of TEC, such as seizures, transient ischemic attacks, and paralysis, are directly related to the severity of the anemia.

## Nursing Assessment and Interventions

### Goal
The patient experiences minimal complications from the disease.

**Assessment:**
- Obtain complete history, including onset of symptoms.
- Assess for signs of bleeding due to thrombocytopenia.
- Assess for fever and other signs of infection and obtain blood cultures if patient is febrile.
- Assess for signs of anemia.
- Review laboratory findings.

**Interventions:**
- If patient is febrile and neutropenic, administer antibiotics immediately.
- Administer blood or platelet transfusions as ordered.
- Monitor laboratory values, especially complete blood count.
- Monitor for increased bleeding and worsening signs of anemia and sepsis.
- Administer prescribed medication regimen as ordered.
- Monitor for side effects of medications.

## Goal
The patient and the family are adequately informed regarding diagnosis, disease, and treatment options.
**Assessment:**
- Assess the patient's and the family's learning styles.
- Assess the patient's and the family's current level of knowledge about the diagnosis.
- Assess the patient's and the family's understanding of the disease's prognosis and treatment options.

**Interventions:**
- Use a communication style that fits the learning style of the patient and the family.
- Provide ongoing instruction and reinforcement of teaching.
- Ensure that the patient and the family understand when and how to contact the healthcare team.
- Ensure that the patient and the family understand signs and symptoms of bleeding, anemia, and infection.
- Ensure that the patient and the family understand the importance of adherence to prescribed medication regimen (e.g., steroids, chelating agents).
- Provide written and verbal information regarding diagnosis and management of illness.
- Emphasize the importance of close follow-up.

## Goal
The patient and the family adjust to diagnosis and prognosis.
**Assessment:**
- Assess the patient's and the family's coping and communication styles.
- Identify the patient's and the family's support systems.
- Assess the patient's and the family's level of coping with the diagnosis and any complications that arise.

**Interventions:**
- Provide ongoing support and education.
- Enlist the help of social workers and psychologists.
- Encourage participation in support groups. Refer the family to national support programs for the various diseases.
- Encourage verbalization of concerns.
- Ensure that support systems are in place if prognosis is grim.

## Expected Patient and Family Outcomes
The child and family can do the following:
- Describe the illness and the treatment options.
- List the possible side effects of treatment.
- Identify signs of bleeding, infection, and anemia.
- Describe available community resources (see **Table 11-3**).
- Demonstrate the skills needed to care for the child at home.
- Explain how and when to contact the healthcare team.

**Table 11-3. Internet Resources for Patients with Bone-Marrow-Failure Syndromes**

Aplastic Anemia & MDS International Foundation, Inc.
www.aamds.org

Fanconi Anemia Research Fund, Inc.
www.fanconi.org

Diamond Blackfan Anemia Foundation, Inc.
www.dbafoundation.org

Diamond Blackfan Anemia Registry
www.dbar.org

National Organization for Rare Disorders, Inc.
www.rarediseases.org

National Cancer Institute: Inherited Bone Marrow Failure
www.marrowfailure.cancer.gov

Clinical Trials Search
www.clinicaltrials.gov

# Shwachman-Diamond Syndrome

*Teresa M. Conte*

## Definition
*Shwachman-Diamond Syndrome* (SDS) is a rare autosomal recessive disease of unknown origin characterized by pancreatic insufficiency, failure to thrive, skeletal abnormalities, and bone-marrow dysfunction.

## Pathophysiology
Patients with SDS have exocrine pancreatic insufficiency in infancy and early childhood. The pancreatic acini cells do not develop and become replaced with fat tissue. The pancreas becomes blocked with fatty tissue, and the digestive enzymes it produces cannot reach the stomach and intestines to assist with digestion. The abnormal functioning of the pancreas leads to malabsorption and malnutrition. As a result of malabsorption, patients develop fatty, foul-smelling stools, stomach pain, and cramping. The condition usually resolves by the age of 4.

Bone-marrow dysfunction is a lifelong component of the disease, with patients experiencing chronic neutropenia. Patients with SDS have neutrophils that can migrate to a site of infection, but once there, they are largely incapable of actually fighting the infection. Recent immunological profiles in patients with SDS have revealed some defects in B cells, T cells, and immunoglobulins. Approximately one third of patients with SDS convert to myelodysplastic syndrome or acute myelogenous leukemia.

## Genetics
The exact cause of SDS is unknown. Scientists have recently discovered a defective gene on chromosome 7 that they believe is responsible for SDS, which has been named the Shwachman-Bodian-Diamond gene.

Although some patients with SDS have immunodeficient expressions, as many as 20% do not, which suggests that there are mutations in the gene that cause variations in some expressions of the disease.

## Incidence and Etiology
SDS occurs in 1 in 20,000 births, is slightly more common in males than in females, and is present in all ethnic groups. It is the second most common cause of pancreatic insufficiency; cystic fibrosis is the most common.

## Clinical Presentation
Infants usually present with weight loss, failure to thrive, diarrhea, steatorrhea, and eczema. Frequent bacterial infections, usually of the respiratory tract and ears, are common. Patients may present with easy bruising, petechiae, bloody emesis, or bloody stools. Webbing of fingers or toes may be present.

## Differential Diagnosis
- Cystic fibrosis
- Pearson syndrome
- Johanson-Blizzard syndrome
- Severe combined immunodeficiency
- Diamond-Blackfan anemia

## Diagnostic
- Complete history and physical exam
- Pancreatic stimulation testing
- Complete blood count with differential
- Serum immunoreactive trypsinogen
- PT/PTT
- Vitamins A, D, and E levels
- Complete metabolic profile
- Seventy-two-hour fecal fat
- Sweat test
- Pancreatic imaging study (ultrasound)
- Bone-marrow aspirate and biopsy with cytogenetics
- Skeletal survey
- Height, weight, and growth.

Expected findings include neutropenia (absolute neutrophil count <1,500 cells/mm$^3$), anemia, thrombocytopenia, pancytopenia, hypocellular bone marrow, negative sweat test, lipid infiltrates in the pancreas, and short height for age.

## Treatment
Symptom management is key for patients with SDS. Malabsorption is treated with pancreatic enzyme replacement. Enzyme replacement is temporary, and patients are usually able to discontinue replacement by age 4 due to the gradual return of a fully functional pancreas.

Fat-soluble vitamins are administered. Neutropenia is treated prophylactically with granulocyte-colony stimulating factors as needed. Prophylactic antibiotics are used occasionally but not widely. Although patients with SDS have a short stature, their growth velocity is normal, so growth hormone replacement is not given. Patients with SDS are prone to dental caries and hypomaturation of teeth, so yearly dental visits are recommended.

## Follow-Up
The patient should be followed by pediatric hematology, oncology, and gastrointestinal providers. Orthopedic and endocrine consults are obtained as needed.

Follow-up should take place every month for the first 1–3 months to assess the efficacy of the treatment plan and to provide anticipatory guidance.

The patient should be reevaluated every 6–12 months. Weight and height measurements should be obtained, and a complete history and physical examination, including developmental assessment, should be completed. A complete blood count with differential, PTT, and complete metabolic panel should be drawn.

Every 1–2 years, fecal fat analysis should be performed to ensure that the functioning of the pancreas has returned to normal. Bone-marrow biopsies with cytogenetics should be done to determine any potential progression to aplastic anemia, myelodysplastic syndrome (MDS), or acute myelogenous leukemia (AML), which increase in incidence after age 10. Sixteen percent of SDS patients progress to MDS or AML. In these cases, allogeneic bone-marrow transplant is the treatment.

## Nursing Assessment and Interventions

### Assessment
- Perform a complete assessment, including vital signs, height, weight, head circumference, and overall appearance.
- Assess the patient's nutritional status, review laboratory values, and interview caregivers about the patient's daily nutritional intake and bladder and bowel habits.
- Assess the patient's developmental level, and consider normal milestones for the patient's age group.
- Assess the caregiver's understanding of SDS, including complications and symptom management.
- If the patient is receiving medications for pancreatic enzyme replacement or colony stimulating factor, assess the caregiver's knowledge of the medications and their comfort level for administering them.
- Assess the patient's and caregiver's ability to cope with the SDS diagnosis.

### Interventions
- Obtain any necessary laboratory work or stool specimens.
- Review patient's nutritional goals with caregivers and provide suggestions for meeting these goals. Provide referral to a pediatric nutritionist if necessary.
- Provide information on infection control. Offer tips to caregivers for prevention of infections during periods of neutropenia. Explain the importance of contacting the healthcare provider if the patient develops a fever or infection.
- Provide information to caregivers about pancreatic enzyme replacement. Stress the importance of compliance with therapy, and offer suggestions on administering and storing the enzymes.
- Provide information on support groups and Internet resources for patients with SDS. Provide information to caregivers regarding a social worker or case manager who can assist with coping and insurance issues.

### Expected Patient and Family Outcomes
- The patient and the family understand the diagnosis and treatment of SDS.
- The patient and the family understand the importance of compliance with symptom management of SDS.
- The patient and the family are compliant with the SDS treatment and will monitor for any adverse effects of the disease or its treatment.

### Additional Resources
- www.shwachman-diamond.org
- www.shwachmandiamondamerica.org

## Chronic Neutropenia

*Karyn J. Brundige*

### Definition
*Neutrophils*, which are also called polys, bands, segs, and granulocytes, are phagocytic white blood cells capable of engulfing and destroying microorganisms. *Neutropenia* is a decrease in the number of neutrophils in the blood and is defined as an absolute neutrophil count (ANC) of less than 1,500 cells/mm$^3$.

The ANC is calculated by multiplying the total white blood cell count (WBCC) by the percentage of neutrophils and bands in the differential. Normal ANC levels vary with age and race; infants have lower ANCs than older children, and individuals of African origin have lower ANCs than Caucasians.

Neutropenia is often classified as mild (ANC 1,000–1,500), moderate (ANC 500–1,000) or severe (ANC <500). Mild-to-moderate neutropenia is associated with an increased risk of developing mild bacterial infections of the skin and mucous membranes. The risk of serious and even life-threatening bacterial infection (e.g., pneumonia, sepsis) increases with the duration and severity of neutropenia. Children with neutropenia are not at increased risk for viral or parasitic infections. Chronic neutropenia is defined as neutropenia lasting longer than 3 months.

### Pathophysiology
Neutropenia may exist from birth (congenital) or develop during life (acquired). Neutropenia may result from malignancy (e.g., acute lymphoblastic leukemia) or hematologic disease (e.g., aplastic anemia), as a side effect of medication or irradiation, or as a symptom of an infectious (e.g., HIV), immunologic (e.g., parvovirus, systemic lupus erythematosus), or metabolic disorder (e.g., Shwachman-Diamond syndrome).

Neutrophils are produced in the bone marrow and released into the bloodstream, where approximately half of the neutrophils freely circulate while the remainder adheres to the vascular surface. In response to acute inflammation, neutrophils migrate from the blood vessels to the site of inflammation by a process termed chemotaxis. Neutrophils survive for only 1–2 days and have an average half-life of 8 hours. Neutropenia occurs when there is either decreased neutrophil production by the bone marrow or increased peripheral destruction. Increased peripheral destruction occurs as a result of the depletion of neutrophil reserves secondary to severe infection or as a result of immune destruction (i.e., the presence of antineutrophil antibodies).

This subsection describes several forms of chronic neutropenia, including severe congenital neutropenia (including Kostmann syndrome), cyclic neutropenia, autoimmune neutropenia, and chronic benign (i.e., idiopathic) neutropenia. Shwachman-Diamond syndrome is discussed in a separate subsection.

### Incidence
Chronic neutropenia is a rare hematologic disorder. Although the true incidence is unknown, estimates indicate approximately 1 case per 200,000 people.

### Clinical Presentation
Often neutropenia is first discovered when a child presents with recurrent fever or infection.

A complete review of systems should focus on the frequency, duration, and severity of infection. Typical signs of infection, such as warmth and swelling, may be absent. A family history of chronic infections or sudden death, especially in infancy, may be an indication of an inherited disorder.

Physical examination should evaluate for the presence of the following:
- Oral mucosa—aphthous ulcers, thrush, periodontal disease (e.g., gingivitis)
- Skin—impetigo, cellulitis, boils, abscesses
- Ears, nose, and throat—upper respiratory infections (e.g., otitis media, sinus infections)
- Lungs—cough, tacyhpnea, adventitious breath sounds, low oxygen saturation
- Gastrointestinal—perirectal and perineal erythema, tenderness, rashes, abscesses
- Lymph nodes—adenopathy, tenderness, erythema

### Diagnosis
The extent of laboratory workup generally depends on the clinical severity and frequency of infections rather than the severity of neutropenia.
- Serial complete blood counts (CBCs): Assess severity and duration of neutropenia; WBCC may be decreased or within normal range; monocytosis and eosinophilia may occur; hemoglobin and platelets are usually normal.
- Bone-marrow evaluation: Exclude malignancy; assess for extent of myeloid differentiation and cytogenetic (i.e., chromosomal) abnormalities.
- Test for possible genetic mutations if indicated.
- Test for neutrophil antibodies if indicated.

### Fever Evaluation
All febrile (temperature of >38.3 °C or 101 °F) children with a history of chronic neutropenia require comprehensive evaluation, including the following:
- History and physical examination (per guidelines listed previously)
- CBC and differential
- Blood cultures

- Urinalysis and urine culture
- Stool culture if diarrhea is present
- Chest X ray if respiratory symptoms are present.

## Treatment

The need for medical intervention depends upon the degree and duration of neutropenia and the incidence of severe infections. Although most forms of chronic neutropenia are responsive to recombinant human granulocyte colony stimulating factor (GCSF; e.g., filgrastim), treatment with GCSF is usually reserved for children with recurrent or severe infections. The dose and frequency of GCSF required to maintain the ANC at >1,000 varies widely; 5–20 mcg/kg/day is usually adequate. Some children, however, may require doses as high as 120 mcg/kg/day, whereas others require only 0.01 mcg/kg/day, or less-than-daily injections.

Severe infections that must be treated aggressively and frequently require inpatient hospital admission for observation and intravenous administration of antibiotics. Antibiotic prophylaxis is discouraged because of the risk for development of resistant organisms. WBC (granulocyte) transfusions are used rarely and only for life-threatening infections, because of both the difficulty in collecting the cells as well as the short life span of mature neutrophils.

## Prognostic Considerations

The majority of children with chronic neutropenia are able to participate in normal activities. In addition to infection, however, chronic neutropenia can predispose children to specific oral and orthopedic complications. Gingivitis and periodontal disease are associated with prolonged neutropenia and may be indications for initiating or adjusting GCSF therapy. Bone demineralization, apparently from underlying disease and not as a result of GCSF therapy, can occur with severe osteopenia or osteoporosis that may increase the risk for fractures. The use of calcium and vitamin D supplements, weight-bearing exercise, and pamidronate (biphosphonate) infusions have been used to prevent and reverse the degree of osteopenia and osteoporosis in children with chronic neutropenia.

A subgroup of children with severe congenital neutropenia and specific genetic mutations have an increased lifetime risk of developing myleodysplastic syndrome (MDS) or acute myelogenous leukemia (AML). New genetic abnormalities, including monosomy 7 and trisomy 21, may precede morphologic abnormalities. These children, therefore, should be monitored with annual bone-marrow aspirate and cytogenetic analysis.

## Congenital Neutropenia

### Severe Congenital Neutropenia

**Definition:** *Severe congenital neutropenia* (SCN) is a heterogeneous group of genetic disorders characterized by ineffective myelopoesis resulting in a selective decrease in the number of mature circulating neutrophils (neutropenia). Dr. Rolf Kostmann first described an inherited form of neutropenia in 1956, reporting on several members of a consanguineous family in Sweden experiencing severe neutropenia, recurrent infections, and, frequently, death in early infancy.

**Pathophysiology and Genetics:** A genetic mutation, either inherited or sporadic, results in impaired myeloid differentiation with few neutrophils maturing beyond the myelocyte stage in the bone marrow (maturation arrest). The resulting neutropenia is generally severe, often with an ANC <100, and is associated with chronic oropharyngeal inflammation, recurrent fevers, and severe infections.

SCN is a genetically heterogeneous disease. Although approximately 30% of SCN, including those of the original Kostmann pedigree, have an autosomal recessive inheritance, the majority of cases (60%) arise as a result of a new autosomal dominant mutation.

*Autosomal-recessive neutropenia (Kostmann syndrome).* Homozygous mutations occur in the HAX-1 gene on chromosome 1. Mutation results in a deficiency of HAX-1, a mitochondrial protein that protects myeloid cells from apoptosis (i.e., programmed cell death).

*Autosomal-dominant neutropenia.* Heterozygous mutations occur in ELA-2, which encodes for neutrophil elastase (elastase mutations). Neutrophil elastase is a protease (enzyme) that is produced during myelopoesis and primarily stored in the granules of neutrophils. The exact pathologic mechanism of the mutated protein remains unclear, but the cellular mechanism appears to be accelerated apoptosis of myeloid progenitor cells.

Less common genetic defects that cause congenital neutropenia have been reported, including rare cases of sex-linked (male) inheritance in a neutropenic variant of Wiscott-Aldrich syndrome and germ-line mutations of the GCSF receptor, which result in severe neutropenia that is resistant to GCSF therapy.

**Incidence:** SCN is a rare hematologic disorder with a frequency estimated at fewer than 1 per 200,000 people.

**Clinical Presentation:** Children present during the first few months of life with fever and recurrent severe bacterial infections, including omphalitis, cellulitis, and perirectal abscess.

**Diagnosis:**
- Serial CBCs: severe neutropenia with ANC <500 and frequently <100
- Bone-marrow evaluation: no evidence of developing neutrophils beyond the promyelocyte/myelocyte stage; annual bone marrow and cytogenetics are used for monitoring for preleukemic transformation
- Genetic testing for possible mutations.

**Treatment:** More than 90% of children with Kostmann syndrome respond to GCSF with an ANC >1,000, although relatively large doses (>8 mcg/kg/day) are required for some children. Bone-marrow transplant from a matched sibling has been successful and is the only curative option.

**Prognostic Considerations:** Before GCSF use, median survival was only 3 years due to death from sepsis and pneumonia. With improved survival as a result of GCSF, MDS and AML have emerged as significant complications. The progression to leukemia appears to begin in the genetic mutation responsible for the neutropenia, which then evolves into GCSF-receptor mutations, monosomy 7, ras oncogene mutations, and, finally, malignancy. MDS or AML arises almost exclusively in the subset of patients with SCN whose illness is caused by ELA-2 mutations; these patients also have lower neutrophil counts and require higher doses of GCSF to achieve a clinical response.

## Cyclic Neutropenia

### Definition
*Cyclic neutropenia* is another type of congenital neutropenia. As the name indicates, this disease is characterized by periodic neutropenia occurring in a 21-day cycle, during which the nadir ANC approaches zero and the peak ANC is normal or near normal. Monocytes cycle but do so in a phase opposite to that of neutrophils. Cyclic neutropenia is also known as cyclic hematopoiesis, because other blood cells, such as platelets or RBCs, may also cycle in recurrent oscillations.

### Pathophysiology
Cyclic neutropenia occurs as a result of fluctuating rates of cell production by the bone-marrow stem cells. Unlike other causes of neutropenia, in this disorder, the appearance of the bone marrow fluctuates during the cycle between a normal appearance and that of severe maturation arrest of neutrophil production. Although all children with cyclic neutropenia have periods of severe neutropenia, the duration varies; some have a low ANC during the entire cycle while others are neutropenic for only a few days.

The most common bacterial infections are of the oral mucosa (e.g., aphthous stomatitis, periodontis) and the upper-respiratory tract (e.g., otitis media, sinusitis). Unlike SCN, life-threatening infections (e.g., sepsis, pneumonia) are infrequent. The severity of bacterial infections correlates with the duration of the neutropenic nadir. Children with cyclic neutropenia show an increased vulnerability to infection with anaerobic bacteria, a fact that suggests impairment in neutrophil function, not just in neutrophil count.

### Genetics
Genetic transmission is autosomal dominant. As with other dominant disorders, sporadic cases commonly arise from new germ-line mutations. Heterozygous mutations of the ELA-2 gene encoding neutrophil elastase (elastase mutations)—genetically similar to the mutations found in autosomal dominant SCN—are responsible for many cases of cyclic neutropenia. The pathologic mechanism of the mutated protein remains unclear.

### Incidence
Cyclic neutropenia is a rare hematological disorder with a frequency estimated at fewer than 1 per 1,000,000 people.

### Clinical Presentation
Although present from birth, the presentation of cyclical neutropenia tends to occur later than that of SCN because the infections are generally less severe. Children typically present with a history of recurrent fever, mouth ulcers, and an excessive number of typical childhood upper-respiratory-tract infections. More severe cases may also include episodes of perirectal cellulitis, pneumonia, or sepsis.

### Diagnosis
Cyclic neutropenia should be considered if infections, especially of the oral mucosa, occur frequently and in 3-week intervals. Serial CBCs, performed at least three times a week for 6 weeks, confirm the cyclical pattern of neutropenia. Marrow examination may show either normal hematopoiesis or maturational arrest in neutrophil production, depending on the timing within the cycle. Genetic testing for elastase mutations may be useful for confirming the diagnosis.

### Treatment
Most cases of cyclic neutropenia respond to 2–3 mcg/kg of GCSF administered every 1–3 days. GCSF does not prevent cycling but does reduce infectious complications by shortening both the cycle length and the duration of neutropenia.

### Prognostic Considerations
Although similar ELA-2 mutations are identified in both cyclic neutropenia and autosomal-dominant SCN, children with cyclic neutropenia are not at increased risk for myeloid malignancies.

## Acquired Neutropenia

### Autoimmune Neutropenia
**Definition:** *Autoimmune neutropenia* (AIN) is a rare disorder caused by increased destruction of neutrophils as a result of autoantibodies directed against neutrophil-specific antigens. AIN is the most common cause of neutropenia in children age 6 months through 4 years.

**Pathophysiology:** An antibody is a protein used by the immune system to identify and neutralize foreign objects such as bacteria and viruses. Each antibody recognizes a specific antigen unique to its target. In autoimmune conditions, the body produces autoantibodies against a protein that normally occurs in the body. Under normal conditions, these antigens are not the target of the immune system. In autoimmune neutropenia, the body makes antibodies against the antigens or proteins on the surface of neutrophils. The body's immune system then attacks its own neutrophils, causing increased destruction. Although neutrophil destruction most commonly occurs in the peripheral blood, targeted granulocytes also may be removed in the bone marrow.

Primary AIN is most commonly seen in children between the ages of 6 months and 4 years; more than 75% of cases occur in children younger than age 3. The etiology is unknown, but there is a possible association with parvovirus B19 infection. Secondary AIN may be associated with autoimmune disorders such as systemic lupus erythematosus or autoimmune lymphoproliferative syndrome. There is no known genetic predisposition to AIN.

Infections are usually mild to moderate; serious infections are uncommon. The neutrophil count may temporarily rise to normal levels during an acute infection.

**Incidence:** AIN is more frequent than SCN, with an incidence of approximately 1 in 100,000 or higher.

**Clinical Presentation:** The majority of children present with mild but chronic infections of the skin and upper-respiratory tract. Physical examination is usually unremarkable; some children present with mild splenomegaly.

**Diagnosis:** Neutropenia may be found only by chance. Daily ANC counts may vary considerably with nadirs less than 500 but without the regular oscillations associated with cyclic neutropenia. Specialized laboratories can perform immunological blood tests for neutrophil-specific antibodies. Because the antibody titer (level) may be quite low, several tests may be required for definitive diagnosis.

Bone-marrow examination is usually not performed if the antibody screen is positive. If it is performed, the bone marrow may show maturational arrest with adequate numbers of early myeloid cells but fewer mature cells. Bone-marrow cytogenetics are normal.

**Treatment:** Children with AIN rarely require treatment for neutropenia. High-dose corticosteroids, intravenous immunoglobulin (IVIG), or GCSF may be administered to temporarily increase the ANC for elective surgery or severe invasive infection. GCSF is the preferred agent due to positive response rates (i.e., 100% for GCSF, 75% for steroids, and 50% for IVIG), specificity, and toxicity profile. Chronic GCSF administration is rarely warranted. Infections usually respond to antibiotics. Prophylaxis is considered in younger children with frequent otitis media to prevent tissue damage.

**Prognostic Considerations:** Spontaneous remission occurs in more than 95% of childhood AIN, usually within 2 years of diagnosis. Disappearance of autoantibodies precedes normalization of the neutrophil count. The detected antibody titer is predictive of both infectious complications and time to remission.

## Chronic Benign (Nonimmune) Neutropenia

**Definition:** A diagnosis of exclusion is used to describe children with chronic neutropenia lacking evidence of immune-mediated disease (i.e., autoneutrophil antibody negative), nutritional deficiency, or myelodysplasia.

**Pathophysiology:** The pathophysiology of the disease is unclear and may be a result of decreased neutrophil production in the bone marrow, excessive neutrophil adherence to the vascular surface (margination), or increased peripheral destruction. A hypothesized etiology is an undiagnosed, underlying inflammatory illness with increased production of cytokines.

**Clinical Presentation:** In the majority of children, chronic benign neutropenia is identified from routine laboratory tests in the absence of any history of infection or other symptoms. When they do occur, they are generally mild and include skin infections, upper-respiratory infections, and diarrhea. Abnormal physical findings are uncommon.

**Diagnosis:** ANC is generally less than 500 but may oscillate; the remainder of the blood count is normal. The bone-marrow findings are generally unremarkable. Although cellularity and degree of maturational arrest may vary, cytogenetics are normal.

**Treatment:** Children with chronic benign neutropenia typically have few severe infections. GCSF or antibiotic prophylaxis is rarely required.

**Prognostic Considerations:** Spontaneous remission within 2 years of diagnosis is common.

## Nursing Assessment and Interventions

The nurse must be knowledgeable about the signs and symptoms of neutropenia and be able to perform a comprehensive history and assessment that focuses on signs of infection (see the discussion under "Clinical Presentation"). Nursing interventions for a child with chronic neutropenia are as follows and depend on the risk and severity of bacterial infection, presence of infectious, comorbid complications, and plan for medical intervention:

- Monitor for complications related to neutropenia (i.e., observe for signs and symptoms of septic shock).
- Protect the child from exposure to infection by advising the child and the family to take the following measures:
  - Maintain good general hygiene, including daily bathing and frequent hand washing.
  - Maintain good oral hygiene, including using antibacterial mouthwash and having regular dental checkups.
  - Remain up to date with routine childhood immunizations.
  - Decrease the child's exposure to individuals with serious infections.
  - Do not use rectal thermometers or suppositories.
- Teach families about neutropenia:
  - Instruct family members about how to protect the child from infection (as previously described).
  - Teach family members to monitor for signs and symptoms of infection.
  - Instruct parents to notify their physician or a responsible healthcare provider immediately if the child develops a fever higher than 38.3°C (101°F) or any signs of infection.
  - Teach families about required laboratory monitoring, including frequency of CBCs and bone-marrow tests.
- Teach families about medical therapies:
  - GCSF administration: Instruct family members about proper administration of GCSF, including sterile technique and rotation of sites to prevent scarring.
  - Antibiotics: Reinforce instructions to complete the entire course of oral antibiotics as prescribed to adequately prevent or treat infection and minimize the development of resistant microorganisms.

## Expected Patient and Family Outcomes

- The child and the family are knowledgeable about neutropenia, the signs and symptoms of infection, and ways to avoid exposure to infection.
- The child has minimal complications related to the neutropenia.

## Additional Resources

- The Neutropenia Support Association, Inc., is a charity that was founded in 1989 to increase awareness and understanding of neutropenia; the Web site contains links to many articles about neutropenia. www.neutropenia.ca/.
- The Severe Chronic Neutropenia International Registry was established in 1994 to collect data for monitoring the clinical course, treatments, and disease outcomes for children and adults with severe chronic neutropenia. http://depts.washington.edu/registry.
- *Understanding severe chronic neutropenia: A handbook for patients and their families* (written for the SCNIR). www99.mh-hannover.de/kliniken/paed_haemonko/scn/handbooks/handbook_en.pdf.

# Immune Thrombocytopenic Purpura

*Phaedra Truglia*

## Definition

*Immune thrombocytopenic purpura* (ITP), also known as idiopathic thrombocytopenic purpura, is a bleeding disorder characterized by decreased platelets. This disease occurs when the immune system produces antibodies against platelets, destroying them primarily within the spleen. It may be classified into acute and chronic categories based on duration rather than clinical findings. Acute ITP is defined as complete resolution of thrombocytopenia within 6 months of onset. Chronic ITP may be defined by the presence of thrombocytopenia for longer than 6 months.

## Pathophysiology

The cause of ITP in children is not known. ITP often follows a recent viral infection; can be drug-induced (e.g., by alcohol, heparin, quinine/quinidine, or sulfonamides); and, in the case of chronic ITP, can be caused by immune disorders (e.g., systemic lupus erythematosus, HIV).

## Incidence and Etiology

ITP is generally considered to be a benign disorder in children. In acute ITP, distribution is relatively equal between males and females. The average age of presentation is between 1–10 years, with a peak incidence between the ages of 2–4 years. Most cases have been found to occur during the winter months.

## Clinical Presentation

- Bruising, petechiae, and/or purpura
- Oral and gingival bleeding
- Epistaxis
- Menorrhagia (in adolescent females)
- Hematuria
- Evidence of intracranial hemorrhage, with possible neurological symptoms
- Signs of gastrointestinal (GI) bleeding
- Thrombocytopenia with no other abnormality in blood counts
- History of recent illness, usually of viral etiology

## Diagnosis

There is no single diagnostic test or study that independently confirms the diagnosis of ITP. Few diagnostic studies other than the history, physical examination (enlarged lymph nodes or spleen), complete blood count, and examination of the blood smear are necessary, provided the patient has isolated thrombocytopenia. Tests used to help with the diagnosis of ITP include the following:

- Complete blood count showing a low platelet count (normal is 150,000/mm$^3$) and mildly elevated platelet size.
- Bone-marrow examination is indicated only if the history, physical examination, blood count (neutropenia, anemia), or blood film is atypical. Bone-marrow aspiration or biopsy appears normal in ITP.
- PTT (coagulation studies) is normal.
- PT (coagulation studies) is normal.
- Platelet-associated antibodies may be detected (predominantly IgG, but IgM and IgA types have also been described).
- Autoimmune screen may be helpful in chronic cases (particularly in adolescent girls).
- A computed tomography scan of the head is warranted if concern exists regarding intracranial hemorrhage.

## Treatment

The treatment of ITP depends on the severity of platelet reduction in the blood. In children, the disease often runs its course without treatment. The main reason for treating children with acute ITP is to prevent intracranial hemorrhage. The treatment of ITP may include the following:

- Observing and monitoring platelet counts (usually with platelets >30,000/mm$^3$)
- Stopping medications that are thought to cause ITP or interfere with platelet function (e.g., aspirin, ibuprofen, and warfarin)
- Treating infections
- Using drug therapy, which may include corticosteroids, Whinrho (anti-D globulin), intravenous gammaglobulin (IVIG), and/or 6-mercaptopurine.
- Splenectomy may be recommended in some instances, because the spleen is the major site of platelet destruction.

## Prognostic Considerations

In some children, the disease often runs its course without treatment. Approximately 83% of children have a spontaneous remission. Fifty percent of children recover in 3 to 4 weeks, 75% in 6 months, and 90% within 12 months. Approximately 2% of patients die.

## Nursing Assessment and Interventions

### Goal

The patient experiences minimal or no bleeding related to ITP.

**Assessment:**
- Assess the presenting symptoms and obtain a complete history (including recent viral infections or illnesses and medications).
- Assess for physical signs of bleeding such as increased bruising, petechiae, epistaxis, neurological changes, and occult blood in urine, stool, and emesis.
- Review laboratory findings.
- Review radiological imaging studies as indicated.
- Review vital signs.

**Interventions:**
- Monitor vital signs frequently (vital signs that may signify increased bleeding include increased heart rate, decreased blood pressure, or both).
- Keep venipunctures, intramuscular injections, and invasive procedures to a minimum.
- Provide instructions on proper mouth care (i.e., use a soft toothbrush or sponge).

### Goal

The patient remains without injury.

**Interventions:**
- Encourage quiet activities. No "rough play."
- Use bedside rails at all times, if hospitalized, to prevent falls.
- Pad crib sides or bedside rails, if hospitalized.
- Assist and supervise child when ambulating.

### Goal

The patient experiences minimal complications or side effects related to treatment.

**Assessment:**
- Assess for side effects related to corticosteroids (e.g., weight gain, change in behavior, GI irritation, metabolic reactions, and cushingoid effects) if indicated.
- Assess for side effects related to IVIG (e.g., fever or chills, nausea or vomiting, urticaria, headaches, hypertension, and generalized malaise) if indicated.
- Assess for side effects related to Whinrho (hemoglobinemia) if indicated.
- Assess for side effects related to 6-mercaptopurine (nausea or vomiting, rash, diarrhea, stomatitis) if indicated.
- Assess for complications related to any surgery performed (e.g., splenectomy).
- Assess for a response to therapy.
- Review laboratory findings.

**Interventions:**
- Provide medication to help alleviate side effects related to treatment.
- Provide comfort measures.
- Educate the patient and the family about potential side effects related to treatment.

### Goal
The patient and the family are adequately informed regarding diagnosis, disease, and treatment.

**Assessment:**
- Assess the patient's and the family's level of knowledge about the diagnosis and disease.
- Assess the patient's and the family's level of knowledge regarding treatment.
- Assess the patient's and the family's learning styles.
- Assess the patient's and the family's understanding of compliance and follow-up.

**Interventions:**
- Communicate with the patient and the family in an appropriate manner.
- Provide the patient and the family with appropriate educational resources and review the material with them (using information sheets from the Internet or the institution, if available).
- Ensure that the family is aware of how and when to call the primary-care provider.
- Encourage the patient and the family to ask questions related to diagnosis, disease, and treatment.
- Emphasize close outpatient follow-up care.
- Emphasize the importance of contacting the physician before changing medications that may increase the risk for ITP or bleeding.

## Expected Patient and Family Outcomes
The patient and the family can do the following:
- Describe ITP.
- Describe how ITP can be treated.
- List the possible side effects (if any) of treatment.
- Describe the schedule of treatment, procedures (if any), and follow-up care.
- Describe the community resources available to them.
- Explain the signs of increased bleeding and how to manage symptoms at home.
- Demonstrate their ability and knowledge regarding when to contact the healthcare team if problems or questions arise.

# Evans Syndrome
*Karyn Brundige*

## Definition
*Evans syndrome* is an uncommon hematologic disorder defined by the simultaneous or sequential combination of autoimmune hemolytic anemia (AIHA) and immune thrombocytopenia-purpura (ITP) in the absence of known underlying etiology; in approximately half of the cases, autoimmune neutropenia also occurs. Dr. Robert Evans and colleagues first described a group of 24 patients with these clinical characteristics in 1951. The disorder has also been termed immune pancytopenia.

## Pathophysiology
Although Evans syndrome appears to be a disorder of both humoral and cellular immune regulation, the exact pathophysiology remains unknown. Hypogammaglobulinemia and other autoimmune problems have been reported in some cases

Autoantibodies may be produced against antigens (proteins) on the surface of erythrocytes, platelets, or neutrophils; the antibodies are cell-type specific and do not cross-react. Immune destruction of red cells, platelets, or neutrophils generally occurs in the peripheral circulation, though targeted cells may also be removed in the bone marrow. Blood-cell production in the marrow (i.e., myelopoeisis) generally compensates for the normal rate of peripheral-cell destruction. If immune destruction occurs at a faster rate than marrow production, peripheral blood levels decrease, resulting in cytopenias.

## Incidence
Evans syndrome is a rare diagnosis; the exact incidence is unknown.

## Clinical Presentation
Children usually present with AIHA or ITP separately or concomitantly. Neutropenia occurs in approximately 50% of cases. The development of the second immune cytopenia may occur months to years after the first cytopenia, thereby delaying diagnosis.

Presenting symptoms of AIHA include pallor, fatigue, jaundice, and, if AIHA is severe, cardiopulmonary failure. Thrombocytopenia is evidenced by petechiae, bruising, and mucutaneous bleeding. Invasive bacterial infections such as sepsis, meningitis, pneumonia, or osteomyelitis may occur if neutropenia is severe. Lymphadenopathy and hepatosplenomegaly may be chronic or intermittent; occasionally it is apparent only during acute exacerbations.

A complete review of systems should focus on signs and symptoms of anemia, hemolysis, thrombocytopenia, and neutropenia, including the frequency, duration, and severity of bleeding and infection:
- General—change in behavior, fatigue, inactivity, malaise

- Skin—pallor, jaundice, bruising, petechiae, purpura
- Ears, nose, and throat—bleeding from the gums or nose; pharyngitis, purulent discharge, sinus tenderness
- Cardiopulmonary—palpitations, dyspnea, dizziness, cough
- Genitourinary—hemoglobinuria (i.e., dark or tea-colored urine); blood in urine, stool, or emesis
- Nervous system—headaches, dizziness, change in level of consciousness.

Physical examination should evaluate for the presence of the following:

- Skin and oral mucosa—pinkness of nail beds, conjunctiva, mucous membranes, and lips; bruising, petechiae, purpura; impetigo, cellulitis, boils, or abscesses; aphthous ulcers, thrush, or periodontal disease
- Eyes—scleral jaundice, scleral bleeding
- Ears, nose, and throat—upper-respiratory infections (e.g., otitis media, sinus infections)
- Heart—tachycardia, cardiac-flow murmurs, hypotension
- Lungs—tachypnea, adventitious breath sounds, hypoxia (i.e., low oxygen saturation); tacyhpnea
- Gastrointestinal—splenomegaly, hepatomegaly; perirectal and perineal erythema, tenderness, rashes or abscesses; blood in stool or emesis
- Genitourinary—blood in urine
- Lymph nodes—adenopathy, tenderness, erythema
- Nervous system—paresthesia, mental activity, and ability studies and to concentrate.

## Diagnosis

Evans syndrome is a diagnosis of exclusion. Other disorders that may present with autoimmune cytopenias (e.g., infections, rheumatologic diseases, malignancies) must be ruled out. Diagnostic studies and tests include

- Complete blood count: anemia, thrombocytopenia, neutropenia, or combined cytopenias; in AIHA, the blood smear may show polychromasia and spherocytes
- Studies consistent with acute hemolysis: elevated reticulocyte count, unconjugated hyperbilirubinemia, and decreased haptoglobin
- Direct Coombs test (direct antiglobulin test): often positive even in the absence of AIHA; may be positive for IgG or complement (C3)
- Antibodies (antierythrocyte, antiplatelet, and antineutrophil): may be positive, but negative test does not exclude the diagnosis
- Serum immunoglobulins and immunoglobulin subclasses: exclude immune deficiencies (e.g., IgA deficiency, common variable immunodeficiency) and use as a baseline prior to immunotherapy
- Antinuclear antibody, double-stranded DNA, and rheumatoid factor: exclude other autoimmune conditions, especially systemic lupus erythematosus
- Bone-marrow evaluation: exclude infiltrative malignancy or aplastic anemia
- Peripheral blood T-cell subsets by flow cytometry: exclude autoimmune lymphoproliferative syndrome (ALPS; see the discussion that follows).

## Autoimmune Lymphoproliferative Syndrome

Recent studies have shown that as many as 50% of patients previously diagnosed with Evans syndrome have autoimmune cytopenias secondary to ALPS. ALPS is a rare disorder that presents in early childhood and is characterized by abnormal lymphocyte survival (defective apoptosis). The majority of patients with ALPS have genetic mutations in the FAS gene; children with Evans syndrome do not have these mutations.

## Treatment

Children with severe anemia or thrombocytopenia require stabilization of cardiopulmonary function; blood or platelet transfusion may be required. Medical management of Evans syndrome is challenging; the syndrome is characterized by periods of both spontaneous and treatment-induced remission and frequent exacerbations. No evidence-based guidelines have been established regarding when to initiate treatment, and no prospective randomized controlled studies for determining optimal treatment regimens have been conducted.

### First-Line Therapy

- Corticosteroids: prednisone 1–4 mg/kg/day; after counts stabilize, wean dose over several weeks
- Intravenous immunoglobulin (IVIG): total of 2 gm/kg in divided doses; higher doses do not usually increase response rate
- Considerations:
  - Steroids are often used as first-line therapy, and IVIG is reserved for patients who fail to respond; relapse occurs when steroids are weaned or patient becomes steroid dependent.
  - IVIG may be preferable to steroids for children younger than 2 years of age for decreasing risk of infection or growth suppression.
  - Thrombocytopenia is generally more responsive to IVIG; AIHA is generally more responsive to steroids.
  - Many patients initially respond to first-line agents but then relapse and require second-line therapy.

### Second-Line Therapy

- Immunosuppressive agents: cyclosporine, mycophenolate mofetil, danazol
- Rituximab (chimeric monoclonal antibody)
- Vincristine
- Splenectomy
- Considerations:
  - Minimal data exist to assist in selection of second-line therapy; age of patient, severity of disease, and short- and long-term side effects of treatment must be considered.
  - Multiagent therapy is often more effective than single-agent therapy.
  - Rituximab induces remission in the majority of patients, but relapse is common 6–12 months after treatment; patients may respond to repeat doses.

### Third-Line Therapy

- Cyclophosphamide
- Alemtuzumab (monoclonal antibody)

- Vincristine-loaded platelets (i.e., platelets harvested by pheresis from healthy ABO-compatible donor, incubated with 5 mg vincristine; excess vincristine removed and platelets resuspended and infused over 30 minutes
- Stem-cell transplant (SCT)
- Considerations:
  – Third-line therapy is reserved for patients with severe relapsing disease despite second-line therapy.
  – SCT may be the only therapy to offer long-term remission (i.e., cure); limited data suggest that allogeneic transplant with human leukocyte antigen-identical donor is superior to autologous SCT; risk of morbidity and transplant-related mortality are high.

## Prognostic Considerations

Unlike most cases of ITP or AIHA that occur in childhood, the clinical course of Evans syndrome is usually chronic, with frequent exacerbations and remissions; occasionally it is fatal. Episodes of ITP appear to occur more frequently and are more difficult to control than AIHA. Long-term survival data are limited; small studies (e.g., a total of 75 patients) have shown mortality rates of 7%–36% with death mainly related to hemorrhage (e.g., gastrointestinal, intracranial) or invasive infection (e.g., pneumonia, sepsis, meningitis). Despite the degree of immune dysfunction, no children in these long-term studies have developed malignancy.

## Nursing Assessment and Interventions

The nurse must be knowledgeable about the signs and symptoms of anemia, thrombocytopenia, and neutropenia, and be able to perform a comprehensive history and assessment focusing on signs of anemia, hemolysis, bleeding, and infection (see the discussion under "Clinical Presentation"). Nursing interventions for a child with Evans syndrome depend on the risk and severity of anemia, bleeding, and bacterial infection and the plan for medical intervention.
- Observe laboratory data for evidence of a decrease in hemoglobin, platelet count, or neutrophil count, and notify the healthcare team.
- Monitor for complications related to anemia:
  – Assess skin for pallor and decreased capillary refill.
  – Assess for decreased energy, fatigue, lethargy, or irritability.
  – Assess for tachycardia, tachypnea, and dyspnea.
  – Assess for headache, hypotension, or syncope.
  – Assess level of consciousness.
- Monitor for complications related to thrombocytopenia:
  – Assess skin, stools, urine, gums, emesis, sputum, and nasal secretions for blood.
- Monitor for complications related to neutropenia:
  – Assess for signs and symptoms of bacterial infection (e.g., pneumonia, meningitis, osteomyelitis, abscess) and septic shock.
- Monitor patient for transfusion complications, including transfusion reactions and volume overload (pulmonary edema).
- Maximize the child's physical tolerance:
  – Provide oxygen, as ordered, when decreased oxygen creates difficult breathing.
  – Provide quiet play activities that promote physical and intellectual development.
  – Promote times for rest and sleep.
- Prevent and decrease the risk of bleeding:
  – Provide a safe environment (e.g., use of helmets, knee pads, and padded cribs).
  – Encourage the use of a soft-bristle toothbrush and electric razor and avoidance of dental flossing.
  – Administer hormonal therapy to inhibit menses (if prescribed).
- Prevent and decrease the risk of infection:
  – Encourage good general hygiene, including daily bathing, oral care, and frequent hand washing.
  – Minimize the child's exposure to individuals known to have serious infections.
  – Do not use rectal thermometers or suppositories.
- Teach the family about hemolytic anemia:
  – Educate about signs and symptoms of worsening anemia, including increased heart rate and respirations, dyspnea, pallor, excessive sleepiness or irritability, headaches, dizziness when standing abruptly, and poor suckling in infants.
  – Educate about signs and symptoms of worsening hemolysis, including abdominal pain, enlarging abdomen, red or dark urine, and jaundice.
  – Review ways to conserve energy and decrease fatigue.
- Teach the family about thrombocytopenia:
  – Educate about signs and symptoms of worsening thrombocytopenia.
  – Review ways to decrease the risk of bleeding.
- Teach families about neutropenia:
  – Educate about signs and symptoms of infection.
  – Review ways to protect the child from infection.
- Educate the patient and the family about the chronic nature of Evans syndrome, which can include periods of remission and exacerbation.
- Educate the patient and the family about medical therapies, rationale for use, potential side effects, and, if parent will administer medications, what to do if a dose is missed.
- Teach the family about postsplenectomy care.
  – Advise that child obtain and wear a medical-alert bracelet.
  – Educate about risks for sepsis and proper response to fever or infection.

## Expected Patient Outcomes

- The child and the family are able to identify the signs and symptoms of anemia, hemolysis, thrombocytopenia, and neutropenia and report them to medical staff.
- The child has minimal complications related to anemia, thrombocytopenia, and neutropenia.

# Thrombosis and Thrombophilia

*Kathy M. Harney*

Thromboembolism in children is rare; however, its incidence is increasing. The rise is attributed to longer survival rates of acute and chronically ill children due in part to advances in medical technology. Anticoagulation practice in the setting of pediatrics is predominantly extrapolated from the adult literature. Despite the upsurge in pediatric thromboembolic events, they are still 100 times less frequent in children than in adults.

## Definition

*Thrombosis* is characterized by the inappropriate formation of a thrombus or clot within the venous or arterial system. *Thrombophilia* is characterized as blood conditions that are associated with an increased tendency to develop thrombus. Thrombophilia may be genetic or acquired or a combination of both.

## Pathophysiology

The pathophysiology of venous thromboembolism is explained by Virchow's triad, which includes stasis, endothelial damage, and hypercoagulability (i.e., alteration in composition of blood).

## Incidence, Etiology, and Genetics

Morgan (2007) reports that 95% of venous thromboembolism in children is due to multiple conditions that may be either congenital or familial, to recurrent events, or to congenital heart disease. It may also be acquired iatrogenically through cancer, trauma or surgery, medications, sepsis, and indwelling central catheters. Known risk factors for thrombosis in the pediatric setting are listed in **Tables 11-4** and **11-5**.

## Clinical Presentation

Thromboembolic events may present with clinical significance or may be incidental findings on radiographic imaging done for an underlying diagnosis. The patient with a deep vein thrombosis (DVT) may present with localized or unilateral pain or tenderness, swelling or edema, discoloration or erythema, poor perfusion, or palpable cords. A positive homans sign is not always predictive of a DVT. If the event is in an upper extremity, internal jugular vein, or superior vena cava, presentation may include the signs listed previously, as well as neck and facial swelling, infection, and neurological changes. In pulmonary emboli (PE), hypoxia, dyspnea, cough, hemoptysis, tachypnea, and tachycardia may be present. There may also be electrocardiogram (EKG) and echocardiogram (ECHO) findings, with concern for right-ventricular dysfunction and pulmonary hypertension. Sinus venous thrombosis or stroke may present with neurological signs and symptoms or papilledema and, in some instances, infection may be present.

## Diagnosis

A diagnostic evaluation begins with a thorough patient history, family history, and physical exam. Evaluation and diagnostic studies should include but are not limited to the following:
- Vital signs, including oxygen saturation:
  - Continuous oxygen saturation monitoring should be considered in the acute setting when PE is suspected.
- Complete blood count with differential
- D-dimer test
- Coagulation studies (e.g., INR/PT/PTT and fibrinogen)
- Factor VIII level
- Hypercoagulation evaluation: appropriate to clinical presentation and history
- Arterial blood gases if PE is suspected (hypoxia/hypocapnia)
- EKG and ECHO when indicated
- Imaging:
  - Doppler ultrasound for diagnosis of DVT is routinely completed in place of venography
  - ECHO to evaluate for cardiac thromboses
  - Appropriate neurological imaging (computed tomography [CT]/magnetic resonance/magnetic resonance venogram)
  - CT angiogram (PE-specific protocols)
  - Baseline ventilation/perfusion scans may be considered.

## Treatment

Treatment options are based on initial clinical presentation, underlying diagnosis, bleeding risks, and age. A heparinoid (e.g., a continuous heparin drip or a low-molecular-weight heparin) routinely is the initial option. Other treatment considerations for the acute setting include thrombolysis, local thrombolytics with or without angioplasty or angiojet, inferior vena cava filter placement, and thromboembolectomy. Direct thrombin inhibitors may be indicated in certain situations (e.g., patients with heparin-induced thrombocytopenia). Depending on the clinical status of the patient, other options may not include anticoagulation but rather observation with serial imaging.

Long-term management includes transition to oral anticoagulants or continued use of a low-molecular-weight heparin, if appropriate, and compression garments when indicated.

### Table 11-4. Acquired Risk Factors Associated with Pediatric Thromboembolic Events

Autoimmune disorders, including antiphospholipid antibody syndrome, IBD, systemic lupus erythematosus

Dehydration

Hyperhomocysteinemia (either acquired or inherited)

Immobility

Indwelling central catheters

Malignancy

Mechanical heart valves

Medications such as L-asparaginase, oral and hormonal contraceptives, high-dose steroids

Myeloproliferative disorders

Nephrotic syndrome

Obesity

Smoking

Surgery

Trauma

### Table 11-5. Inherited Risk Factors Associated with Pediatric Thromboembolic Events

**Factor V Leiden (FVL)** in the Caucasian population is the most common inherited disorder predisposing to thrombosis risk. Approximately 5%–8% of Caucasians are heterozygous for FVL and 0.1% are homozygous. FVL is a point mutation in gene for factor V, allowing resistance to the effects of protein C.

**Prothrombin gene mutation 20210A** incidence in the Caucasian population is estimated to be 2%–3%. Thought to cause higher-than-normal levels of plasma prothrombin.

**Antithrombin III deficiency** involves impaired neutralization of thrombin. The deficiency may be associated with other disease entities, such as nephrotic syndrome, protein-losing enteropathy, and the use of L-asparaginase.

**Protein C deficiency** is inherited in an autosomal-dominant manner. Protein C is a vitamin-K-dependent protein, and it acts as a natural anticoagulant when the protein is activated. Although rare, homozygous or compound-heterozygous patients with severe protein C deficiency may present with purpura fulminans or diffuse intravascular coagulation in the neonatal period.

**Protein S deficiency** also increases risk for thrombosis, because protein S is a vitamin-K-dependent protein and it acts as a cofactor to protein C.

**Homocysteine** is an amino acid. Hyperhomocysteinemia may be genetic or acquired. Elevated levels are associated with arterial vascular disease and stroke and with recurrent thrombosis. Elevated homocysteine levels are influenced by intake of folate, vitamin B 12, and vitamin B 6. Inherited hyperhomocysteinemia may be the result of the common polymorphism in the methyltetrahydrofolate reductase gene.

**Lipoprotein(a)** elevated levels have been associated with an increased risk for atherosclerotic disease and venous thrombosis. When levels are elevated, fasting cholesterol panels should be completed.

Adapted from "Pediatric Thrombosis," by C. Hoppe & A. Mastunaga, 2002, *Pediatric Clinics of North America, 49*, pp. 1257–1283.

## Prognostic Considerations

Goldenberg, Knapp-Clevenger, and Manco-Johnson (2004) found that elevated plasma factor VIII levels and/or D-dimers at the time of presentation and again after 3 or 6 months of anticoagulation therapy suggested poor outcomes. Poor outcomes included persistent thrombus, recurrent thrombus, and postthrombotic syndrome (PTS).

PTS consists of limb discomfort and includes findings such as stasis, swelling, skin discoloration, and stasis ulcers or infection. As noted previously, certain risk factors may include an elevation in factor VIII or D-dimer, occlusive thrombi, persistence of thrombi, and number of veins involved.

## Nursing Assessment and Interventions

### Goal
The patient experiences minimal complications related to the thromboembolic event.

**Assessment:**
- Assess presenting symptoms and obtain a complete history, including the incidence and duration of symptoms; predisposing factors (e.g., trauma, recent surgery, oral contraceptive use, smoking); personal bleeding history; and family history.
- Perform a complete physical examination.
- Review imaging and laboratory findings.
- Assess for discomfort and degree of pain.

**Interventions:**
- Monitor vital signs and continued oxygen saturation; monitor for any changes in cardiorespiratory evaluation (e.g., tachycardia, shortness of breath, chest pain).
- Obtain baseline coagulation studies and complete blood count (CBC) if not previously completed.
- Initiate appropriate anticoagulation as ordered—a low-molecular-weight heparin or unfractionated heparin is routinely prescribed prior to starting warfarin.
- Provide pain medication as needed, remembering to avoid nonsteroidal antiinflammatory drugs.
- Monitor for signs and symptoms of bleeding—test emesis, urine, and stool for occult blood.
- Obtain appropriate levels (e.g., anti-Xa/INR) through a non-exposed heparin access to assess adequate dosing of anticoagulant.

### Goal
The patient experiences minimal complications related to anticoagulation therapy.

**Assessment:**
- Assess for bleeding related to anticoagulation therapy.
- Assess for clot extension.
- Assess for hypoxia.
- Monitor for adequate pulses and perfusion of affected extremities.
- Ensure there are no signs of heparin-induced thrombocytopenia while patient is on a heparinoid.
- Assess nutritional habits and identify vitamin K intake, because foods high in vitamin K can block the effect of oral anticoagulants.
- Ensure that appropriate laboratory monitoring of anticoagulation therapy is in place.
- Assess the need for a subcutaneous catheter device.

**Interventions:**
- Check CBC.
- Test emesis, urine, and stool for occult blood.
- Assess skin for ecchymosis and petechiae.
- Elevate affected extremity.
- Provide pain medication as needed.
- Measure for gradient compression garment after swelling subsides.
- Encourage early ambulation and physical therapy as tolerated after anticoagulation is initiated.
- Schedule and document routine monitoring of anticoagulation levels.
- Assess nutritional intake.
- Place a subcutaneous catheter device if indicated.

## Goal

The patient and the family are adequately informed regarding diagnosis, disease, and treatment and have appropriate support.

**Assessment:**
- Assess the patient's and the family's level of knowledge about the diagnosis and disease.
- Assess the patient's and the family's level of knowledge about treatment.
- Assess the patient's and the family's learning styles.

**Interventions:**
- Communicate with the patient and the family in an appropriate style.
- Educate the patient and the family about the importance of consistent nutritional intake while on an oral anticoagulant. Provide educational information regarding vitamin-K-containing food items.
- Educate the patient and the family about anticoagulation medication and anticoagulation precautions (e.g., avoiding contact sports) as well as signs and symptoms of bleeding and clot extension.
- Provide appropriate educational resources to the patient and the family and review the material with them.
- Ensure availability of community resources or nursing.
- Ensure that the family knows when and how to contact the healthcare team.
- Encourage the patient and the family to ask questions related to the diagnosis, disease, and treatment.

## Expected Patient and Family Outcomes

The patient and family can do the following:
- Describe diagnosis and the plan of care.
- Describe any risk factors, acquired or inherited, that have been identified.
- Describe possible side effects of the event and the therapy.
- Explain the importance of follow-up and routine anticoagulation monitoring.
- Describe the schedule of therapy, follow-up imaging, laboratory monitoring, and appointments.
- Describe the importance of maintaining a consistent diet while on an oral anticoagulant. List some vitamin-K-containing foods.
- Describe a situation that would warrant a phone call to the healthcare team or an emergency hospital visit.
- Describe available community resources.
- Explain the importance of wearing a medical alert bracelet or identifier.
- Explain how and when to contact the healthcare team if problems or questions arise.

## References

Goldenberg, N., Knapp-Clevenger, R., & Manco-Johnson, M. (2004). Elevated plasma factor VIII and D-dimer levels as predictors of poor outcomes of thrombosis in children. *New England Journal of Medicine, 351,* 1081–1088.

Morgan, J. (2007). Perioperative venous thrombosis in children: Is it time for primary prophylaxis? *Pediatric Anesthesia, 17,* 99–100.

# Hemolytic-Uremic Syndrome

*Leticia Valdiviez*

## Definition

*Hemolytic-uremic syndrome* (HUS) is characterized by microangiopathic anemia, thrombocytopenia, and acute renal failure. In children, it is the most common cause of acute renal failure. The syndrome may follow an episode of diarrhea, the use of some drugs (e.g., cyclosporine), malignancy, or glomerulopathies, or it may be idiopathic.

## Incidence and Etiology

HUS was first described in 1955. The annual incidence is approximately 1 in 100,000 people and may be increasing. In the United States, 354 E. coli 0157:H7-associated HUS cases were reported between 1982 and 2002. In patients infected with a Shiga-toxin-producing strain of E. coli, HUS occurs in 5%–15% of cases. Other pathogens that can cause HUS include salmonella and *Campylobacter jejuni*. Worldwide, a higher incidence of HUS is found in South Africa, Holland, and Argentina. HUS has also been associated with severe pneumococcal infections.

HUS occurs in all races; however, it is less common in the African-American population. Males and females are affected equally; however, females may be more severely affected.

HUS can be either diarrhea associated (D+) or nondiarrhea associated (D-). The clinical courses and prognoses differ for each. D- HUS may follow a respiratory illness but does not follow a prodromal illness. D+ HUS is more common in the summer months and in early fall. D- HUS is not season associated, is seen in adults, and occurs sporadically. D+ HUS usually occurs in children age 7 months to 6 years. There is no age predilection for D- HUS.

Risk factors for development of HUS after colitis include young age, infection with the E. coli strain, administration of antiperistaltic agents or antibiotics, and a high fever or a high leukocyte count.

## Genetics

HUS has several genetic forms. Familial HUS accounts for 5%–10% of the cases. Genetically induced cases of HUS usually are preceded by a diarrheal illness. They often are recurrent and associated with a guarded long-term prognosis regarding maintenance of normal kidney function. The best-studied genetic variant of HUS involves mutations in one of the short consensus repeat segments of the gene for factor H, a protein that regulates complement.

## Pathophysiology

D+ HUS is usually preceded by a colitis caused by Shiga-toxin-producing E. coli. It is structurally related to ricin and cholera toxin. Inflammation of the colon leads to systemic absorption of the Shiga toxin and lipopolysaccharide from the gastrointestinal (GI) tract. These toxins bind to globotriaosylceramide, a glycolipid receptor molecule on the surface of the endothelial cells in the gut and kidney. Occasionally they bind to other organs. The damaged endothelial cells of the glomerular capillaries release vasoactive and platelet-aggregating substances. The endothelial cells swell, and fibrin is deposited on the injured vessel walls.

This swelling and microthrombi formation within the glomerular capillaries produce a localized intravascular coagulopathy. The glomerular filtration rate is reduced, and renal insufficiency ensues. Erythrocytes are damaged and fragmented as they flow through the glomerular capillaries. This leads to microangiopathic hemolytic anemia. Hemolysis can also be due to lipid peroxidation.

The resulting thrombocytopenia is thought to be the result of platelet destruction, increased consumption, liver and spleen sequestration, and intrarenal aggregation. Shiga toxin also binds to activated platelets.

Other factors contributing to thrombocytopenia include
- Abnormalities of antiplatelet-aggregating agents (prostaglandin I2)
- Abnormalities of platelet-aggregating agents (thromboxane A2)
- Abnormal von Willebrand factor multimers.

## Clinical Presentation
The clinical course of HUS can vary. Severity of symptoms can range from subclinical to life threatening.

Patients with D+ HUS may experience several days of diarrhea (with or without vomiting), followed by weakness, lethargy, irritability, and pallor. Bloody diarrhea is present in 80%–90% of the cases. The patient may also experience restlessness, oliguria, edema, and macroscopic hematuria. The clinical picture may resemble that of someone with symptoms of acute abdomen.

### Hematologic Symptoms
Hemolysis is present in all patients with HUS. It can proceed rapidly, causing a rapid fall in hematocrit. Platelet counts usually fall below 40,000/mm$^3$. The degree of thrombocytopenia does not correspond with the severity of the HUS. As a result of the thrombocytopenia, the patient may have petechiae, purpura, and oozing from venipuncture sites. Overt bleeding is less common.

Thrombi can form in a number of organs. Thrombotic ischemia can occur in the gut, with the colon most severely affected. The central nervous system (CNS) can also suffer ischemic damage, producing neurologic manifestations.

Despite severe hematologic abnormalities, many children can maintain relatively normal renal function.

### Renal Symptoms
Acute renal insufficiency usually begins with the onset of hemolysis. Frequent, watery stools may mask a decreasing urine output. Oliguria generally develops 1 day to 2 weeks after the onset of diarrhea in D+ HUS. If renal insufficiency is not recognized and treated, hyponatremia, hyperkalemia, severe acidosis, ascites, edema, pulmonary edema, and hypertension can occur within days of the initial illness. Oliguria lasts about a week in 60% of patients.

### Central-Nervous-System Symptoms
D- HUS tends to be associated with a greater number of neurologic symptoms than D+ HUS. Patients often present with sudden onset of lethargy and irritability. Other CNS findings may include ataxia, coma, seizures, cerebral swelling, hemiparesis, and other focal neurologic signs. The changes may be caused by ischemia from microthrombi or by the effects of hypertension, hyponatremia, or uremia.

### Gastrointestinal Symptoms
As described previously, D+ HUS is preceded by diarrhea. GI symptoms may improve as other HUS symptoms present. Intestinal necrosis can be a life-threatening complication. Mild pancreatic involvement is common but also can be severe and lead to insulin-dependent diabetes, and rarely, exocrine dysfunction. Jaundice may also be present.

### Infection
Five percent to twenty percent of patients present with fever. The presence of fever, leukocytosis, or both is a prognostic indicator of the risk of developing more severe HUS. Rectal prolapse can occur in 10% of cases, and 2% of patients may need surgery for gangrene.

### Cardiovascular Symptoms
Congestive heart failure can occur. The nurse should be alert for physical signs and symptoms, including hypertension, pallor, lethargy, irritability, abdominal pain, peripheral edema, petechiae, purpura, or oozing from venipuncture sites.

## Diagnosis
HUS is a clinical diagnosis. The classic diagnostic criteria are microangiopathic hemolytic anemia, thrombocytopenia, and acute renal failure following an episode of bloody diarrhea. Diagnosis may not be as clear if there is no history of diarrhea. Other related conditions, such as thrombotic thrombocytopenic purpura, bilateral renal-vein thrombosis, and lupus must be ruled out. Other similar disorders that must be ruled out include disseminated intravascular coagulation, cavernous sinus hemangioma, and vasculitic disorders. **Table 11-6** shows common laboratory tests used to daignose HUS along with their results.

White blood cells are usually increased in the blood of a patient with HUS. Activated neutrophils are believed to damage endothelial cells by releasing elastase and producing free radicals. Elastase is a catabolic enzyme that promotes endothelial detachment. Monocytes may also be stimulated to release cytokines, such as interleukin-1 and tumor necrosis factor.

Von Willebrand factor frequently is abnormal in amount and character.

### Imaging and Other Studies
A chest X ray may be ordered to detect pulmonary congestion or edema. An electrocardiogram can detect effects of hyperkalemia.

If biopsies are obtained, renal histologic analysis may reveal swollen glomerular endothelial cells. Thrombi may be observed in capillaries and arterioles. Tissue biopsies of the gut may reveal microangiopathy with cell injury, thrombosis, submucosal edema, and hemorrhage.

## Treatment
- Supportive care is the mainstay of therapy. Some patients with acute renal failure require dialysis.
- Anticonvulsants are indicated if the patient develops seizures. Intravenous immunoglobulin (IVIG) may hasten recovery in patients with thrombocytopenia and oliguria and reduce CNS sequelae. However, IVIG has not been shown to be effective for the treatment of familial HUS.

### Table 11-6. Laboratory Tests Commonly Used to Diagnose Hemolytic-Uremic Syndrome

| Test | Expected Result with Hemolytic Uremic Syndrome (HUS) |
|---|---|
| Activated partial thromboplastin time | Normal |
| Bicarbonate concentration | Decreased (acidosis) |
| Bilirubin level | Increased |
| Blood smear | Fragmented blood cells |
| Blood urea nitrogen/creatinine ratio | Elevated |
| Calcium | Decreased |
| CBC | Thrombocytopenia, anemia, elevated WBC with a left shift |
| Coombs | Positive in S pneumoniae-associated HUS |
| Fibrin degradation products | Increased |
| Fibrinogen | Normal or increased |
| Lactate dehydrogenase | Elevated |
| Liver enzymes (alanine transaminase/aspartate aminotransferase) | Elevated |
| Phosphorous | Elevated |
| Potassium | Elevated (renal failure/hemolysis) |
| Protein/albumin | Mildly decreased |
| Prothrombin time | Normal |
| Reticulocyte count | Elevated |
| Serum haptoglobin | Decreased |
| Sodium | Decreased (fluid overload) |
| Triglyceride levels | Increased |
| Uric acid | Elevated (acute renal failure, dehydration, cell breakdown) |
| Urinalysis | Protein, heme, bilirubin, red blood cells, white blood cells, casts |

- Antihypertensives and diuretics may be useful for controlling hypertension and fluid overload. Corticosteroids, plasma infusions, plasmapheresis, furosemide, and captopril do not affect the outcome of HUS.
- Hemoglobin should be maintained above 7 gm/dL. Platelet transfusions are recommended for symptomatic bleeding and prior to surgical procedures but may worsen the thrombotic complication of the illness.
- Anticoagulant and thrombolytic agents have not been found to be beneficial in HUS. Aspirin and diprydamole may have little clinical significance.
- Oral diets should be low in sodium and high in calories. If the patient experiences continued diarrhea, colitis, or abdominal pain, total parenteral nutrition may need to be initiated.

## Prognostic Considerations

In 1955, HUS was nearly always fatal. By the 1990s, the mortality rate had decreased to 3%–5%. This improvement is attributed to better management of hypertension and acute renal failure with use of preemptive dialysis. The mortality rate in underdeveloped countries remains high at approximately 70%. Patients with hereditary HUS have a worse prognosis, with mortality rates greater than 90% in patients with autosomal-dominant disease and 60%–70% in patients with the autosomal-recessive form.

In general, patients with D+ HUS have a better outcome than patients with D- HUS. HUS has also been associated with severe pneumococcal infections and carries a poorer prognosis than those caused by E. coli. Although most patients' renal function returns to normal, some have persistent renal failure. Twenty-five percent of patients with HUS suffer lasting renal impairment.

## Nursing Assessment and Interventions

### Goal

The patient experiences minimal complications related to the onset of acute renal failure.

**Assessment:**
- Assess for urine output.
- Monitor intake and output.
- Weigh patient daily.
- Monitor frequency and amount of stools.
- Monitor heart rate and blood pressure.
- Assess for changes in level of consciousness.

**Interventions:**
- Restrict fluids to insensible losses and output.
- Monitor electrolytes.
- Administer diuretics as needed.
- Use fluids that do not have added potassium.

### Goal

The patient experiences minimal complications related to the onset of altered blood-cell counts.

**Assessment:**
- Observe laboratory data for changes in the complete blood count.

- Report hemoglobin of <7 gm/dL.
- Observe for petechiae, purpura, and oozing from puncture sites.
- Assess skin color for pallor.
- Assess for decreased energy, fatigue, irritability, or lethargy.
  **Interventions:**
- Administer blood products as needed.
- Administer platelet transfusions as needed.
- Monitor for signs and symptoms of fluid overload.

## Goal
The patient and the family are adequately informed regarding the patient's diagnosis, disease, and treatment.
  **Assessment:**
- Assess the patient's and the family's level of knowledge about the disease and its treatment.
- Assess the patient's and the family's learning styles.
- Assess how well the patient and the family understand the role of the healthcare team.
  **Interventions:**
- Communicate with the patient and the family in an appropriate style.
- Provide the patient and the family with educational material and review it with them.
- Ensure that the patient and/or the family knows how and when to notify the healthcare team.
- Encourage the patient and the family to ask questions regarding the diagnosis and treatment.

## Expected Patient and Family Outcomes
The patient and family can do the following:
- Describe HUS and the plan of care.
- List the signs and symptoms that require notification of the healthcare team.
- Describe the schedule of treatment, procedures, and follow-up care.

# Paroxysmal Nocturnal Hemoglobinuria

*Colleen Nixon*

## Definition
*Paroxysmal nocturnal hemoglobinuria* (PNH) is an acquired, life-threatening, rare hematologic disorder characterized by the clinical triad of hemolytic anemia, pancytopenia, and thrombosis. PNH results from a nonmalignant clonal hematopoietic stem-cell disorder characterized by an acquired somatic mutation of the X-linked chromosome within the glycosylphosphatidylinositol (GPI) PIGA gene.

## Classification
The International PNH Interest Group organizes PNH clones into three separate subgroups based on presentation, clinical symptoms, and disease progression.

### Classic PNH
The patient with classic PNH typically has clinical symptoms of intravascular hemolysis, including anemia, an increased reticulocyte count, increased lactate dehydrogenase (LDH), and decreased serum haptoglobin levels. In addition, there is evidence of major populations of PNH type III red blood cells (RBCs), meaning there is complete GPI deficiency. The patient shows no evidence of another underlying bone-marrow abnormality.

### PNH in the Setting of Another Specified Bone-Marrow Disorder
Patients in this group have laboratory values and symptoms consistent with hemolysis, as well as an existing bone-marrow abnormality or a history of marrow disease (e.g., PNH/aplastic anemia or PNH/myelodysplastic syndrome).

### Subclinical PNH
Patients in this group do not have clinical or laboratory data consistent with hemolysis. Subclinical PNH (PNH-sc) is seen predominately in patients with bone-marrow failure syndromes, primarily aplastic anemia and refractory anemia-myelodysplastic disease.

Children with PNH frequently present with PNH-sc (i.e., class 3 PNH) in conjunction with bone-marrow-failure syndromes.

## Pathophysiology
PNH is a nonmalignant clonal hematopoietic stem-cell disorder characterized by an acquired somatic mutation on the X-linked chromosome within the phosphatidylinositol glycan complementation class A (PIGA) gene. This mutation prevents GPI anchor synthesis, resulting in proteins, which are normally bound to the cell surface by GPI anchors, to be deficient. As a result, patients with PNH have stem cells with a partial deficiency (i.e., PNH type II cells) or a complete deficiency (i.e., PNH type III cells) of GPI-anchored proteins. The GPI-anchor deficiency causes the cells to become more vulnerable to attack by the complement system (i.e., the part of the immune system that destroys bacteria), resulting in hemolysis, thrombosis, and bone-marrow failure. Intravascular hemolysis, a chief manifestation of this disease, is caused by a partial or complete absence of the GPI-anchored complement regulatory proteins CD 55 and CD 59 on erythrocytes. Patients with PNH have platelets that are also deficient in GPI-anchored proteins. The lack of CD 59 causes platelets to have an increased sensitivity to complement-mediated lysis, leading to increased thrombotic risk.

## Incidence
PNH is a rare disorder and the prevalence data are inexact. This impreciseness is due in part to the technique with which PNH is diagnosed. When flow cytometry is used to make the diagnosis, all patients with the presence of PNH clones, including patients with PNH-sc, are included in the prevalence data. Using high-flow cytometry, data were extrapolated to determine the incidence of PNH to be approximately 8,000–10,000 in North America and Western Europe. The incidence of patients with clinical PNH (i.e., patients with evidence of hemolysis) is estimated to be approximately 1,000–2,000 patients, or 3–5 million persons in the United States (C. Parker, personal communication, February 19, 2008).

PNH can be diagnosed at any age, but occurs predominately during adulthood; the average age at diagnosis is 30–45 years. Although well-documented cases of pediatric PNH are limited, it is estimated that approximately 10% of patients with PNH are younger than 21 years at the time of diagnosis. Nishimura and colleagues (2004) found males and females to be equally affected. Hillmen and colleagues (2006) report a median survival of 10 years from the time of PNH diagnosis. The development of the worldwide patient registry and the use of consistent testing are essential for obtaining comprehensive epidemiologic data to appreciate the true prevalence of PNH.

## Clinical Presentation

PNH is an uncommon disease, and in children, the disease is often misdiagnosed and incorrectly managed. A literature review from 1967 to 2005 found only 51 cases of pediatric PNH in which presentation, treatment, and outcomes were documented. This demonstrates how little is known about the presentation in children with PNH, their response to therapy, and their long-term survival rate (van den Heuvel-Eibrink, 2007). In early case reports, it appeared that pediatric and adult patients with PNH presented with similar signs and symptoms, such as hemolysis, bone-marrow failure, and thrombosis. In adults with classic PNH, gross hemoglobinuria was reported in approximately 35% of patients, whereas in pediatric patients, the occurrence of hemoglobinuria at presentation is approximately 15%–20%. Findings obtained through the use of flow cytometry show that adult patients reportedly present with a higher incidence of bone-marrow failure and a lower incidence of hemoglobinuria, which is similar to the pediatric presentation. Thrombotic events occurring at presentation are uncommon; they are reported in approximately 5% of patients. Patients who present with venous thrombosis involving the mesenteric or portal veins, cerebral veins, or dermal veins should be evaluated for PNH, particularly if there are simultaneous cytopenias or evidence of intravascular hemolysis or both. Patients can also present with gastrointestinal (GI) problems, such as episodic abdominal pain, dysphagia, and erectile dysfunction. All patients who present with aplastic anemia should be screened for PNH at diagnosis and at least yearly thereafter.

## Diagnosis

The most rapid and reliable test used for diagnosing PNH is high-resolution flow cytometry analysis, using antibodies directed against GPI-anchors. This test replaces the acid Ham and sucrose lysis tests as the gold standards for diagnosis. The resulting analysis yields more than a positive or negative result; it also identifies the percentage of cells that are abnormal. To best manage the anemia of PNH, it is important to determine the percentage and type of lacking RBCs. For patients with PNH, the larger the percentage of abnormal clones, the greater the associated risk of hemolysis or thrombotic events. The use of flow cytometry identifies small PNH clones that previously would have been undetectable. To best evaluate the percentage of GPI-anchor erythrocyte deficiency, flow cytometry analysis should be obtained prior to transfusions or at least no later than 1 month after transfusion.

Other important tests necessary to confirm the PNH diagnosis include a thorough history and physical, complete blood count (CBC), reticulocyte count, haptoglobin levels, urinalysis, and liver-function tests, particularly LDH and bilirubin (fractionated).

Bone-marrow biopsy, aspirate, and cytogenetics that evaluate cellularity, clonality, and dysplasia are required for complete disease classification.

## Treatment

Because of the rarity of PNH, this illness often is not considered in the differential diagnosis when a patient presents with hemoglobinuria, abdominal pain, or anemia. Parker and colleagues (2005) have identified patients with other disorders who may be at risk for PNH, even when hemoglobinuria is not present. Patients who present with one or more of the following conditions must be screened to avoid a delay in treatment: hemoglobinuria; Coombs-negative hemolytic anemia; aplastic anemia; refractory anemia-myelodysplastic syndrome; thrombosis development in the hepatic, abdominal, cerebral or dermal veins; and GI complaints with symptoms of intravascular hemolysis.

Treatment strategies for PNH differ based on presentation, clinical symptoms, and disease progression. Patients who present with persistent bone-marrow failure syndromes receive therapy to correct the underlying marrow abnormality. Stem-cell transplantation is the only curative option, but this strategy must be weighed against the potential morbidity and mortality.

Because children often present with PNH-sc, matched sibling donor or matched unrelated donor stem-cell transplantation is the current recommended treatment for children with bone-marrow failure syndromes with PNH clones. The conditioning regimen is determined based on the underlying disease. For patients without a matched sibling donor, other treatment options are considered, including immunosuppressive therapy using prednisolone, antithymocyte globulin, and cyclosporine.

The therapy for patients with classic PNH (typically adults) involves supportive care with transfusions as needed, supplemental folic acid for patients with hemolysis, and, if necessary, thrombosis treatment. Currently, there is no standard of treatment for adults or children who have thromboembolic events. For this group of patients, stem-cell transplantation is the only curative treatment, and the recommendations concerning eligibility for this treatment are not as clear. Potential candidates for transplantation include patients who have aplastic anemia, bone-marrow refractory, hemolytic anemia, life-threatening complications, and those who are transfusion dependent.

The development of eculizumab, a monoclonal antibody that prevents terminal complement activation, has proven to be effective at reducing intravascular hemolysis, thereby decreasing the number of blood transfusions required. Other benefits for patients treated with eculizumab include increased quality of life (as measured by the European Organisation for Research and Treatment of Cancer QLQ-C30 scale) with improvements (i.e., some complete resolution) in fatigue, dyspnea, dysphagia, abdominal pain, and erectile dysfunction. It is unclear whether eculizumab reduces the risk of thrombosis development in patients with PNH. Patients seem to tolerate the drug well; the most common side effects are headache, nasopharyngitis, back pain, cough, and nausea. Eculizumab can increase the risk of meningococcal infections, so patients should be vaccinated with a meningococcal vaccine at least 2 weeks before receiving the first dose of eculizumab and must be revaccinated according to current medical guidelines. Patients should be monitored closely for early signs of meningococcal infections, evaluated immediately if infection is suspected, and treated with antibiotics if necessary. The safety and efficacy in patients younger than 18 years have not been determined. Treatment options for children and adults continue to be determined based on presentation, the type of PNH, and the trajectory of the illness. Healthcare providers must educate patients and families about the importance of participating in the Global PNH Registry (www.pnhregistry.com).

## Nursing Assessment and Interventions

### Goal
The patient experiences minimal complications related to the onset of disease.

**Assessment:**
- Assess the presenting symptoms and obtain a complete history, including signs of anemia (e.g., headache, fatigue, shortness of breath, pallor, bounding pulse); bleeding; thrombotic events; GI problems (e.g., episodic abdominal pain and dysphagia); genitourinary problems (e.g., gross hemoglobinuria); and fever.
- Perform a complete physical examination to determine the possible source of bleeding (e.g., bruising, petechiae, purpura); pain (location, onset, duration, past pain experience, alleviating interventions); presence of murmur; respiratory compromise; and neurological changes.
- If fever is present, determine possible source of infection.
- Review laboratory findings.

**Interventions:**
- If patient is febrile, administer antibiotics without delay.
- Administer aggressive intravenous hydration, pain medications, and RBC or platelet transfusions (or both) as ordered.
- Monitor CBC and differential count, blood and other cultures, vital signs, and pulse oximetry readings.
- Monitor frequently for development of new complications, such as neurological changes, respiratory deterioration, ineffectively managed pain, and fever.

### Goal
The patient and the family are adequately informed regarding the diagnosis, disease, and treatment.

**Assessment:**
- Determine the patient's and the family's learning styles.
- Assess the patient's and the family's level of knowledge about the diagnosis, complications, treatment options, and prognosis.
- Determine whether the patient is eligible to receive eculizumab.
- Assess the patient's and the family's understanding of compliance and follow-up.
- Assess the patient's and the family's knowledge and understanding of the multidisciplinary team members and their roles in treatment.

**Interventions:**
- Use communication techniques that fit the patient's and the family's learning styles.
- Provide ongoing instruction and reinforcement of instruction to the patient and the family. Understand normal blood counts and know when transfusions are indicated.
- Provide the patient and the family with appropriate educational resources, and review the material with them (using information sheets from the Internet or the institution if available).
- Ensure that the family is aware of how and when to call the primary-care provider.
- Encourage the patient and the family to ask questions related to the diagnosis, disease, and treatment.
- If the patient is to receive eculizumab, ensure that he or she is vaccinated with a meningococcal vaccine at least 2 weeks before receiving the first dose of eculizumab. Revaccinate according to current medical guidelines.
- Patients should be monitored closely for early signs of meningococcal infections, evaluated immediately if infection is suspected, and treated with antibiotics if necessary.
- If patient is receiving eculizumab, review side effects of medication (e.g., headache, nasopharyngitis, back pain, cough, and nausea) and when to report these side effects to the healthcare provider.
- Emphasize close outpatient follow-up care.
- Ensure that patients with PNH participate in the Global PNH Registry.

## Expected Patient and Family Outcomes
The child and the family can do the following:
- Describe PNH and the plan of care.
- List the expected and possible side effects of therapy.
- Outline methods for preventing infection.
- Describe the schedule of treatment, procedures, and follow-up care.
- Describe available community resources.
- Demonstrate the skills needed to care for the child at home.
- Explain how and when to contact the healthcare team if problems or questions arise.

## References
Hillmen, P., Young, N., Shubert, J., Brodsky, R., Socie, G., Muus, P., et al. (2006). The complement inhibitor eculizumab in paroxysmal nocturnal hemoglobinuria. *New England Journal of Medicine, 355,* 1233–1243.

Nishimura, J. I., Kanakura, Y., Ware, R. E., Shichishima, T., Nakakuma, H., Ninomiya, H., et al. (2004). Clinical course and flow cytometric analysis of paroxysmal nocturnal hemoglobinuria in the United States and Japan. *Medicine, 83,* 193–207.

Parker, C., Omine, M., Richards, S., Nishimura, J., Bessler, M., Ware, R., et al. (2005). Diagnosis and management of paroxysmal nocturnal hemoglobinuria. *Blood, 106,* 3699–3709.

van den Heuvel-Eibrink, M. M. (2007). Paroxysmal nocturnal hemoglobinuria in children. *Pediatric Drugs, 9,* 11–16.

# Hemophilia

*Rhonda Fritz*

*Hemophilia* is a genetic disorder characterized by a deficiency or absence of clotting factors that results in prolonged bleeding. It is caused by the inheritance of a functional defect in the factor VIII or IX protein that has an X-linked inheritance pattern.

## Classification

Hemophilia is classified according to the missing or deficient protein. Hemophilia A is known as factor VIII deficiency or classical hemophilia. Hemophilia B is known as factor IX deficiency or Christmas disease.

## Incidence

It is estimated that hemophilia occurs in 1 in 5,000 male births. Eighty percent to 85% of those with hemophilia have hemophilia A, and 10%–15% have hemophilia B.

## Inheritance

The clinical manifestations of hemophilia have been recognized since biblical times. The *Talmud,* the ancient text of Jewish law, did not allow circumcision of a baby boy who had two older brothers who died as a result of bleeding from circumcision.

Known as the "royal disease" in Europe, all of the affected males of European royal families were direct descendants of Queen Victoria of England. In the United States, the inheritance pattern of hemophilia was first described in the early 1800s.

The genes responsible for hemophilia were identified and cloned during the 1980s.

## Genetics

Hemophilia is a sex-linked recessive disorder. The abnormal gene responsible for hemophilia is carried on the X chromosome. Males have only one X chromosome and thus, if affected, express the trait. The Y chromosome found in males primarily determines gender and does not contain genes that make clotting factor. Females carry two X chromosomes and thus, if affected, do not express the trait. If the defect exists in the female's X chromosome, it can be masked by the presence of a normal gene on the second X chromosome. In this case, the female is considered a carrier with the potential to pass on the disease to her offspring.

Obligate carriers include all daughters of men with hemophilia (a male can pass on his X chromosome only to a daughter), one son and another relative with hemophilia, or two or more sons with hemophilia.

Approximately 30% of the cases have no family history. This may be due to a new mutation that arises during the development of the mother's egg cells. Germline mosaicism occurs when the mother's eggs carry the mutation; however, it is not present on the genes in her other cells.

If an egg is fertilized by an X-bearing sperm with a mutation occurring on the factor VIII (FVIII) or factor IX (FIX) gene on an X chromosome in an egg, the male offspring will have hemophilia. If an egg is fertilized by an X-bearing sperm, the female offspring will be a carrier. If a mutation occurs in an X-bearing sperm, the female offspring also will be a carrier.

## Genetic Counseling

If there is a family history of hemophilia, genetic counseling is advisable prior to carrier testing or conception. Included in the counseling are the psychosocial aspects, hemophilia care, cost and insurance issues, and reproductive option choices. Reproductive choices prior to conception include contraception, gamete intrafallopian transfer, abortion following chorionic villus sampling, in vitro fertilization and sex selection, and adoption.

## Clinical Presentation

Clinical presentation includes bleeding from circumcision, multiple raised bruises without known trauma, prolonged mouth bleeding, and prolonged oozing after a finger or heel stick; follow-up laboratory studies are required.

Approximately 30% of children present with bleeding from circumcision; 1%–2% present with intracranial hemorrhage. Many children present when reaching developmental milestones (e.g., crawling, pulling to stand) and become easily injured (e.g., with increased bruising, swelling, redness at joints, or mouth bleeding).

## Sites of Bleeding

### Joint

The primary site of bleeding is the synovium that lines the joint. Initially, patients can detect a tingling sensation or warmth in the area, followed by increased pain and decreased range of motion as the bleeding progresses. If left untreated, the bleeding continues to fill the joint space. Repeated bleeding into the same joint (i.e., target joint) can lead to chronic joint disease. A target joint is defined as three bleeds into the same joint during a 6-month period. Over time, chronic joint arthropathy can develop.

**Chronic Joint Arthropathy:** The synovial membrane releases plasmin to break down the blood protein. Because it does not differentiate between proteins, it also breaks down the cartilage protein in the process. This destroys the synovium and subsequently, hemosiderin (from iron-containing compounds in the blood) collects in the joint cartilage and synovial membrane and evolves into chronic inflammation. The inflammation can eventually lead to synovitis and, ultimately, narrowing of joint space, bone erosion, and cyst formation, limiting range of motion and leading to chronic arthritis and disability. Early treatment or prophylaxis can help prevent long-term joint damage.

### Muscle

Muscle is the second most frequent site of bleeding in hemophilia; the bleeding often is difficult to find as it is deep in the muscle and not in a closed space. Large-muscle bleeds can result in major blood loss and severe muscle contractures due to fibrosis and atrophy. Symptoms reported occasionally include a vague description of pain with movement.

### Mouth

Bleeding from the oral mucosa or frenulum due to trauma can be difficult to control and can result in large blood-volume loss. The actual amount may be overlooked because of the intermittent nature of the bleed or swallowing of blood. Assess for pallor, lethargy, nausea, vomiting, or abdominal pain.

### Gastrointestinal
Gastrointestinal bleeding can be serious and requires aggressive factor replacement and careful blood-count monitoring. There is the potential for significant blood loss and shock

### Hematuria
Blood in the urine can occur spontaneously in hemophilia. Painless episodes have no known cause and typically do not produce significant blood loss. Repeated episodes should be evaluated. Hematuria occurring after trauma or associated with pain should be carefully evaluated.

### Laboratory Studies
Studies should include PT and PTT. The PTT measures deficiencies on the intrinsic pathway. FVIII and FIX deficiencies are disorders of the intrinsic pathway of coagulation; therefore, PT will be normal and PTT will be prolonged. If the PTT is prolonged, the diagnosis is confirmed by low or absent FVIII or FIX.

### Levels of Severity
The distinguishing feature of hemophilia is deep bleeding into the joints and muscles that typically corresponds to the level of disease severity.

Severe hemophilia is characterized by frequent bleeding episodes. Spontaneous bleeding can occur without known trauma. Children with moderate hemophilia usually bleed after minor trauma, and bleeding typically is not spontaneous. Mild hemophilia is characterized by bleeding from trauma or surgery.

### Treatment
Major bleeds are corrected with 100% factor replacement; minor bleeds with 50% replacement. Mucous-membrane bleeding, such as mouth bleeds, are also treated with antifibrinolytic agents (**Table 11-7**).

### Prophylaxis
Prophylaxis is a program for preventing bleeding episodes and, ultimately, long-term joint damage.

A 5-year, multicenter trial found prophylaxis initiated between 6 and 30 months of age to be effective for the prevention of joint bleeding, structural joint damage, and frequency of bleeding in boys with FVIII deficiency (Manco-Johnson et al., 2007).

### Primary Prophylaxis
Primary prophylaxis consists of regular infusions of FVIII or FIX with the goal of preventing joint bleeding. It is usually started in children with severe hemophilia. The goal is to keep the factor level greater than 1%. To accomplish this, those with FVIII deficiency generally require 50% replacement every other day, and those with FIX deficiency require 50% replacement 2–3 times a week. The difference between the frequency of infusions depends on various practices. One practice depends on the half-life of the two factor deficiencies: FVIII half-life is 10–12 hours; FIX half-life is 24 hours. In Canada, an escalating dose model is used, wherein the patients are infused once a week, and the frequency of infusions are increased according to the bleeding pattern.

---

### Figure 11-7. Treatment for Hemophilia

**Recombinant Factor VIII Concentrates**
The recombinant products are derived from Chinese hamster ovary or baby-hamster kidney cells that have been transfected with the human factor VII, VIII, or IX gene. They also undergo a combination of viral clearance and inactivation steps to ensure safety and purity. There are many different brands of recombinant factor VIII on the market.

**First Generation**
**Recombinate** is the first-generation recombinant factor VIII product and is stabilized with added human albumin.

**Advanced Generation**
Advanced-generation products include **Helixate FS** and **Kogenate FS,** which are stabilized with sucrose. **Refacto** is a B-domain-deleted factor VIII product. Human serum albumin is used in cell culture, but the product is albumin-free in the final formulation. **Advate** is an advanced-generation product that is not exposed to albumin at any point during the manufacturing process. **BeneFIX** is a recombinant-factor IX product formulated without albumin, as is **Novo VII,** a product for the treatment of inhibitors and patients deficient in factor VII.

**Plasma-Derived FVIII and FIX Products**
Produced from large pools of donor plasma and concentrated for factors VIII or IX. The donors are rigorously screened and the human plasma is tested for blood-borne viruses such as HIV and hepatitis A, B, and C.

**Desmopressin (DDAVP)** is a synthetic vasopressin analog that increases plasma FVIII and vWf levels. It is used as a treatment for patients with mild-to-moderate FVIII deficiency. Patients are tested to determine response to guide therapy. The nasal form, **Stimate**, can be kept refrigerated in the home and used for bleeding episodes. Side effects include facial flushing, transient headaches, nausea, and abdominal cramps. DDAVP should be used with caution in patients with a history of venous thrombosis or cardiac diagnosis, because reports of thrombotic events exist. It is not administered in children younger than 2 years or in elderly patients because both groups are at risk for water intoxication, hyponatremia, and seizures. Tachyphylaxis can occur when DDAVP is administered on a daily basis and typically is not administered longer than 2–3 days. Patients are instructed to limit fluid intake for 24 hours following DDAVP treatment to avoid hyponatremia.

**Antifibrinolytic Agents**
**Aminocaproic acid (Amicar)** is an antifibrinolytic agent effective in situations in which fibrinolysis plays a role, such as mucous-membrane bleeding. It can be used alone or in conjunction with factor concentrates or DDAVP. It is particularly useful for surgeries such as tonsillectomies or dental extractions; it is also used in conjunction with DDAVP or clotting factor. Contraindicated in the presence of disseminated intravascular coagulation, hematuria, prothrombin complex concentrates, or activated prothrombin complex concentrates because of the risk of thrombotic complications.

Opinions also differ regarding when to start prophylaxis, and the practice continues to evolve. Some providers believe that there is an increase of inhibitor development when factor is introduced at a young age. In addition, venous access is often a barrier to compliance with prophylaxis in young children. Starting prophylaxis at a later age may prevent the need for a central line, which has the potential for infection, deep vein thrombosis, and mechanical dysfunction. On the other hand, starting factor before the first joint bleed occurs may help prevent long-term joint damage.

### Secondary Prophylaxis
Secondary prophylaxis is started after repeated bleeding into the same joint (i.e., target joint). It is often done on a short-term basis.

## Inhibitors
Inhibitors are antibodies that develop in response to clotting factor and can cause serious complications. Inhibitors neutralize or destroy circulating FVIII or FIX. Approximately 20%–33% of those with hemophilia A develop inhibitors, and 1%–6% of those with hemophilia B develop them. Inhibitors are measured with a Bethesda inhibitor assay and are classified as high responders (>5 Bethesda units [BUs]) or low responders (<5 BUs).

Inhibitors tend to develop during childhood; the average age is 12 years. The risk is greatest during the first 50 exposures to recombinant FVIII. Studies of children receiving recombinant FVIII have shown inhibitor development at an average age of 1–2 years after approximately 10 treatments. Potential risk factors include type and severity of hemophilia, family history of inhibitors, and ethnic origin. Theories of inhibitor development include age at first exposure to clotting factor; route, intensity, and method of FVIII administration; modification of the immune response to FVIII through breast-feeding or inflammatory response; and type of FVIII product infused.

A clinical sign of inhibitor development is bleeding with poor response to factor infusion. Patients are instructed to contact their physician if bleeding is not adequately resolved after factor administration, and an inhibitor level should be checked. Laboratory signs include peak FVIII or FIX levels without the corresponding increase in factor level and a positive inhibitor level (measured in BUs).

Management of inhibitors includes treatment with bypassing agents such as activated prothrombin complex concentrates (e.g., activated prothrombin complex concentrate [APCC], FVIII-inhibitor bypassing activity), porcine FVIII, or recombinant factor VIIa (FVIIa). APCCs contain factors II, VII, IX, and X. They are plasma derived and virally deactivated. No factor level is achieved.

Activated recombinant FVII is thought to provide a burst of tissue factor at the local bleeding site. No factor level is achieved. It is short acting and requires that infusions be repeated every 2–3 hours.

Patients with FIX inhibitor are at risk for anaphylaxis when exposed to FIX. There is also a risk of developing nephrosis with ongoing treatment with FIX.

## Immune Tolerance
Attempts to overwhelm the inhibitor are conducted through immune-tolerance regimens. Success is determined by the eradication of the inhibitor, loss of anamnestic response, and the return of normal response to factor both clinically and by laboratory studies.

Inhibitor studies are ongoing. Variability exists among immune-tolerance treatment regimens throughout the world. With some variability, standard practice in the United States is administration of an infusion of 100 U/kg daily.

## Comprehensive Care
The care of patients with hemophilia requires a comprehensive healthcare team that uses a family-centered approach to providing optimal care for the individual with hemophilia and support for his family. The primary goals are minimizing complications from bleeding and treatment, reducing school and work absences, and minimizing lifestyle disruptions.

The functions of the hemophilia treatment center (HTC) staff include diagnosis and evaluation of individuals with bleeding disorders; treatment of bleeding episodes and complications; coordination of care; education of the patient and the family; outreach to the community; advocacy; and research and data collection.

HTCs located throughout the United States are supported in part by grants from the Maternal and Child Health Bureau of the U.S. Department of Health and Human Services and by the Centers for Disease Control and Prevention.

## Nursing Assessment and Interventions
### Goal
The patient experiences minimal complications from joint bleeding and long-term joint damage is prevented.

**Assessment:**
Early joint bleeding:
- Obtain an accurate history, including any prior joint bleeds and their frequency.
- Determine when symptoms first started.
- Note any limping or favoring of the joint.
- Assess patient's range of motion.
- Note reports of pain.

**Interventions:**
- Rest, ice, compression, elevation (RICE)
- Early treatment; evaluate response
- Involve parents and child in the process.
- Determine when to wean factor by clinical response.
- Advise family to contact the HTC if patient does not respond to the factor.
- Evaluate the frequency of bleeding into joint, and consider prophylaxis for frequent bleeds.
- If breakthrough bleeding occurs while patient is on prophylaxis, consider kinetic studies to determine factor utilization as well as inhibitor check.
- Evaluate the need for muscle strengthening for affected joint after bleed is resolved.

**Assessment:**
Late or severe joint bleeding:
- Obtain an accurate history, including any prior joint bleeds and their frequency.
- Assess for swelling, warmth, and pain.
- Evaluate for muscle bogginess, atrophy, and weakness, as well as range of motion.

- Differentiate between chronic arthropathy and acute joint bleeding.
- Pain assessment should distinguish between chronic pain and arthritis and acute bleed pain.
  
  **Interventions:**
- RICE
- Early treatment; evaluate response
- Involve physical therapist and orthopedist.
- Magnetic resonance imaging, if indicated
- Evaluate need for brace or surgery, such as synovectomy, and level of commitment on the part of the patient.
- Pain management
- Provide support and education to the patient and family.

## Expected Patient and Family Outcomes

The patient and the family can do the following:
- Verbalize understanding of the disease process.
- Identify signs and symptoms of bleeding episodes.
- Demonstrate administration of factor infusions.
- State when and how to notify the healthcare team.
- Verbalize understanding of injury-prevention strategies.

### Reference

Manco-Johnson, M. J., Abshire, T. C., Shapiro, A. D., Riske, B., Hacker, M. R., Kilcoyne, R., et al. (2007). Prophylaxis versus episodic treatment to prevent joint disease in boys with severe hemophilia. *New England Journal of Medicine, 357*, 535–544.

# Von Willebrand Disease

*James E. Munn*

## Definition

*Von Willebrand disease* (vWD) is an inherited bleeding disorder that results from quantitative (i.e., low or absent levels) or qualitative (i.e., impaired functioning) defects of von Willebrand factor (vWf), a multimeric glycoprotein required for normal hemostasis.

## Pathophysiology

VWf serves two major roles in hemostasis. First, it is necessary for platelet adhesion to sites of vascular injury and platelet aggregation during conditions of high shear stress (e.g., high blood flow in small vessels). Second, vWf circulates as a noncovalent complex with factor VIII; it protects factor VIII from proteolysis through the body's normal enzymatic processes. Deficiencies or dysfunctions of vWf result in a tendency toward bleeding, and, by contrast, high levels or increased function might lead to thrombotic concerns.

Manufactured in endothelial cells and megakaryocytes, vWf is required in both primary and secondary hemostasis. Stored in Weibel-Palade bodies found in endothelial cells and platelet α-granules, vWf can be released when needed and is an acute-phase reactant. Levels are elevated during advanced pregnancy, with increased stress, and when inflammatory processes are present.

The disorder was first described by Erik A. von Willebrand in 1926, when he wrote about a large family cohort from the Åland Islands near Finland. The family presented with numerous episodes of mucosal bleeding. The index patient was a young girl who, at age 13, eventually died of a massive hemorrhage during her fourth menstrual cycle. Since both sexes of this family were affected by mucosal bleeding, Dr. von Willebrand, who originally termed this disease hereditary pseudohemophilia, correctly deduced that the disorder was different from hemophilia and was autosomally inherited. The same type of clinical disorder was reported by several Americans in 1928.

The vWf protein was identified by Zimmerman and colleagues in 1971, and cDNA cloning of the molecule was achieved in 1985.

## Subtypes

Nomenclature for vWD has changed over the years, and the current classification lists six subgroups: type 1, type 2 (with four subtypes), and type 3. Types 1 and 3 represent quantitative deficiencies in vWf. Accounting for about 70%–80% of diagnosed cases, vWD type 1 results when lower than normal levels of vWf are present in circulation. Type 3, however, is the complete absence of vWf and is rare. Type 2 (representing about 20%–30% of vWD cases) results from qualitative defects in vWf and has been subdivided into four categories: 2A, 2B, 2M, and 2N.

The vWf glycoprotein is composed of multimers (i.e., protein segments of low, intermediate, and high molecular weights). Defects related to the vWf molecule give rise to the type 2 subtypes. They can be distinguished as follows:
- Type 2A—loss of intermediate and high-molecular-weight multimers.
- Type 2B—loss of high-molecular-weight multimers with hyperaffinity to platelet binding (often resulting in thrombocytopenia).
- Type 2M—all multimers present except hypoaffinity to platelet binding. The Vicenza variant shows extra-large multimers.
- Type 2N—the Normandy variant; multimers are generally normal but unable to bind to factor VIII (resulting in low factor VIII levels).

## Prevalence, Incidence, and Etiology

Considered the most common inheritable bleeding diathesis in humans, vWD is prevalent in about 1%–2% of the population. Prevalence rates are higher in countries where consanguineous marriages are common. Incidence rates are not affected by race, religion, socioeconomic status, or age but appear to show a slight predominance in females, most likely due to menstrual bleeding concerns at diagnosis. Often, a positive family history augments diagnosis in infants and toddlers because of the autosomal-dominant inheritance pattern found in most types of vWD.

Decreased amounts or impaired functioning of vWf remains the primary cause of vWD; however, acquired vWD has been reported. Acquired vWD generally occurs when an antibody (i.e., inhibitor) to vWf occurs, as seen in some lymphoproliferative disorders, some forms of congenital cardiac disease, uremia, Wilms' tumors, systemic lupus erythematosus, hypothyroidism, and the use of some drugs (e.g., valproic acid). Treatment or removal of the underlying condition usually corrects the bleeding symptoms in these individuals.

## Genetics

Most forms of vWD are inherited in an autosomal-dominant pattern. Located on the tip of the p arm of chromosome 12, the vWf gene is about 180 kilobases long, as vWf is a complex molecule. Multimeric subunits add to the molecule's complexity, and more than 50 genotypes have been identified.

The breakdown of inheritance by vWD type is
- Type 1—autosomal dominant
- Type 2A—usually autosomal dominant
- Type 2B—autosomal dominant
- Type 2M—autosomal dominant
- Type 2N—autosomal recessive
- Type 3—usually autosomal recessive; however, some homozygous or compound heterozygous inheritances of type 1 have occurred.

## Clinical Presentation

Although theoretically, bleeding can occur wherever there is a blood vessel, the most common presentation in vWD is mucocutaneous bleeding; for example, epistaxis, ecchymoses/hematomas, menorrhagia, gastrointestinal (GI) or genitourinary (GU) bleeding, hemorrhage after childbirth or dental extractions, and postoperative wound bleeding. In some cases of vWD (such as type 3), intramuscular and intraarticular bleeds, such as those seen in some hemophilia patients, can occur.

Interestingly, vWD exhibits a heterogeneous bleeding pattern within the same family. This phenotypic variability, or incomplete penetrance, can be affected by blood type (e.g., ABO grouping), estrogen levels, liver disease, and stress. Also, vWf levels increase with age, so mild symptoms may diminish over time.

**Table 11-8** lists the vWD types, inheritance patterns, diagnostic test results, and clinical presentations.

## Diagnosis

Although vWD is the most common inherited bleeding disorder, the diagnosis can be difficult to make. Because hormone levels, stress, exercise, and blood group can affect vWf levels, diagnosis of vWD often requires more than one set of blood tests.

As with all diagnostic approaches, a thorough history and physical should precede any blood work. Care should be taken to assess personal and family history of bleeding, because families may consider their bleeding patterns to be "normal."

Attention to frequency of bleeding and bruising; areas affected (usually mucous membranes); precipitating events (e.g., trauma, surgery, dental procedures.); amount of blood loss noted; length of time required to control bleeding; alleviating measures employed; and use of doctors' offices, hospitals, or emergency rooms for care must be considered. Assessment of menorrhagia in adolescent females should include length of menstrual periods, number and types of hygiene products used, frequency of pad or tampon changes, amount of saturation noted with each change, and whether the individual exhibits signs or symptoms of excessive blood loss (e.g., dizziness, shortness of breath, pallor, lethargy, tachycardia). Menstrual bleeding diaries are helpful for elucidating blood loss.

The most common laboratory tests used to diagnose vWD include
- Factor VIII assay
- vWf antigen level
- vWf activity (ristocetin cofactor activity)
- Multimer analysis.

Other laboratory tests that can assist with diagnosis include
- a PTT
- Bleeding time
- Complete blood count, including platelet count and differential
- ABO blood grouping (type-O patients have a lower-than-expected vWf Ag)
- Platelet functional analyzer testing
- Ristocetin-induced platelet aggregation study (for type 2B)
- Factor VIII binding assay (for type 2N).

## Prognostic Considerations

With the use of appropriate treatment products, life expectancy is normal for patients with vWD. Determining which patients will bleed most or require frequent treatment is impractical for each type of vWD because of the phenotypic variability within individuals and between family members. Patients with type 3 and some individuals with type 2 require a vWf-replacement product. Bleeding episodes should be assessed for minor, major, or life- or limb-threatening status and treated based on the evaluation.

## Treatment

The primary goal of vWD treatment is to stop or prevent bleeding while concurrently minimizing or eliminating treatment and bleeding complications. Treatment is based on the bleeding site, severity, target joint status (usually for patients with type 3), type of vWD diagnosed, and age, and may be episodic (i.e., whenever bleeding occurs) or prophylactic (i.e., to prevent bleeding). Therapeutic interventions can be classified into either nonreplacement or replacement therapy:

- Nonreplacement therapy:
  - 1-desamino-8-D-arginine vasopressin (DDAVP)—stimulates a rise in circulating vWf. May be given intravenously (IV), intranasally, or subcutaneously. The intranasal form is contraindicated in children younger than 2 years. Because dilutional hyponatremia can be a severe side effect, fluid restrictions should be enforced with DDAVP use. Not generally used in patients with type 2B.
  - Antifibrinolytic agents—prevention of clot lysis by plasmin (aminocaproic acid and tranexamic acid)—IV and orally. Avoid use of these agents when hematuria is present.
  - Hormone use—often estrogen-containing oral contraceptives or Mirena IUD
  - RICE
- Replacement therapy:
  - Cryoprecipitate—seldom used since the advent of vWf-containing factor VIII concentrates
  - Platelet transfusion—rarely used but has been successful as an adjuvant to vWf-containing factor VIII concentrates in some patients
  - vWf-containing factor VIII concentrates—all plasma derived and with specific U.S. Food and Drug Administration-approved uses (e.g., Humate-P, Alphanate, Koate-DVI)

Table 11-8. vWD Type, Inheritance, Diagnostic Results, and Clinical Findings

| vWD Type | Multimer Analysis | Ristocetin Cofactor Activity | vWf Antigen | FVIII | Inheritance Pattern | Clinical Bleeding Presentation | Other |
|---|---|---|---|---|---|---|---|
| 1 | Normal distribution | Usually low | Usually low | Usually normal; can be low | Autosomal dominant | Usually mucocutaneous | Accounts for 70%–80% of diagnosed cases of vWD |
| 2A | Abnormal; loss of intermediate and high molecular weight (MW) multimers | Markedly low | Usually low or normal | Usually normal; can be low | Usually autosomal dominant | Usually mucocutaneous | Most common Type 2 subtype |
| 2B | Abnormal; loss of high MW multimers | Markedly low | Usually low or normal | Usually normal; can be low | Usually autosomal dominant | Usually mucocutaneous | Ristocetin induced platelet aggregation to confirm diagnosis; hyperaffinity to platelet binding |
| 2M | Normal distribution/Vicenza variant; shows extra-large multimers | Usually low | Usually low or normal | Usually normal; can be low | Autosomal dominant | Usually mucocutaneous | Hypoaffinity to platelet binding |
| 2N | Normal distribution; occasional abnormal pattern | Usually normal; can be low | Usually normal; can be low | Markedly low | Autosomal recessive | Usually mucocutaneous | FVIII binding assay to confirm diagnosis |
| 3 | Absent | Not detectable | Not detectable | Markedly low | Usually autosomal recessive; can be autosomal dominant | Can bleed in muscles and joints | Requires IV-replacement therapy |

— Because of potential blood-borne virus transmission associated with plasma-derived products, viral-attenuation techniques are employed during the screening, processing, manufacturing, and formulating of vWf-containing factor VIII replacement products. vWf concentrates that have no exposure to blood and eliminate the risk of virus transmission are in development. In fact, clinical trials of a recombinant-derived, blood- and plasma-free vWf concentrate are being designed.

## Nursing Assessment and Interventions

### Goal
The patient experiences minimal complications related to bleeding.

**Assessment:**
- Review the patient's vWD type, if known, and usual treatment modalities.
- Ascertain whether patient had tried the usual course of treatment and control of bleeding was not achieved.
- Assess presenting bleeding episode and obtain a complete history, including precipitating cause (e.g., trauma, surgery, dental procedure, menses, gastrointestinal (GI) or genitourinary (GU) bleeding, environmental conditions or allergens, spontaneous bleed); duration of bleeding; individual and family history; site of bleeding; severity of bleeding; and initial symptoms (e.g., pain, swelling, redness, warmth, neurological changes, menstrual blood loss documented by a bleeding diary, fevers, lethargy, abdominal cramping, loss of range of motion [ROM] of affected extremity).
- Perform a complete physical examination to determine the presence of dizziness, pallor, petechiae, infection, neurologic changes, hematomas or ecchymoses, epistaxis, intramuscular bleeding, intraarticular bleeding, hematuria, melena, amount of menstrual blood loss, and loss of mobility or ability to perform activities of daily life (ADL).
- Assess level of pain.
- Review laboratory findings.
- Review radiological imaging studies as indicated.
- Review surgical reports as indicated.
- Assess venous access as indicated.

**Interventions:**
- Administer appropriate treatment modality based on bleeding episode, laboratory and radiological findings, and child's age.
- Administer treatment prior to scans, procedures, imaging studies, and sutures.
- Treat bleeds at the onset of symptoms and with appropriate product.
- Encourage yearly comprehensive evaluations at a treatment center or doctor's office.
- Provide pain medication as needed.
- Provide comfort measures.
- Encourage exercise to help build muscles and protect joints.
- Assess joint range of motion measurements regularly as indicated.
- Monitor for signs of compromise—neurological, respiratory, and hemodynamic.
- Monitor complete blood count, with platelets and differential, for hemorrhage and infection.

- Monitor appropriate coagulation studies for effectiveness of treatment measures.
- Utilize adjunctive therapies (e.g., crutches, walkers, wheelchairs, ace wraps, kinesiotaping, orthotic adaptive equipment, protective dental gear) as needed for decreased movement, loss of mobility, prevention of reinjury, and inability to perform ADL.
- Teach home or self-infusion as a treatment option when indicated.
- Discuss venous access options (e.g., central venous access devices, peripherally inserted central catheters, arteriovenous fistulas) when venous access is poor or difficult.
- Readjust treatment plan from episodic care to prophylaxis as needed.

### Goal
The patient experiences minimal complications related to treatment.

**Assessment:**
- Assess for exposure to blood-borne viruses (presence of flu-like symptoms, lethargy, abdominal distension or discomfort, right-upper-quadrant pain, recurrent opportunistic infections, jaundice, hepatosplenomegaly, esophageal varices, thrombocytopenia).
- Assess for development of inhibitors (inability to control bleeding with usual vWf containing factor VIII concentrate, increased bleeding or bruising despite treatment-product use).
- Assess for venous-access-device complications (e.g., infection, mechanical malfunction, catheter-related thrombosis, presence of collateral circulation, signs of superior vena cava syndrome) as indicated.
- Assess for surgery-related complications (e.g., increased bleeding, poor wound healing, infection).
- Review laboratory findings as indicated.
- Review imaging studies as indicated.
- Review surgical and pathology reports as indicated.

**Interventions:**
- Administer hepatitis A and B vaccines.
- Test for antibody (inhibitor) formation as indicated.
- Test regularly for blood-borne infections.
- Refer patient for alternative venous access as indicated.
- Obtain cultures and radiographic imaging as needed for suspected venous access device complications (e.g., infection or extraluminal thrombosis) and initiate therapy (e.g., antibiotics, antipyretics) as indicated.
- Administer declotting medications (alteplase, urokinase) as indicated for suspected venous-access-device intraluminal thrombosis.
- Review all results of laboratory and radiological studies with the patient and the family.
- Refer patient to infectious diseases or hepatologic specialists for positive viral laboratory findings as indicated.
- Educate the patient and the family about treatment complications, including signs and symptoms of infection and thrombosis, as well as treatment-product safety profiles.
- Provide instruction on proper venous-access-device care.

### Goal
The patient and the family experience minimal emotional stress and are adequately informed regarding the diagnosis of vWD and available treatment options.

**Assessment:**
- Review the patient's and the family's history of bleeding.
- Assess the patient's and the family's knowledge regarding bleeding disorders, specifically vWD.
- Assess the patient's presenting symptoms, including precipitating cause (e.g., trauma, surgery, dental procedure, menses, GI or GU bleeding, environmental conditions or allergens, spontaneous bleed); duration, site, and severity of bleeding; and initial symptoms (e.g., pain, swelling, redness, warmth, neurological changes, menstrual blood loss documented by a bleeding diary, fevers, lethargy, abdominal cramping, loss of ROM of affected extremity).
- Perform a complete physical examination to determine presence of dizziness, pallor, petechiae, signs of infection, neurological changes, hematomas or ecchymoses, epistaxis, intramuscular bleeding, intraarticular bleeding, hematuria, melena, amount of menstrual blood loss, and loss of mobility or ability to perform ADL.
- Assess level of pain.
- Review laboratory findings.
- Review radiological imaging studies as indicated.
- Review surgical reports as indicated.
- Assess venous access as indicated.
- Review inheritance pattern of bleeding within the family.
- Determine the family's coping strategies and support systems available to them.

**Interventions:**
- Monitor for signs of compromise—neurological, respiratory, hemodynamic.
- Explain laboratory and imaging results to the patient and the family.
- Provide the patient and the family with honest answers.
- Provide comfort measures.
- Administer appropriate treatment modality based on bleeding episode, laboratory and radiological findings, and child's age.
- Administer treatment prior to scans, procedures, imaging studies, and sutures.
- Provide pain medication as needed.
- Provide education to the patient and the family that is age appropriate, specific to the diagnosis, and incorporates the best learning style of each individual.
- Reassure the patient and the family about available treatment strategies.
- Coordinate ongoing care and learning in a variety of settings—hospital, home, school, camp, consumer educational meetings, and family support groups.
- Introduce the patient and the family to a variety of supportive individuals, organizations, and foundations to minimize feelings of isolation.
- Refer the patient and the family to community services as needed.
- Illustrate inheritance of vWD using family pedigree whenever possible.

- Encourage the patient and the family to ask questions related to the diagnosis, the disease, and the treatment of vWD.
- Solicit and utilize the patient's and the family's input in the development of an ongoing care plan.

## Expected Patient and Family Outcomes
The child and the family can do the following:
- Describe their specific vWD diagnosis, treatment, inheritance, and plan of care.
- List types of bleeding episodes (e.g., mucous membrane, soft tissue, muscle, joint) and products and strategies used for treating each.
- Describe the signs and symptoms of bleeding and when to treat them.
- Compare and contrast minor, major, and life- or limb-threatening bleeds and how to manage each.
- Explain how and when to contact the healthcare team if problems or questions arise.
- Demonstrate appropriate home or self-infusion skills needed for treatment as indicated.
- Outline methods for prevention and treatment of bleeding complications.
- Formulate a plan of care with the treatment team that takes into account vWD diagnosis, age and maturity of the child, type and frequency of treatment needed for controlling or preventing bleeding and that maximizes adherence to the established plan.
- List available community and family resources.

## Bibliography

### Autoimmune Hemolytic Anemia
Gehrs, B. C., & Friedberg, R. C. (2002). Autoimmune hemolytic anemia. *American Journal of Hematology, 69*(4), 258–271.
King, K. E., & Ness, P. M. (2005). Treatment of autoimmune hemolytic anemia. *Seminars in Hematology, 42*(3), 131–136.

### Sickle-Cell Disease
Driscoll, C. M. (2007). Sickle cell disease. *Pediatrics in Review, 28*(7), 259–268.
Miller, S. T., Sleeper, L. A., Pegelow, C. H., Enos, L. E., Wang, W. C., Weiner, S. J., et al. (2000). Prediction of adverse outcomes in children with sickle cell anemia. *New England Journal of Medicine, 342,* 83–89.
Vichinsky, E. P. (2004). Pulmonary hypertension in sickle cell disease. *New England Journal of Medicine, 350,* 857–859.

### Thalassemia
Cappellini, M. D., Bejaoui, M., Agaoglu, L., Porter, J., Coates, T., Jeng, M., et al. (2007). Prospective evaluation of patient-reported outcomes during treatment with deferasirox or deferoxamine for iron overload in patients with s-thalassemia. *Clinical Therapeutics, 29,* 909–917.

### Glucose-6-Phosphate Dehydrogenase Deficiency
Lanzkowsky, P. (2005). *Manual of pediatric hematology and oncology* (4th ed., pp. 153–157). Burlington, MA: Elsevier Academic Press.
Luzzatto, L. (2003). Glucose-6-phosphate dehydrogenase deficiency and hemolytic anemia. In D. G. Nathan, S. H. Orkin, D. Ginsburg, & A. T. Look (Eds.), *Hematology of infancy and childhood* (6th ed., pp. 704–725). Philadelphia: W.B. Saunders.

### Hereditary Spherocytosis
Alter, B. P., & D'Andrea, A. D. (2003). Inherited bone marrow failure syndromes. In R.I . Handin, S. E. Lux, & T. P. Stossel (Eds.), *Blood: Principles and practice of hematology* (2nd ed., pp. 209–272). Philadelphia: Lippincott Williams & Wilkins.
Bolten-Maggs, P. H. (2004). Hereditary spherocytosis: New guidelines. *Archives of Disease in Childhood, 89,* 809–812.

### Bone-Marrow-Failure Syndromes
Alter, B. P., & Young, N. S. (2003). Inherited bone marrow failure syndromes. In D. G. Nathan, S. H. Orkin, D. Ginsberg, & A. T. Look (Eds.), *Hematology of infancy and childhood* (6th ed., pp. 280–365). Philadelphia: W.B. Saunders.
Hillman, R. S., Ault, K. A., & Rinder, H. M. (2005). *Hematology in clinical practice* (4th ed.). New York: McGraw Hill.

### Shwachman-Diamond Syndrome
Federman, N., & Sakamoto, K. (2005). The genetic basis of bone marrow failure syndromes in children. *Molecular Genetics and Metabolism, 86,* 100–109.
Grinspan, Z., & Pikora, C. (2005). Infections in patients with Shwachman-Diamond Syndrome. *The Pediatric Infectious Disease Journal, 24*(2), 179–181.
Rothbaum, R., Perrault, J., Vlachos, A., Cippoli, M., Alter, B., Burroughs, S., et al. (2002). Shwachman-Diamond syndrome: Report from an international conference. *The Journal of Pediatrics, 141,* 266–270.

### Chronic Neutropenia
Ancliff, P. J. (2003). Congenital neutropenia. *Blood Reviews, 17,* 209–216.
Carlsson G., Andersson, M., Putsep, K., Garwicz, D., Nordenskjold, M., Henter, J., et al. (2007). Kostmann syndrome or infantile genetic agranulocytosis, part one: Celebrating 50 years of clinical and basic research on severe congenital neutropenia. *Acta Paediatrica, 95,* 1526–1532.
Carlsson G., Melin, M., Dahl, N., Ramme, K. G., Nordenskjold, M., Palmblad, J., et al. (2007). Kostmann syndrome or infantile genetic agranulocytosis, part two: Understanding the underlying genetic defects in severe congenital neutropenia. *Acta Paediatrica, 96*(6), 813–819.
Christensen, R., & Calhoun, D. (2004). Congenital neutropenia. *Clinics in Perinatology, 31,* 29–38.

### Immune Thrombocytopenic Purpura
Klassen, R. J., Blanchette, V. S., Barnard, D., Wakefield, C. D., Curtis, C., Bradley, C. S., et al. (2007). Validity, reliability and responsiveness of a new measure of health related quality of life in children with immune thrombocytopenic purpura: The Kids' ITP Tools. *The Journal of Pediatrics, 150,* 510–515.
Sevier, N., & Houston, M. (2005). Chronic refractory ITP in children: Beyond splenectomy. *Journal of Pediatric Oncology Nursing, 22,* 145–151.

Silverman, M. A. (2007, January 18). *Idiopathic thrombocytopenic purpura.* Retrieved October 15, 2007, from www.emedicine.com/emerg/topic282.html.

## Evans Syndrome

Evans, R. S., Takahashi, K., Duane, R. T., Payne, R., & Liu, C. (1951). Primary thrombocytopenic purpura and acquired hemolytic anemia. *Archives of Internal Medicine, 87*(1), 48–65.

Norton, A., & Roberts, I. (2006). Management of Evans syndrome. *British Journal of Haematology, 132*(2), 125–137.

Shvidel, L., Sigler, E., Shtalrid, M., & Berrebi, A. (2006). Vincristine-loaded platelet infusion for treatment of refractory autoimmune hemolytic anemia and chronic immune thrombocytopenia: Rethinking old cures. *American Journal of Hematology, 81*(6), 423–425.

Teachey, D. T., Manno, C. S., Axom, K. M., Andrews, T., Choi, J. K., Greenbaum, B. H., et al. (2005). Unmasking Evans syndrome: T-cell phenotype and apoptotic response reveal autoimmune lymphoproliferative syndrome (ALPS). *Blood, 105* (6), 2443–2448.

Zecca, M., Nobili, B., Ramenghi, U., Perrotta, S., Amendola, G., Rosito, P., et al. (2003). Rituximab for the treatment of refractory autoimmune hemolytic anemia in children. *Blood, 101*(10), 3857–3861.

## Thrombosis and Thrombophilia

Blumenstein, M. (2007). Early ambulation after acute deep vein thrombosis: Is it safe? *Journal of Pediatric Oncology Nursing, 24,* 309–313.

Bonduel, M. (2006). Oral anticoagulation in children. *Thrombosis Research, 118,* 85–94.

Goldenberg, N., Knapp-Clevenger, R., & Manco-Johnson, M. (2004). Elevated plasma factor VIII and D-dimer levels as predictors of poor outcomes of thrombosis in children. *New England Journal of Medicine, 351,* 1081–1088.

Manco-Johnson, M. (2005). Etiopathogenesis of pediatric thrombosis. *Hematology, 10*(Suppl. 1), 167–170.

Manco-Johnson, M. (2006). Postthrombotic syndrome in children. *Acta Haematologica, 115,* 207–213.

Monglae, P., Chan, A., Massicotte, P., Chalmers, E., & Michelson, A. D. (2004). Antithrombotic therapy in children: The seventh ACCP conference on antithrombotic and thrombolytic therapy. *Chest, 126,* 645–687.

Young, G. (2006). Diagnosis and treatment of thrombosis in children: General principles. *Pediatric Blood and Cancer, 46,* 540–546.

## Hemolytic-Uremic Syndrome

Biega, T., & Prauner, R. *Hemolytic-uremic syndrome.* Retrieved November 24, 2007, from www.emedicine.com/ped/topic960.htm.

Brandt, J., Wong, C., Mihm, S., Roberts, J., Smith, J., Brewer, E., et al. (2002). Invasive pneumococcal disease and hemolytic uremic syndrome. *Pediatrics, 110,* 371–376.

Glaser, L. G. (n.d.) *Hemolytic uremic syndrome.* Retrieved December 7, 2007, from www.medstudents.com.br/pedia/pedia5.htm.

## Paroxysmal Nocturnal Hemoglobinuria

Araten, D. J., & Luzzato, L. (2006). The mutation rate in PIG-A is normal in patients with paroxysmal nocturnal hemoglobinuria (PNH). *Blood, 108*(2), 734–736.

Hill, A., Richards, S. J., & Hillmen, P. (2007). Recent developments in the understanding and management of paroxysmal nocturnal haemoglobinuria. *British Journal of Haematology, 137,* 181–192.

Hill, A., Ridley, S. H., Esser, D., Oldroyd, R. G., Cullen, M. J., Kareclas, P., et al. (2006). Protection of erythrocytes from human complement-mediated lysis by membrane-targeted recombinant soluble CD59: A new approach to PNH therapy. *Blood, 107*(5), 2131–2137.

Richards, S. J., Hill, A., & Hillmen, P. (2007). Recent advances in the diagnosis, monitoring, and management of patients with paroxysmal nocturnal hemoglobinuria. *Cytometry. Part B, Clinical Cytometry, 72B,* 291–298.

## Hemophilia

Butler, R. B., McClure, W., & Wulff, K. (2003). Practice patterns in haemophilia A therapy: A survey of treatment centres in the United States. *Haemophilia, 9,* 549–554.

DiMichele, D. (2004). *Inhibitors in hemophilia: A primer.* Montreal, Canada: World Federation of Hemophilia.

DiMichele, D. (2007). Inhibitors to Factor VIII: Epidemiology and treatment. In C. A. Lee, E. E. Berntorp, & W. K. Hoots (Eds.), *Textbook of hemophilia* (pp. 64–70). Malden, MA: Blackwell Publishing.

Kasper, C. K., & Buzin, C. H. (2007). *Genetics of hemophilia A and B.* King of Prussia, PA: The CSL Behring Foundation for Research and Advancement of Patient Health.

Manco-Johnson, M. J., Abshire, T. C., Shapiro, A. D., Riske, B., Hacker, M. R., Kilcoyne, R., et al. (2007). Prophylaxis versus episodic treatment to prevent joint disease in boys with severe hemophilia. *New England Journal of Medicine, 357,* 535–544.

Ross, J. (2004). *Perspectives of hemophilia carriers.* Montreal, Canada: World Federation of Hemophilia.

## Von Willebrand Disease

Manco-Johnson, M., Nuss, R., Lear, J., Wiedel, J., Geraghty, S. J. Hacker, M., et al. (2002). Von Willebrand disease and other inherited bleeding disorders in children with hemophilia. *Journal of Pediatric Hematology/Oncology, 24*(7), 534–539.

# Index

Note: Page numbers followed by *f* refer to figures; page numbers followed by *t* refer to tables.

## A

ABO types, matching, 64
Absolute granulocyte count, 65
Absolute neutrophil count (ANC), 65–66, 101, 102, 122, 298, 304–307
ABVD (adriamycin, bleomycin, vinblastine, dacarbazine) regimen, 26
ABVE-PC (adriamycin, bleomycin, vincristine, etoposide, prednisone, cyclophosphamide) regimen, 26
Access to care, 202–203
Acquired aplastic anemia, 297–298, 298*t*
Acquired neutropenia, 306–307
ACTH deficiency, 254
Actinomycin D. *See* Dactinomycin.
Acupuncture, 116
Acute chest syndrome, 289
Acute graft versus host disease (AGVHD), 104–105
Acute hemolytic anemia, 295, 296–297
Acute lymphoblastic leukemia (ALL), 15–19, 16*t*, 17*t*, 55*f*, 74
Acute myelogenous leukemia (AML), 16*t*, 17*t*, 55*f*
Acute nonlymphoblastic leukemia, 17*t*
Acute promyelocytic leukemia (APML), 17
Acute radiation dermatitis, 143*t*
Acute renal failure, 107
Acyclovir (Zovirax), 103, 124, 134
Adenoviral vectors, 113
Adenovirus infections, 108
Adhesions, abdominal, 264
Adjuvant chemotherapy, 76
Adolescents (12–20 years)
    assessment of pain in, 151*t*
    caloric needs, 170*t*
    cancers among, 54*f*
    concept of death, 228
    development of, 147*t*, 191–194, 217
    enteral products, 172*t*
    osteosarcoma in, 36
    outcomes of education, 219
    psychological preparation for procedures, 163*t*
    risk factors for cancer in, 13*t*
    teaching, 216*t*, 218*t*
Adrenocorticotropin deficiency, 254
Adriamycin. *See* Doxorubicin.
Adrucil. *See* 5-Fluorouracil.
Adult cancers, characteristics of, 12*t*
Adult education
    characteristics of learners, 220*t*
    guidelines for, 220*t*
    outcomes of, 221
Adults
    caloric needs, 170*t*
    enteral products, 172*t*
Advate, 321*t*

Age/aging
    assessments appropriate for, 14–15
    late reproductive system effects and, 267
    normal hematocrit levels, 63*t*
    normal hemoglobin values, 63*t*
    normal MCH levels, 63*t*
    normal MCV levels, 63*t*
    osteosarcoma survival and, 38*t*
    psychosocial effects and, 275
    respiratory system damage and, 261–262
Agranulocytes, 63
Airway/breathing, postoperative, 93
Albumin solutions, 180
Alemtuzumab (Campath), 101, 110*t*
Alkaline phosphate, serum, 37
Alkeran. *See* Melphalan.
Alkylating agents, 76, 77*t*, 100, 266. *See* specific agents.
Allogeneic stem cell transplantation, 98, 98*t*
Allopurinol (Zyloprim), 85*t*, 153
Alopecia, 96, 158
Aloxi (palonestron), 141*t*
Alpha-fetoprotein (AFP), 56, 70
Alpha-interferon, 23
Alpha thalassemia, 292–293
American Cancer Society, 277
American College of Surgeons, 7
American Nurses Credentialing Center Magnet Recognition Program, 7
Americans with Disabilities Act (ADA), 276, 278
Amethopterin. *See* Methotrexate.
Amicar (aminocaproic acid), 321*t*
Amifostine (Ethyol), 85*t*
Aminocaproic acid (Amicar), 321*t*
Aminoglycoside antibiotics, 130, 176*t*. *See also* specific antibiotics.
Aminopterin, 73
Amphotericin B (Fungizone), 103, 134
Amputation, 39, 144–145, 270
Anaphylaxis, 158
Anaplastic astrocytoma, 28
Anaplastic large-cell lymphoma (ALCL), 20, 21, 23
ANC. *See* Absolute neutrophil count.
Ancestry, 202
Anemia, 64–65. *See also specific* conditions.
    after stem cell transplantation, 102
    bone-marrow suppression and, 122
    medical management, 122
    during terminal phase of disease, 231
Anesthesia, 93
Angiogenesis, sustained, 14
Angiogenesis inhibitors, 30
Aniridia, 44
Ann Arbor staging classification, 26

Anorexia/early satiety, 171*t*, 232. *See also* specific side effects.
Anthracyclines, 18, 90, 136, 260, 263. *See also* specific agents.
Anthropomorphic measurements, 170
Antibiotics. *See also* specific antibiotics.
    after surgery, 93
    assessments, 94
    classes of, 176*t*–177*t*
    description, 76–77
    examples, 77*t*
    interventions, 94
    ototoxicity, 130
    principles of therapy using, 178*t*
    prophylactic, 133
    side effects of, 176*t*–177*t*
Antiemetics, 73, 139, 140*t*, 141*t*
Antifungal agents, 177. *See also* specific drugs.
Anti-GD2 monoclonal antibodies, 35
Antigrowth signals, 13–14
Antimetabolites, 77, 77*t*, 100. *See also* specific agents.
Antipneumocystis agents, 177
Antithrombin III deficiency, 313*t*
Antiviral agents, 177. *See also* specific agents.
Anxiety, 232
*APHON Counts*, 6
Aplastic anemia, 17, 297–300
Aplastic crisis, 289
Appetite-stimulant medications, 171–172
Aprepitant (Emend), 140*t*, 141*t*
Ara-C. *See* Cytarabine.
Ara-G (nelarabine), 84*t*
Aranesp (darbepoetin alfa), 109
Arsenic trioxide (Trisenox), 78*t*, 110*t*
Arthrodesis, 39
Artifical nutrition, 172
Askin's tumor, 40
Asparaginase, 18
Asparaginase (Elspar), 78*t*, 138
Assessments. *See also* specific cancers; specific conditions; specific therapies.
    diagnostic, 70
    goals of, 14–15
    standards of care, 4
Association of Cancer Online Resources (ACOR), 279*t*
Association of Pediatric Hematology/Oncology Nurses (APHON), 4, 6–8, 225
Association of Pediatric Oncology Nurses (APON), 3, 4–6
Astrocytomas, 28, 30
Ataxia telangiectasia, 17, 20
Ativan (lorazepam), 141*t*, 231
Audiograms, 130*f*
Autoimmune hemolytic anemia (AIHA), 286–288
Autoimmune lymphoproliferative syndrome (ALPS), 310–311
Autoimmune neutropenia (AIN), 306–307
Autologous stem cell transplant donors, 98, 98*t*
Autonomy, principle of, 241
Avascular necrosis, 271, 290
Avastin (bevacizumab), 110*t*
Ayurvedic medicine, 116
Azoospermia, 267

## B

Bactrim (trimethoprim and sulfamethoxazole, Septrax, Co-trimoxizole), 87*t*
Basic fibroblast growth factor (bFGF), 14
Basophils, function of, 63
B-cell lymphomas, classification, 20
BCNU (carmustine), 30, 66*t*, 79*t*
Bcr-abl, 110
BEACOPP (bleomycin, etoposide, adriamycin, cyclophosphamide, vincristine, prednisone, procarbazine) regimen, 26
Beckwith-Wiedemann syndrome, 44, 48, 55–56
Bectumomab (ImmuRaid-LL2), 109
Behavioral changes, 128–129
Benadryl (diphenylhydramine), 141*t*
Beneficence, principle of, 241
BeneFIX, 321*t*
Benzodiazepines, 231
Bereavement, 229, 235–237
Best Pharmaceuticals for Children Act–2002, 74
Beta thalassemia, 292–293
Bevacizumab (Avastin), 110*t*
Bexxar (tositumomab and I-131), 110*t*
Beyond the Cure, 279*t*
Bilirubin, 62
Biochemical markers, 16
Biologic agents, 30
Biological safety cabinets, 89
Biologic response modifiers (BRMs), 108–112
Biopsies, 70, 92
Biotherapeutic agents, 89, 110*t*
Bladder, 96, 266
Bladder dysfunction, 266
Bleeding, 231
Bleomycin (Blenozane), 54, 56, 261, 262
Bleomycin sulfate (Blenoxane), 78*t*
Blood, whole, 62, 179
Blood cells
    normal parameters, 63
    origin of, 62–63
Blood products, 178–182
    complications of, 123
    definition, 178
    indications, 179
    sources of components, 179
    types of, 179–181
Bloom syndrome, 17
"Blueberry muffin" sign, 33
Body-based practices, 115
Bone
    effects of radiation therapy on, 96, 258, 270
    late effects of cancer, 259
Bone marrow
    aspiration of, 18, 29, 70
    blood cell formation by, 62

signs of NHL, 21
stem cell harvesting from, 99
suppression of, 101–102
Bone-marrow-failure syndromes, 297–302, 302t
Bone-marrow suppression, 122–123
Bone marrow transplantation, 35, 258, 263, 264
Bone scans, 29, 72
Bortezomib (Velcade), 110t
Brachytherapy, 95
Brain
anatomy of, 29f
effects of radiotherapy, 95
imaging of, 29
Brainstem astrocytomas, 30
Brain stem auditory-evoked responses, 130
Brainstem gliomas, 28
Brain tumors, 28–31
Bromocriptine, 254
Burkitt's lymphoma (BL), 20, 21, 23
Burkitt's-like lymphoma (BLL), 20, 21
Busulfan (Myleran)
characteristics of, 78t
effect on fertility, 267
history of, 73
neutropenia caused by, 66t
pulmonary toxicity, 261
Bystander effect, 113

## C

Cachexia, 145
Caloric needs, 170t
Campath (alemtuzumab), 101, 110t
Camptosar. *See* Irinotecan.
Camptothecins, 77
Cancer. *See also* Childhood cancers *specific* Cancers.
acquired capabilities of, 13–14, 13f
susceptibility genes, 12–13
Cancer Legal Resource Center, 277
Candida infections, 134
Candlelighters Childhood Cancer Foundation, 277, 278
Capillary-leak syndrome, 103–104
Capromab pentomab (ProstaScint), 109
Carbepenems, 176t
Carboplatin (Paraplatin)
characteristics of, 78t
interventions for extravasation, 91t
late effects of, 266
neutropenia caused by, 66t
in non-Hodgkin's lymphoma, 23
in pediatric brain tumors, 30
in relapsed/recurrent kidney tumors, 47
subconjunctival, 53
Cardiac complications, 132–133
Cardiomyopathies, 260
Cardiovascular system, late effects on, 249t, 260–261
Caring, definition of, 208
Carmustine (BCNU), 30, 66t, 79t
Carotid artery disease, 258

Cataracts, 108, 256
"Cathie face," 300
CCNU. *See* Lomustine.
CDKN2A deletions, 41
CeeNU. *See* Lomustine.
Cell cycle, 13–14, 13t, 76, 76f, 77t
Cell therapy, 112–115
Central hypoventilation, 33
Central line bacteremia, 174t
Central nervous system (CNS)
complications, 126–130
effects of radiotherapy, 95
late effects of cancer, 246–253, 247t
prophylactic therapy, 18, 19, 23
second malignancies, 273
symptoms of NHL, 21
tumors of, 10, 28–32, 31, 55t
Central venous access devices (CVADs), 165–167
Central venous lines, 90
Cephalosporins, 176t
Cerebellum, astrocytomas, 30
Cerebral vascular accidents (CVAs), 289. *See also* Stroke.
Cerebrospinal fluid, ICPs and, 28
Cerebrovascular complications, 258–259
Certification, APHON, 7
Certified pediatric oncology nurses (CPON), 224–225
Cerubidine (daunomycin), 136
Cetuximab, 111
CEV (carboplatin, etoposide, vincristine) regimen, 53
CH 14.18 chimeric MoAb anti-GD2, 110t
Chemical or reactive hepatitis, 137–138
Chemoreceptor trigger zone (CTZ), 138
Chemotherapeutic agents. *See also* specific agents; specific regimens.
cardiovascular changes, 260
characteristics of, 78t–87t
classification of, 76–77
emetogenic potential of, 139t
late effects, 256–257, 263–264
safe handling of, 89–90
side-effects, 73–74, 77
skin reactions and, 142, 143t
Chemotherapy. *See also* specific cancers; specific drugs.
conditioning regimens, 100
history of, 73–74
infertility and, 267
late effects, 245–261
overcoming resistance to, 88t
principles of, 75–76
types of, 76
Chemotherapy agents, 77t
Chest X-rays, 18
Chicken pox (varicella zoster), 124, 125t
Childhood cancer
characteristics of, 12t
clinical trials, 74–75
common concerns, 222
educational priorities, 222–224

epidemiology of, 10–15
etiology, 11
history of treatment for, 2
incidence, 10–11, 11t
late effects, 245–261, 247t–251t
mortality rates, 10–11, 11t
overview, 10
patterns of, 11
risk factors, 11
symptoms suggestive of, 71t
trends, 11t
Childhood Cancer Survivor Study (CCSS), 279t
Children, risk factors, 13t, 146
Children's Cancer Group (CCG), 2
Children's Cancer Study Group, 73
Children's Cause for Cancer Advocacy (CCCA), 279t
Children's Oncology Group (COG), 2, 74
Chiropractic care, 115, 116
Chlorpromazine (Thorazine), 140t, 141t
Cholelithiasis, 264, 290
CHOP (cyclophosphamide, doxorubicin, vincristine, prednisone) regimen, 23
Chromosomal abnormalities, 17t, 40
Chronic graft versus host disease (AGVHD), 105–106, 108. See also Graft versus host disease (GVHD).
Chronic myeloid leukemia (CML), 15, 16
Chronic neutropenia, 304–307
Cisplatin (Platinol)
characteristics of, 79t
cranial nerve deficits after, 127
in germ cell tumors, 56
GI complications, 135
interventions for extravasation, 91t
late effects of, 266
in nasopharyngeal carcinoma, 54
for neuroblastoma, 35
neutropenia caused by, 66t
for osteosarcoma, 38
in pediatric brain tumors, 30
Cis-retinoic acid, 23
Citrovorum factor (leucovorin calcium, folinic acid, Welcovin), 87t
Cladribine, 79t
Classroom visits, 207
Clear-cell sarcoma of the kidney, 43, 47
Clinical trials
minority groups and, 203
phases of, 74–75
regulatory requirements, 75
review of investigational protocols, 222
Clofarabine, 74, 79t
Clostridium septicum, 156
Clotrimazole (Mycelex), 134
Clotting concentrates, 181
Codman's triangle, 37
Cognitive deficits, 128–129, 146, 246, 251–253, 290
Collaboration, professional standard for, 4, 6
Collegiality, 4, 6

Colonoscopy, 93
Combination chemotherapy. *See also* Chemotherapy; specific agents; specific regimens.
definition, 76
history of, 73
late effects of, 266
radiation sensitivity and, 96
Comfort measures, 223, 233t
Common Terminology Criteria for Adverse Events, 134
Communication
assessment of coping skills, 15
facilitation of, 223
psychosocial effects and, 275
Compazine (prochlorperazine), 140t, 141t
Compensated hypothyroidism, 255
Complementary and alternative medicine (CAM), 115–116
Complete blood counts (CBCs), 18, 70
Comprehensive Omnibus Budget Reconciliation Act, 277
Computerized tomography (CT) scans, 72
Conditioning therapy regimens, 23, 100–101
Conformal radiation therapy, 95
Congenital aplastic anemia, 298–300
Congenital mesoblastic nephroma, 44
Congenital neutropenia, 305
Connective tissue, 258, 259
Consolidation chemotherapy, 18
Constipation, 136–137, 171t, 232
"Consumer Guide for Getting and Keeping Health Insurance," 277
Coordination of care, 4
Coping skills, 15, 197, 223, 275
COPP/ABV (cyclophosphamide, vincristine, prednisone, procarbazine, adriamycin, bleomycin, vinblastine) regimen, 26
COPP (cyclophosphamide, vincristine, procarbazine, prednisone) regimen, 26
Cord blood collection, 100
Coronary artery disease, 260, 261
Corticosteroids, 18, 77, 80t, 251
Cosmegen. *See* Dactinomycin.
CPT-11. *See* Irinotecan.
Cranial nerve deficits, 28, 127–128
Cranial nerves, 127f, 128t
Cranial radiation therapy (XRT), 23
Craniopharyngioma, 28, 30
Cryoprecipitates, transfusion, 180
Cryptorchidism, 56
Culturally-sensitive care, 202–204
Cutaneous infections, 175t
Cyclic neutropenia, 306
Cyclin-dependent kinases (CDKs), 14
Cyclins, 14
Cyclophosphamide (Cytoxan)
characteristics of, 80t
effect on fertility, 267
for Ewing's sarcoma family of tumors, 41
for fibrosarcoma, 55

in germ cell tumors, 56
history of, 73
late effects of, 266
in nasopharyngeal carcinoma, 54
for neuroblastoma, 35
neutropenia caused by, 66t
for non-Hodgkin's lymphoma, 23
for pediatric brain tumors, 30
pulmonary toxicity, 261
for rhabdomyosarcoma, 50
Cyclosporine (Sandimmune), 107, 266
Cystitis, 267
Cytarabine (ara-C, cytosine arabinoside, Cytosar-U)
characteristics of, 23, 80t
cranial nerve deficits after, 127
GI complications, 135–136
intrathecal, 18
neutropenia caused by, 66t
Cytogenetics, 16–17, 70
Cytokines, 109–110, 111
Cytomegalovirus (CMV), 108, 181
Cytomegalovirus (CMV) pneumonitis, 106
Cytosine arabinoside, 261
Cytovene (ganciclovir), 103
Cytoxan. See Cyclophosphamide.

## D

Dacarbazine (DTIC), 55, 80t, 91t
Daclizumab (Zenapax), 110t
Dactinomycin (Actinomycin D, Cosmegen)
characteristics of, 80t
for Ewing's sarcoma family of tumors, 41
for fibrosarcoma, 55
in germ cell tumors, 56
history of, 73
interventions for extravasation, 91t
neutropenia caused by, 66t
radiation sensitivity and, 263
for rhabdomyosarcoma, 50
Dactylitis, 289
Damage response genes, 12–13
Darbepoetin alfa (Aranesp), 109, 123
Dasatinib (Sprycel), 110t
Daunomycin (Cerubidine), 66t, 91t, 136
Daunorubicin (daunomycin and doxorubicin), 81t
Death. See also Terminal care; Terminally-ill children.
approaching, 230t
children's concept of, 223, 228–229
Debridement, 92
Debulking, 92
Decadron (dexamethasone), 140t
Deltasone (prednisone), 73
Dental injury. See Oral cavity; Teeth.
Dermatitis, 143t. See also Skin.
Desmopressin (DDAVP), 126–127, 254, 321t
Desquamation, 96
Dexamethasone (Decadron), 18, 140t, 141t

Dexrazoxane (Zinecard), 73, 87t
DHAD (mitoxantrone, Novantrone), 84t
Diabetes insipidus (DI), 126–127, 254
Diagnosis, standards of care, 4
Diagnostic procedures, 70–73
Diamond-Blackfan anemia, 17, 300–301
Diarrhea, 135–136, 171t
Diazepam (Valium), 231
Dietary adaptations, 171
Dietary supplementation, 171
Diffuse large B-cell lymphoma, 20, 21
Diffuse pontine gliomas, 30
Diflucan (fluconazole), 103, 134
Digestive tract, 95–96. See also Gastrointestinal complications; Gastrointestinal tract.
Dihydrofolate reductase gene, 114
Diphenylhydramine (Benadryl), 141t
Disseminated intravascular coagulation (DIC), 156
DNA, structure of, 11–12
DNA-binding agents, 90
DNA repair, 12–13
Docetaxel (Taxotere), 81t
Documentation
in clinical trials, 75
investigational drug recordkeeping, 75
Donor lymphocyte infusions (DLI), 114
Dopamine antagonists, 140t
Double effect, principle of, 241
Down syndrome, 17
Doxorubicin (Adriamycin)
clinical trials, 73
in combination regimens, 73
for Ewing's sarcoma family of tumors, 41
for fibrosarcoma, 55
in germ cell tumors, 56
GI complications, 136
interventions for extravasation, 91t
intrathecal, 18
in nasopharyngeal carcinoma, 54
neutropenia caused by, 66t
in non-Hodgkin's lymphoma, 23
for osteosarcoma, 38
for rhabdomyosarcoma, 50
Drainage tubes, 93
DTIC (dacarbazine), 80t
Dysgeusia, 171t
Dyskeratosis congenita (DKC), 300
Dysphagia, 96
Dyspnea, 231

## E

Ears, 248t, 256
Eculizumab, 318
Educating the Child with Cancer, 278
Education. See also Health teaching.
health promotion, 278–279
issues for cancer survivors, 276–277

priorities, 222–224
psychosocial effects and, 275
resources, 207t
standard for, 4
Electrocardiograms, 72
Elitek (rasburicase), 153
Elspar (asparginase), 78t, 138
Elutriation, 100
Emend (aprepitant), 140t, 141t
Employee Retirement and Income Security Act, 276
Employment problems, 276–277
Encephalitis, 128
Endocrine glands, 96, 108
Endocrine-hypothalamic-pituitary axis, 247t
Endocrine system abnormalities, 131–132
End-of-life care. *See also* Terminal care; Terminally-ill children.
    family response to, 198
    importance of parents' communication, 223
    pain management, 229–231
    physical care, 229–233
    self-care interventions for nurses, 211
Endoscopy/colonoscopy, 93
Energy medicine, 115–116
Engraftment, definition, 101
Enteral nutrition, 172–173
Enteral products, 172t
Enteritis, 264
Environmental exposures, 17
Eosinophils, function of, 63
Ependymoma, 28, 30
Epidemiology, 10–15
Epidophyllotoxins, 77
Epirubicin, 91t
Epoetin (Epogen, Procrit, erythropoietin), 62, 64, 109, 123, 296
Epogen (erythropoietin, epoetin, Procrit), 62, 109, 296
Epratuzumab, 110t
Epstein-Barr virus, 20, 54
Epstein-Barr virus-lymphoproliferative disease (EBV-LPD), 114
Equianalgesic conversions, 153t
Erlotinib (Tarceva), 110t, 111
Erythema, 96
Erythropoietin (epoetin, Epogen, Procrit), 62, 64, 109, 123, 296
Esophagitis, 134–135, 174t
Esophagus, 96
*Essentials of Pediatric Heamatology/Oncology Nursing: A Core Curriculum*, 7
Ethical dilemmas, 241–242, 242t
Ethics, professional standard for, 4–5, 6
Ethnicity, 202
Ethnic populations, demographics of, 101
Ethyol (amifostine), 85t
Etoposide (VP-16, VePesid)
    characteristics of, 81t
    for Ewing's sarcoma family of tumors, 41
    for fibrosarcoma, 55
    interventions for extravasation, 91t
    in nasopharyngeal carcinoma, 54
    for neuroblastoma, 35

    neutropenia caused by, 66t
    in non-Hodgkin's lymphoma, 23
    for osteosarcoma, 38
    in pediatric brain tumors, 30
    in relapsed/recurrent kidney tumors, 47
    for rhabdomyosarcoma, 50
Evaluation, standards of care, 4
Evans syndrome, 309–311
Ewing, James, 40
Ewing's sarcoma family of tumors (ESFT), 40–43, 41t, 42f, 55t
Exostosis, 270
External beam radiation, 95
Extramedullary relapse, 19
Extraosseous Ewing's sarcoma (EES), 40
Extravasation, interventions for, 91t
Eyes, late effects on, 256–257

# F

Factor VIII concentrates, recombinant, 321t
Factor V Leiden (FVL), 313t
Familial adenomatous polyposis, 55–56
Familial factors, 17
Families
    assessments, 14–15
    common concerns, 14
    culture and, 203
    definition of, 197–199
    dynamics within, 200, 201
    educational resources for, 207t
    education of, 219, 219t, 220t, 221t, 222
    immunizations, 126t
    learning needs, 224
    management styles, 189t
    psychosocial effects on, 275
    resources for, 199–202, 237
Family and Medical Leave Act of 1993, 276
Family-centered care, 233
Fanconi anemia, 17, 298–299, 299f
Fatigue, radiation therapy and, 95
Fenretinide, 35
Fertile Hope, 279t
Fertility preservation, 132
Fever, 231–232, 289
Fibrosarcoma, 54–55
Fibrosis, 262
FICA (faith, importance, influence, community, and address) tool, 204
Fidelity, principle of, 241
Financial burdens, 200, 201
Fluconazole (Diflucan), 103, 134
Fludarabine, 81t
Fluid balance, 30, 93–94
5-Fluorouracil (5-FU, fluorouracil, Adrucil), 54, 73, 81t, 135
Folic acid antagonists, 2, 73
Folinic acid (leucovorin calcium, citrovorum factor, folinic acid, Welcovin), 87t
Follicle-stimulating hormone (FSH), 146
Food and Drug Administration (FDA) guidelines, 75

# Index

Foundations Series, 7
Fractures, pathological, 37, 270
French-American-British Cooperative Group (FAB) classification system, 16, 16t
Fresh-frozen plasma transfusion, 180
Fungal infections, 103, 134
Fungizone (amphotericin B), 103, 134
Furosemide (Lasix), 30, 130

## G

Gallstones, 290
Ganciclovir (Cytovene), 103
Gardasil, 111
Gastrointestinal complications, 103, 134–140. *See also* Nutritional complications.
Gastrointestinal tract, late effects on, 250t, 263–265
G-CSF (granulocyte colony-stimulating factor, Neupogen), 73, 109, 122–123, 300
Gefitinib (Iressa), 110, 111
Gemcitabine, 81t
Genes, 11–13
Gene therapy, 112–115
Genetic mutations, 273
Gene transfer, 113, 114
Genitourinary system, late effects, 250t, 265–267
Gentuzumab ozogamicin (Mylotarg), 110t
Germ-cell gene transfer, 113
Germ cell tumors, 55t, 56
Gift giving, 211
Gleevac (imatinib mesylate), 82t, 110
Glioblastoma of the brainstem, 28
Glucocorticoids, 140t
Glucose-6-phosphate dehydrogenase deficiency (G6PDD), 294–296
GM-CSF (granulocyte-macrophage colony-stimulating factor, Leukine), 109
Gonadotropin deficiency, 254
Graft failure, 104
Graft versus host disease (GVHD), 114
    after stem cell transplantation, 103, 104–105
        prevention of, 100, 106t
        staging and grading, 105t
        transfusions and, 123
        treatment of, 106t
        xerophthalmia and, 257
Grandparents, needs of, 234
Granisetron (Kytril), 140t, 141t
Granulocyte colony-stimulating factor (G-CSF, Neupogen), 73, 109, 122–123, 300
Granulocyte-macrophage colony-stimulating factor (GM-CSF, Leukine), 39, 109, 122–123, 300
Granulocytes, 63, 65, 180
Graves' disease, 255, 256
Grief, 223, 228–229, 237–239
Grief work, 228–229
Groshong central venous catheter, 165, 166f
Growth and development, 146–148, 147t, 163t, 290

Growth factors (Neupogen), 73
Growth hormone deficiency, 253, 254
Growth signals, cancer and, 13

## H

Hand and foot syndrome, 289
Hazardous drugs, classification of, 89
Head and neck, 21, 248t, 258–260
Healing touch, 116
Healthcare professionals
    ethical dilemmas, 241–242
    grief of, 237–238
    moral distress, 239–241
Health insurance, 276–277
Health Insurance Portability and Accountability Act, 277
Health maintenance, 278–279
Health promotion, 4, 278–279
Health teaching, 4. *See also* Education.
Healthy People 2010, 202
Hearing, late effects on, 248t, 256–257
Heart, 96, 132–133
Heavy metals, 100, 130
Helixate FS, 321t
Hematocrit, 63t, 64
Hematology, 285–328
Hematopoietic cells, 16, 96
Hematopoietic growth factors, 109, 111
Hematopoietic hierarchy, 62f
Hematopoietic stem cell transplantation (HSCT). *See also* Stem cell transplantation.
    biotherapeutic agents used in, 110t
    complications of, 101–107, 102t
    conditioning regimens, 100–101
    discharge planning after, 107
    diseases treated with, 99t
    donor evaluation, 100
    for dyskeratosis congenita, 301
    engraftment of, 102t
    for Fanconi anemia, 299–300
    infectious complications, 103t
    late effects, 108
    outpatient follow-up, 107–108
    patient evaluation, 100
    types of, 98–99
Hematopoietic system
    components of, 15
    late effects of cancer, 252t, 271–272
Hemihypertrophy, 44
Hemoglobin E trait, 293
Hemoglobin H disease, 292
Hemoglobins, 62, 63t, 64
Hemolytic-uremic syndrome (HUS), 314–317, 316t
Hemophilia, 320–323, 321t
Hemorrhagic cystitis, 107, 142, 175t
Hemosiderin, 62
Heparin (Liquaemin), 99
Hepatic fibrosis, 263, 264

Hepatitis, 137–138, 264
Hepatitis B vaccine, 111
Heptatoblastoma, 55–56
Herceptin (trastuzumab), 39, 110t, 111
Hereditary retinoblastoma, 36, 37t
Hereditary spherocytosis, 296–297
Herpes simplex virus (HSV), 124
Herpes zoster (shingles), 124–125
Herrick, James, 288
Hickman® Dual-Lumen catheter, 166f
High-dose chemotherapy with stem-cell rescue (HDC/SCR), 35
History, 2–3, 73–74
HLA typing, 98, 179–180
HN2. See Mechlorethamine.
Hodgkin's lymphoma, 25–28, 55t
Home environments, 199–201
Homocysteine, 313t
HOPE tool, 204
Hormone replacement therapy, 269
Hormones, 77, 77t, 131
Horner syndrome, 33, 127
Hospice care, pediatric-focused, 234–235
Human chorionic gonadotropin, 56
Human genome, 12
Human lymphocyte antigens (HLA), 98, 179–180
Human papilloma virus (HPV), 111
HumaSPECT (Tc-99 votumumab), 109
Hycamtin (topotecan), 50, 85t
Hydeltra-T.B.A. See Prednisone.
Hydrocephalus, shunts for, 29f
Hydrocortisone, 254
Hydrops fetalis, 292
Hydroxyurea (Hydrea), 66t, 81t
Hydroxyzine (Vistaril/Atarax), 141t
Hyperalimentation, 173
Hyperfractionated radiation treatment, 30
Hyperleukocytosis, 153–154
Hyperprolactemia, 254
Hyperthyroidism, 255, 256
Hypothalamic-pituitary axis (HPA), 253–255
Hypothyroidism, 255, 256

# I

Ibritumomab tiuxetan In-111 (Zevalin), 109, 110t
ICE (ifosfamide, carboplatinum, etoposide) regimen, 23, 47
Idamycin (idarubicin), 82t, 91t
Idiopathic thrombocytopenic purpura (ITP), 307–308
Ifex. See Ifosfamide.
Ifosfamide (isophosphamide, Ifex)
  characteristics of, 82t
  cranial nerve deficits after, 127
  for Ewing's sarcoma family of tumors, 41
  for fibrosarcoma, 55
  interventions for extravasation, 91t
  late effects of, 266
  in non-Hodgkin's lymphoma, 23
  for osteosarcoma, 38
  for rhabdomyosarcoma, 50

Ilorazepam (Ativan), 231
Imaging studies, diagnostic, 71–73
Imatinib mesylate (Gleevac), 82t, 110, 110t
Immune pancytopenia, 309–311
Immune system
  impairment of, 123–126
  late effects of cancer, 252t, 272–273
Immune thrombocytopenic purpura, 307–309
Immunizations, 125, 126t
Immunodeficiency, 123–124
Immunoglobulin G (IgG) infusions, 103
Immunophenotyping, 16, 70
Immunosuppression, 108
Immunosuppressive agents, 106t. See also specific agents.
Immunotherapy, 35, 101, 114
ImmuRaid-LL2 (bectumomab, LymphoScan), 109
Implanted venous access devices (IVAD), 166
Implementation, standards of care, 4
Individuals with Disabilities Education Act of 1990, 278
Induction chemotherapy, 18, 19
Infants (birth–1 year)
  assessment of pain in, 151t
  with CNS tumors, 29
  concept of death, 228
  development of, 147t, 186, 216–217
  enteral products, 172t
  outcomes of education, 219
  preparation for procedures, 163t
  risk factors of treatment, 146
  teaching strategies, 216t, 218t
Infections
  blood counts in, 65
  impaired immune system and, 123–125
  late effect of HSCT, 103, 103t, 108
  late effects of cancer, 272–273
  risk factors, 174–175
  in sickle-cell disease, 289
  during terminal phase of disease, 231–232
  treatment of, 173–178, 174t–175t
Infertility, 267
Infliximab (rituximab, Rituxan), 23, 110t
Informed consent, 75
In non-Hodgkin's lymphoma, 23
Insertional oncogenesis, 114
Insurance problems, 276–277
Intelligence scores, 146
Intensity-modulated radiation therapy (IMRT), 95
Interferon (Intron A, Roferon-A), 82t
Interferons, 109, 111
Intergroup Rhabdomyosarcoma Study Group (IRSG), 2, 50t, 73
Interleukin 11 (oprelvekin, Neumega, IL-11), 122, 123
Interleukins, 109, 111
International Classification of Childhood Cancer (ICCC), 11
International neuroblastoma staging system (INSS), 34t
Interpersonal caring relationships, 209
Interventions. See specific cancers; specific therapies.
Interventions, goals of, 14–15. See also specific cancers; specific conditions.

# Index

Intestinal fibrosis, 264
Intracranial pressures (ICPs), 28
Intralobar nephrogenic rests (INLR), 44
Intraoperative radiation therapy (IORT), 95
Intravenous immunoglobulin (IVIG), 124, 125$t$
Intron A (interferon, Roferon-A), 82$t$
Invasive procedures, diagnostic, 70–71
Investigational drugs
    recordkeeping, 75
Iressa (gefitinib), 110, 111
Irinotecan (CPT-11, Camptosar)
    characteristics of, 82$t$
    in neuroblastoma, 35
    in pediatric brain tumors, 30
    for rhabdomyosarcoma, 50
Irradiated blood products, 181
Irritant drugs, extravasation, 91$t$
Isophophamide. *See* Ifosfamide.
Isopto-Hyoscine (scopolamine hydrobromide), 231
IV tubing, safe handling of, 89

## J
Jamshidi needles, 70
*Journal of Pediatric Oncology Nursing (JOPON)*, 7
*Journal of the Association of Pediatric Oncology Nurses (JAPON)*, 7
Justice, principle of, 241

## K
Kidneys
    effect of radiation therapy on, 96
    late effects on, 266
    renal complications, 140–141
    in sickle-cell disease, 290
    treatment, 267
    tumors of, 43–48
Klinefelter syndrome, 17
Knudson's two hit theory, 52
Kognate FS, 321$t$
Kübler-Ross, Elisabeth, 235
Kytril (granisetron), 140$t$, 141$t$

## L
Laboratory tests, diagnostic, 70
Lactic dehydrogenase, serum, 37
Lance Armstrong Foundation/LIVESTRONG™, 279$t$
Lapatinib, 111
Large-cell lymphomas, 23
Large intestine, effects of radiation, 96
Lasix (furosemide), 30, 130
Late effects, 245–261
Leadership, professional standard for, 6
Learning
    critical periods for, 222–224
    principles of, 219–220
    problems with, 278
Legal concerns, in terminal care, 243

Leg ulcers, 290
Leucovorin calcium (Wellcovorin, citrovorum factor, folinic acid), 87$t$
Leukemias, 15–20, 273
Leukine (granulocyte-macrophage colony-stimulating factor, GM-CSF), 109
Leukocyte-reduced blood products, 181
Leukoencephalopathy, 246, 252
Leukoria, 52
Lifestyle changes, 222, 279
Li-Fraumeni syndrome, 37, 37$t$, 48, 55–56
Limb-length discrepancies, 270
Limb salvage procedures, 38–39, 144–145
Lipoprotein a, 313$t$
Liposomes, 113
Liquaemin (heparin), 99
Liver
    chemical or reactive hepatitis, 137–138
    effect of radiation therapy on, 96
    enzyme baseline, 18
    late effects on, 250$t$, 263–264
L-MTP-PE (mifamurtide), 111
Local-control irradiation, 101
Lomustine (CCNU, CeeNU), 30, 66$t$, 83$t$
Long-term Follow-up Guidelines for Survivors of Childhood, Adolescent, and Young Adult Cancers, 273, 279$t$
Lorazepam (Ativan), 141$t$
Loss of heterozygosity (LOH), 12, 45
Low-dose, involved field radiation therapy (LD-IRTR), 26
L-PAM. *See* Melphalan.
Lumbar punctures (LP), 18, 70–71
Lungs
    effect of radiation therapy on, 96
    late effect of HSCT, 108
Luteinizing hormone (LH), 146
Lymphatic system, 62
Lymphoblastic lymphoma (LL), 20–21, 23
Lymphocyte-depleted Hodgkin's lymphoma (LDHL), 25
Lymphocyte-rich classical Hodgkin's lymphoma (LRCHL), 25
Lymphocytes, 63, 96
LymphoScan (bectumomab, ImmuRaid-LL2), 109

## M
Macrocytic anemia, 299
Macrolide antibiotics, 176$t$
Magnetic resonance angiography (MRA), 29
Magnetic resonance imaging (MRI), 29
Maintenance therapy, 18
Malabsorption, 145
Malignant hepatic tumors, 55–56
Manipulative-based practices, 115
Mannitol (Osmitrol), 30
Massage, 116
Mass effects, 28
Maternal factors, 17
Matulane (procarbazine), 84$t$
Maximally-tolerated dose (MTD), 74

Mean corpuscular hemoglobin (MCH), 63t
Mean corpuscular volume (MCV), 63t
Mechlorethamine (nitrogen mustard, Mustargen, HN2), 73, 83t, 91t, 136
Medical coverage, 200, 201
Medical Information Bureau, 277
Medical records, 75
Medulloblastoma, 28, 30
Melanoma, 55t
Melphalan (Alkeran, L-PAM, L-sarcolysin), 66t, 73, 83t
Memorial Sloan-Kettering Cancer Center, 2
Meningitis, 128, 175t
6-mercaptopurine (Purinethol, 6-MP), 18, 66t, 73, 83t, 264
Mesna (Mesnex), 73, 87t
Metaiodobenzylguanidine (MIBG) scans, 34
Metastasis, 14
Methotrexate (MTX, Mexate, Amethopterin)
    characteristics of, 83t
    in combination regimens, 73
    GI complications, 136
    hepatic dysfunction and, 264
    history of, 73
    intrathecal, 18
    late effects of, 266
    in nasopharyngeal carcinoma, 54
    in non-Hodgkin's lymphoma, 23
    for osteosarcoma, 38
    pulmonary toxicity, 261
    radiation sensitivity and, 246
Methylphenidate (Ritalin), 252
Metoclopramide (Reglan), 141t
Mexate. See Methotrexate.
Midazolam (Versed), 231
Mifamurtide (L-MTP-PE), 111
Military service applications, 276–277
Mind-body medicine, 115
Mineralocorticoids, 254
Minimally-invasive surgery, 92
Minimal residual disease (MRD), 19
Minority status, 202
Mitomycin, 91t
Mitoxantrone (Novantrone, DHAD), 84t, 91t
Mixed cellularity Hodgkin's lymphoma (MCHL), 25
Mixed hypothyroidism, 256
Monoclonal antibodies, 109, 111
Monocytes, function of, 63
Monosomy 7, 17
Mood alterations, 128
MOPP (mechlorethamine, Oncovin, prednisone, procarbazine) regimen, 73
Moral distress, 239–241
Moyamoya disease, 258
6-MP. See Mercaptopurine.
MTX. See Methotrexate.
Mucositis, 134–135, 171t, 174t
Multidisciplinary teams, 224
Multidrug resistant-1 gene, 113
Multimodal therapies, 76

Murphy Ann Arbor System, 22
Musculoskeletal complications, 143–145
Musculoskeletal system, late effects, 252t, 269–271
Mustargen. See Mechlorethamine.
Mycelex (clotrimoxazole), 134
Mycostatin (nystatin), 134
Myelodysplasia, therapy-related, 271
Myelodysplastic syndrome, 17
Myleran (busulfan), 73, 78t
Mylotarg (gentuzumab ozogamicin), 110t

## N

Naloxone, 152
Nasopharyngeal carcinoma, 54
National Children's Cancer Society, 278
National Coalition for Cancer Survivorship, 277
National Wilms' Tumor Study (NWTS) Group, 2, 46t, 73
Nausea and vomiting, 138–140
    chemotherapy and, 73, 138
    interventions, 171t
    pathophysiology of, 139t
    radiation therapy and, 96
    during terminal phase of disease, 232
Necrotizing gingivitis, 174t
Nelarabine (ara-G), 84t
Neoadjuvant chemotherapy, 76
Nephroblastomatosis, 44
Nephrogenic rests, 44
Neumega (interleukin 11, IL-11, oprelvekin), 122, 123
Neuopogen (granulocyte colony-stimulating factor, G-CSF), 73, 109, 122–123, 300
Neuroblastoma, 32–36,
Neurocognitive deficits. See Cognitive deficits.
Neuroendocrine dysfunction, 146
Neurofibromatosis, 17, 33, 48
Neuropathic pain, 148
Neutropenia, 65–66
    acquired, 306–307
    after stem cell transplantation, 102
    bone-marrow suppression and, 122
    chemotherapy agents as cause of, 66t
    chronic, 304–307
    congenital, 305
    cyclic, 306
    medical management, 122–123
Neutrophils, 63, 65
Nilotinib, 110t
Nitrogen mustard. See Mechlorethamine.
Nitroreductase, bacterial, 114
Nitrosureas, 100, 261
NK-1 antagonists, 140t
"No blood return" algorithm, 169f
Nodular lymphocyte-predominant Hodgkin's lymphoma (NLPHL), 25
Nodular sclerosis Hodgkin's lymphoma (NSHL), 25
Non-DNA binding agents, 90
Non-Hodgkin's lymphoma (NHL), 20–24, 55t
Nonmaleficence, principle of, 241

# Index

Nonprofessional relationships, 209t
Novantrone (mitoxantrone, DHAD) characteristics of, 84t
Novo VII, 321t
Nulasta (pegfilgrastim), 110, 122–123
Nurse-patient relationships, 208–212
Nursing assessments. *See* specific cancers; specific conditions.
*Nursing Care of Children and Adolescents with Cancer*, 7
Nursing interventions. *See* Interventions.
Nutrition, alterations in, 145
Nutritional assessments, 169–170
    anthropomorphic measurements, 170
    identifying at-risk patients, 173
    interventions, 170–173
    laboratory values, 170
Nutritional complications, 145–146. *See also* Gastrointestinal complications.
Nutritional support, 169–173
Nuvion (vizilizumab), 110t
Nystatin (Mycostatin), 134
N-myc oncogene, 12, 33

## O

Occlusive-cerebral vasculopathy, 258
Occupational Safety and Health Administration (OSHA), 89–90
OEPA (vincristine, etoposide, prednisone, adriamycin) regimen, 26
Oncogenes, description, 12
Oncologic emergencies, 153–158
Oncology Nursing Certification Corporation (ONCC), 7, 225
Oncology Nursing Society (ONS), 225
Oncorvin. *See* Vincristine.
Ondansetron (Zofran), 73, 140t, 141t
Oophoropexy, 269
Ophthalomology, 248t
Opioids, weaning from, 153t
OPPA (vincrisitine, prednisone, procarbazine, and adriamycin) regimen, 26
Oprelvekin (Neumega, interleukin 11, IL-11), 122, 123
Opsomyoclonus, 33
Oral Assessment Scale, 134
Oral cavity, 134, 135t
Oral mucosa, 96
Oregovmomab Tc-99 (OvaRex), 109
Osmitrol (mannitol), 30
Osteopenia, 270
Osteoporosis, 270
Osteosarcoma, 36–40, 37t, 38t, 55t
Ototoxicity, 130–131
Outcomes identification, 4, 15
OvaRex (Tc-99 oregovmomab), 109
Ovarian tumors, 56
Ovaries, 96, 251t, 268–269
Oxaplatin, 91t
Oxygen supplementation, 231
Oxygen therapy, monitoring of, 262

## P

Paclitaxel (Taxol), 84t, 91t
Paget's disease, 36
Pain
    assessment by stage, 151t
    definition, 148
    effects of, 150t
    equianalgesic conversions, 153t
    locations of, 152t
    medications for, 149t
    processes underlying, 148–150
    quality of, 152t
    types of, 148, 152t
    unrelieved, 150, 150t
    Wong-Baker Faces Pain Rating Scale, 152t
Pain crisis, 289
Pain management, 151–153
    after surgery, 93
    assessments, 94
    for children dying of cancer, 229–231
    equianalgesic conversions, 153t
    interventions, 94
    oral cavity complications, 135
    psychological preparation for procedures, 162–164
    sedation for procedures, 164–165
*Pain Management in Children with Cancer*, 7
Palliative care, educational priorities, 223
Palliative surgery, 92
Palonestron (Aloxi), 141t
Pancreatitis, 138
Parainfluenza virus, 108
Paraplatin. *See* Carboplatin.
Parents, 234, 235–236
Paroxysmal nocturnal hemoglobinuria (PNH), 317–319
Pathological fractures, 37, 270
Patient-controlled analgesia (PCA), 152
Patients, common concerns, 14
Pediapred. *See* Prednisone.
Pediatric Chemotherapy and Biotherapy Program, 7
Pediatric Exclusivity Provision, 74
Pediatric hematology/oncology nurses, 2–6, 224–225, 237–239
Pediatric Oncology Group (POG), 2, 73
*Pediatric Oncology Nursing: Scope and Standards of Practice*, 4, 7
*Pediatric Tumor Series: Handbooks for Families*, 7
Pegfilgrastim (Nulasta), 110, 122–123
Pelvis, late effects on, 266
Penicillins, extended-spectrum, 176t
Pericarditis, 260
Perilobar nephrogenic rests (PLNR), 44
Peripherally inserted central catheters (PICCs), 166, 166f
Peripheral neuropathy, 247t, 252
Peripheral primitive neuroectodermal tumors, 40–43
Peripheral stem-cell collection, 99–100
Peripheral venous access, 90
Perirectal abscesses, 175t
Perirectal cellulitis, 137, 175t
PermCath central venous catheter, 165
Per-Q-Cath® PICCs, 166f

Personal protective equipment, 89
P53 mutations, 36, 40, 44
Phantom pain, 148
Phenergan (promethazine), 141t
Phenothiazines, 140t
Philadelphia chromosome-positive leukemia, 16
Photosensitivity, 142
Planet Cancer, 279t
Planning, standards of care, 4
Plant alkaloids, 77t, 100
Plant-derived products, 77
Plasma, fresh-frozen, 180
Plasma protein fractions, 180
Platelets, 63, 67–68, 122, 179–180. *See also* Thrombocytopenia
Platinol. *See* Cisplatin.
Pneumocystic pneumonia, 108
*Pneumocystis carinii* pneumonia, 123–124
Pneumonia, 174t
Pneumonitis, 133, 262
Positioning, for surgery, 93
Positron emission tomography (PET) scans, 29, 72
Posterior fossa symptoms, 28
Posterior fossa syndrome, 29, 129–130
Postoperative management, 93
Postremission therapy, 19
P16/p14ARF deletions, 41
Precocious puberty, 253, 254
Prednisone (Deltasone, Pediapred, Hydeltra-T.B.A.), 18, 23, 73, 140t
Preemptive analgesia, 152
Preoperative management, 93
Preschoolers (3–5 years)
    assessment of pain in, 151t
    caloric needs, 170t
    concept of death, 228
    developmental stages, 147t
    development of, 188–189, 217
    enteral products, 172t
    outcomes of education, 219
    psychological preparation for procedures, 163t
    teaching strategies, 216t, 218t
Priapism, 289–290
Procarbazine (Matulane), 84t
Prochlorperazine (Compazine), 140t, 141t
Procrit (erythropoietin, epoetin, Epogen), 109
Professional Boundaries for Registered Nurses, 209
Professional practice evaluation, 4, 5
Professional relationships, 209t
Professonal performance standards, 4–5
Promethazine (Phenergan), 141t
ProstaScint (capromab pentomab), 109
Prostate gland, 266
Protein S deficiency, 313t
Protein tyrosine kinase inhibitors (PTKIs), 110–111
Protein tyrosine kinases (PTKs), 110–111
Prothrombin gene mutation 20210A, 313t
Proton radiation therapy, 95
Pseudoaddiction, 152

Pseudomembranous colitis, 175t
Pseudomonas aeruginosa, 156
Psychological concerns, 271
Psychosocial care, 233–235, 271
Psychosocial issues, 185–213
    educational, 227–278
    personal-emotional, 275–276
    political-social, 276–277
Publications, APHON, 7
Pulmonary edema, 106–107, 262
Pulmonary fibrosis, 133–134
Pulmonary hemorrhages, 106
Pure red-cell aplasia, 300–301
Purinethol. *See* Mercaptopurine.

## Q
Quality of practice, standard for, 4

## R
Race
    AML and, 17
    APML and, 17
    Ewing's sarcomas, 41t
    risk of cancer and, 202
    tumors of the kidney and, 43
Radiation parotitis, 95
Radiation recall, 142
Radiation therapy (RT)
    cardiovascular effects, 260
    cataracts and, 256
    for CNS tumors, 30
    conditioning regimens, 100
    cranial nerve deficits after, 127
    for Ewing's sarcoma family of tumors, 41
    GI complications, 136
    infertility and, 267
    for kidney tumors, 47
    late effects of, 245–261, 266, 269–271
    low-dose, involved field, 26
    methods of delivery, 95
    for neuroblastoma, 35
    in non-Hodgkin's lymphoma, 23
    osteosarcoma risk and, 37t
    ototoxicity, 130
    planning process, 95
    principles, 94–97
    for rhabdomyosarcoma, 50
    second malignancies and, 273
    side effects, 95–96
    skin changes and, 142, 143t
Radiologic imaging, diagnostic, 72
Radionucleotide delivery, 35
Range of movement (ROM) limitations, 144
Rare tumors of childhood, 54–58
Rasburicase (Elitek), 153
Rb gene, 12
Recombinate, 321t

# Index

Red blood cells (RBCs, erythrocytes), 62, 63, 64, 122, 179. *See also* Anemia.
Reed-Sternberg cells, 25
Reese-Ellsworth classification of retinoblastoma, 52*t*
Refacto, 321*t*
Regional chemotherapy, 76
Reglan (metoclopramide), 141*t*
Rehabilitation Act of 1973, 206, 278
Relapses
 educational priorities, 223
 family response to, 198
Relationships
 boundaries, 209–210
 educational priorities about, 223
 nurse/patient, 208–212
Religion, 204
Renal cell carcinoma, 44
Renal complications, 140–141
Renal failure, 18, 107
Renal impairment, 290
Renal insufficiency, 266
Renal medullary carcinoma, 44
Renal toxicity, 107
Reproductive organs, 96, 251*t*, 267. *See also* Ovaries; Testes.
Research, professional standard for, 6
Resection, complete, 92
Resource utilization, 6
Respiratory depression, 152
Respiratory system, late effects, 249*t*, 261–263
Resting energy expenditure (REE), 169, 170*t*
Restlessness, 232
Reticulocytes, 64
Retinoblastoma, 12, 52–54
Retinoic acids, 84*t*
Retinoid compounds, 35
Retinopathy, 290
Retroviral vectors, 113
Retroviral-viremia, 114
Rhabdomyosarcoma (RMS), 48–51, 50*t*, 55*t*
Rhinorrhea, 174*t*
Rhomboid tumor of the kidney, 44, 47
Rh typing, 64
Risk factors, 13*t*
Ritalin (methylphenidate), 252
Rituals, use of, 234
Rituximab (infliximab, Rituxan), 23, 110*t*
Robotics, surgical, 93
Roferon-A (interferon, Intron-A), 82*t*
Rotationplasty, 39
Rothmund-Thompson syndrome, 37*t*

## S

Sacrococcygeal teratomas, 56
Safety, handling chemotherapy agents, 89–90
Salivary glands, 95–96, 258, 259
Salvage therapy, 23
Sanctuary therapy, 76
L-Sarcolysin. *See* Melphalan.

Scatter radiation, 270
School-age children (6–12 years)
 assessment of pain in, 151*t*
 caloric needs, 170*t*
 concept of death, 228
 development of, 147*t*, 189–191, 217
 enteral products, 172*t*
 outcomes of education, 219
 psychological preparation for procedures, 163*t*
 teaching strategies, 216*t*, 218*t*
School nurses, 224
Schools
 absenteeism, 278
 attendance, 205–208
 reentry, 205–208
School staff, 207, 224
Schwachmann-Diamond syndrome (SDS), 302–304
Schwachmann syndrome, 17
Scoliosis, 146, 270
*Scope and Standards of Pediatric Oncology Nursing Practice*, 4
Scope of Practice and Outcome Standard of Practice for Pediatric Oncology Nurses, 4
Scopolamine hydrobromide (Isopto-Hyoscine), 231
Screening
 importance of, 279
 for second malignancies, 274*t*
 for sickle cell disease, 290
Secondary malignancies, 108, 273–274, 274*t*
Sedation, 93, 164–165, 164*t*
Seizures, 231
Self-advocacy, importance of, 277
Self-care interventions, 211
Self-evaluation, standard for, 4
Septic shock, 155–156
Septrax (Bactrim, trimethoprim and sulfamethoxazole, Septrax, Co-trimoxizole), 87*t*
Serotonin receptor antagonists, 140*t*
Serum chemistries, diagnostic, 70
Shingles (herpes zoster), 124–125
Shock, 155–156
Shunts, hydrocephalus, 29*f*
Siblings
 dealing with death, 228
 immunizations, 126*t*
 needs of, 198, 234
 of terminally-ill children, 223
Sickle-cell disease (SCD), 288–292, 289*f*, 291*t*
Sickle-cell hemoglobinopathy, 44
Sickle-cell pain, 152
Side effects, 121–160
 of antibiotics, 176*t*–177*t*
 of biotherapeutic agents, 111
 education on, 222
 of gene therapy, 114
 of radiation therapy, 95–96
Sinusitis, 174*t*

Skin
 altered integrity of, 142–143
 effect of radiation therapy on, 96
 function of, 142
 infections, 175t
 late effects of cancer, 252t, 259
 radiation-induced vascular injury, 258
Slipped capitofemoral epiphysis, 270
Small intestine, 96
Sodium bicarbonate, 153
Solid tumors, 10
Somatic-cell gene transfer, 113
Somatic pain, 148
Somnolence syndrome, 95
Spinal cord, effects of radiotherapy, 95
Spinal cord compression, 157
Spinal cord tumors, 31
Spine, imaging of, 29
Spiritual beliefs, 234
Spirituality, 204
Splenectomy, 272–273
Splenic sequestration, 289
Sprycel (dasatinib), 110t
St. Jude Children's Research Hospital, 2, 22, 22t, 73
Staging, surgical, 92
Standards of care, 4
Standards of Pediatric Oncology Nursing Practice (APON), 4
Stem cell-product purging, 100
Stem cells, collection of, 99–100
Stem cell transplantation, 23, 98t, 101. *See also* Hematopoietic stem cell transplantation (HSCT).
Stereotactic radiosurgery, 95
Stomach, radiation therapy and, 96
Stomatitis, 134
Strictures, abdominal, 264, 267
Stroke, 258, 289
Supportive care, 30, 161–183
Surgery. *See also* specific cancers.
Surveillance Epidemiology and End Results (SEER) program, 10–11, 11
Surviving and Moving Forward, 279t
Survivorship, web resources for, 279t
Syndrome of inappropriate antidiuretic hormone secretion (SIADH), 157–158
Syngeneic stem cell transplantation, 98, 98t
Synovial sarcoma, 56–57

# T

Tacrolimus (Prograf), 107
Tarceva (erlotinib), 110t, 111
Taste buds, 258, 259
Taste changes, 171t
Taxanes, 90, 127
Taxol (paclitaxel), 73, 84t
Taxotere (docetaxel), 81t
T-cell depletion, 100
T-cell lymphomas, 20
Teachers, communication with, 207

Teeth, 96, 249t, 258, 259
Telomerases, 14
Telomeres, 14
Temozolomide (Temodar), 30, 84t
Teniposide (VM-26, Vumon), 66t, 85t
Teratomas, 56
Terminal care, 241–242, 242t, 243
Terminal events, 229
Terminal illness, dimensions of, 229
Terminal periods, 229
Terminal phases, 229
Terminally-ill children
 ethical dilemmas in care, 242t
 physical care of, 229–233
 psychosocial care, 233–235
Testes, 96, 251t, 267–268
Testicular tumors, 56
Thalassemia, 292–294
Therapeutic touch, 116
6-Thioguanine (6-TG), 73
Thioguanine (6-thioguanine, 6-TG), 85t, 264
Thioplex (triethylenethiophosphoramine thiotepa), 30, 66t, 85t
Thiopurine-S-methyltransferase gene, 74
Thiotepa (triethylenethiophosphoramine, Thioplex), 30, 66t, 85t
Thorazine (chlorpromazine), 140t, 141t
Thrombocytopenia, 67–68, 102–103, 122, 299
Thromboembolic events, 312t, 313t
Thrombophilia, 312–314
Thrombosis, 312–314
Thrush, oral, 124
Thyroid cancer, 55t
Thyroid gland, 248t, 255–257
Thyroiditis, 255, 256
Thyroid stimulating hormone, 254
Thyroxin replacement therapy, 254
Tissue invasion, 14
Tissue tolerance doses (TTDs), 95, 96
Toddlers (1–3 years)
 assessment of pain in, 151t
 caloric needs, 170t
 concept of death, 228
 development of, 147t, 187–188, 217
 enteral products, 172t
 outcomes of education, 219
 psychological preparation for procedures, 163t
 teaching strategies, 216t, 218t
Topoisomerase inhibitors, 73, 136
Topotecan (Hycamtin), 35, 50, 66t, 85t
Tositumomab and I-131 (Bexxar), 110t
Total body irradiation (TBI), 23, 100, 258, 261, 269
Total parenteral nutrition, 173
Trace-element deficiencies, 145
Transfusions, 64, 123, 264. *See also* Blood products.
Transient erythroblastopenia of childhood (TEC), 301
Transient radiation myelopathy, 95
Trastuzumab (Herceptin), 39, 110t, 111
Treatments, principles of, 70
Tricyclic antidepressants, 149–150

Triethylenethiophosphoramine (thiotepa, Thioplex), 30, 66*t*, 85*t*
Trimethoprim and sulfamethoxazole (Bactrim, Septrax, Co-trimoxizole), 87*t*
Trisenox (arsenic trioxide), 110*t*
Trisomy 8, 40
Trisomy 12, 40
Trisomy 21, 17
TrkA gene, 33
Tru-Cut needles, 92
Tumor lysis syndrome (TLS), 19, 154–155, 154*f*
Tumor markers, diagnostic, 70
Tumor suppressor genes, 12
Tunneled external devices, 165
Typhlitis, 156–157, 175*t*
Tyrosine kinase inhibitors, 111

## U
Ultrasound imaging, diagnostic, 72
Upper gastrointestinal endoscopy/colonoscopy, 93
Ureter, late effects on, 266
Urethra, late effects on, 266
Uric acid, 18
Urinalysis, diagnostic, 70
Urinary tract, 96
Urinary tract infections, 175*t*
U.S. Department of Defense, 276
Uterus, late effects on, 266

## V
Vaccines, 111, 126*t*
VAC (vincristine, dactinomycin, cyclophosphamide) regimen, 50–51
Vagina, late effects on, 266
Valcyclovir, 103
Valium (diazepam), 231
Valvular damage, 260
VAMP (vincristine, adriamycin, methotrexate, prednisone) regimen, 26
Varicella zoster (chicken pox), 108, 124, 125*t*
Vascular changes, late effects, 258–260
Vascular endothelial growth factor (VEGF), 14, 110
Vascular endothelial growth factor receptor (VEGFR), 110
Vasoactive intestinal peptide (VIP), 33
VBL. *See* Vinblastine.
VCR. *See* Vincristine.
Velban. *See* Vinblastine.
Velcade (bortezomib), 110*t*
Veno-occlusive disease, 104
Venous access devices, 92, 222
Ventriculoperitoneal shunt infections, 175*t*
VePesid. *See* Etoposide.
Versed (midazolam), 231
Vesicants, 90–92, 91*t*
Vinblastine (VLB, vincaleukoblastine, Velban), 23, 66*t*, 85*t*, 91*t*, 127
Vinca alkyloids, 77*t*, 90
Vincaleukoblastine. *See* Vinblastine.

Vincristine (VCR, Oncovin), 18
  characteristics of, 86*t*
  in combination regimens, 73
  cranial nerve deficits after, 127
  for Ewing's sarcoma family of tumors, 41
  for fibrosarcoma, 55
  in germ cell tumors, 56
  interventions for extravasation, 91*t*
  in nasopharyngeal carcinoma, 54
  for neuroblastoma, 35
  in non-Hodgkin's lymphoma, 23
  in pediatric brain tumors, 30
  for rhabdomyosarcoma, 50
Vinorelbine, 85*t*, 91*t*
Viral vectors, 113
Visceral pain, 148
Vision, late effects on, 256–257
Vistaril/Atarax (hydroxyzine), 141*t*
Vitamin deficiencies, 145
Vizlizumab (Nuvion), 110*t*
VM-26 (teniposide, Vumon), 85*t*
Vomiting. *See* Nausea and vomiting
Von Willebrand disease (vWD), 323–327, 325*t*
Votumumab Tc-99 (HumaSPECT), 109
VP-16 (etoposide). *See* Etoposide (VP-16, VePesid).
Vumon (teniposide, VM-26), 85*t*

## W
Wellcovorin (leucovorin calcium, citrovorum factor, folinic acid), 87*t*
*When Your Child Has Cancer*, 7
White blood cells (WBCs), 63, 65, 96
Wilms' tumor (WT), 2, 43, 45*t*, 46–47, 46*t*
Wiskott-Aldrich syndrome, 20
Wong-Baker Faces Pain Rating Scale, 152*t*
World Health Organization (WHO), 16*t*, 20, 25
Wound care, 94

## X
Xerophthalmia, 257

## Y
Young adults (18–25 years), 194–197

## Z
Zenapax (daclizumab), 110*t*
Zerostomia, 171*t*
Zevalin (ibritumomab tiuxetan In-111), 109, 110*t*
Zinecard (dexrazoxane), 87*t*
Zinsser-Engman-Cole syndrome, 300
Zofran (ondansetron), 140*t*, 141*t*
Zovirax (acyclovir), 134
Zyloprim (allopurinol), 85*t*, 153